Diagnostic Neuroradiology

Wu-Chung Shen

Diagnostic Neuroradiology

A Practical Guide and Cases

Springer

Wu-Chung Shen
Professor of Radiology
Department of Medical Imaging, China Medical University Hospital
College of Medicine, China Medical University
Taichung
Taiwan

ISBN 978-981-15-4050-9   ISBN 978-981-15-4051-6 (eBook)
https://doi.org/10.1007/978-981-15-4051-6

This Springer imprint is published by the registered company Springer Nature Singapore Pte Ltd.
The registered company address is: 152 Beach Road, #21-01/04 Gateway East, Singapore 189721, Singapore

This book is dedicated to my beloved wife, Mei Yun Shen-Liu. I appreciate her for taking care of my family and me, as well as supporting my devotion to radiology and medical education.

Foreword 1

I am glad that Professor Wu-Chung Shen has been invited by Springer Nature to author this new neuroimaging textbook. Professor Shen has published several highly acclaimed neuroradiology textbooks in Chinese. In this textbook written in English, Professor Shen has endeavored to enrich its substantive and pedagogical content. I am thus honored to write a preface for his book.

I am a pediatric neurologist. When I was the Director of the Pediatric Department of China Medical University Hospital (CMUH), I invited Professor Shen to regularly teach imaging and case discussion with young residents and medical students. Professor Shen is a skilled educator who has a wealth of teaching materials for improving young physicians' image reading abilities. Since Professor Shen became the director of the School of Medicine and dean of the College of Medicine of China Medical University, he has made prominent contributions to reform and improve medical education. He has been repeatedly voted as Excellent Faculty and Most Popular Faculty among students.

The China Medical University and Healthcare System is world-class and comprises 16 hospitals and a medical university. In Shanghai Jiao Tong University's 2019 Academic Ranking of World Universities, China Medical University was ranked 308th, only second to National Taiwan University among Taiwan universities and first among private universities in Taiwan. According to Times Higher Education's 2019 Asia University Rankings, China Medical University was ranked 60th among universities in Asia, third among Taiwan universities, and first among Taiwan's private universities.

We have vigorously developed characteristic healthcare services and achieved international standards in fields such as stroke treatment, organ transplantation, cardiovascular disease treatment, cancer treatment, plastic and reconstructive surgery, minimally traumatic surgery, reproductive medicine, and international health. In recent years, we have developed cutting-edge precision medicine, cell therapies, and artificial intelligence applications and also facilitated development in the biomedical industry. With aims to develop a world-class university and network of medical centers and to create world-class and cutting-edge biomedical parks, we established the Hsinchu Health Industry Park and Taichung Shuinan International Health Industrial Park.

With patient-centered healthcare as our core philosophy, we provide top quality healthcare services and constantly purchase the latest medical equipment, such as those for computed tomography, magnetic resonance imaging, positron emission tomography, and angiography from major manufacturers in Europe and the United States. These advanced instruments enable Professor Shen to collect much valuable data for teaching and research. In addition, Professor Shen's published radiology books, which were written in Chinese, have been popular and highly acclaimed among young physicians.

I admire Professor Shen's meticulous and persistent pursuit of his ideals. He has invested additional effort to write this book in English. I believe that this book will be very helpful for young physicians and medical students worldwide. Through the book, the world can gain insight to Taiwan's high-quality healthcare services. I also welcome scholars from all over the world to visit the China Medical University and Healthcare System for academic exchange.

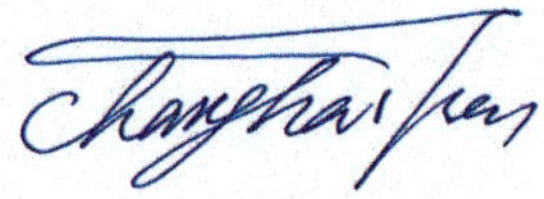

Chang-Hai Tsai
Chairman of China Medical University and Healthcare System
Taichung, Taiwan

Foreword 2

I am a neurosurgeon at the China Medical University Hospital (CMUH), who has worked with neuroradiologist Professor Wu-Chung Shen for a long time. The Departments of Neurology, Neurosurgery, Radiology, Pathology, and Rehabilitation in CMUH regularly hold joint discussion sessions to discuss pedagogically valuable clinical cases that have been difficult to treat and diagnose. In particular, Professor Shen's insightful exposition of patients' images during the discussion sessions has considerably benefitted all participating physicians, particularly young physicians and medical students.

The CMUH is a medical center with 2200 beds that mainly treats patients in emergency or critical conditions. The CMUH values the use of various examination instruments, such as those for computed tomography (CT), magnetic resonance imaging (MRI), positron emission tomography, and angiography. Much has been invested in hardware and software for the provision of immediate updates. Besides, most of the new instruments are accompanied with new software, such as those for computed tomography angiography, CT-perfusion, diffusion weighted imaging, magnetic resonance spectroscopy, and functional MRI. I want to extend my appreciation to Professor Shen and colleagues of the medical imaging department for their effective use of new technologies. Their practice has become a reference for various departments' clinicians and has enabled clinicians to diagnose and treat patients rapidly and accurately.

Taiwan's National Health Insurance (NHI) system offers Taiwanese people convenient and high-quality healthcare. Similar to the NHI database which provides big data for medical researchers, the CMUH has also established its own large database where personal information is meticulously de-identified. We have encouraged colleagues to utilize valuable data for teaching and research in dissertations or books. I have observed that young physicians and medical students are adroit in interpreting images, where such skill is attributable to the teaching provided by excellent radiologists such as Professor Shen. I am glad that world-renowned Springer Nature has invited Professor Shen to author a neuroimaging textbook and share pedagogically valuable cases with young physicians and medical students worldwide. The CMUH has attracted numerous young physicians worldwide to learn by observation. I hope the book published by Springer Nature can show Taiwan's high-quality healthcare to the rest of the world. I also welcome more young physicians to CMUH to learn and join scientific researches.

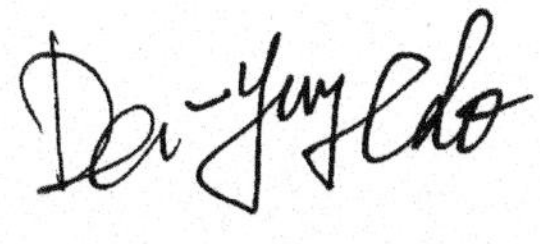

Der-Yang Cho, MD
Superintendent
China Medical University Hospital
Taichung, Taiwan

Acknowledgments

All the images are provided by the database of China Medical University Hospital (CMUH), Taichung, Taiwan, and every image is carefully de-identified. All the illustrations are produced by Hsiu-Chen Lu, senior executive officer, Educational Resources Section of CMUH and Wu-Chung Shen, the author of this book.

Contents

Introduction

For the past 40 years, I have been a radiologist; my greatest joy is teaching the medical students, who rotate into the Department of Medical Imaging every 2 weeks to a month, and young residents who are recruited every year. I often feel an urgent need to impart knowledge of basic image interpretation to the students and resident physicians and also to guide them in applying such knowledge to clinical practices. Over the past 40 years, substantial technological advances have been made in medical imaging devices, particularly those for computed tomography (CT), magnetic resonance imaging (MRI), and angiography. Although the examination speed, image resolution, and diagnosis accuracy of the devices have been improved drastically, these improvements have also increased the complexity of image interpretation content. Such complexity is not only challenging to learners, but teachers as well.

Written based on my 40 years of teaching experience, this book is targeted for medical students and residents. The first chapter covers the fundamental CT and MRI anatomy of the brain and lists basic and commonly seen anatomical positions in clinical applications. The second chapter covers basic concepts required for CT and MRI interpretation, including CT grayscale, which is known as the basic language of CT, as well as various MRI pulse sequences, contrast medium enhancement concepts, mass effect, brain tissue edema, hydrocephalus, and brain tissue atrophy. Chapter 3 covers head injuries and Chapters 4 and 5 cover strokes. These chapters are the highlights of this book. Clerks who join the radiology department for only 2 weeks should familiarize themselves with interpreting images of head injuries and strokes. Because head injuries, intracerebral hemorrhage, subarachnoid hemorrhage, and brain infarction comprise 70% of emergency cases, students who can interpret images of these cases are capable of interpreting most CT and MRI images. After students become familiar with images of head injuries and strokes, they may naturally develop skills for interpreting images of tumors and infections in the central nervous system (CNS). Alternatively, interns or senior clerks who join the radiology department for a month should familiarize themselves with intracranial tumors (Chap. 6), CNS infections (Chap. 7), and spinal diseases (Chap. 8) images. These chapters constitute the underlying framework of this book.

The title of this book is *Diagnostic Neuroradiology: A Practical Guide and Cases*. It uses numerous empirical clinical cases to illustrate CNS diseases and provides interpretations of the illustrated images. This book focuses on CT and MRI images. Each case represents a typical slide for teaching. All X-ray, CT, MRI, and angiography images were collected from practical clinical cases. This book contains ample medical images, all of which are from meticulously de-identified practical cases. All contents were extracted from the large database established by the China Medical University Hospital in Taichung, Taiwan. These databases, including the National Health Insurance Research Database of Taiwan and the databases established by various teaching hospitals, are key components to Taiwan's high-quality healthcare system, which has been ranked highly among countries.

MRI pulse sequences are complex. In addition to the axial section, the sagittal and coronal sections are often presented altogether. Therefore, notes for the pulse sequences as well as the sagittal and coronal sections (with the axial section unspecified) have been added on each MRI image to aid readability. In contrast, notes have not been attached to CT images because readers are familiar with the images; CT images are relatively simple and most commonly encountered in clinical practice.

In 1995, I published a neuroradiology textbook, a book that was written in Chinese. The book has been a favorite textbook among medical students and young physicians. I also manage a website called *Uncle Shen's Teaching Site* that provides pedagogical resources for students. For more than 20 years, I have played multiple roles as radiologist, department director, college dean, and vice superintendent of teaching in the hospital. Because of the demands of these administrative positions, I could not author a new book. After I left my administrative positions, Springer-Nature Co., to my surprise, invited me to write a new book. This invitation has greatly motivated me to compile data for authoring this book.

The fundamentals of CNS diseases have not changed since I became a radiologist more than 40 years ago. However, advances in technology and healthcare have drastically improved our knowledge, tests, and treatments of these diseases. I hope this book can aid medical students, young physicians, and medical staff in other relevant medical fields in conducting clinical diagnosis and therapeutic decision-making based on image interpretation.

1 Brain Neuroimaging Anatomy

Abstract

Understanding the brain imaging anatomy of CT and MRI is crucial in diagnosing various central nervous system diseases. This chapter briefly introduces the essential anatomic locations of the brain parenchyma and subarachnoid space (SAS). Brain parenchyma includes the centrum semiovale, corpus callosum, basal ganglion, brainstem, cerebellum, and corticospinal tract. SAS includes the ventricles, cisterns, fissures, and several sulci.

Understanding the anatomy of images resulting from computed tomography (CT) (Fig. 1.1) and magnetic resonance imaging (MRI) of the brain (Figs. 1.2, 1.3, and 1.4) is essential for interpreting brain imaging.

1. It is crucial to understand not only the anatomy of the most commonly used axial sections but also the anatomy of coronal and sagittal sections.
2. In addition to the brain parenchyma, the anatomy of subarachnoid spaces is also crucial for the interpretation of brain images.
3. Besides, the cranial bones, skull base, paranasal sinuses, mastoid, and cervical spine should be observed.
4. The brain parenchyma includes frontal, temporal, parietal, and occipital lobes, the basal ganglion, corpus callosum, brainstem, and cerebellum.
5. The subarachnoid space (SAS), also known as cerebrospinal fluid (CSF) space, contains the following:
   - Ventricles: Lateral, third, and fourth ventricles, and the aqueduct.
   - Cisterns: Suprasellar and quadrigeminal cisterns and others.
   - Fissures: Sylvian and interhemispheric fissures and others.
   - Sulci: Central and parieto-occipital sulci and others.

Figures 1.1. 1.2, 1.3, and 1.4 include the basic anatomical structures for the interpretation of brain imaging; all parts have detailed anatomical terms, but these are not described in detail in this book.

1.1 Brain Parenchyma

1.1.1 Centrum Semiovale and Corona Radiata

Above the lateral ventricle, the subcortical white matter present in frontoparietal lobes is collectively referred to as the centrum semiovale (Fig. 1.5).

In a CT image, the gray matter appears gray, and the white matter appears slightly darker; hence, the two can be distinguished.

The centrum semiovale contains a vital structure called the corona radiata, which is a prominent white matter fiber. The corticospinal tract, which is responsible for motor conduction, is passed down by the cortical motor cortex via the corona radiata and then down to the internal capsule.

The corona radiata can be distinguished using MRI T2WI and FLAIR. It is white matter, but the signal is slightly whiter than that for other white matter.

1.1.2 Corpus Callosum

The corpus callosum is the largest white matter structure in the human brain and is approximately 10 cm long (Fig. 1.6). Its most crucial function is to connect the left and right cerebral hemispheres. The structure is divided as follows, from front to back:

- Rostrum
- Genu
- Body—a thin part in the posterior of the body called the isthmus
- Splenium

W.-C. Shen, *Diagnostic Neuroradiology*, https://doi.org/10.1007/978-981-15-4051-6_1

Along the upper edge of the corpus callosum, there is a large piece of gray matter called the cingulum or cingulate cortex, which is part of the limbic system.

1.1.3 Basal Ganglion and Thalamus

In neurology, the basal ganglia are vital anatomical structures. They are located deep in the brain, connecting the cerebral cortex, hypothalamus, and brainstem (Fig. 1.7).

In the brain, gray matter is situated in the outer layer, white matter is situated in the inner layer, and the basal ganglion is situated deep in the brain, but it is gray matter; hence, it is also called deep gray matter.

The basal ganglion contains the putamen, caudate nucleus, and globus pallidus.

The putamen and globus pallidus are collectively known as the lentiform nucleus.

The lentiform nucleus and caudate nucleus are collectively called corpus striatum.

The broad basal ganglion also contains the subthalamic nuclei and substantia nigra of the midbrain.

1.1.4 Brain Stem

1.1.4.1 Midbrain

The left and right cerebral peduncles are visible on CT and MRI cross-sections; consequently, the midbrain looks like a croissant.

On MRI, T2WI, FLAIR, and SWI images, the red nucleus and substantia nigra in the midbrain are visible, but MRI cannot display the third cranial nerve nucleus and many nerve bundles in the brainstem (Fig. 1.8).

When a transtentorial herniation occurs, the midbrain is compressed and deformed (see Chap. 2).

1.1.4.2 Pons

On CT and MRI cross-sections, the pons appears as an apple shape (Fig. 1.9).

1.1.4.3 Medulla Oblongata

It contains the bilateral pyramids and inferior cerebellar peduncles (Fig. 1.10).

The pyramid is a stop of the corticospinal tract; thus, this tract is also called the pyramidal tract.

1.1.5 Corticospinal Tract

The corticospinal tract is the most critical motor pathway that controls the movement of various parts of the body (Fig. 1.11).

A motor command from the motor cortex of the frontal lobe is passed down to the corona radiata and then to the brain stem via the posterior limb of the internal capsule.

The first stop of the brain stem is the cerebral peduncle of the midbrain.

It goes down the front part of the pons, then down to the pyramid of the medulla oblongata, and then crosses the spinal cord from left and right.

Because it passes through the pyramid, it is also called the ***pyramidal tract.***

From the motor cortex, any segment of the corticospinal tract that has a lesion can cause weakness in the contralateral limb.

In MRI, T2WI, and FLAIR images, the corticospinal tract appears slightly whiter than surrounding tissues.

1.1.6 Cerebellum

The cerebellum is connected to the brainstem by three cerebellar peduncles (Fig. 1.12):

- Superior cerebellar peduncle → midbrain
- Middle cerebellar peduncle → pons
- Inferior cerebellar peduncle → medulla oblongata

The cerebellum is divided into three lobes:

- Anterior lobe
- Posterior lobe
- Flocculonodular lobe

In the middle is the cerebellar vermis, and both sides are the cerebellar hemispheres.

The outer layer of the cerebellum is a gray matter called the cortex.

The inner layer of the cerebellum is white matter called the medulla, which is also known as "arbor vitae cerebellum," which is named for its branched, tree-like appearance.

The dentate nucleus is the largest among the many nuclei present in the cerebellum. It can be observed using MRI, T2WI, and FLAIR. It is especially apparent in SWI; it is easy to have physiological calcification.

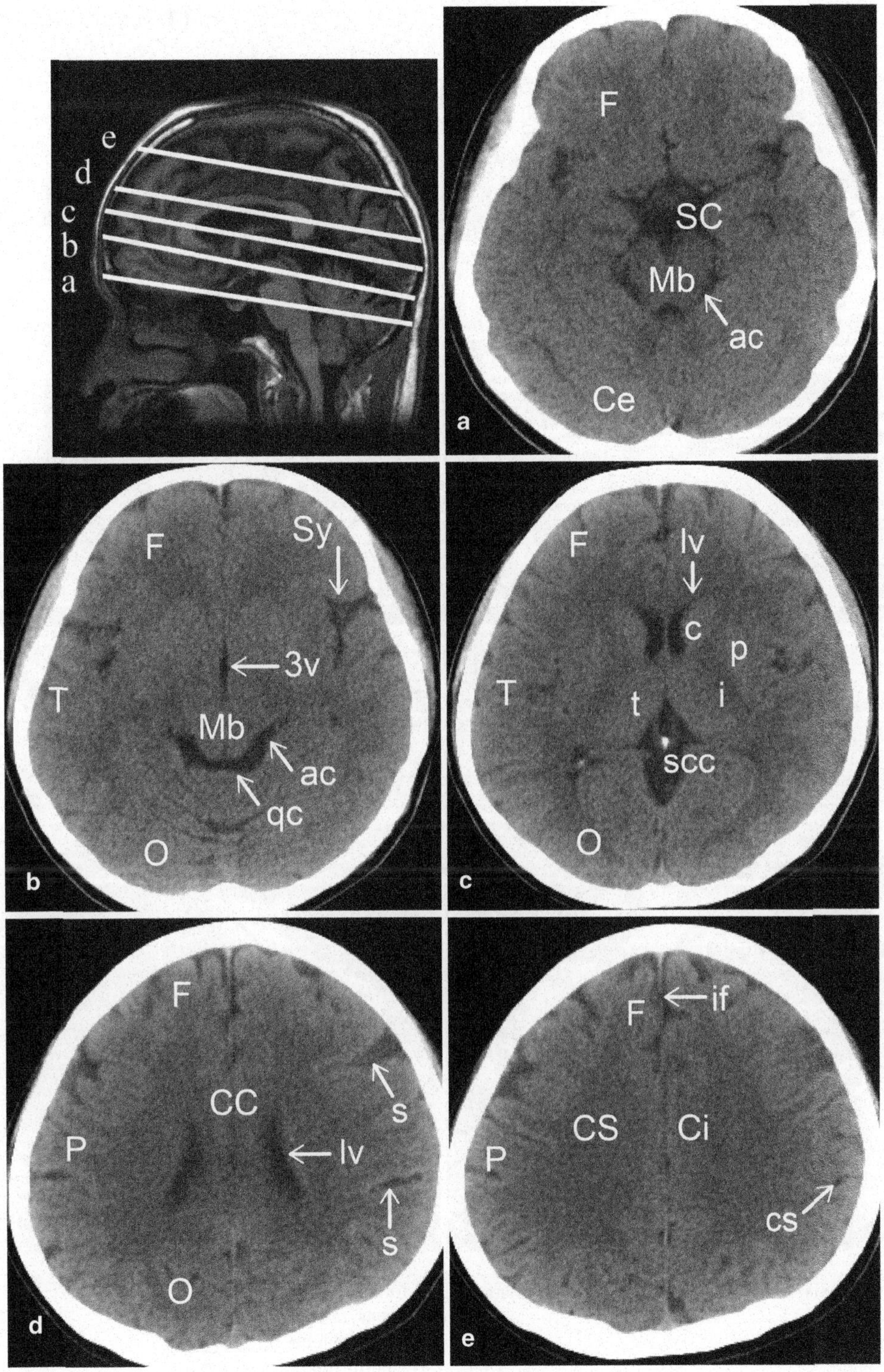

Fig. 1.1 CT—axial sections of normal brain and subarachnoid spaces
F: frontal lobe
Mb: midbrain
T: temporal lobe
SC: suprasellar cistern
Ce: cerebellum
Sy: Sylvian fissure
O: occipital lobe
3v: third ventricle
qc: quadrigeminal cistern
ac: ambient cistern
lv: lateral ventricle
scc: supracerebellar cistern
c: caudate nucleus
p: putamen
t: thalamus
i: internal capsule
CC: corpus callosum
s: sulcus
if: interhemispheric fissure
P: parietal lobe
Ci: cingulum
cs: central sulcus
CS: centrum semiovale

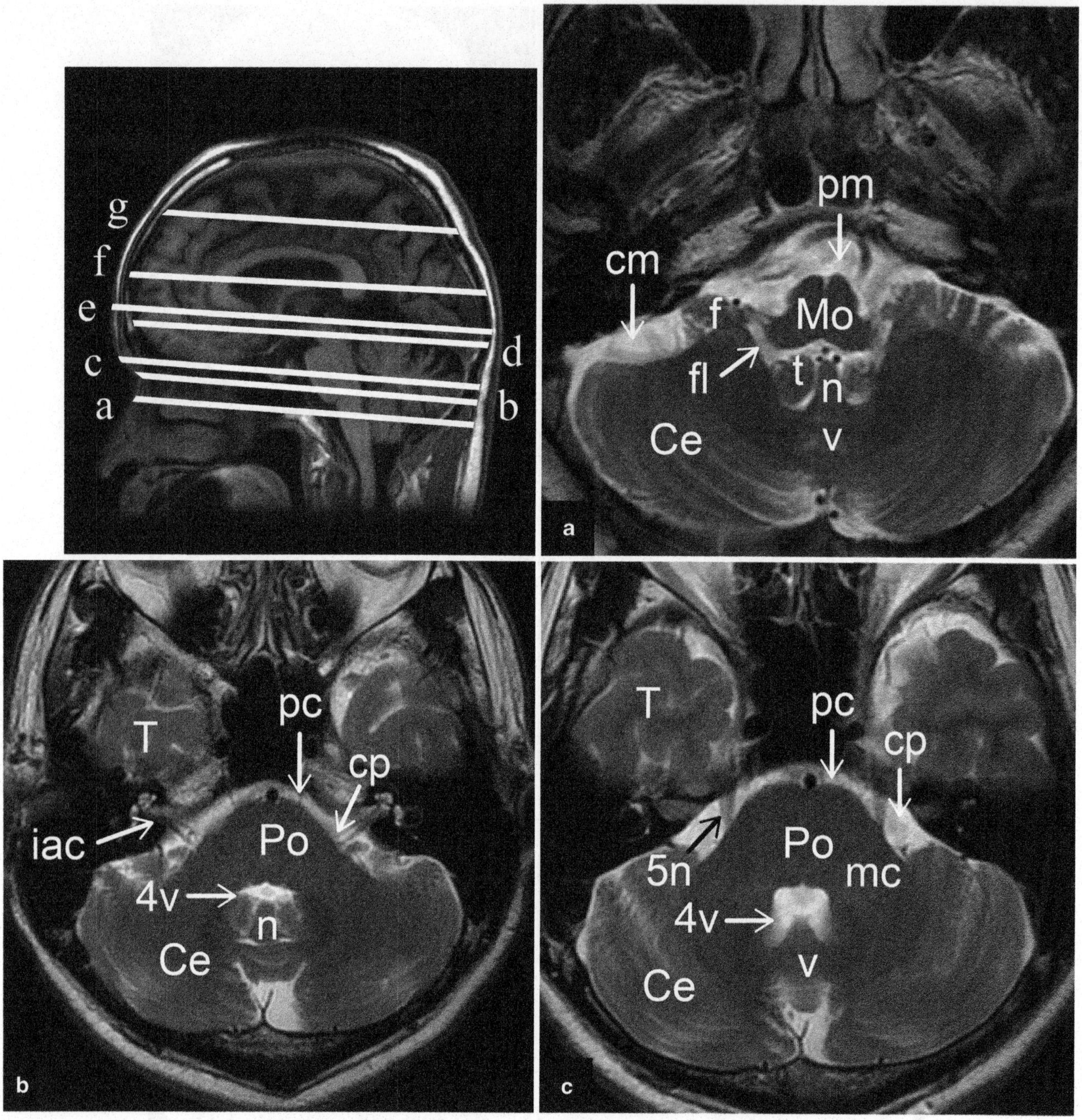

Fig. 1.2 MRI, T2WI—axial sections of normal brain and subarachnoid spaces
Mo: medulla oblongata
Ce: cerebellar hemisphere
f: flocculus
t: tosnsil
v: vermis
n: nodule
cm: cerebellomedullary cistern
pm: premedullary cistern
fl: foramen of Luschka
Po: pons
T: temporal lobe
4v: fourth ventricle
iac: internal auditary canal
cp: cerebellopontine angle cistern
pc: prepontine cistern
mc: middle cerebellar peduncle
5n: trigeminal nerve

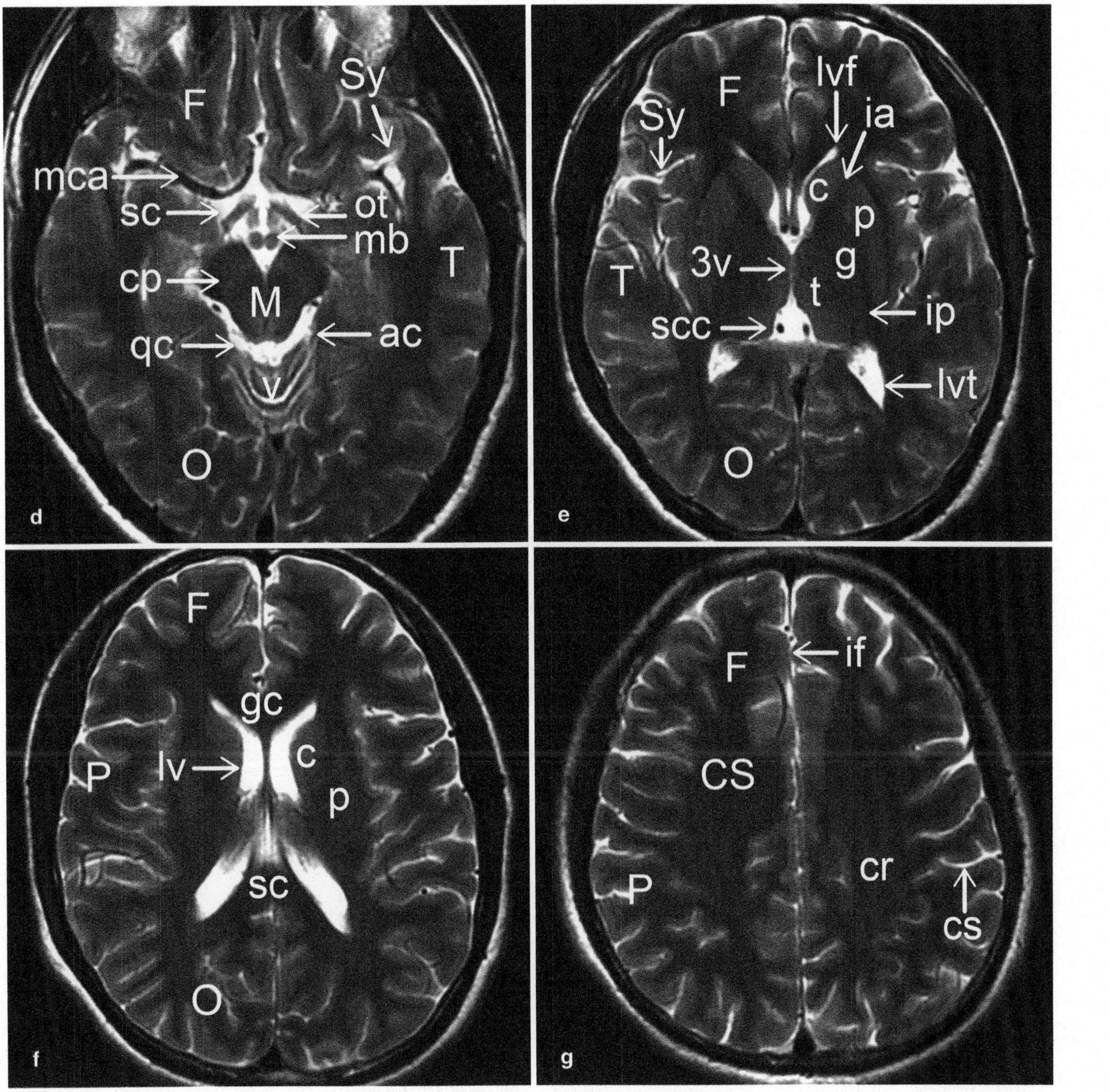

Fig. 1.2 (continued)
M: midbrain
F: frontal lobe
T: temporal lobe
O: occipital lobe
cp: cerebral peduncle
mb: mammillary body
mca: middle cerebral artery
sc: suprasellar cistern
ot: optic tract
Sy: Sylvian fissure
qc: quadrigeminal cistern
ac: ambient cistern
3v: third ventricle
lv: lateral ventricle
lvf: frontal horn of lateral ventricle
lvt: trigone of lateral ventricle
scc: supracerebellar cistern
c: caudate nucleus
p: putamen
g: globus pallidus
t: thalamus
ia: anterior limb of internal capsule
ip: posterior limb of internal capsule
P: parietal lobe
gc: cgenu of corpus callosum
sc: splenium of corpus callosum
CS: centrum semiovale
cr: corona radiata
if: interhemispheric fissure
cs: central sulcus

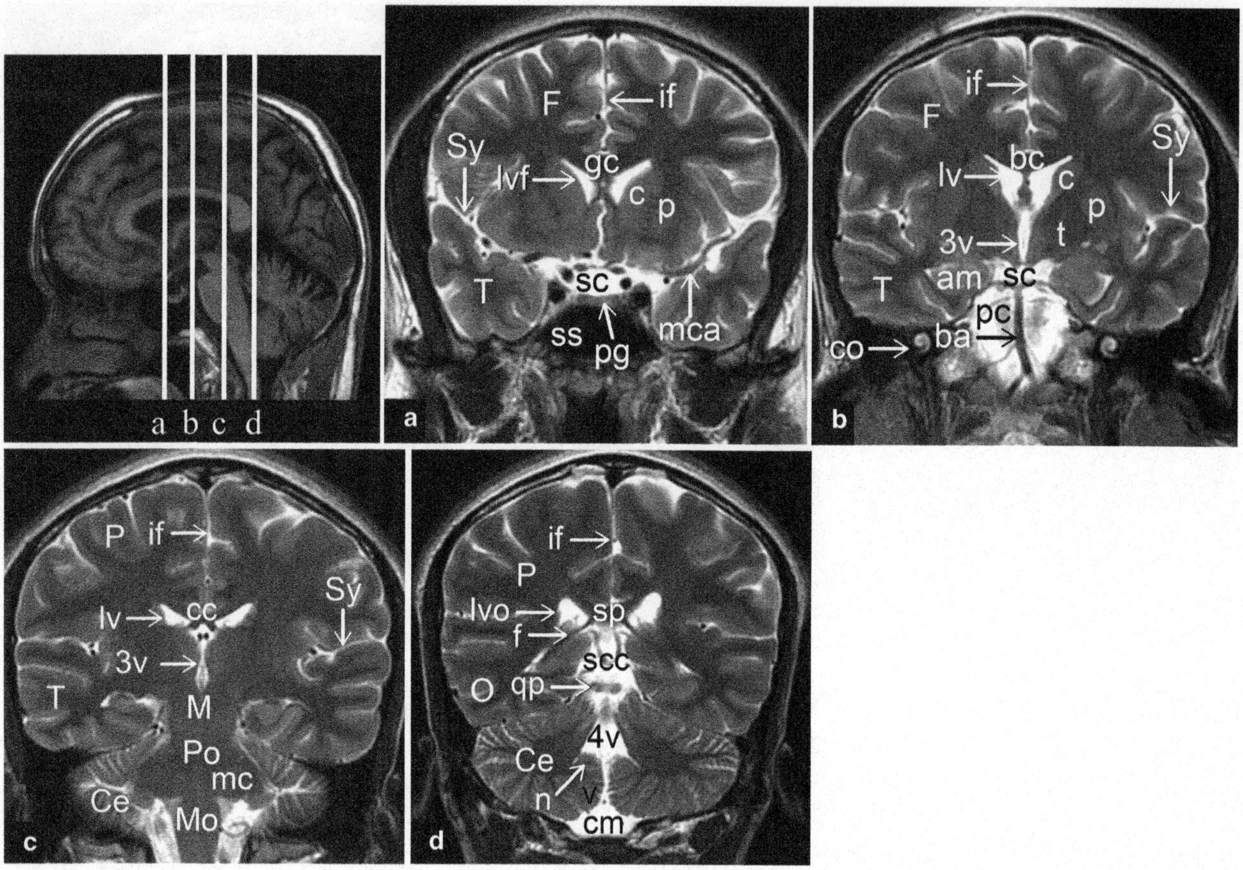

Fig. 1.3 MRI, T2WI—coronal sections of normal brain and subarachnoid spaces
F: frontal lobe
T: temporal lobe
if: interhemispheric fissure
Sy: Sylvian fissure
lvf: frontal horn of lateral ventricle
c: caudate nucleus
p: putamen
gc: genu of corpus callosum
pg: pituitary gland
sc: suprasellar cistern
mca: middle cerebral artery
ss: sphenoid sinus
3v: third ventricle
t: thalamus
lv: lateral ventricle
pc: prepontine cistern
bc: body of corpus callosum
am: amygdala
ba: basilar artery
co: cochlea
P: parietal lobe
cc: corpus callosum
M: midbrain
Po: pons
Mo: medulla oblongata
Ce: cerebellum
mc: middle cerebellar peduncle
O: occipital lobe
sp: splenium of corpus callosum
lvo: occipital horn of lateral ventricle
f: fornix
4v: fourth ventricle
v: vermis
scc: supracerebellar cistern
qp: quadrigeminal plate
cm: cisterna magna
n: nodule

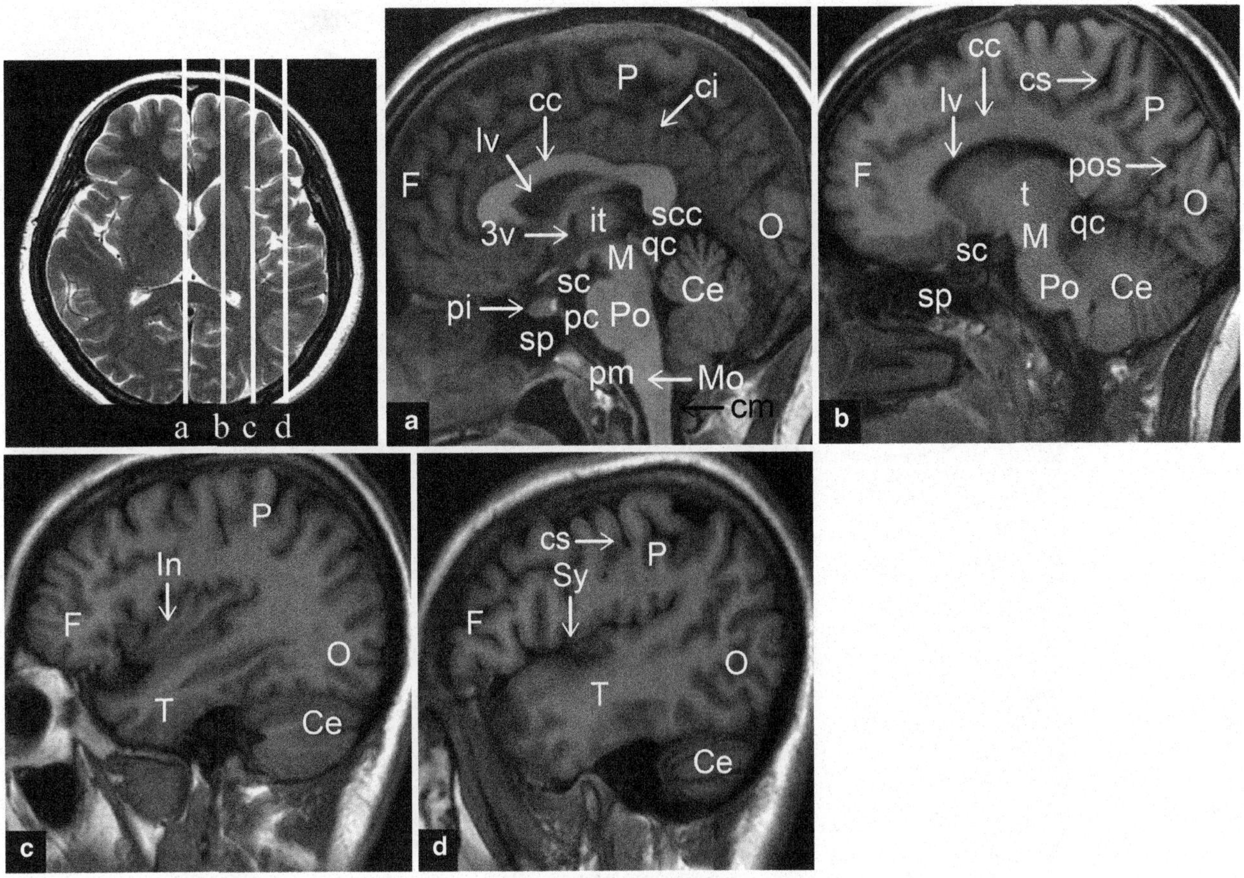

Fig. 1.4 MRI, T1WI—sagittal sections of normal brain and subarachnoid spaces
F: frontal lobe
P: parietal lobe
O: occipital lobe
3v: third ventricle
it: inter-thalamic adhesion
lv: lateral ventricle
cc: corpus callosum
M: midbrain
Po: pons
Mo: medulla oblongata
ci: cingulum
sc: suprasellar cistern
pi: pituitary gland
qc: quadrigeminal cistern
scc: supracerebellar cistern
sp.: sphenoid sinus
pc: prepontine cistern
pm: premedullary cistern
cm: cisterna magna
t: thalamus
cs: central sulcus
pos: parieto-occipital sulcus
T: temporal lobe
Ce: cerebellum
In: insular cortex
Sy: Sylvian fissure

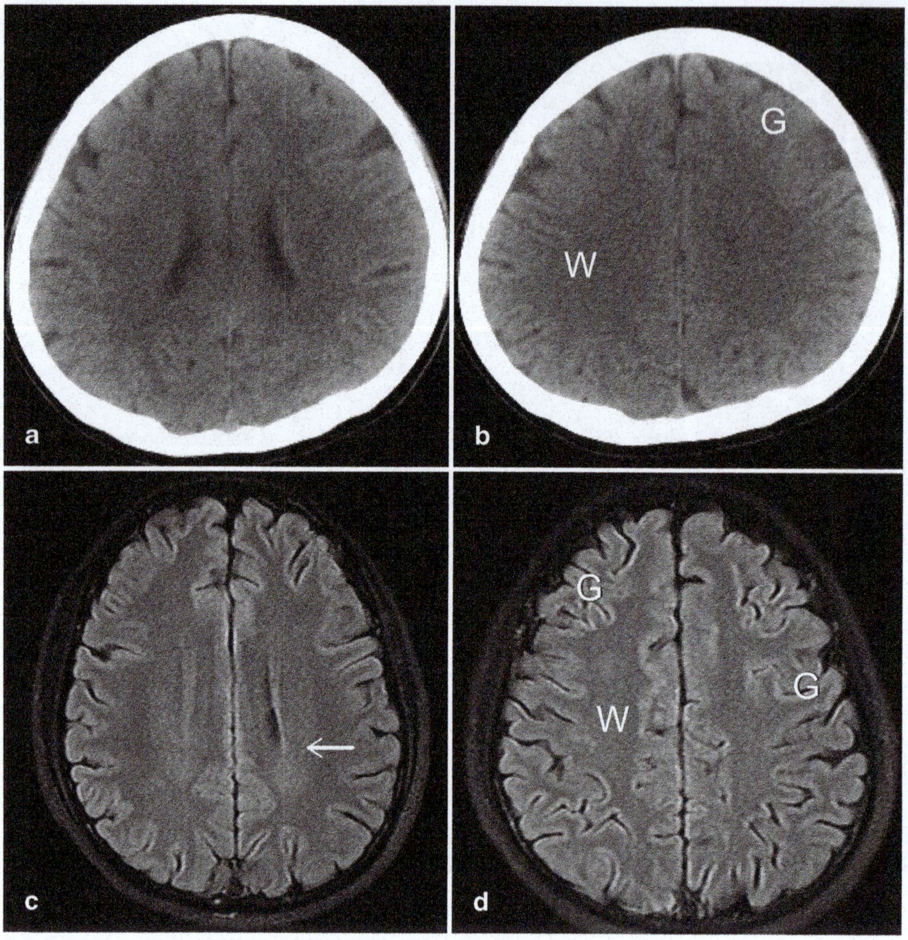

Fig. 1.5 Centrum semiovale and corona radiata. (**a**, **b**) CT: gray matter appears gray, white matter appears mildly gray-dark, and they can be distinguished. (**c**, **d**) MRI, FLAIR: gray matter appears gray, white matter appears gray-dark, and they can be distinguished. Corona radiata (arrow) can be distinguished in the FLAIR because its signal is slightly higher than that of other white matter

G: gray matter
W: white matter
arrow: corona radiata

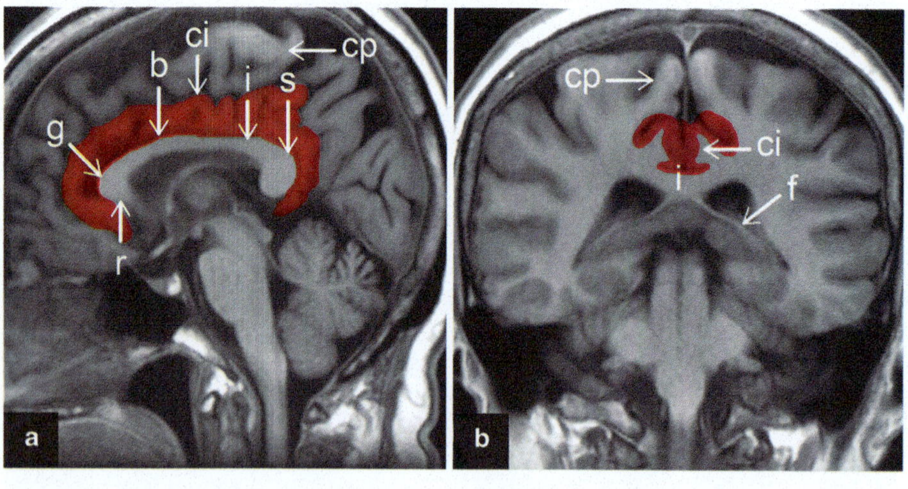

Fig. 1.6 Corpus callosum and cingulum. MRI, T1WI (**a**) sagittal (**b**) coronal
r: rostrum
g: genu
b: body
s: splenium
i: isthmus
ci: cingulum (red color)
cp: cortex of parietal lobe
f: fornix

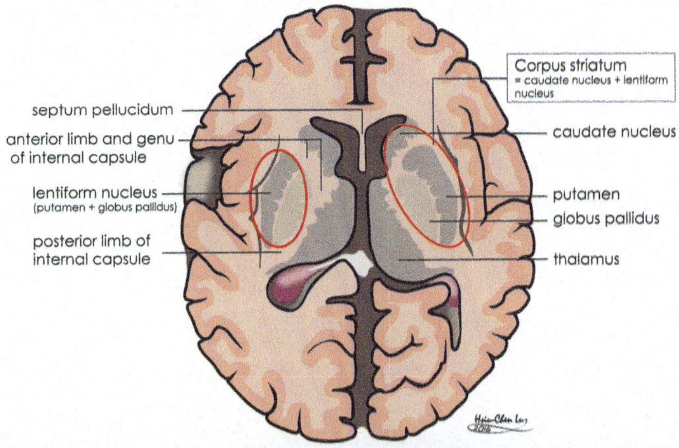

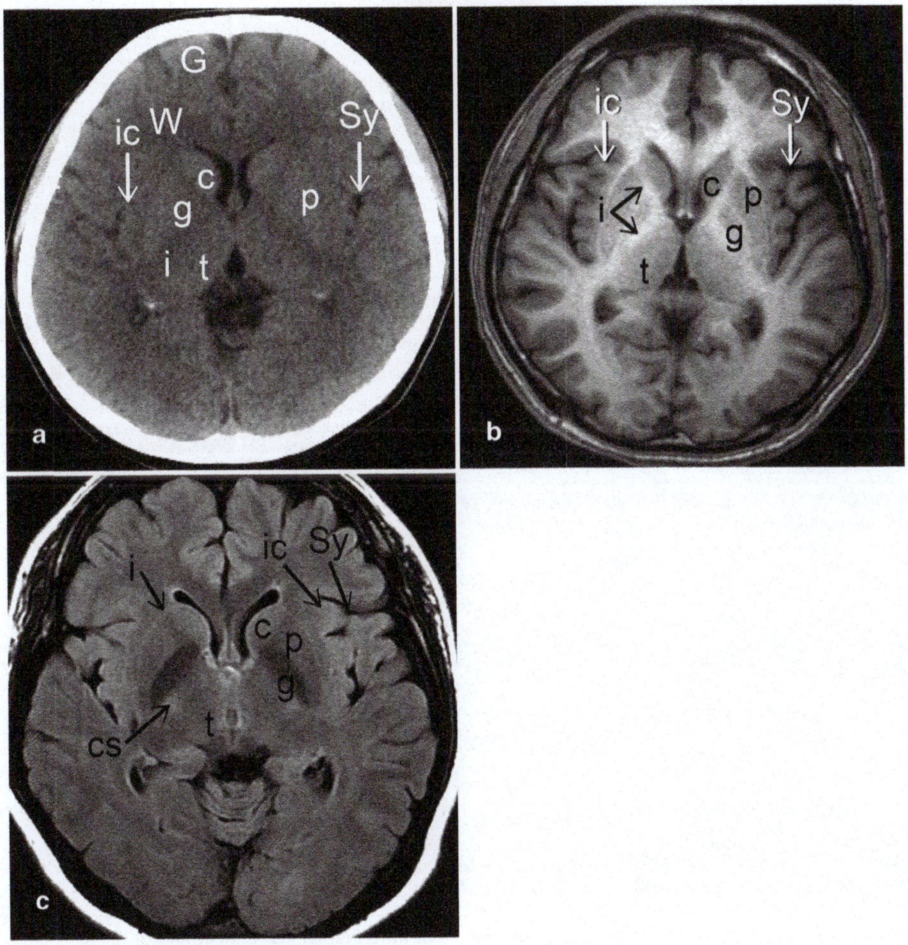

Fig. 1.7 Basal ganglia. (**a**) CT of basal ganglia, (**b**) MRI T1WI, (**c**) MRI FLAIR: *G* gray matter, gray, *W* white matter, slightly darker. The gray matter is in the outer layer, and the white matter is in the inner layer. Deep inside the bilateral Sylvian fissures (Sy), the apparent gray matter structures are the basal ganglia and thalami (t). Between the two is the internal capsule (i), which is white matter and is obviously darker in CT. Putamen (p) and globus pallidus (g) are not easily distinguishable in CT images. (**b**, **c**) MRI: globus pallidus is slightly darker on FLAIR, due to iron content

c: caudate nucleus
p: putamen
g: globus pallidus
t: thalamus
i: internal capsule
ic: insular cortex
Sy: Sylvian fissure
cs: corticospinal tract in the posterior limb of internal capsule

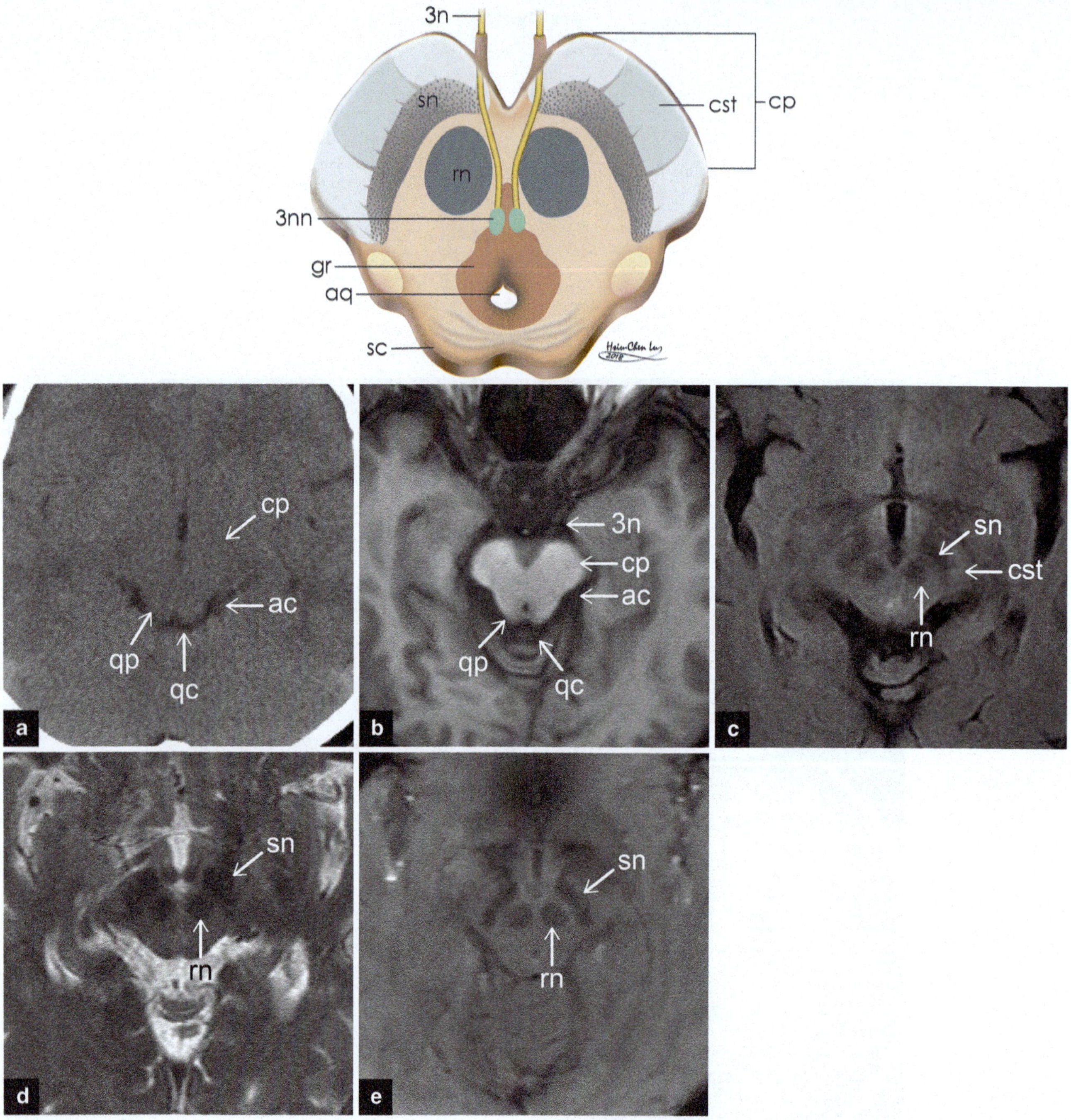

Fig. 1.8 Midbrain. (**a**) CT: only shows the shape of the midbrain. (**b**) MRI, T1WI: can see the shape of midbrain more clearly than in a CT image. (**c–e**) MRI, FLAIR, T2WI, SWAN: can see the red nucleus and substantia nigra clearly

cp: cerebral peduncle
cst: corticospinal tract
rn: red nucleus
sn: substantia nigra
3n: third cranial nerve, oculomotor nerve
3nn: nucleus of third cranial nerve
aq: aqueduct
gr: periaqueductal gray matter
sc: superior colliculus
qp: quadrigeminal plate
qc: quadrigeminal cistern
ac: ambient cistern

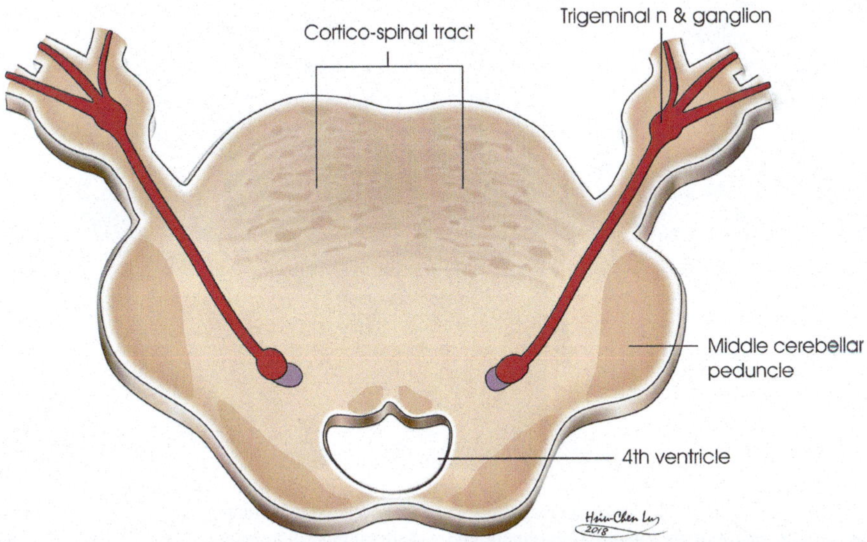

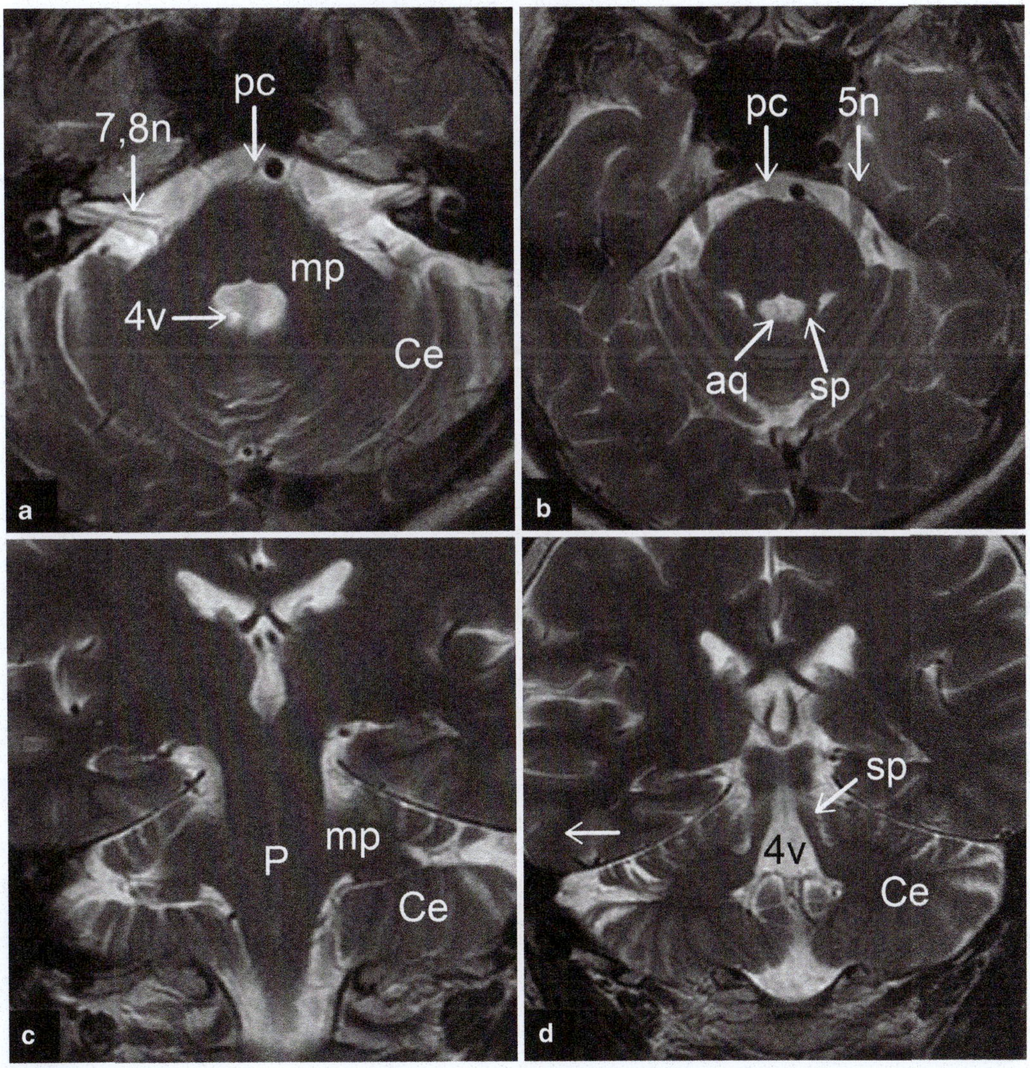

Fig. 1.9 Pons MRI: T2WI (**a**, **b**) axial and (**c**, **d**) coronal sections
a: inferior part of pons
b: superior part of pons
sp.: superior cerebellar peduncle
mp: middle cerebellar peduncle
pc: prepontine cistern
7,8n: seventh and eighth cranial nerves
5n: fifth cranial nerve
4v: fourth ventricle
aq: aqueduct
Ce: cerebellar hemisphere
P: pons

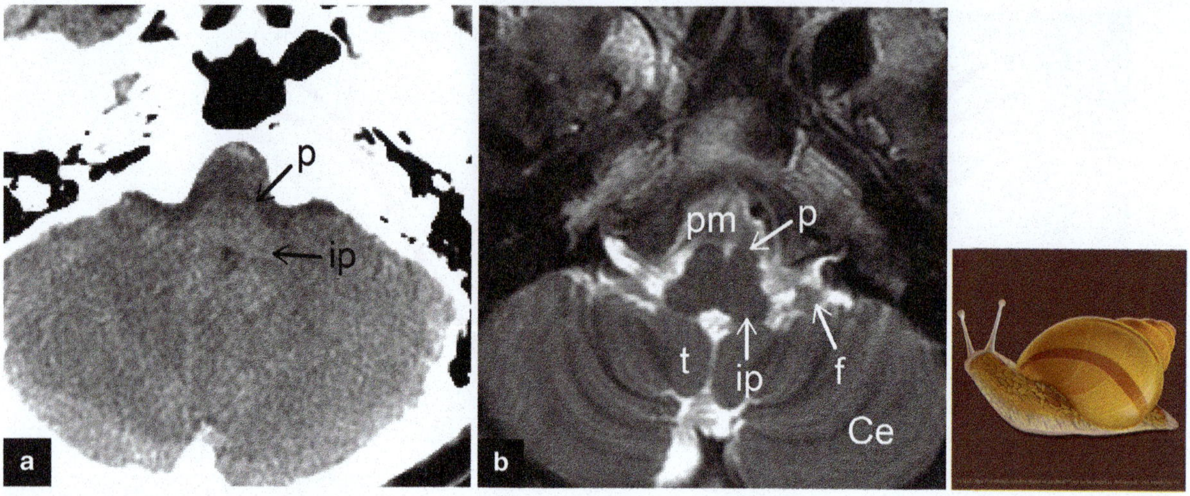

Fig. 1.10 Medulla oblongata. (**a**) CT: medulla oblongata is unclear in CT. (**b**) MRI, T2WI: can see the shape of the medulla oblongata and surrounding structures. The entire medulla oblongata appears as a snail. The pyramid is a stop for the corticospinal tract that conveys movements. Hence, the corticospinal tract is also called the pyramidal tract
p: pyramid
ip: inferior cerebellar peduncle
Ce: cerebellar hemisphere
f: flocculus
t: tonsil
pm: premedullary cistern

Fig. 1.11 Corticospinal tract (pyramidal tract). MRI of corticospinal tract: (**a–d**) FLAIR, axial (**e**, **f**) T2WI, axial and coronal: (**a**) Corona radiata level: the corticospinal tracts are in the corona radiate, which is in the subcortical white matter of frontoparietal lobes—within the centrum semiovale. In FLAIR, the corona radiata appears slightly white (arrows). (**b**) Basal ganglion level: the corticospinal tracts pass through the posterior limbs of internal capsules, manifesting as a small white point (arrows). g: globus pallidus. (**c**) Midbrain level: the corticospinal tracts (arrows) pass through the cerebral peduncles. s: substantia nigra. (**d**) Pons level: the corticospinal tracts are slightly white on both sides of the pons. (**e**) Medulla oblongata level: the corticospinal tracts pass through the pyramid (p). (**f**) T2WI, coronal section: the entire corticospinal tract (arrows)

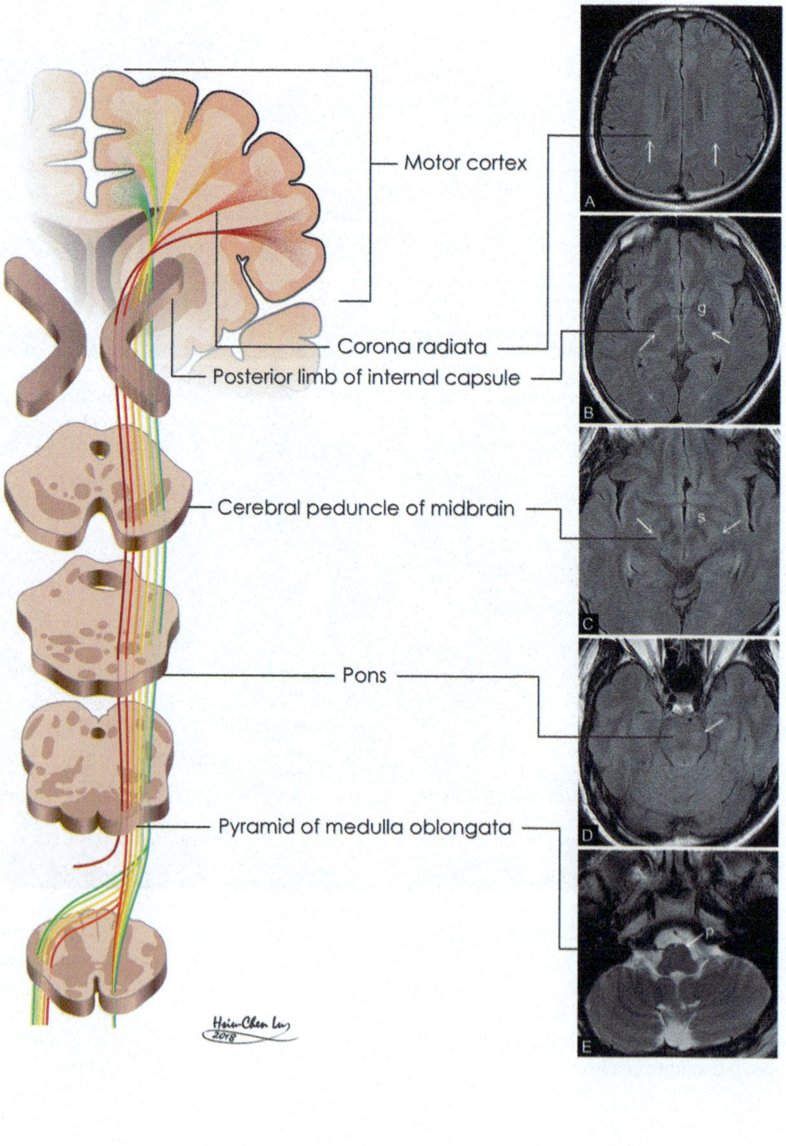

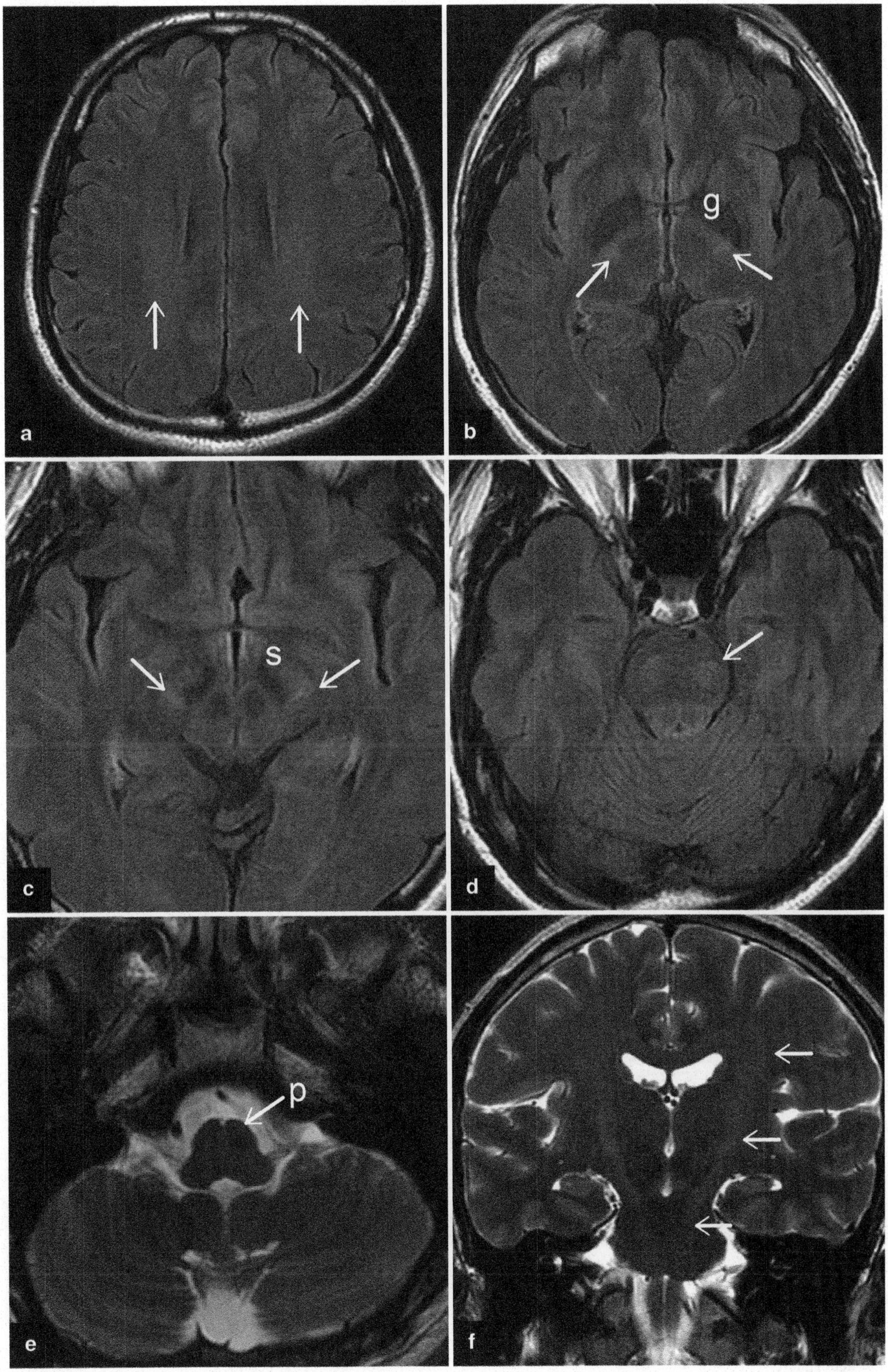

Fig. 1.11 (continued)

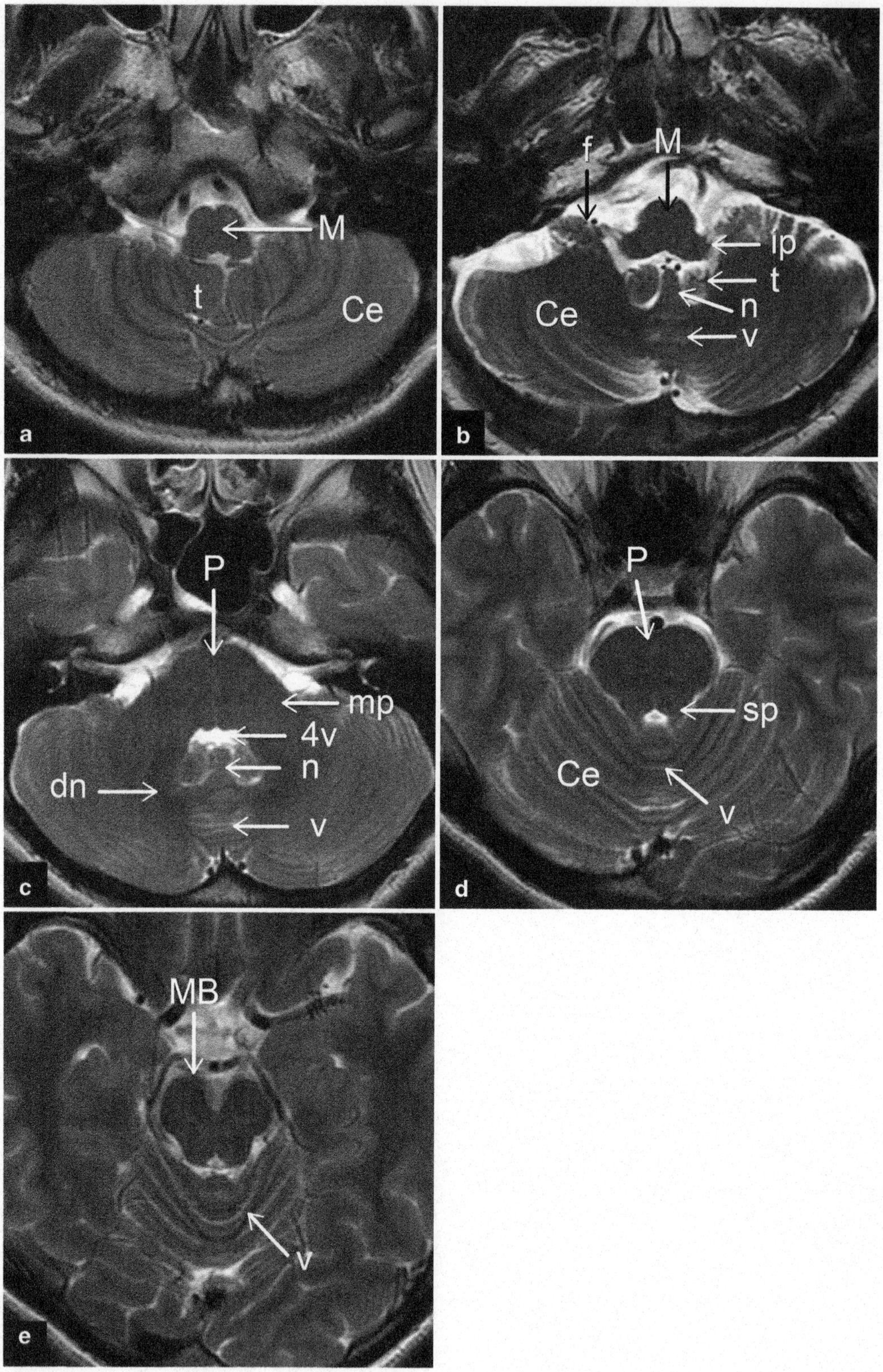

Fig. 1.12 Cerebellum. T2WI, axial sections
M: medulla oblongata
P: pons
MB: midbrain
Ce: cerebellar hemisphere
v: vermis
t: tonsil
f: flocculus
n: nodule
dn: dentate nucleus
ip: inferior cerebellar peduncle
mp: middle cerebellar peduncle
sp.: superior cerebellar peduncle
4v: fourth ventricle

1.2 Subarachnoid Space

Subarachnoid space (SAS), also known as cerebrospinal fluid space (CSF space), contains the following anatomies:

The ventricles, cisterns, fissures, and sulci, which are connected from the skull to the entire spinal canal. The whole brain and spinal cord are immersed in the CSF to keep lubricating. These constructs are just different names and are communicating with each other.

The CSF space is essential when interpreting CT and MRI images because they can help to identify the anatomy of the brain tissue.

The SAS itself, which may have many diseases, such as subarachnoid hemorrhage (SAH; Chap. 4), meningitis (Chap. 7), and pneumocephalus (Chap. 3).

Moreover, when reading the mass effect, whether CSF spaces are compressed and deformed or have disappeared must be checked. In the interpretation of brain tissue atrophy, whether the CSF spaces in the vicinity have widened is important (Details in Chap. 2).

1.2.1 Ventricles

The ventricles (Fig. 1.13) include the following:

- Lateral ventricles—right and left lateral ventricles
- Third ventricle (3rd ventricle)
- Fourth ventricle (4th ventricle)
- Aqueduct connects the third and fourth ventricles

The ventricles have choroid plexus to produce CSF.

1.2.1.1 Lateral Ventricle

Includes:

- Ventral horn or frontal horn
- Posterior horn or occipital horn
- Trigone
- Inferior horn or temporal horn

Inferior Horn or Temporal Horn

Usually, the temporal horns are small and have a slit-like shape. When slight hydrocephalus occurs, temporal horns become most sensitive and expand slightly, appearing as two beards (Figs. 1.14, 2.27, and 2.28).

Foramen of Monro

A small hole between the two lateral ventricles is called the interventricular foramen or foramen of Monro, and it also connects to the third ventricle.

Septum Pellucidum

A transparent membrane between the anterior horns of the bilateral lateral ventricles commonly used in anatomical terms. The following situations may affect the septum pellucidum:

(a) When an anterior communicating artery aneurysm ruptures, it may have a hematoma here (Figs. 4.41 and 4.43).
(b) Typically, the septum pellucidum is located in the midline, but after a mass effect, it shifts to one side (see Chap. 2).
(c) A cavity, which is called the ***cavum septum pellucidum*** or fifth ventricle, sometimes extends back to the splenium of the corpus callosum, which is called the ***cavum vergae*** or sixth ventricle (Fig. 1.15). However, the sixth ventricle can also exist alone. The fifth and sixth ventricles are normal variations and are not connected to the lateral or third ventricle.

1.2.1.2 Third Ventricle

On the transverse section of a CT or MRI image, the normal third ventricle appears as a slit. When mild hydrocephalus is present, the third ventricle is most sensitive, expands slightly, and exhibits an oval shape (Figs. 2.27 and 2.28).

1.2.1.3 Cerebral Aqueduct (Sylvian Aqueduct)

It links the third and fourth ventricles; it is located in the posterior of the pons and goes up through the midbrain into the third ventricle.

Because of its slenderness, the aqueduct is readily apparent in the MRI sagittal section, but it is not easy to identify in the CT and MRI axial sections. When SAH occurs, the aqueduct turns white on CT images (Figs. 1.14, 4.20, and 4.21).

1.2.1.4 Fourth Ventricle

The fourth ventricle is located behind the pons and medulla oblongata and in front of the cerebellum. It connects to the third ventricle via the aqueduct and to the cisterna magna from below via the foramen of Magendie.

The fourth ventricle connects to bilateral cerebellopontine (CP) angle cisterns via bilateral lateral apertures of the fourth ventricle, which is also known as the foramen of Luschka.

The fourth ventricle also has a choroid plexus that produces CSF, which is located above the cerebellar tonsil.

The fourth ventricle appears as a diamond in a coronal section (Fig. 1.3d).

1.2.2 Cisterns

We must know several essential cisterns.

1.2.2.1 Suprasellar Cistern

Located above the sella turcica, it presents a pentagon shape. It is an essential anatomical structure. The suprasellar cistern is preceded by the frontal lobe, besides it is the bilateral temporal lobes, and behind it is the brainstem (pons and midbrain).

When there is a strong intracranial mass effect that may cause uncal herniation or central herniation, the brain tissue herniates into this cistern. Moreover, when the mass effect is more severe and causes transtentorial herniation, the distortion or even disappearance of the cistern is observed (see Chap. 2, Figs. 2.20, 2.21, 2.22, 2.23, and 2.24).

SAH is caused by an aneurysm rupture; this cistern is filled with blood, which spreads to other CSF spaces (Chap. 4).

1.2.2.2 Quadrigeminal Cistern

It is located behind the midbrain and exhibits a smiling mouth shape on CT and MRI axial sections.

When a transtentorial herniation occurs, this cistern distorts or even disappears (see Chap. 2, Figs. 2.20, 2.22, 2.23, and 2.24).

1.2.2.3 Supracerebellar Cistern

It is located behind the quadrigeminal cistern and above the cerebellum.

1.2.2.4 Ambient Cistern

It is located in front of the quadrigeminal cistern and beside the bilateral cerebral peduncles.

1.2.2.5 CP Angle Cistern (Cerebellopontine Angle Cistern)

It is the subarachnoid space observed in the posterior fossa, located outside the cerebellum and pons.

1.2.2.6 Prepontine Cistern

This cistern is located in front of the pons.

1.2.2.7 Cisterna Magna (Cerebellomedullary Cistern)

It is located behind the medulla oblongata and under the cerebellum.

1.2.3 Fissures

1.2.3.1 Sylvian Fissure

The Sylvian fissure is also known as the lateral sulcus or lateral fissure (Figs. 1.1, 1.2, 1.3, and 1.4).

It is the earliest sulcus to develop during the embryonic period.

It is a crucial anatomical boundary, with the frontal lobe in front, temporal lobe in the lower back, parietal lobe in the upper back, and basal ganglia on the inside.

The Sylvian fissure appears as a Y-shape in CT and MRI axial sections.

The branches of the middle cerebral artery are present within this fissure.

SAH usually appears in the Sylvian fissure and is easily identifiable on CT images (Chaps. 3 and 4).

1.2.3.2 Interhemispheric Fissure

The interhemispheric fissure (Figs. 1.1, 1.2, and 1.3), also known as the medial longitudinal fissure, is a split between bilateral cerebral hemispheres, with a falx in the middle; the main trunks of bilateral anterior cerebral arteries are located in this fissure.

In the interhemispheric fissure, it is easy to have SAH and even subdural hematoma (Chap. 3).

1.2.4 Sulci

The surface of the brain is covered with numerous sulci; some of them are named. In this book, we only mention the two most essential sulci, namely the central sulcus and parieto-occipital sulcus.

1.2.4.1 Central Sulcus of Rolando

It is a crucial anatomical landmark (Figs. 1.1e and 1.2g). In front of this sulcus is the frontal lobe, and behind it is the parietal lobe. The primary motor cortex is in front of it, and the primary somatosensory cortex is behind it.

1.2.4.2 Parieto-Occipital Sulcus

This sulcus is located between the parietal lobe and the occipital lobe (Fig. 1.4b).

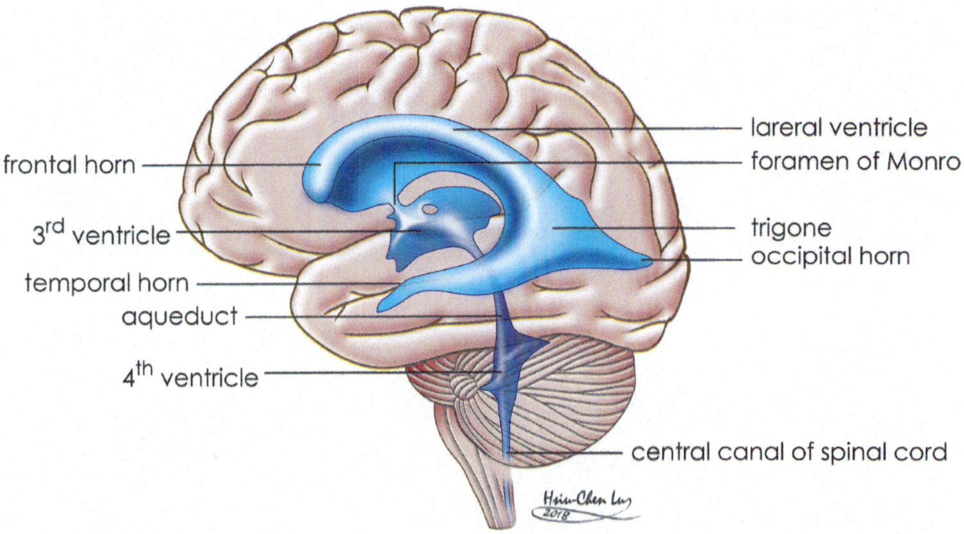

Fig. 1.13 The ventricles

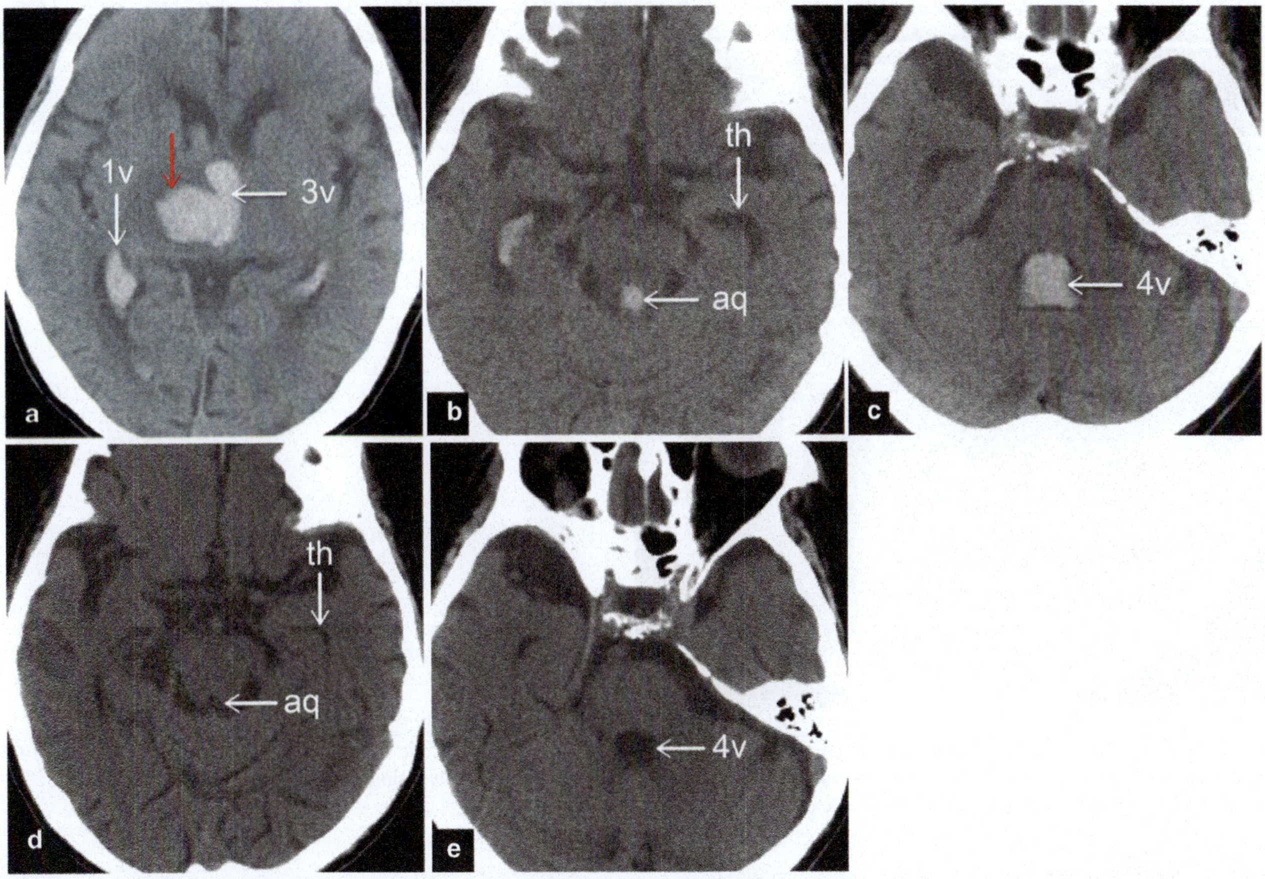

Fig. 1.14 M/72, Thalamic hemorrhage with intraventricular hemorrhage (IVH). (**a–c**) CT: an acute hematoma (red arrow) in the right thalamus due to hypertension; the hematoma ruptures into the third ventricle (3v) and lateral ventricle (lv), and flows to the fourth ventricle (4v) via the aqueduct (aq). The SAH causes mild hydrocephalus; the bilateral temporal horns (th) are slightly dilated. (**d**, **e**) Compare with the CT from 1 year ago: the fourth ventricle containing CSF appears dark (4v), the aqueduct (aq) is too small to be recognized, and the temporal horns (th) are slit-like

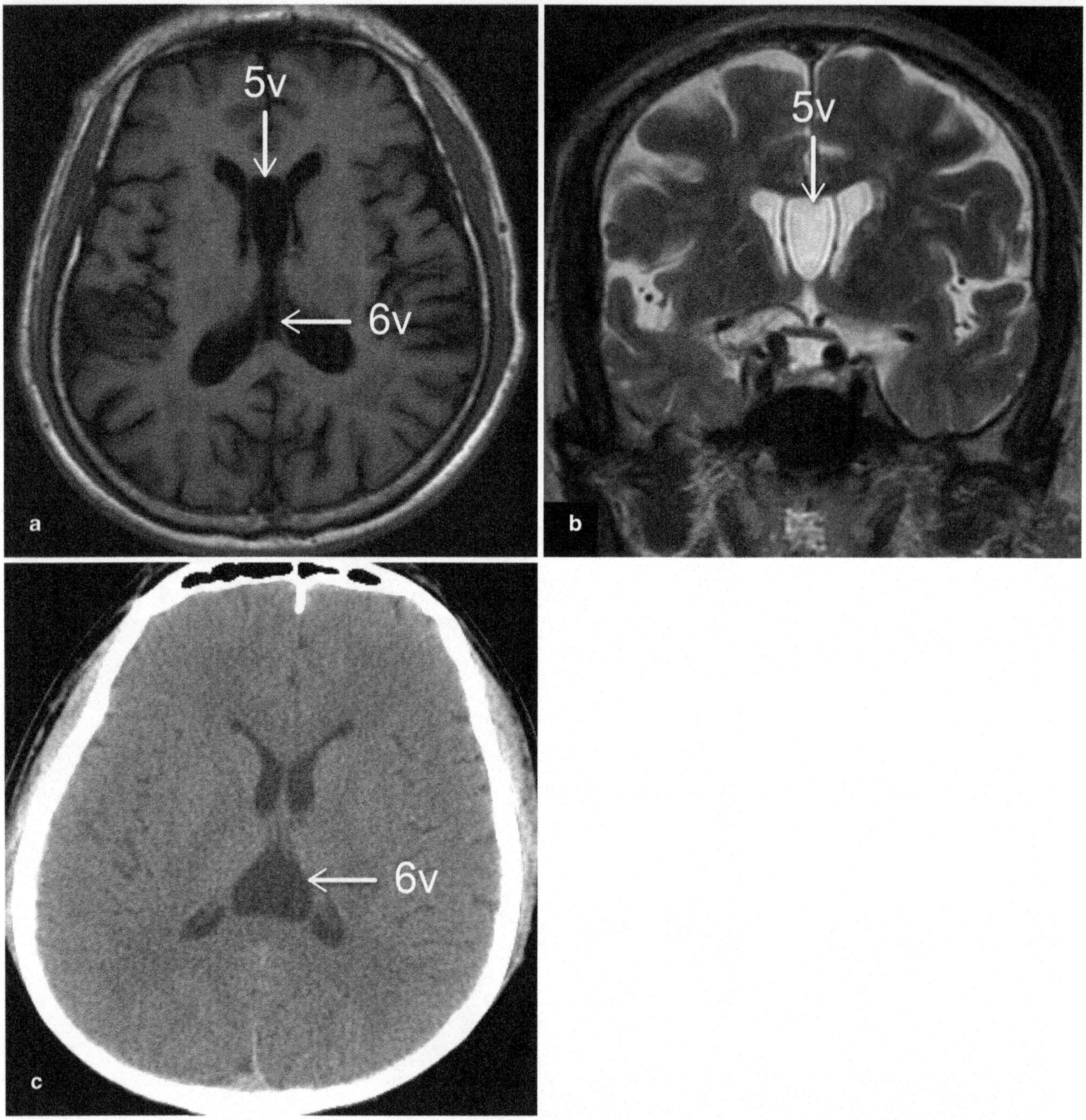

Fig. 1.15 Cavum septum pellucidum and cavum vergae. (**a**) MRI, T1WI, axial (**b**) T2WI, coronal: the cavum septum pellucidum (fifth ventricle, 5v) sometimes extends back to the splenium of the corpus callosum and forms the cavum vergae (sixth ventricle, 6v). (**c**) CT: another case has only a single cavum vergae (sixth ventricle)

2 Basics of Interpretation of Brain CT and MRI

Abstract

Several basic concepts are crucial for using CT and MRI in diagnosing central nervous system diseases. Familiarity with the densities of normal structures and pathology is the first step to interpret the CT images. In addition, familiarity with MR pulse sequences and signal intensity of normal structures and pathologies is essential to interpret the MR images. Normal brain tissue has no contrast medium enhancement because of the blood–brain barrier. Non-brain tissue structures such as vessels, falx, and tentorium and most pathologies can be enhanced by contrast medium. Most "active lesions" have a mass effect. For severe mass effect, several kinds of brain tissue herniations occur. There are five patterns of intracranial hemorrhages exist. The hydrocephalus may be divided as obstructive and communicating. For mild hydrocephalus, dilatations of the third ventricle and temporal horns of the lateral ventricle are most sensitive. Three kinds of brain tissue edema, namely cytotoxic and vasogenic and interstitial, are noted, and MRI DWI is crucial to distinguish them. The diagnosis of brain atrophy sees the widening of subarachnoid spaces. CT for Wallerian degeneration can identify only the atrophy of cerebral peduncle in the late-stage. MRI long TR images can show hyperintensity along the course of the corticospinal tract.

2.1 CT Grayscale

The CT grayscale is also known as the Hounsfield scale (Table 2.1). It is a tool used to interpret CT results.

In CT, the water attenuation value to X-rays is set to 0 Hu (Hounsfield units). Water in the human body includes the cerebrospinal fluid (CSF) and urine. The attenuation value of such fluids (approximately 4–6 Hu) is slightly higher than that of water, and these fluids appear dark in the CT image (Fig. 2.1). The matter with a Hu attenuation value lower than that of water includes fat (−20 to −120 Hu) and air (−1000 Hu) (Fig. 2.2). The attenuation values and colors of normal tissues are displayed in Table 2.1.

Table 2.1 CT grayscale

Tissue and pathology	Hu	Density
Metal		Artifacts generated
Bone cortex	1000–1800	White
Bone marrow	400–800	White; dark gray on bone window
Calcification	100–500	White
Hematoma (acute)	60–90	White
Soft tissue	35–45	Gray
Soft tissue edema	15–30	Dark gray, with mass effect
Soft tissue necrosis (e.g., encephalomalacia)	10–20	Dark gray
Body fluid (e.g., CSF)	4–6	Dark
Water	0	Dark
Fat	−20 to −120	Dark
Air	−1000	Dark

Bone appears white (Fig. 2.1), and the bone cortex cannot be distinguished from bone marrow. Therefore, the area should be adjusted to the bone window when necessary. On the bone window, bone marrow appears dark gray, whereas the bone cortex appears white.

Intracerebral hematoma (ICH) appears white (60–90 Hu) when it is fresh and in the acute stage. The hematoma becomes absorbed and gradually diluted over time. Within about 40–60 days, the hematoma may appear dark gray (20–30 Hu) and cannot be distinguished from cerebral edema (Fig. 2.3).

Only ICH appears white. Acute hematoma in another body part will not appear as white, as does ICH.

Brain tissue edema appears slightly dark gray with mass effect when it is in the early period. As the mass

W.-C. Shen, *Diagnostic Neuroradiology*, https://doi.org/10.1007/978-981-15-4051-6_2

effect increases over time, the color becomes even darker (Fig. 2.4). If the edema does not disappear, the brain tissue gradually necroses. In the chronic stage, the original edema area becomes encephalomalacia, and the CT image is dark and reveals brain tissue atrophy.

Calcification in the brain, physiological or pathologic, is easily identified (Fig. 2.5) and should not be confused with ICH. Physiological calcification is generally bilaterally symmetric. Some brain tumors and arteriovenous malformations (AVMs) contain calcifications.

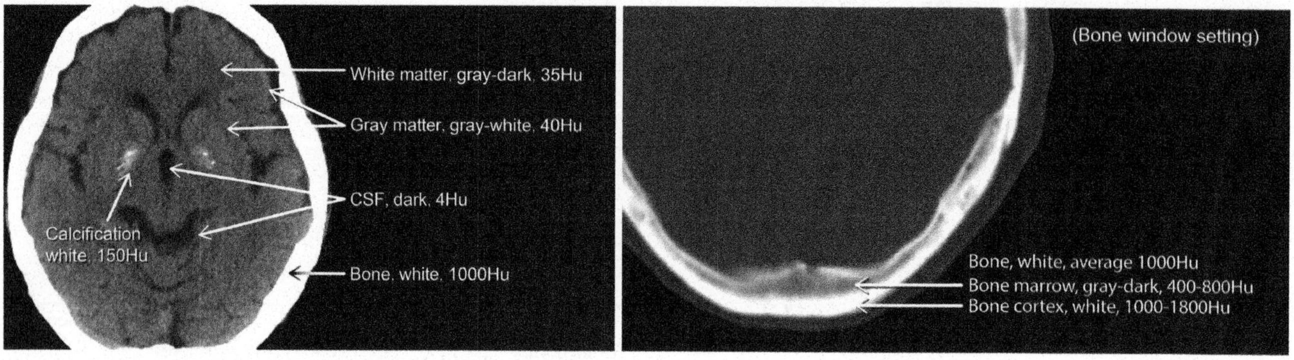

Fig. 2.1 CT of brain and cranium of a healthy 70-year-old man

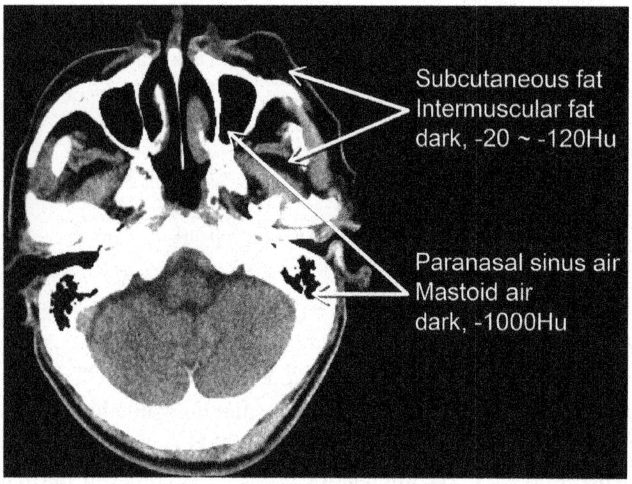

Fig. 2.2 Normal paranasal sinuses and mastoids

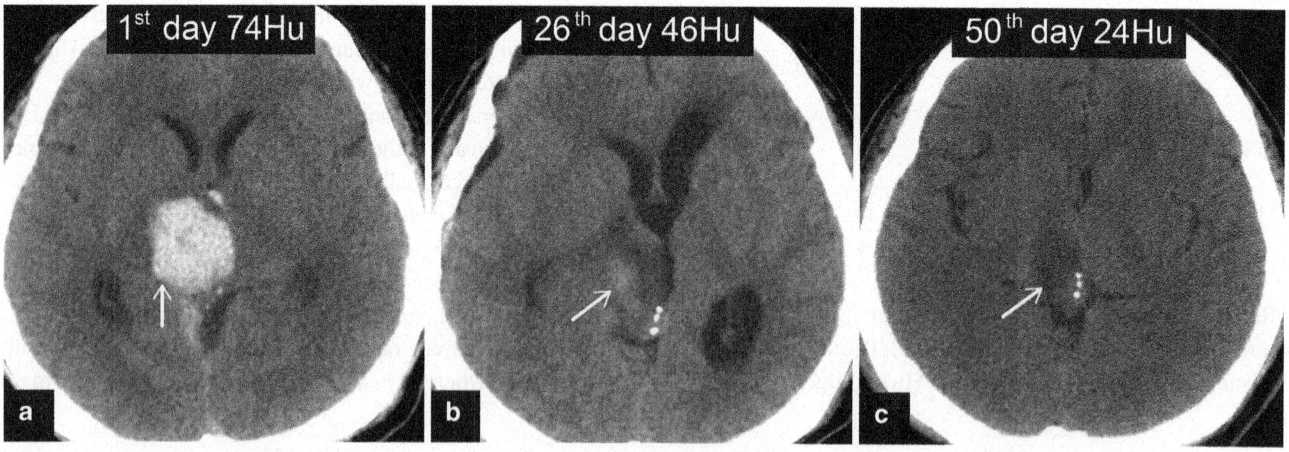

Fig. 2.3 M/47, intracerebral hematoma (ICH), and its evolution. CVA due to right thalamic hemorrhage. On CT, fresh ICH appears white ([**a**] acute stage), fades over time ([**b**] late subacute stage), and becomes dark gray ([**c**] late subacute stage). The ICH is easily mistaken for brain tissue edema when it turns dark gray (**c**)

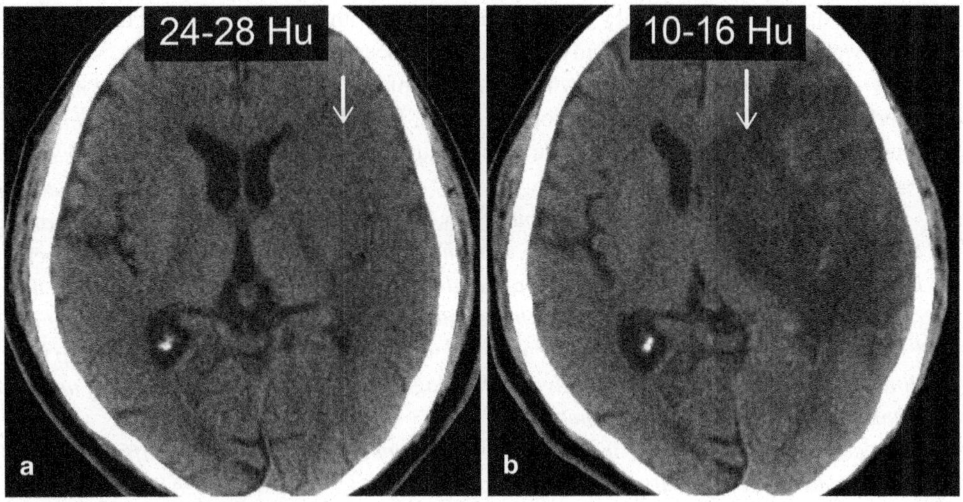

Fig. 2.4 M/73, acute brain tissue edema due to MCA infarction. Acute brain tissue edema shows mass effect in addition to dark gray density (note: sulci have disappeared). (**a**) On the first day of infarction, it is in the very early stage of brain tissue edema, density slightly decreases to dark gray (24–28 Hu), and the mass effect is weak. (**b**) On the fourth day of infarction, brain tissue edema peaks, density darkens (10–16 Hu), and the mass effect is strong

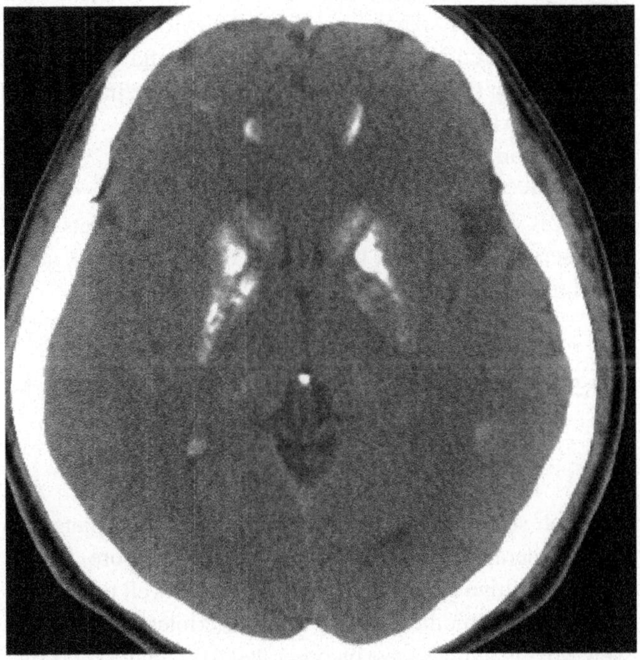

Fig. 2.5 F/39, Calcifications. Patient with hyperparathyroidism. Calcification in the bilateral corpus striata. Calcification: 100–500 Hu. Calcification is white and usually bilaterally and symmetrically

2.2 MRI Pulse Sequences

The number of available MRI pulse sequences has increased with the advancement of MRI instruments, resulting in shorter examination time, improved image resolution, and strengthen functionality. Therefore, MRI instruments must be continually updated in both their hardware and software to meet user needs. Not all pulse sequences are used in routine examinations; some are applied only in specific diseases. Figure 2.6 illustrates the color (signal intensity) of routine pulse sequences employed in regular clinical examinations.

2.2.1 Spin Echo Sequences

The spin echo sequence is the most fundamental and commonly used MRI sequences; it includes the following:

- ***T1-weighted image (T1WI)***

  Images with a short repetition time (TR) and short echo time (TE) are necessary for routine MRI examinations. In a T1WI, CSF appears dark; white matter appears slightly gray (mild hyperintensity), and the gray matter appears slightly dark (mild hypointensity). Fat appears white (hyperintensity). Cerebral edema appears dark gray. Subacute hematoma-containing methemoglobin appears white. Protein-containing cysts appear white.
- ***T2-weighted image (T2WI)***

  The T2WI is obtained using long TR and long TE, CSF appears white (hyperintensity). Brain tissue edema appears gray-white (mild hyperintensity). And a slight increase in water content, such as demyelination and gliosis, also appear gray-white in T2WI.
- ***Proton-density-weighted image (PDWI)***

  A PDWI is an image obtained using long TR and short TE; this has similar effects to those in a T2WI but removes the flowing CSF signals. The current MRI, PDW is no longer used, replaced by FLAIR.

2.2.2 Inversion Recovery Sequences

- ***Fluid-attenuated inversion recovery (FLAIR)***

  A FLAIR image is a type of T2WI from which the signal intensity of flowing CSF has been removed (attenuated), and appears dark. Only brain tissue lesions with static water—such as edema, demyelination, and encephalitis—show high signals (gray-white). A lack of CSF interference facilitates the observation of lesions. FLAIR images are also one of the most basic pulse sequences in routine MRI examinations.

CSF signals of a sulcus with a lesion, if any, might not be completely attenuated. For example, in meningitis and leptomeningeal metastasis, CSF is impure and referred to as dirty CSF. In FLAIR images, sulcal hyperintensity may be observed (Fig. 2.7) [1]. *This sign, combined with injection of contrast medium, is conducive to the diagnosis of meningitis and leptomeningeal metastasis.*

In certain situations, CSF is clean, but sulcal hyperintensity nonetheless appears in a FLAIR image. Thus, sulci around the tumor, sulci in the cerebral infarction area, sinus thrombosis, and sulci near vascular diseases (e.g., AVM and AV fistula) may exhibit the white FLAIR signals of a sulcus [1, 2].

- ***Short tau inversion recovery (STIR), also named short inversion time (TI) inversion recovery (STIR)***

  STIR is used to suppress fat signals. STIR is routinely used in MRI of spine examination.

2.2.3 Gradient Echo Sequences (GREs)

- ***T2*WI***

  $T2^*$WI is used to detect minerals in the brain, such as calcium, iron, copper, etc. It is very sensitive to the detection of intracranial hemorrhage. Both old and new hemorrhage show very dark signals. In the new MRI instrument, T2*WI has been replaced by SWI.
- ***Fat-suppression imaging sequence***

  This sequence can be used when obtaining both T1WIs and T2WIs. It is often used in MRI of orbits and skull base examinations to suppress the fat signal. It is also used in T1WI with Gadolinium enhancement to avoid the fat from interfering with the enhanced lesion.

2.2.4 Diffusion-weighted imaging (DWI)

DWI has become the routine MRI pulse sequence for imaging the brain. It is also used in abdomen, pelvis, and prostate examinations. DWI is mainly used in acute brain infarcts which cause acute cytotoxic edema. Cytotoxic edema of the brain tissue hinders the Brownian motion of water molecules in brain tissue. This restricted diffusion of water molecules results in strong DWI signals and white appearance (Fig. 2.8). Water molecule diffusion restriction does not occur in other conditions, such as peritumoral white matter edema and increased water in brain tissue caused by demyelination; thus, the signals are unaffected (no signal change in DWI).

Besides, the following is observed for DWI:

1. *The solid part of most brain tumors, benign or malignant, appears slightly white in DWI, whereas hemangioblastoma with abundant vessels appears dark in DWI (Fig. 6.19).*
2. *Cystic change and necrosis of tumors exhibit signals similar to that of CSF, namely dark in DWI and white in the apparent diffusion coefficient (ADC) map* (Fig. 2.9).
3. *Pus in a brain abscess has strong diffusion restriction; hence, the pus appears white in DWI and has a low ADC showing dark in the ADC map* (Fig. 2.10). *This is a crucial difference from the signals of tumor cystic change or necrosis.*

- ***Apparent diffusion coefficient (ADC)***

  The ADC is a consequence of DWI, quantifies the diffusion coefficient of water molecules. The resulting image is called an ADC map. A lower coefficient indicates a darker signal. Therefore, the cytotoxic edema of acute infarction appears white in DWI and dark in the ADC map (Fig. 2.6e); the pus appears white in DWI and dark in ADC map (Fig. 2.10).
- ***Diffusion tensor imaging***

  This imaging method enables observation of how nerves in the brain connect. This technique lets MRI observe the diffusion behavior of water molecules in the white matter area.

2.2.5 Susceptibility-Weighted Imaging (SWI), or Susceptibility-Weighted Angiography (SWAN)

SWI can sensitively detect focal magnetic field changes in some minerals such as iron and calcium. Therefore, SWI is highly sensitive to new and old bleeding, as well as the contrast between middle arteries, veins, arterioles, and venules. New MRI machines have incorporated SWI, and SWI is thus used in routine examinations (Fig. 2.6f).

2.2.6 MR Angiography (MRA)

MRA comprises several techniques:

- Time-of-flight angiography: MRA can be performed without a contrast medium. This MRA is a routine examination item in MRI.
- Phase-contrast imaging is commonly used in MR venography, if necessary.
- Contrast-enhanced MRA.

  Injection of contrast media in MRA can save on examination time and obtain images with high resolutions. However, because this technique requires the injection of a contrast medium, it is not included in routine examinations.

2.2.7 MR Spectroscopy (MRS)

The MRS currently available in clinical practice employs hydrogen 1 and is called proton magnetic resonance spectroscopy. Using MRS within MRI, metabolites in the brain, including normal brain tissues (Fig. 2.11) and metabolites in the lesion region (Figs. 2.9 and 2.10), can be detected, which is explained as follows.

2.2.7.1 N-Acetyl Aspartate (NAA) (2.0 ppm)

NAA exists in neurons rather than glial cells and is a marker of neuron integrity. The NAA level decreases if a disease destroys neurons, such as stroke, multiple sclerosis, and brain tumor. Metastasis (Fig. 2.9) and tumors that do not contain neurons (e.g., meningioma) result in low NAA levels. No NAA is present in a brain abscess (Fig. 2.10).

2.2.7.2 Creatine (Cr) (3.0 and 3.9 ppm)

Cr has two waveforms at 3.0 and 3.9 ppm. Generally, the signal at 3.0 is observed.

Because Cr is stable, it can be used as a standard value.

Cr level is reduced in most brain diseases.

2.2.7.3 Choline (Cho) (3.2 ppm)

Cho is a main component of cell membranes, and the Cho level is increased in diseases with high cell membrane conversions such as ischemia, demyelination, tumors, and inflammation.

The Cho level of malignant tumors is notably increased.

2.2.7.4 Myo-Inositol (mI) (3.3 and 3.6 ppm)

mI is a metabolite of astrocytes. In normal neonatal brain tissues, low-grade astrocytoma, gliosis, acute demyelination, and schwannoma, the mI level is increased.

In any disease that destroys astrocytes—such as ischemia, tumor, and demyelination—the mI level is decreased.

2.2.7.5 Glutamate/Glutamine (Glx) (2.3 ppm)

Glx is the neurotransmitter released by neurons.

Hepatic encephalopathy and other acute diseases such as stroke, demyelination, and epilepsy cause the Glx level to increase.

2.2.7.6 Lactate (Lac) (1.3 ppm)

Lac does not exist in normal brains except for those of neonates. It is a product of anaerobic metabolism. Increased Lac level represents anaerobic glycolysis.

In cerebral infarction area, and in malignant tumor necrosis (Figs. 6.5, 6.24, and 6.25), pus (Figs. 7.11 and 7.12), encephalitis (Figs. 7.19 and 7.22), the glycolysis makes the oxygen demand increased, the Lac level is elevated.

2.2.7.7 Lipid (Lip) (0.9 and 1.3 ppm)

When cells are destroyed, Lip is increased in processes such as tumor necrosis (Figs. 2.9, 6.5, 6.6, 6.24, and 6.25) and abscess (Figs. 2.10, 7.11, 7.12, and 7.15). The central nervous system lymphoma is a solid mass without necrosis, but its Lip level is increased (Fig. 6.15), possibly because of the deformation of lymphoid cells [3].

Other metabolites:

In pus, MRS reveals succinate (2.4 ppm), acetate (1.99 ppm), alanine (1.5 ppm), Lac/Lip (1.3 ppm), and amino acid (0.9 ppm) (Fig. 2.10, 7.11, and 7.12).

- MRS is not included in routine MRI examinations. It is conducted when necessary.
- ***MRS techniques:***

  MRS is mostly used to perform single-voxel MRI on the lesion region of interest to clarify the waveforms of various metabolites. If the lesion covers a large region, multivoxel MRS (Fig. 6.5) can be conducted; however, the image will be relatively difficult to interpret.

  In routine examinations, single-voxel MRS is often employed in the detection of various metabolite waveforms, with a short TE needed (20–40 ms). An intermediate TE (125–144 ms) is required when necessary, and Lac, alanine, and amino acid are inverted to facilitate their distinction from Lip (Figs. 6.24, 6.25, 7.11, 7.12, 7.19, and 7.22).
- ***How Can Lac Be Distinguished from Lip?***

  Lac and Lip are present in numerous brain lesions. They sometimes exist simultaneously. Because both their signals are generally at 1.3 ppm and thus overlap, they are commonly labeled jointly as Lac/Lip (Fig. 6.5). However, they are distinguishable if the signals are observed carefully.

  1. The Lac signal normally may have doublet peaks (Fig. 7.19), whereas the Lip signal has a single peak.
  2. In an MRS image obtained using an intermediate TE (125–144 ms), the Lac signal is inverted (Fig. 6.24, 6.25, 7.11, 7.12, 7.19, and 7.22), but the Lip signal is not (Fig. 2.9, 2.10, 6.6, 6.24, 6.25, 7.11, 7.12, and 7.15). This difference makes them distinguishable.

2.2.8 Functional MRI (fMRI)

In fMRI, a small variation in blood flow throughout brain tissue under-stimulation is employed to detect the activity of the cerebral cortex.

The new 1.5T and 3T MRI pulse sequences used in routine brain examinations include the following:

T1WI, T2WI, FLAIR, DWI (including ADC map), T2*WI or SWI (either one), and MRA (Fig. 2.6).

Routine pulse sequences for spine examination include the following:

T1WI, T2WI, and T2 STIR (Chap. 8)

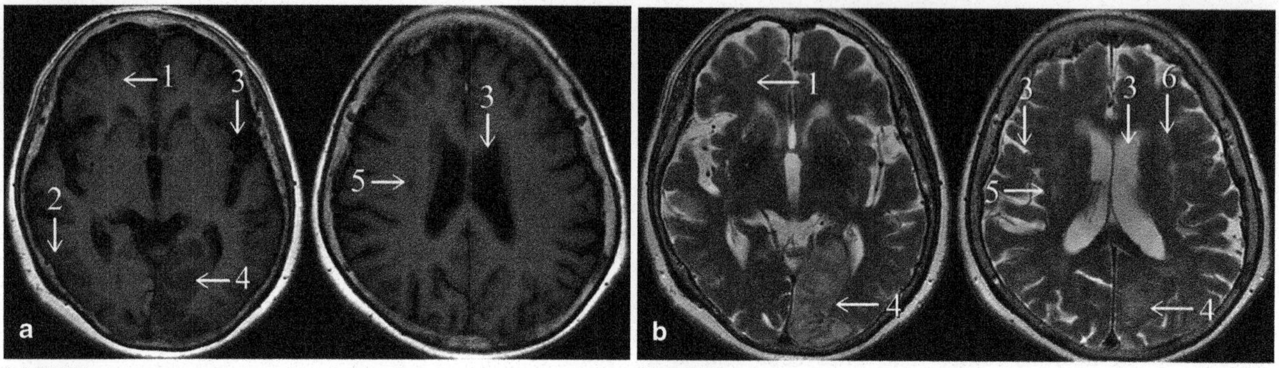

(a) T1W1
1. white matter: gray-white
2. gray matter: gray-dark
3. CSF: dark
4. edema: gray-dark
5. chronic infarct: gray-dark

(b) T2W1
3. CSF: white
4. edema: gray-white
5. chronic infarct: gray-white
6. leukoaraiosis (demyelination): gray-white

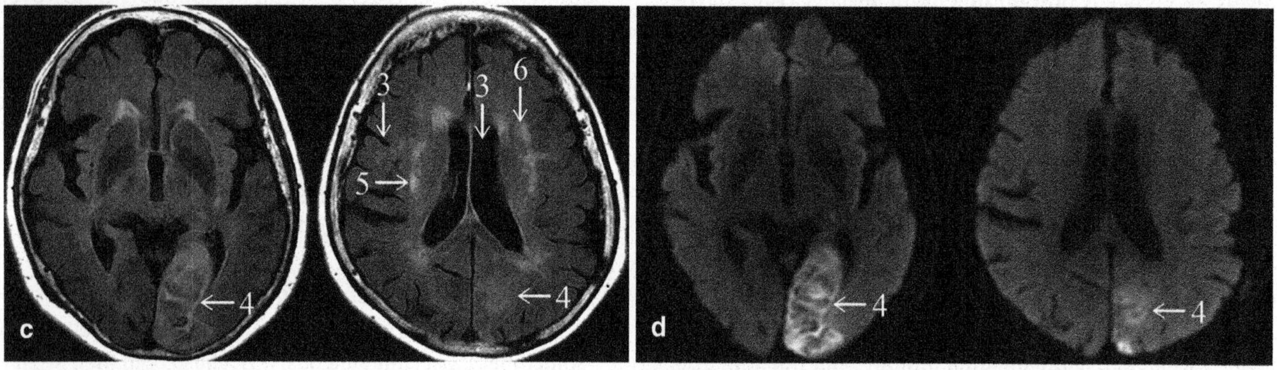

(c) FLAIR (T2 FLAIR)
3. CSF: dark
4. edema: gray-white
5. chronic infarct: gray-white
6. leukoaraiosis (demyelination): gray-white

(d) DW1
Infarction edema: white
Only acute infraction edema has water-diffusion restriction and is bright (very white). Other including chronic infarct and leukoaraiosis, lack a signal change.

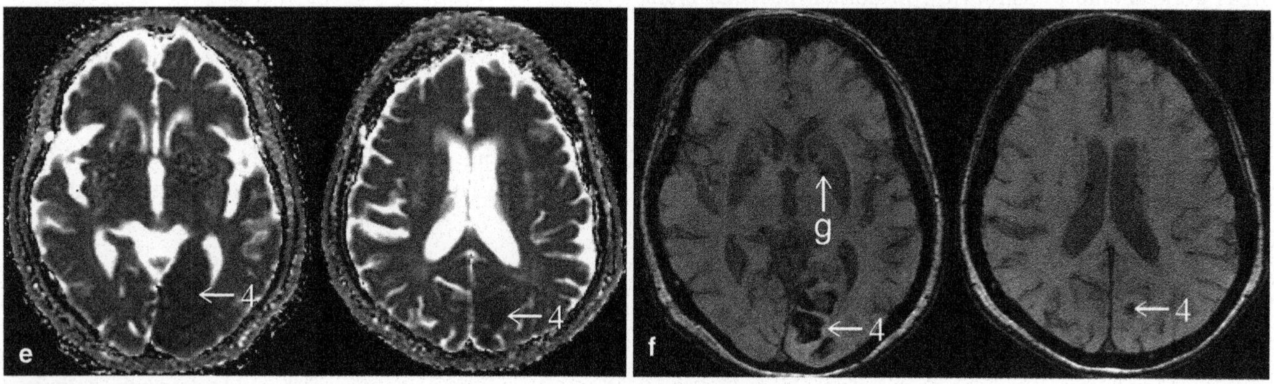

(e) ADC
Infarction edema: dark
ADC reflects the water-diffusion coefficient. Cytotoxic edema has a low efficient and is dark (4).
The remaining chronic infarct and leukoaraiosis are as gray-white as T2W1

(f) SWI (SWAN)
hemorrhagic transformation (4); dark
g: globus pallidus small calcification : dark

Fig. 2.6 Signal intensity (color) of the routine pulse sequences of MRI of the brain. F/85, Lt. PCA acute infarction with hemorrhagic transformation in the left occipital lobe

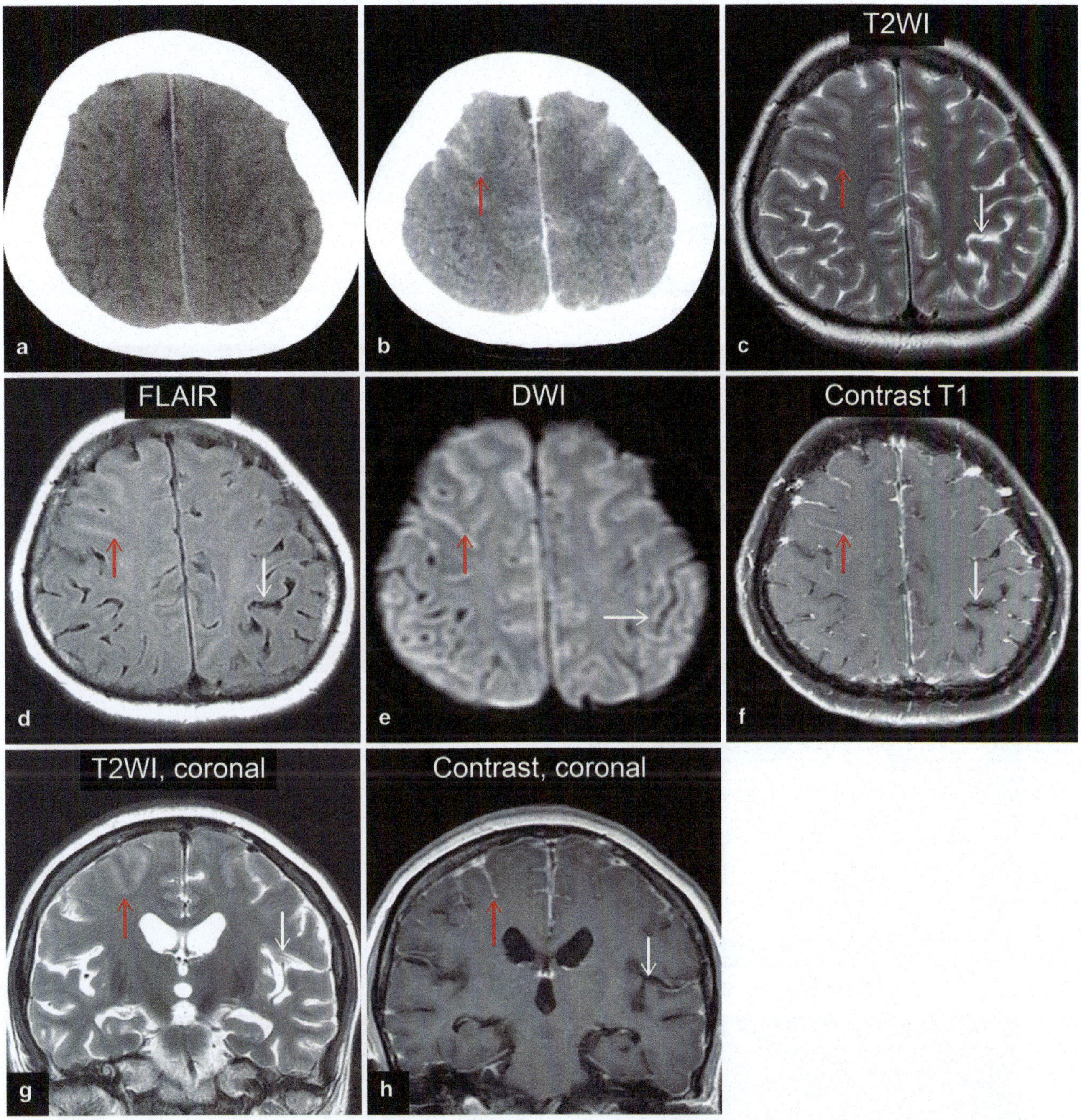

Fig. 2.7 F/53, Leptomeningeal metastasis in the bilateral frontal lobes. A patient with Merkel cell carcinoma received CT and MRI examinations for headache, vomiting, and fever. (**a**) CT: The sulci in the bilateral frontal lobes are unclear. (**b**) Contrast CT: Sulci exhibit linear enhancement (red arrow). (**c**) MRI and T2WI: The sulci (red arrow) in the front of the bilateral frontal lobes appear gray-white, are unlike normal sulci (white arrow), which are white because of CSF. (**d**) In FLAIR: The sulci are not attenuated and appear gray-white (red arrow) in contrast to normal sulci (white arrow), which are dark. (**e**) DWI: similar findings to those of FLAIR. (**f**) Contrast T1WI: Abnormal sulci have linear enhancement (red arrow). (**g**) T2WI, coronal, and (**h**) contrast T1, coronal: comparison of differences between sulci with leptomeningeal infiltration (red arrows) and normal sulci (white arrow). The microscopic examination of CSF revealed malignant cells. Therefore, this is leptomeningeal metastasis, not meningitis

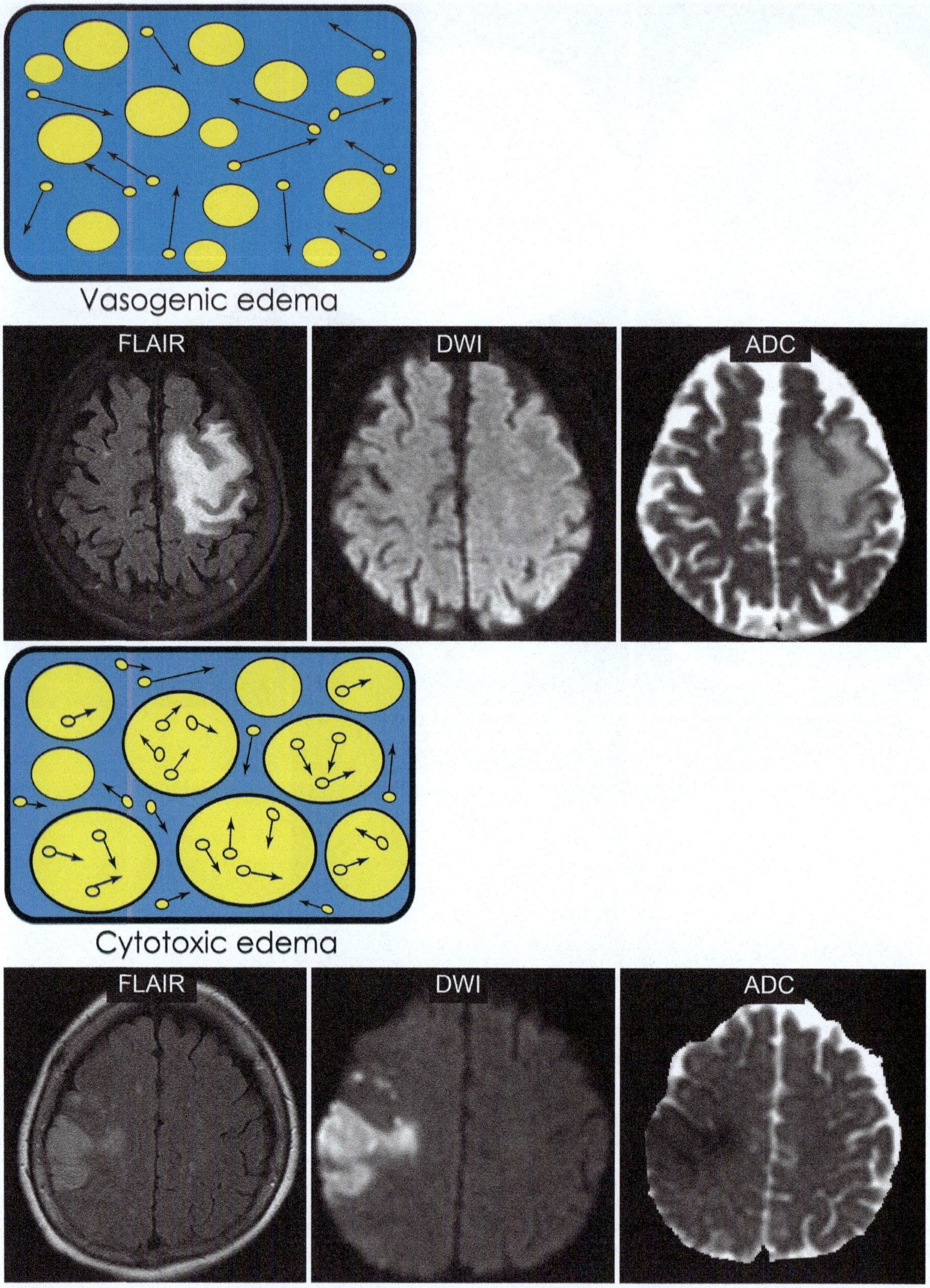

Fig. 2.8 The signal intensity of two kinds of brain tissue edema. **Vasogenic edema**: Although the water content in the brain tissue edema has increased, the astrocytes and neurons are not swollen, and water molecule movement (diffusion) remains free. In FLAIR, the edema appears gray-white. The DWI does not show signal change, but the ADC presents a high signal due to water increase. **Cytotoxic edema**: Water content has increased in the brain tissue edema and is intracellular. Water is present in astrocytes and neurons and causes these cells to swell. The swollen cells inhibit water molecule movement (diffusion restriction). In FLAIR, the edema appears gray-white. The diffusion restriction shows a high signal on DWI. ADC reflects the reduction in diffusion coefficient and presents hypointensity (low signal)

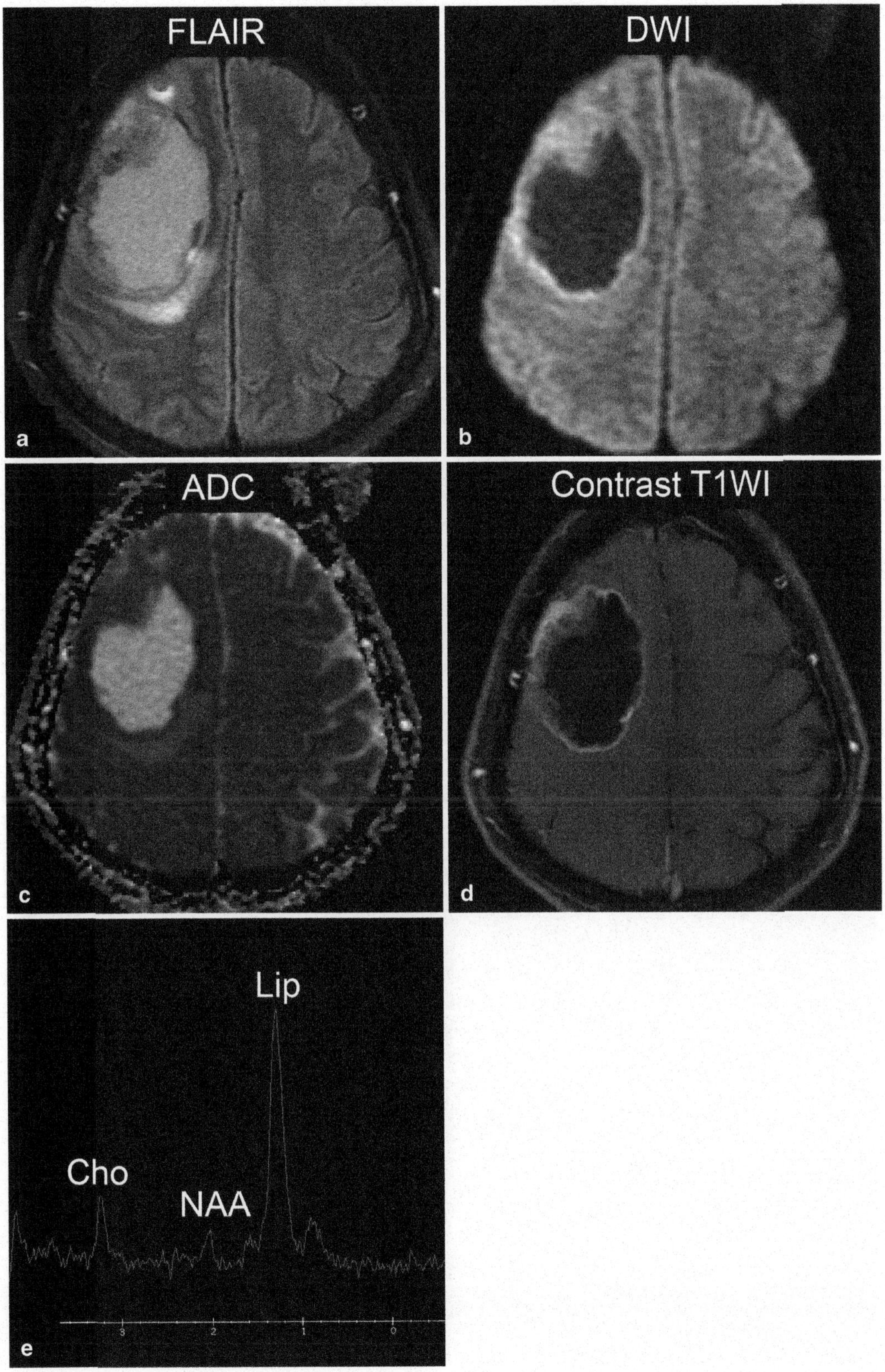

Fig. 2.9 F/50, Metastasis. A breast cancer patient suffered a severe headache for 1 month. (**a–d**) MRI: a tumor mass in the right frontal lobe, with severe central necrosis, the necrotic area contains fluid, no diffusion restriction, hyperintensity on FLAIR, hypointensity (dark) on DWI, and hyperintensity on ADC, and with ring enhancement. (**e**) MRS (TE 144 ms): MRS of the necrotic part. NAA: 2.0 ppm, much reduction. Cr: 3.0 ppm, not present. Cho: 3.2 ppm, slightly reduction. Lip: 1.3 ppm, very high level of lipid

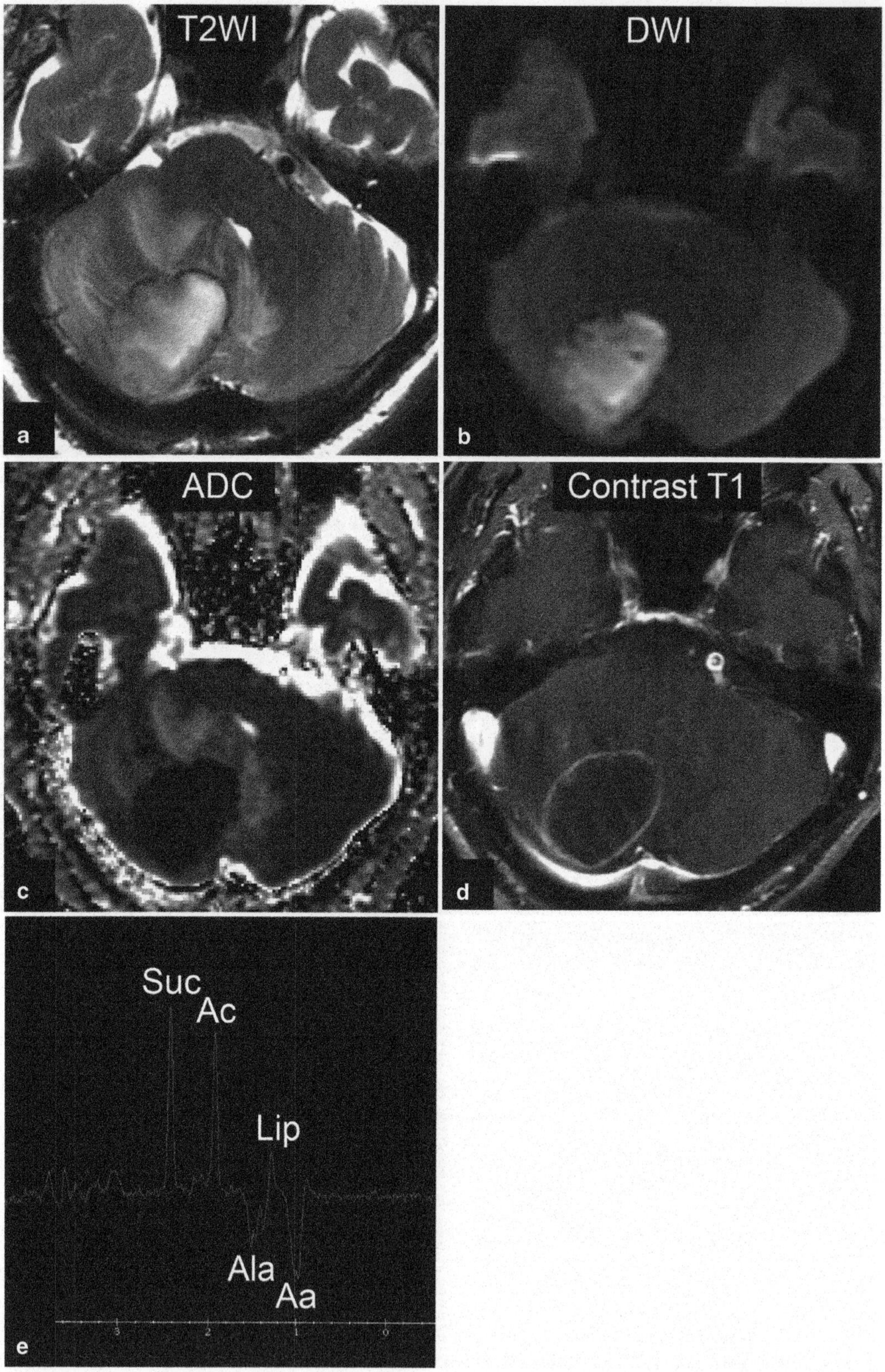

Fig. 2.10 M/74, MRS of a cerebellar abscess. (**a**–**c**) Cystic mass in the right cerebellum. The content is slightly white (hyperintensity) on T2WI, bright (hyperintensity) on DWI, and very dark (hypointensity) on ADC, indicating that the diffusion restriction is strong. This is a characteristic of pus. (**d**) Contrast T1WI: ring enhancement of the cystic mass. (**e**) MRS (144ms): The following abnormal metabolites are present: Suc: succinate (2.4 ppm), Ac: acetate (1.99 ppm), Ala: alanine (1.5 ppm), Lip: lipid (1.3 ppm), and Aa: amino acid (0.9 ppm). NAA, choline, and creatinine, which should be present in normal brain tissue, are absent

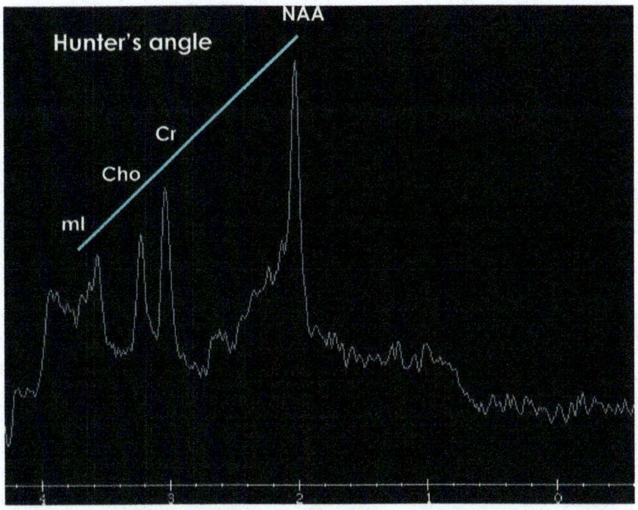

Fig. 2.11 Normal MRS of brain tissue. NAA: N-acetylaspartate (NAA): resonates at 2.0 ppm (neuronal marker), Cr: creatine: 3.0 ppm (energy metabolism), Cho: choline: 3.2 ppm (cell membrane marker), mI: Myo-inositol: 3.5 mm (glial cell marker does not easily appear in adults), NAA/Cr ratio: 2.0 < 1.6 abnormal. NAA/Chol ratio: 1.6 < 1.2 abnormal. Chol/Cr ratio: 1.2 > 1.5 abnormal. Typical standard MRS, mI-Cho-Cr-NAA, are connected to form Hunter's angle

2.3 Contrast Media Enhancement

CT is conducted by intravenously administering an iodinated contrast medium (Fig. 2.12). MRI is conducted by intravenously administering a gadolinium contrast medium (Fig. 2.13).

After the injection of the contrast medium, the brain tissue is not enhanced because of the blood–brain barrier (BBB).

Normal intracranial structures that can be enhanced include the following (Figs. 2.12 and 2.13):

Arteries: such as ICA, MCA, ACA, and PCA.

Veins: internal cerebral vein and venous sinuses such as cavernous sinus, straight sinus, transverse sinus, and superior sagittal sinus.

Non-brain tissues: tentorium, falx, intraventricular choroid plexus, and the pituitary gland.

If BBB disruption occurs, the disrupted region of brain tissues is enhanced. A common situation is that cerebral infarction is enhanced during the hyperemia period (Fig. 2.14).

Low-grade intracerebral tumors, such as low-grade astrocytoma, have a wholesome BBB, show no enhancement. The intracerebral tumors showing enhancement are possibly malignant.

Because of no BBB, the extra-axial brain tumors, such as meningioma and acoustic schwannoma, always have well enhancement (Chap. 6).

Vessel diseases, such as AVM and aneurysm, are a vascular disease, contrast medium can directly enter the lesions, so have strong enhancement (Chap. 4).

Generally, for the same lesions, the MRI enhancement is more explicit than CT enhancement.

Enhancement of contrast medium occurs not only in brain tissues and tumors but also in the subarachnoid spaces and other parts.

1. *Leptomeningeal enhancement* (Fig. 2.7)*, which refers to the linear enhancement of CSF spaces, such as sulci and cisterns. This type of enhancement occurs in meningitis (Chap. 7) and meningeal metastasis (Chap. 6).*
2. *Pachymeningeal enhancement* (Fig. 2.15) *is observed in intracranial hypotension and chemical or aseptic meningitis.*

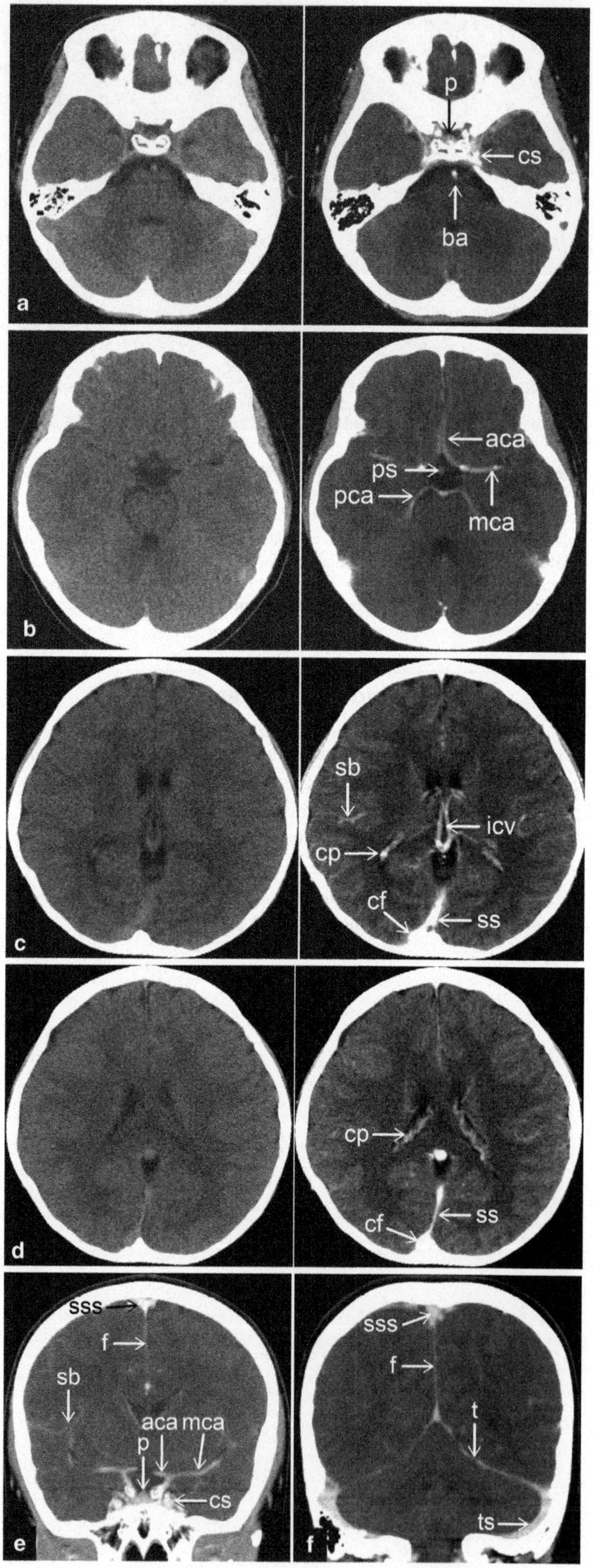

Fig. 2.12 Normal brain enhancement
(**a–d**): Left: plain CT
Right: contrast CT
(**e, f**) Contrast CT, coronal views
mca: middle cerebral artery
aca: anterior cerebral artery
pca: posterior cerebral artery
ps: pituitary stalk
p: pituitary gland
cs: cavernous sinus
ba: basilar artery
cp: choroid plexus of the lateral ventricle
ss: straight sinus
icv: internal cerebral vein
cf: confluence of sinus
sb: Sylvain branches of MCA
f: falx
t: tentorium
sss: superior sagittal sinus
ts: transverse sinus

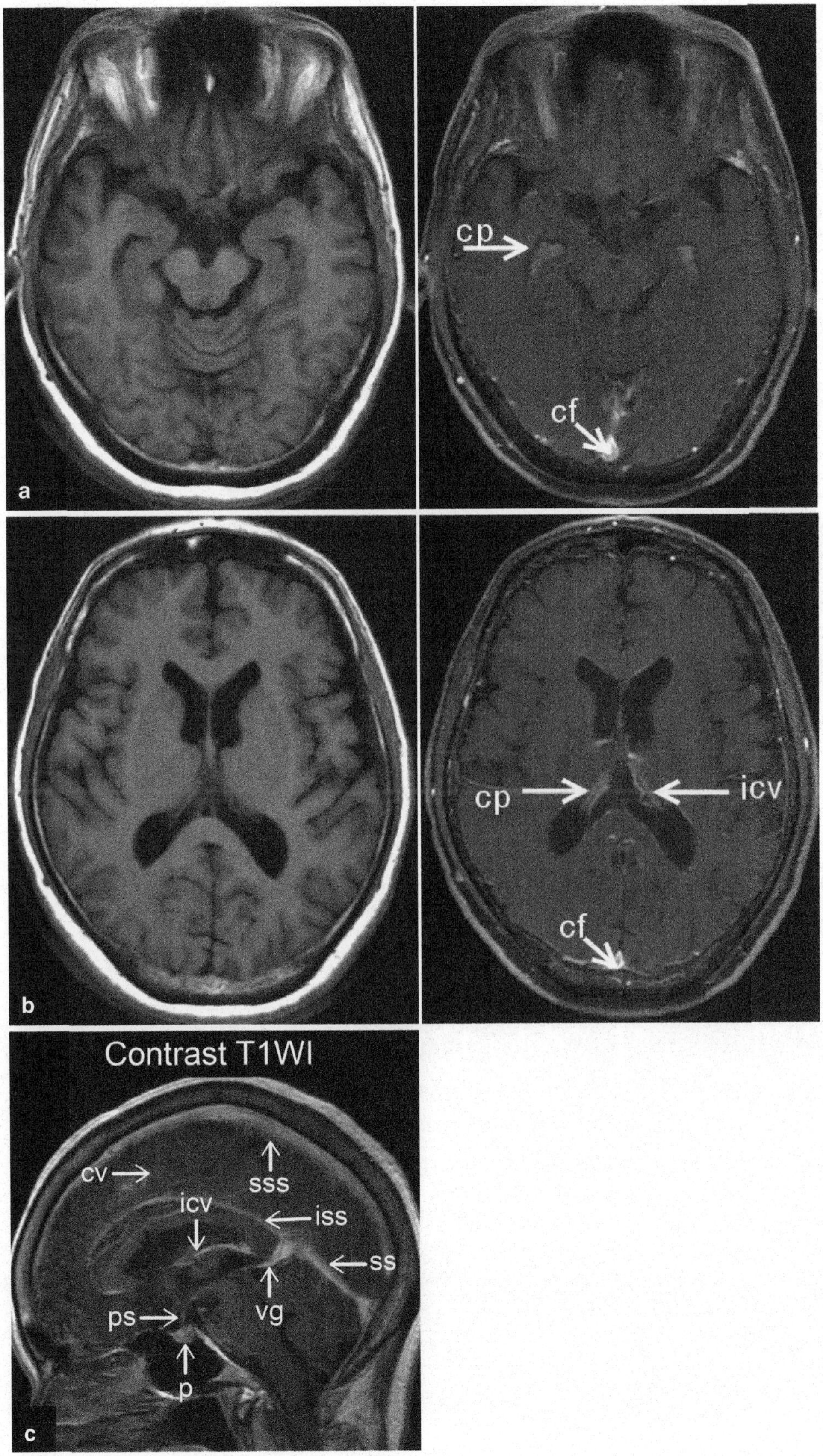

Fig. 2.13 MRI enhancement in normal brain. (**a**, **b**) left: T1W1, right: contrast T1W1. (**c**) contrast T1W1, sagittal. *cp* choroid plexus of the lateral ventricle, *icv* internal cerebral vein, *cf* confluence of sinus, *sss* superior sagittal sinus, *iss* inferior sagittal sinus, *ss* straight sinus, *vg* vein of Galen, *cv* cortical vein, *p* pituitary gland, *ps* pituitary stalk

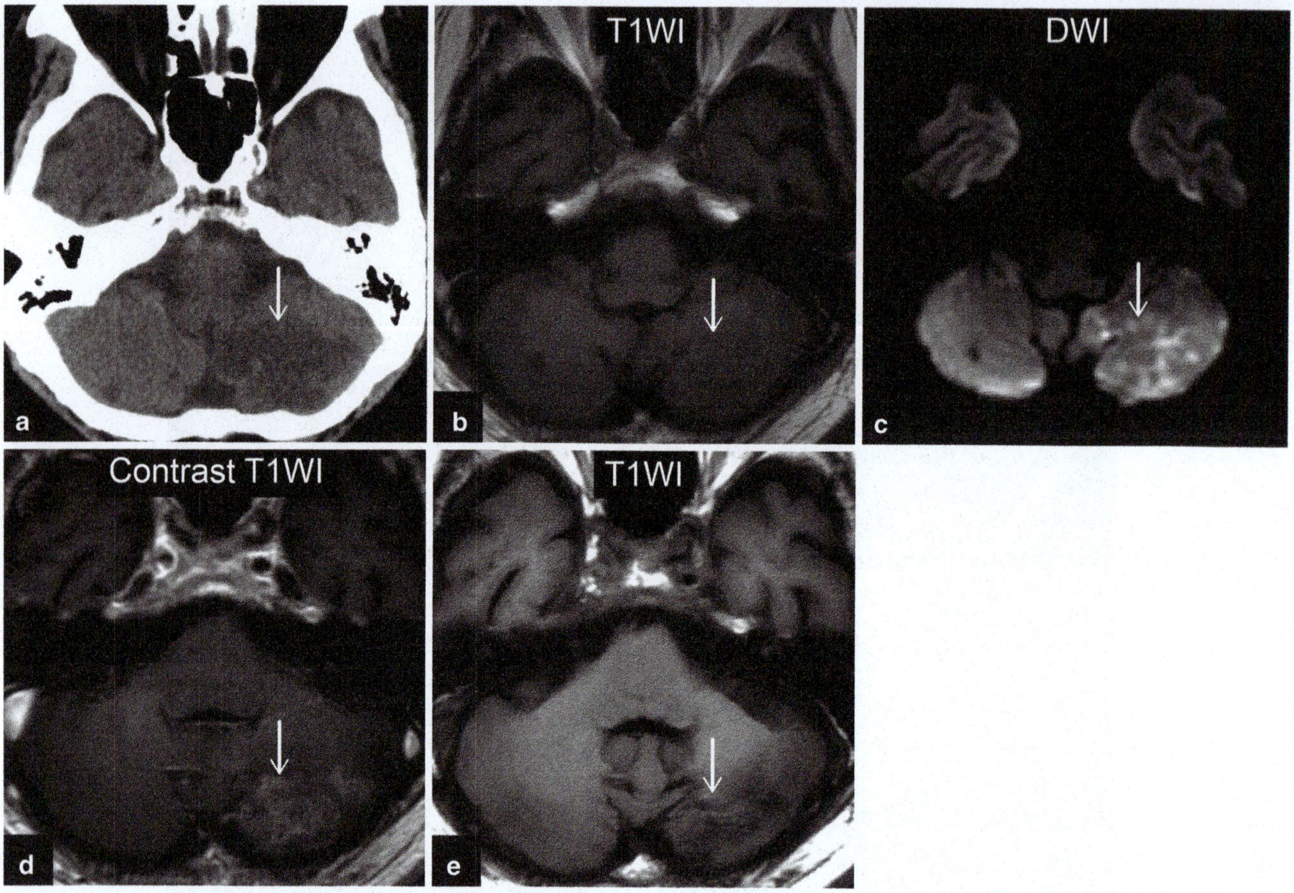

Fig. 2.14 M/79, Contrast enhancement in a cerebellar infarction area. The patient complained of dizziness and unsteady gait for a few days, but the actual symptoms onset time was unknown. (**a**) CT: An area of brain tissue edema (arrow) in the left cerebellum suspected to be an acute infarction. (**b**) T1WI: this area with mild hypointensity (arrow) in T1WI. (**c**) DWI: heterogeneous hyperintensity that is not as bright as typical cytotoxic edema of acute infarction. Thus, the contrast medium was administrated. (**d**) Contrast T1WI: abnormal enhancement in this area (arrow), suspected to be the blood–brain barrier (BBB) destruction stage of infarction. Tumor infiltration, however, cannot be ruled out. (**e**) Follow-up MRI 4 months later, T1WI: This area has become necrotic and atrophic (arrow) after 4 months. Thus, this is an infarction, not a tumor

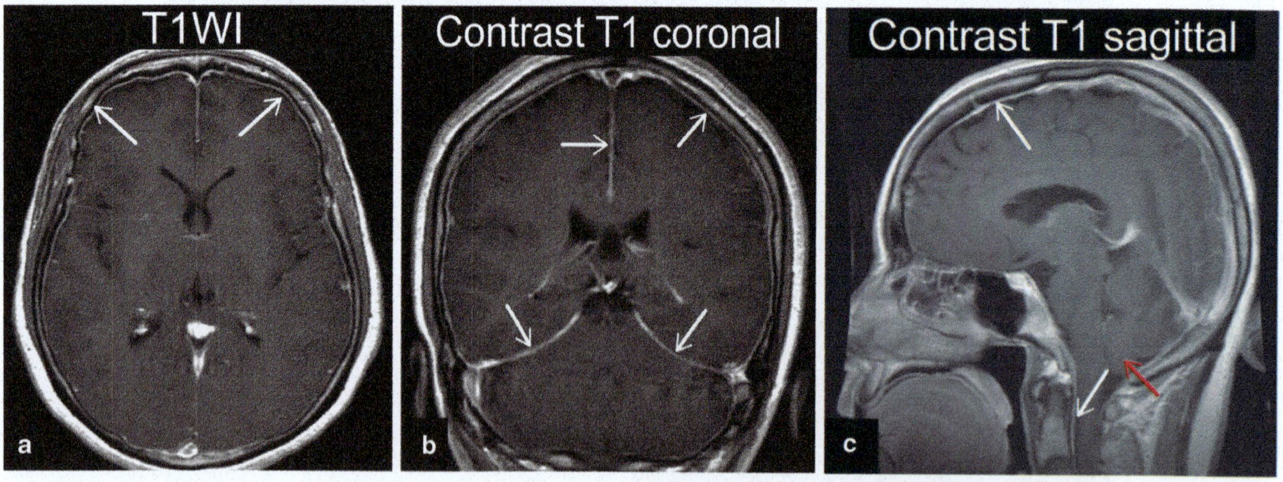

Fig. 2.15 F/49, Intracranial hypotension with pachymeningeal enhancement. Severe headache for a week. (**a**, **b**) MRI, contrast T1WI: Linear enhancement of the dura outside the cerebral hemispheres and the cerebellar tentorium and falx (white arrows). No enhancement in the cerebral or cerebellar sulci. Thus, the above characteristics indicate pachymeningeal enhancement. (**c**) Contrast T1WI, sagittal: In addition to linear enhancement of the dura (white arrows), mild downward herniation of the cerebellar tonsil (red arrow) is noted. This is a sign of intracranial hypotension

2.4 Mass Effect

During the interpretation of CT and MRI images, the mass effect concept is critical. Tumors, hematomas, and cerebral edema can create the mass effect of compression of brain tissue (Figs. 2.16, 2.17, 2.18, 2.19, 2.20, 2.21, 2.22, 2.23, 2.24, and 2.25). Generally, the mass effect occurs when lesions are active.

The interpretation of the mass effect is based on compression of the subarachnoid space. The related signs are as follows:

1. Subarachnoid structures such as ventricles, cisterns, fissures, and sulci around the lesion are compressed and changed to be smaller or completely disappeared (Figs. 2.4, 2.16, and 2.17).
2. Medial structures such as falx and spectrum pellucidum are shifted to the contralateral side (Figs. 2.16, 2.22, and 2.24).
3. If the foramen of Monro is compressed, the CSF of the contralateral ventricle has poor circulation, and the contralateral ventricle may be slightly dilated (Figs. 2.22, 2.23, and 2.24).
4. When the mass effect compresses the third or fourth ventricle or the cerebral aqueduct, hydrocephalus develops (Fig. 2.18).
5. When the mass effect occurs bilaterally, the frontal horns of the lateral ventricles are compressed to form the shape of rabbit ears (Fig. 2.19).
6. A strong mass effect may cause herniation of brain tissue, including the following types (Fig. 2.20): subfalcine herniation (Figs. 2.22 and 2.24), central herniation (Fig. 2.21), uncal herniation (Figs. 2.22, 2.23, and 2.24), transtentorial herniation (Figs. 2.22, 2.23, and 2.24), and tonsillar herniation (Figs. 2.18 and 2.25).

2.4.1 Interpretation of Brain Herniation

Brain herniation is usually an emergency condition; therefore, CT is urgently required. Health professionals must learn how to interpret brain herniation in CT scans.

2.4.1.1 CT

- **Uncal herniation:** The suprasellar cistern is deformed or wholly disappeared (Figs. 2.22, 2.23, and 2.24) because the uncus has slipped into the suprasellar cistern. Uncal herniation may compress the MCA and cause MCA infarction.
- **Transtentorial herniation:** The quadrigeminal cistern is deformed or wholly disappeared (Figs. 2.22, 2.23, and 2.24) because the uncus has slipped into the suprasellar cistern and further downward, passing through the tentorium cerebelli and thereby compressing and distorting the brain stem. Therefore, the quadrigeminal cistern behind the midbrain may be disappeared. Such herniation may compress the PCA and cause PCA infarction (Fig. 3.31; Chap. 3).

  Observation of the suprasellar cistern and quadrigeminal cistern is crucial. If the cisterns are deformed or disappeared (Figs. 2.22, 2.23, and 2.24), uncal or transtentorial herniation may have occurred.
- **Subfalcine herniation or cingulate herniation:** The cingulate gyrus under the frontal lobe is inclined to the other side (Figs. 2.22 and 2.24), thereby compressing the ACA and causing ACA infarction (Fig. 3.31; Chap. 3).

2.4.1.2 MRI

Because MRI is not suitable for emergency brain examinations, herniation is less likely to be observed using MRI than using CT. However, MRI does show the herniations as mentioned above more clearly than CT. In particular, tonsillar herniation can be directly observed in the sagittal section of an MRI image (Figs. 2.15, 2.18, and 2.25). This herniation may compress the vertebral artery or branches, causing infarction.

- **Peripheral Brain Tissue Atrophy**

  In contrast to the mass effect, an old lesion with peripheral brain tissue atrophy may make the adjacent ventricles, cisterns, fissures, and sulci dilated (Fig. 2.17).

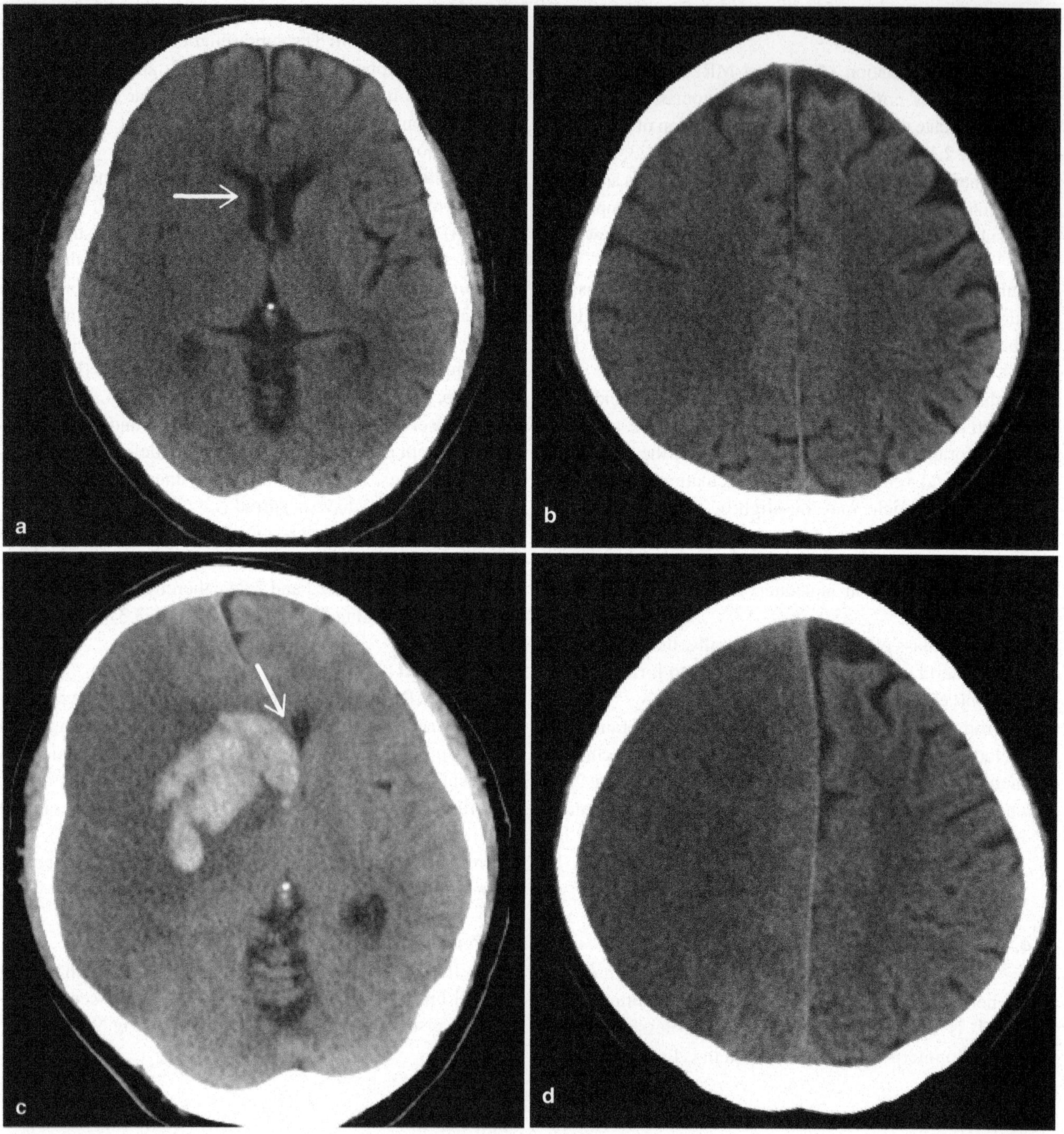

Fig. 2.16 M/65, MCA infarction edema causes mass effect. (**a**, **b**) CT performed 10 h after the onset of stroke symptoms: visible early brain tissue edema. The brain edema has caused mild mass effect, the right lateral ventricle is slightly compressed (arrow), and the right cerebral sulci have been obliterated. (**c**, **d**) On the third day of CT: additional evidence of infarction edema, which combines hemorrhagic transformation. The brain tissue edema and hematoma strengthen the mass effect, the right ventricle is completely flattened, the cerebral sulci have entirely disappeared, and the midline (septum pellucidum) has shifted to the left (arrow). The sulci of the contralateral left hemisphere shrink when the mass effect is strong

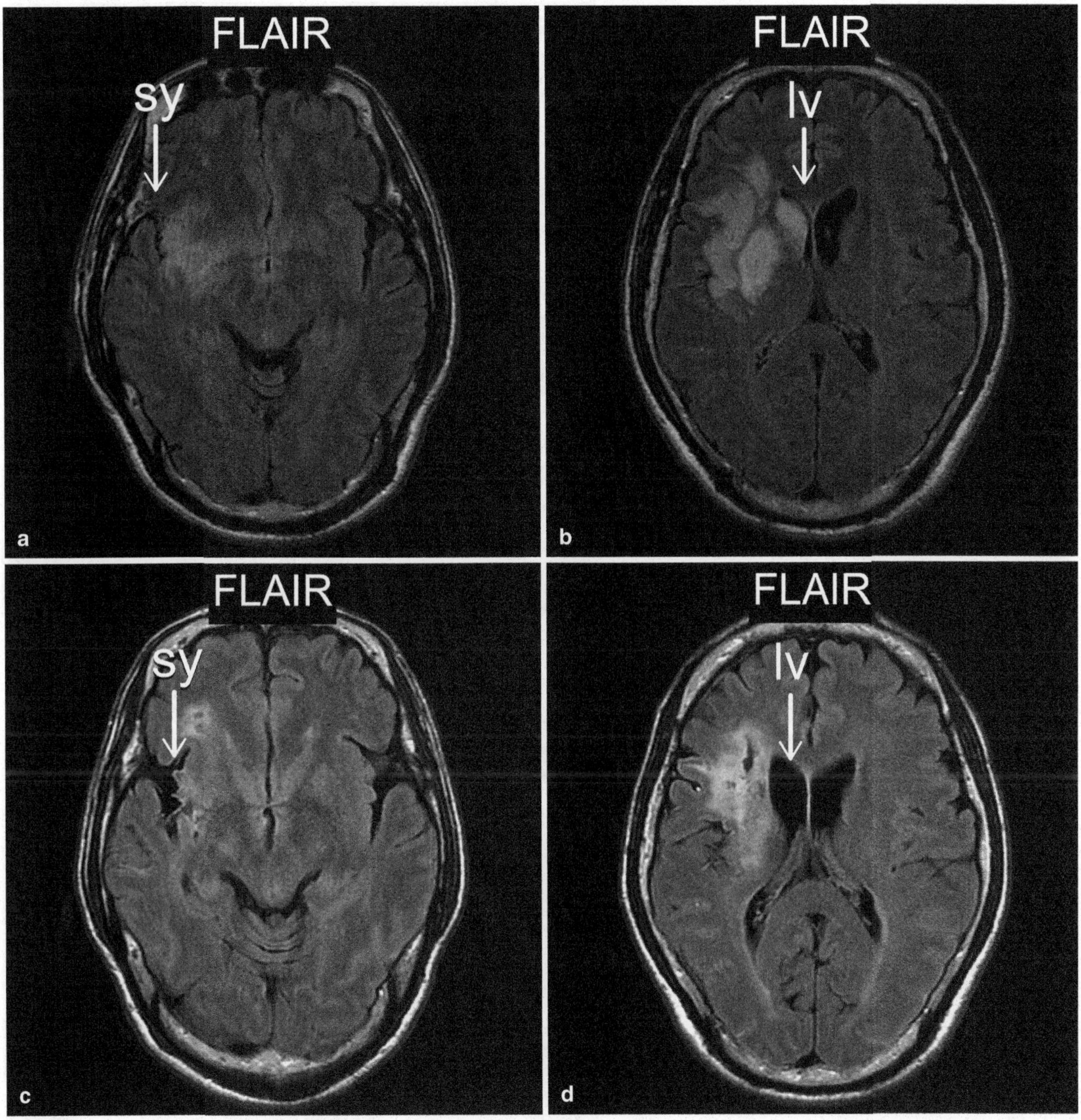

Fig. 2.17 M/55, Basal ganglion infarction, mass effect, and atrophy. (**a**, **b**) MRI, FLAIR: Hyperintensity in the right putamen, caudate nucleus, and insular cortex indicates that this is acute infarction edema. The edema causes a mass effect, and the right lateral ventricle (lv) and Sylvian fissure (sy) are compressed and squashed. (**c**, **d**) MRI, 3 months later, FLAIR: It changed into chronic infarction. The infarct area remains hyperintense and exhibits some necrotic cystic change. Chronic infarction lacks mass effect; by contrast, brain tissue is somewhat atrophic, the lateral ventricle (lv) and Sylvian fissure (sy) slightly dilate

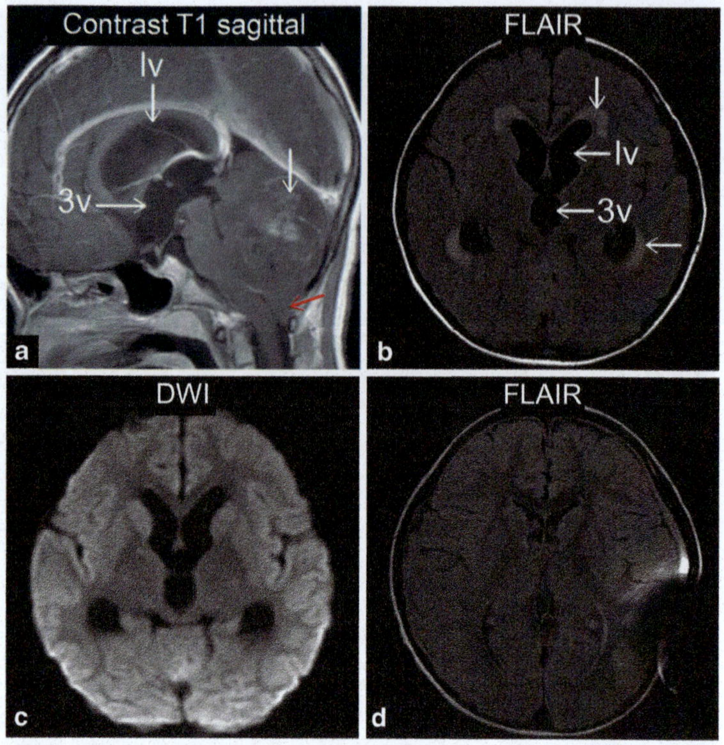

Fig. 2.18 F/7, Cerebellar medulloblastoma causes hydrocephalus. (**a**) MRI, contrast T1WI: The tumor (arrow) in the cerebellar vermis causes a mass effect, compresses the fourth ventricle and aqueduct, and induces obstructive hydrocephalus. The third ventricle (3v) and bilateral lateral ventricles (lv) are dilated. There is also tonsillar herniation (red arrow). (**b**) FLAIR: There is periventricular hyperintensity (arrows); this is transependymal CSF resorption due to severe and acute hydrocephalus and is a type of interstitial edema. (**c**) DWI: No signal change is observed because the interstitial edema lacks diffusion restriction. (**d**) After the surgical removal of this tumor, hydrocephalus and the periventricular interstitial edema disappeared

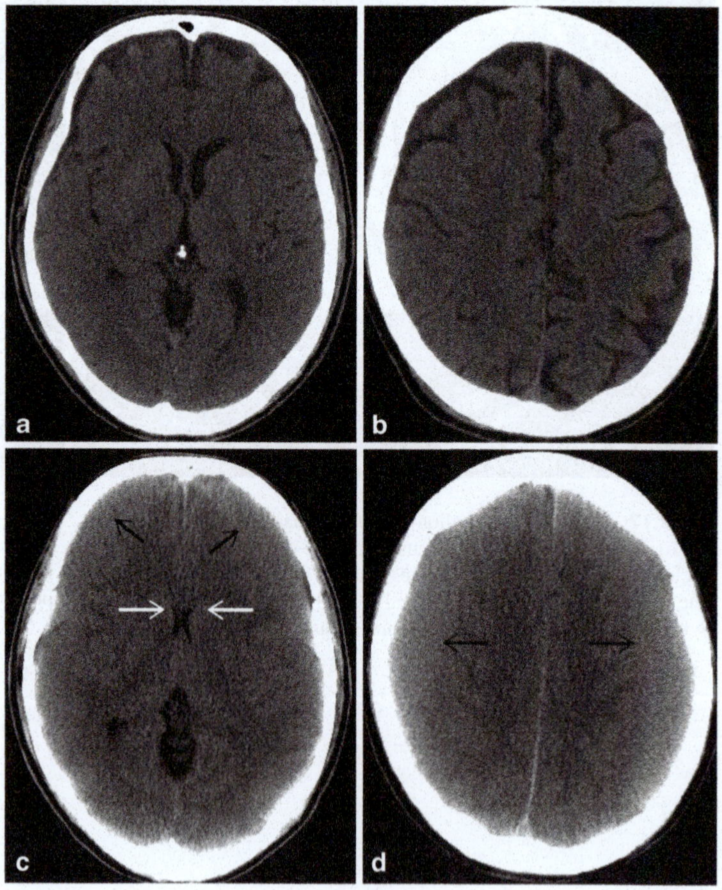

Fig. 2.19 M/67, Bilateral chronic subdural hematomas cause mass effect. (**a**, **b**) CT: CT for an acute head injury that shows no intracranial hematoma or brain tissue edema. Brain cortical atrophy is present, and the cortical sulci are widened. (**c**, **d**) After 1.5 months, the patient experienced severe headaches and awkward hand and feet movement. CT shows two isodense chronic subdural hematomas (SDHs, black arrows) on both sides. The cerebral cortical sulci have disappeared, and the bilateral lateral ventricles are compressed and appear bicornuate or rabbit ears shape (white arrows) because of the mass effect produced by the bilateral chronic subdural hematomas

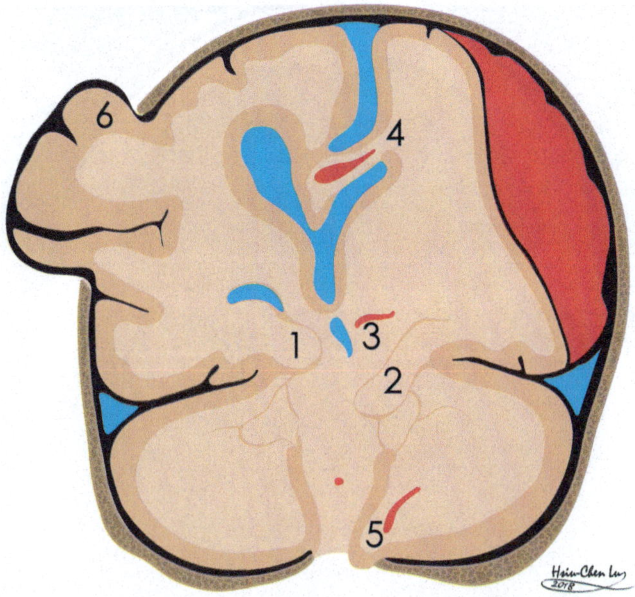

Fig. 2.20 Brain tissue herniations. Six types of brain tissue herniations caused by the severe mass effect: 1. Uncal herniation. 2. Transtentorial herniation (Transtentorial herniation always combine with uncal herniation). 3. Central herniation. 4. Subfalcine or cingulate herniation. 5. Tonsillar herniation. 6. External herniation

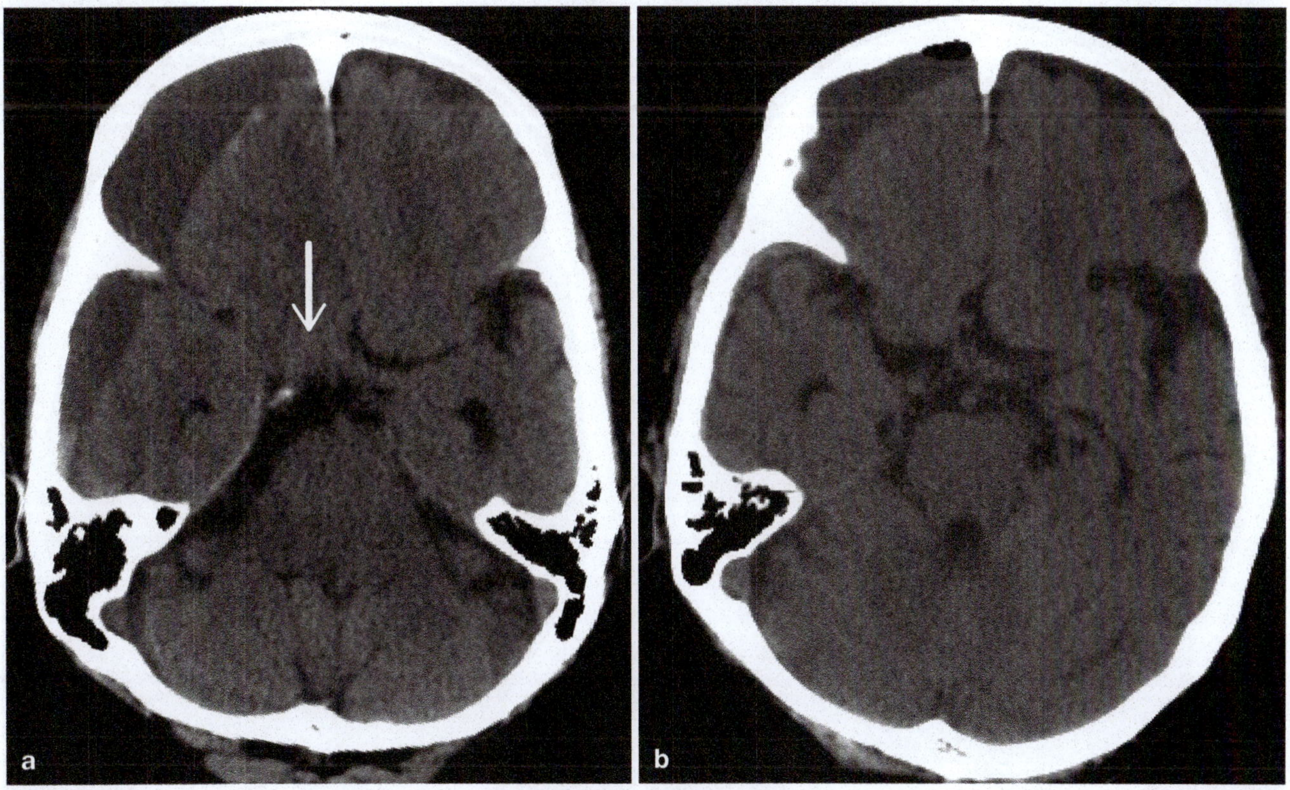

Fig. 2.21 F/85, Subdural effusion (SDE) causes central herniation. (**a**) CT: SDE in the right frontotemporal region creates a considerable mass effect. The brain tissue of the frontal lobe slides into the suprasellar cistern (arrow), thus deforming the pentagonal shape of the suprasellar cistern, this is a central herniation. (**b**) CT after surgery: SDE shrinks after drainage, the mass effect drastically decreases, and the suprasellar cistern returns to a pentagonal shape

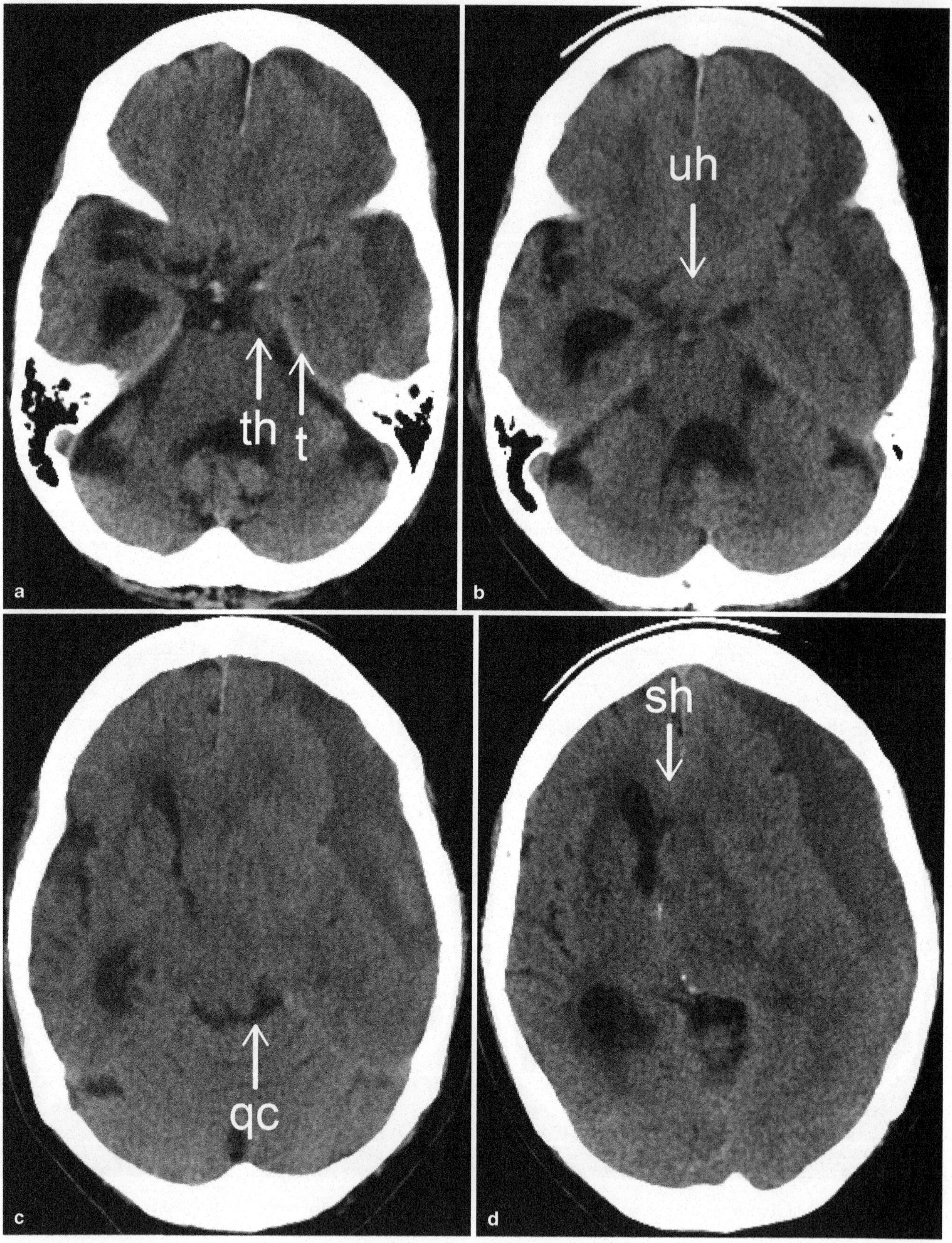

Fig. 2.22 F/81, Chronic SDH causes uncal/transtentorial herniations. (**a–c**) CT: Hypodense chronic SDH on the left side that creates a significant mass effect. The uncus of the temporal lobe slips into the suprasellar cistern and slightly falls toward the tentorium (t), representing uncal/transtentorial herniations (uh/th). The suprasellar cistern and quadrigeminal cistern (qc) are deformed due to these two herniations. (**d**) CT: The strong mass effect also causes subfalcine herniation (sh)

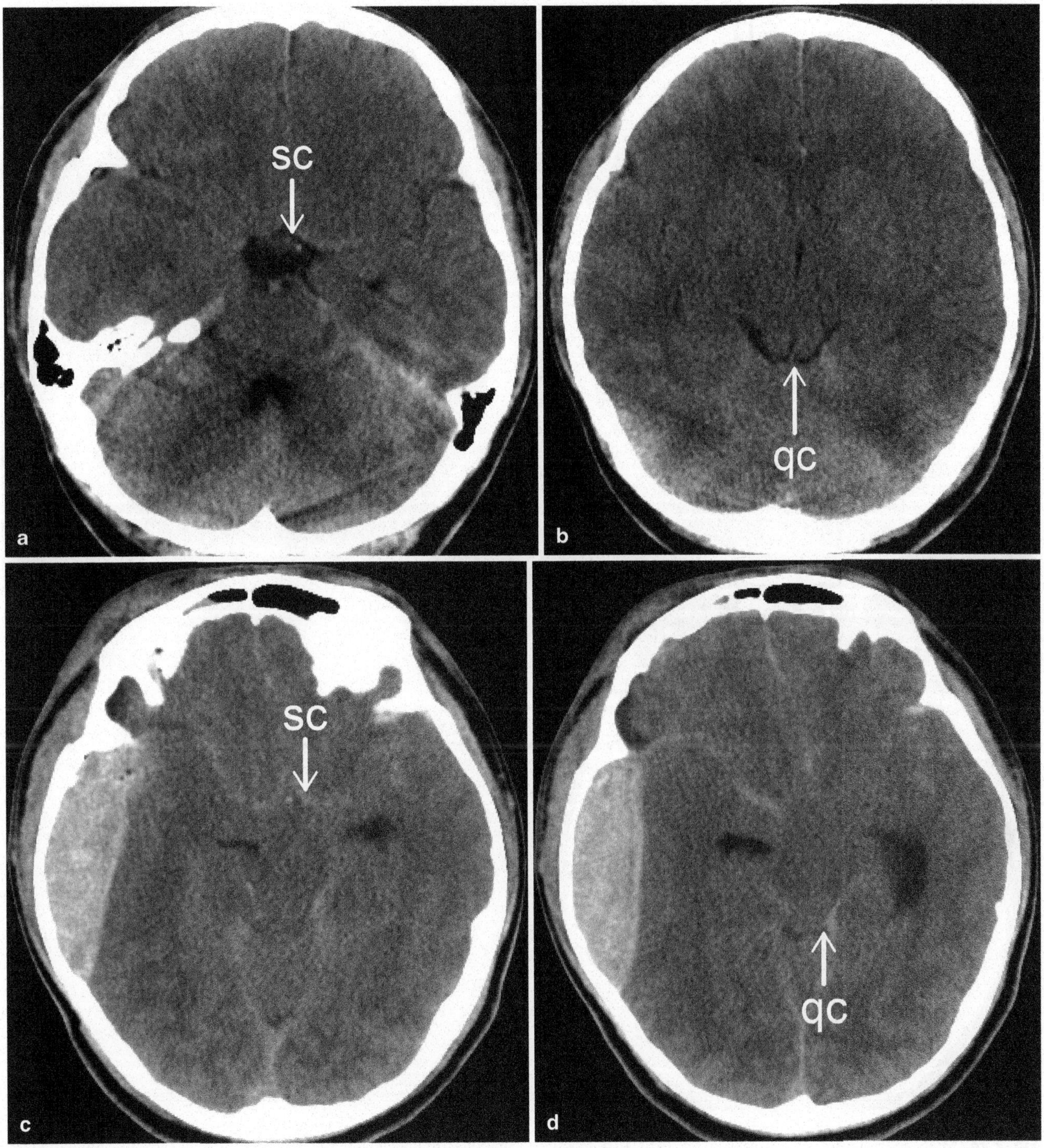

Fig. 2.23 M/18, Epidural hematoma (EDH) causes uncal/transtentorial herniations. (**a, b**) Emergency CT immediately after head injury: no visible bleeding or cerebral edema. The suprasellar cistern (sc) has a pentagonal shape, and the quadrigeminal cistern (qc) has a bow shape. (**c, d**) After 6 h, the patient suddenly became comatose. Repeat CT: shows a massive EDH on the right side that causes a strong mass effect. The disappearance of the suprasellar (sc) and quadrigeminal (qc) cisterns represents uncal/transtentorial herniations

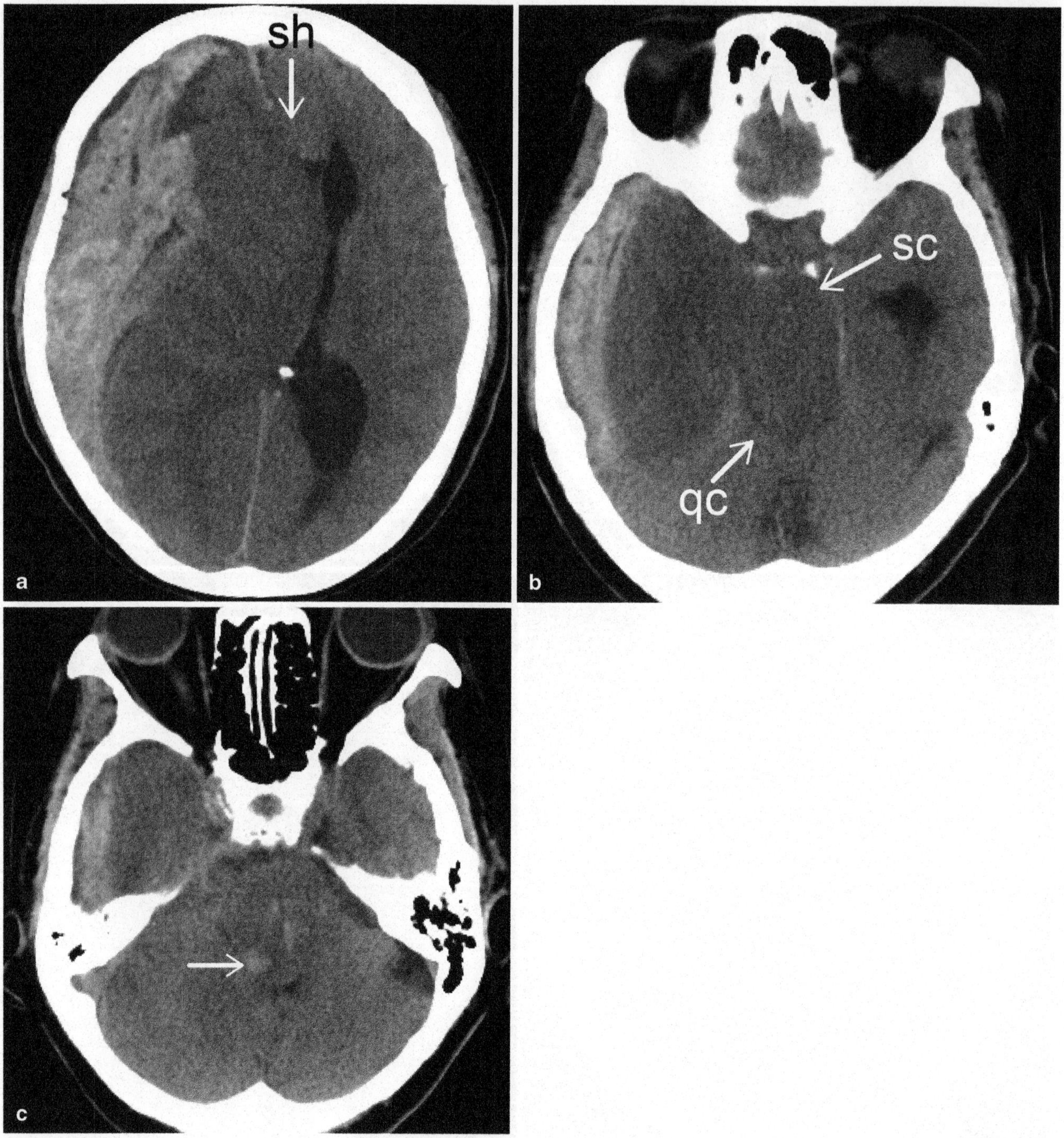

Fig. 2.24 M/46, SDH causes strong mass effect. (**a**) CT: A massive acute SDH creates a strong mass effect with midline left shifting and subfalcine herniation (sh). (**b**) The disappearance of suprasellar cistern (sc) and quadrigeminal cistern (qc) represents uncal/transtentorial herniations. (**c**) Petechial hemorrhages in the pons (arrow), a kind of Duret hemorrhages, are caused by herniation hitting the brain stem. It is a sign of poor prognosis

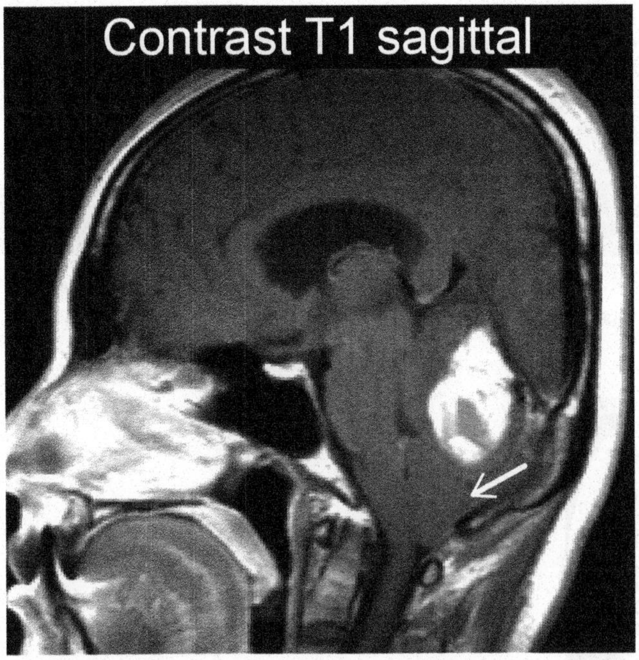

Fig. 2.25 F/34, Cerebellar vermis tumor causes tonsillar herniation. MRI, contrast T1WI, sagittal: A tumor mass is enhanced in the cerebellar vermis. It creates a mass effect and causes the cerebellar tonsil to slip downward (arrow). This is tonsillar herniation

2.5 5H, Five Types of Intracranial Hemorrhages

Intracranial hemorrhage has five types (Fig. 2.26):

1. **Intracerebral hemorrhage and intracerebral hematoma (ICH)**

   ICH is a commonly used term for brain tissue hemorrhage or a hematoma in the brain tissue. The hemorrhage or hematoma may be in the cerebral lobes, cerebellum, basal ganglion, brainstem, and corpus callosum. It can also be called **intraparenchymal hemorrhage or hematoma (IPH).** The causes of this type of hemorrhage are mostly an external injury to the head (Chap. 3) and a cerebrovascular accident (CVA; Chap. 4). CVA-induced intracerebral hemorrhages comprise the following.

   (a) Deep hemorrhage is hemorrhage at the putamen, caudate nucleus, thalamus, and the brainstem. The leading cause is hypertensive stroke.

   (b) Lobar hemorrhage is hemorrhage at the cortex/subcortex of frontal, parietal, occipital, or temporal lobes. The leading cause is amyloid angiopathy. AVM and tumor bleeding are also common causes.

2. **Subdural hematoma (SDH)**
3. **Epidural hematoma (EDH)**

   SDH and EDH are both extracerebral and are mainly caused by head injury (Chap. 3). Other causes include AVM, aneurysm, and AV fistula. Because hematoma is generally present during observation of CT and MRI imaging, SDH and EDH are referred to as subdural or epidural "hematoma," not subdural or epidural "hemorrhage."

4. **Subarachnoid hemorrhage (SAH).**

   SAH is referred to as" hemorrhage" rather than subarachnoid "hematoma" because hematoma does not form from SAH.

   SAH is further divided as follows:

   (a) Primary SAH or spontaneous SAH is mainly caused by a ruptured aneurysm (Sect. 4.3 of Chap. 4).

   (b) Secondary SAH develops from ICH flowing into the subarachnoid space.

   (c) Traumatic SAH is caused by head injury (Chap. 3).

5. **Intraventricular hemorrhage (IVH).**

   Most instances of IVH result from ICH breaking into ventricles or from a head injury. The incidence of primary IVH is low. AVM rupture is a cause of primary IVH (Chap. 4).

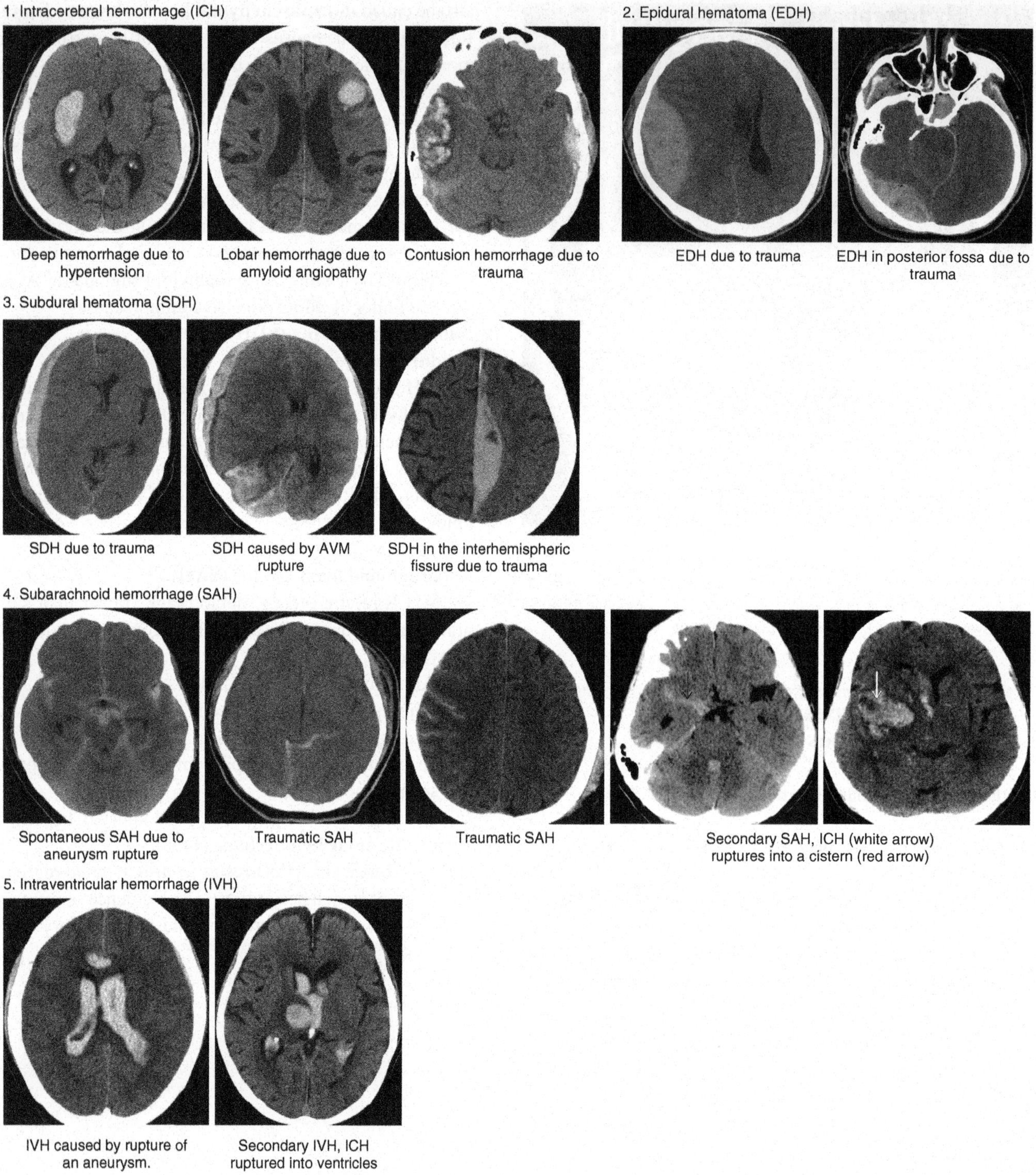

Fig. 2.26 5H: Five types of intracranial hemorrhages

2.6 Hydrocephalus

The classification of hydrocephalus according to the causes is of three types:

1. **Obstructive hydrocephalus**
   (a) An intraventricular tumor causes an obstruction.
   (b) An extra-ventricular lesion compressing the ventricle—especially compression on the foramen of Monro, third ventricle, cerebral aqueduct, or fourth ventricle (Fig. 2.18)—may cause hydrocephalus.
   (c) The intraventricular hemorrhage (IVH) may obstruct the third ventricle or cerebral aqueduct and causes hydrocephalus.
2. **Communicating hydrocephalus**
   (a) SAH: Acute SAH results in poor subarachnoid CSF circulation and soon produces mild acute hydrocephalus (Figs. 2.27 and 2.28). SAH subsequently induces subarachnoid adhesion and results in chronic communicating hydrocephalus (Fig. 2.28).
   (b) Meningitis causes subarachnoid adhesion, resulting in hydrocephalus (Fig. 2.29).
   (c) Subarachnoid tumor infiltration, such as leptomeningeal metastasis, causes hydrocephalus (Chap. 6).
3. **CSF overproduction**
   CSF overproduction is a rare type of communicating hydrocephalus. Most instances are a papilloma of the choroid plexus of the ventricle, which continuously secretes CSF and causes communicating hydrocephalus.

Interpretations of hydrocephalus include the following notifications:

1. **Mild hydrocephalus**
   The third ventricle and temporal horns of lateral ventricles are most sensitive to ventricular expansion (Figs. 2.27 and 2.28). The normal third ventricle is a linear shape. During hydrocephalus, the third ventricle becomes oval in form. The temporal horns of the lateral ventricles can barely be seen in young people but are slightly larger and look like commas in older adults. The temporal horns of the lateral ventricles expand notably during mild hydrocephalus. The third ventricle and temporal horns thus dilate slightly, appearing in images as having a big nose and large mustache (Fig. 2.27).
2. **Moderate hydrocephalus**
   The ventricles are significantly dilated, easy to interpret (Fig. 2.28), but must pay attention to distinguish between communicating and obstructive hydrocephalus. If it is obstructive, finding out the location and cause of the obstruction is essential.
3. **Acute and severe hydrocephalus**
   In acute and severe hydrocephalus, transependymal CSF resorption occurs, this is a kind of interstitial edema. In CT, this is called periventricular lucency (darkening beside the ventricle; Fig. 2.29). In MRI, long TR images have periventricular hyperintensity (whitening beside the ventricle; Fig. 2.18), but no signal change on DWI because interstitial edema has no diffusion restriction.
4. **Brain-atrophy-induced ventricle expansion**
   Not all ventriculomegaly entail hydrocephalus, during brain atrophy, the ventricles may expand (Fig. 2.32). For brain atrophy, all the subarachnoid spaces including ventricles, sulci, cisterns, fissures are dilated.

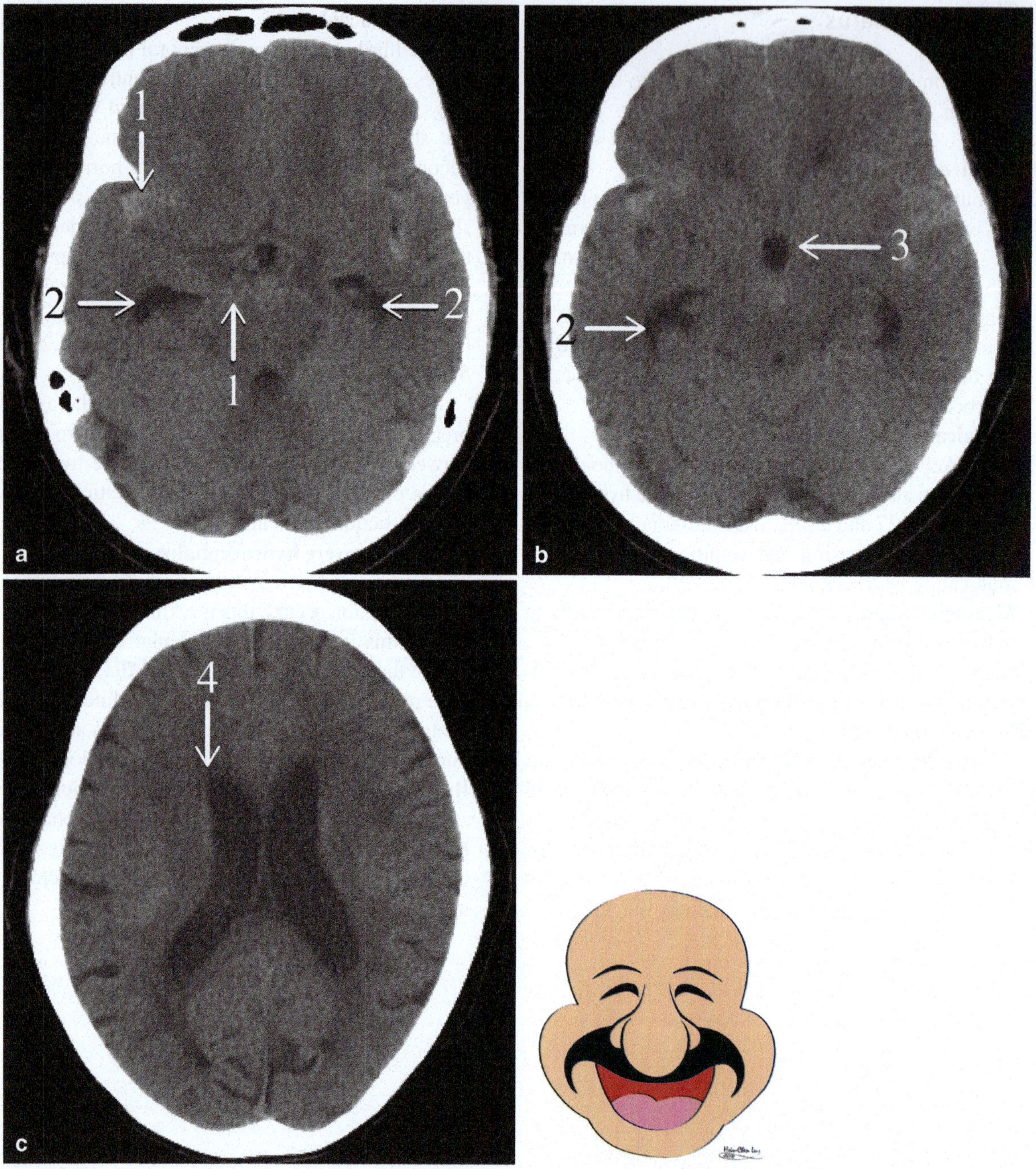

Fig. 2.27 F/76, SAH causes mild hydrocephalus. (**a–c**) CT: small amount of SAH in the suprasellar cistern and Sylvian fissure (1). The bilateral temporal horns are slightly dilated (2) and appear similar to two beards. The dilated third ventricle (3) seems similar to a large nose. This feature is a sign of mild hydrocephalus. Classifying this feature as mild hydrocephalus by looking at the lateral ventricle (4) is difficult

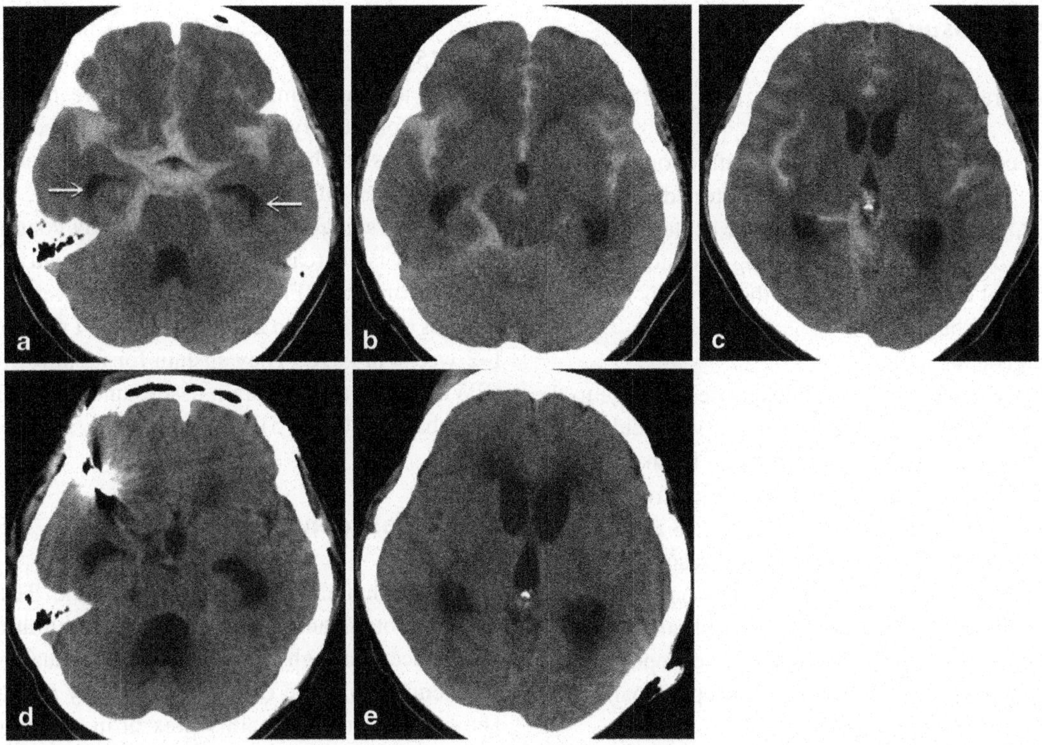

Fig. 2.28 F/59, SAH causes hydrocephalus. (**a–c**) CT: diffuse SAH. The slight enlargement of the temporal horns (arrows) of the bilateral lateral ventricles represents the presence of mild hydrocephalus caused by SAH. SAH may complicate CSF circulation, thus causing mild hydrocephalus. (**d**, **e**) CT after 5 months: All ventricles are dilated. This is communicating hydrocephalus, which is a sequela caused by SAH. SAH may cause subarachnoid space adhesion and complicate CSF circulation, thus causing communicating hydrocephalus

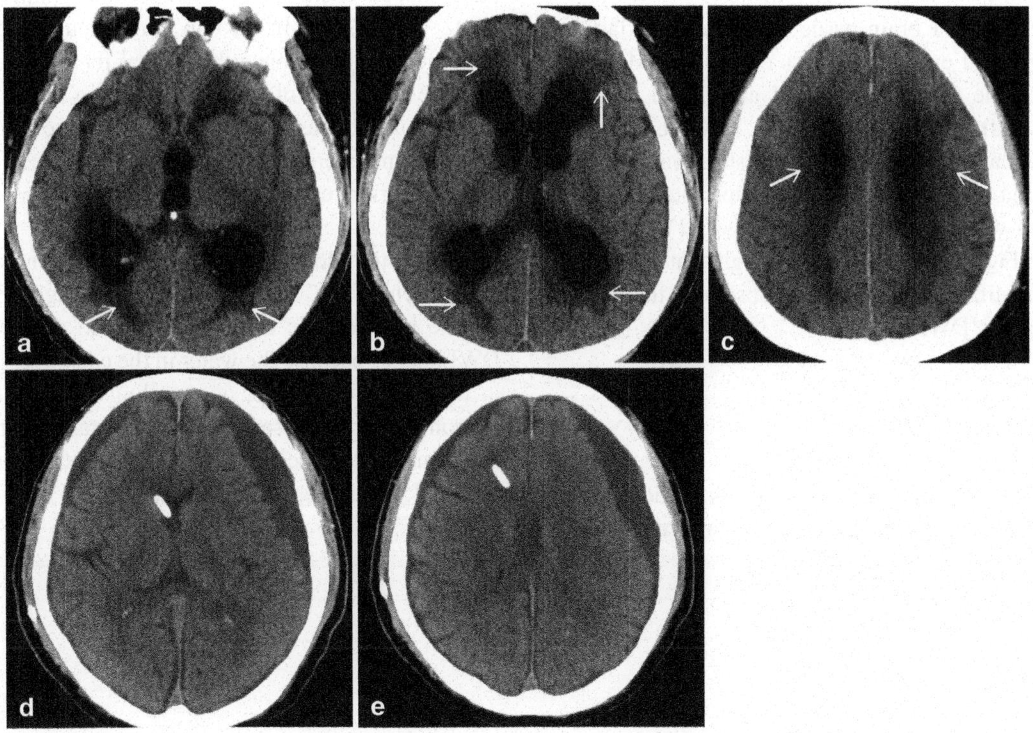

Fig. 2.29 M/62, Meningitis causes hydrocephalus. (**a–c**) CT: Each ventricle is dilated; this is communicating hydrocephalus caused by meningitis. The brain tissue surrounding the ventricle is dark, this is interstitial edema (arrows) induced by acute and severe hydrocephalus, which causes transependymal CSF resorption. (**d**, **e**) Follow-up CT after V-P shunt drainage: The ventricles have shrunk, and the interstitial edema has disappeared. Nonetheless, subdural effusions appear outside the cerebral hemispheres

2.7 Brain Tissue Edema

Four types of brain edema exist [4]:

1. Cytotoxic edema occurs in ischemic infarction (Chap. 5).
2. Vasogenic edema, or named white matter edema, perifocal edema, generally has a lesion in the center—such as a tumor, cerebral abscess, or absorbing hematoma—causing peripheral brain tissue edema, the edema is mainly in white matter (Chaps. 6 and 7).
3. Interstitial edema

   Acute and severe hydrocephalus causes damage to the ependymal lining. CSF permeates the ventricular wall and accumulates in the periventricular brain tissue, to form interstitial edema, which is also called transependymal CSF resorption or migration (Figs. 2.18 and 2.29).
4. Combined edema, cytotoxic edema, and vasogenic edema concurrently present. The following conditions may cause combined edema, such as cerebral contusion, venous infarction, hypoxic–ischemic encephalopathy, toxic encephalopathy, hypertensive encephalopathy, and encephalitis (Chaps. 3, 5, and 7).

Among the four types of brain tissue edema, cytotoxic edema and vasogenic edema are the most clinically important because they cause significant mass effect and neurologic symptoms. Besides, cytotoxic edema may gradually result in brain tissue necrosis and atrophy.

The four types of brain tissue edema appear dark gray in CT images and exhibit the mass effect. The MRI T1WI is similar to the CT image. T2WI and T2-FLAIR show hyperintensity from all types of edema. However, only cytotoxic edema causes water diffusion restriction and brightens the edema area in DWI images (hyperintensity, white) (Fig. 2.8). In vasogenic (Figs. 2.8, 2.30, 2.31) and interstitial edema (Fig. 2.18) regions, although water content is increased, no diffusion restriction is observed, therefore, no signal change on DWI.

2.7.1 Cytotoxic Edema

Brain tissue edema induced by ischemic infarction is a type of cytotoxic edema; it thus involves cell swelling caused by water entering astrocytes and neurons in the ischemic brain tissue [5].

DWI and ADC mapping in MRI are the most suitable methods for identifying cytotoxic edema because astrocytes and neurons in the edema regions swell and cause intercellular water diffusion restriction. In DWI, these regions have strong signals and appear white. By contrast, the ADC coefficient is decreased in these regions, and the ADC map thus appears dark (Figs. 2.6 and 2.8). However, these signal changes only maintain 2–3 weeks in DWI and approximately 1–2 weeks in ADC. They sustain for months in FLAIR and T2WI images until the brain tissues undergo necrosis or cavitary changes (Chap. 5).

2.7.2 Vasogenic Edema

Tight endothelial junction rupture of the BBB results in plasma protein entering vessels and infiltrating extracellular spaces through the BBB, thereby causing extracellular edema. This type of edema generally develops rapidly. The water content is mainly present in white matter. Water infiltrates the fiber tracts of white matter and eventually affects gray matter.

Similar to cytotoxic edema, vasogenic edema appears dark gray in CT images and exhibits the mass effect. The critical indicator of vasogenic edema is the white matter that forms palm-shaped edema. Once we see the palm-shaped white matter edema, we must do an intravenous injection of contrast medium to enhance the central focal lesion (Fig. 2.30) because the density of central focal lesion is similar to normal brain tissue, not easy to distinguish. In some situations, vasogenic edema is present without the central focal lesion, such as in posterior reversible encephalopathy syndrome (PRES) (Fig. 2.31).

Vasogenic edema also appears hypointensity on T1WI, hyperintensity on T2WI and FLAIR images. The primary feature is vasogenic edema exhibits no signal variation in DWI images because the water in the edema region increases in the interstitial space, no swelling of the astrocytes and neuron cells, so causes no diffusion restriction (Figs. 2.8, 2.30, and 2.31). Their appearance in ADC is similar to that in T2WI, appearing hyperintensity.

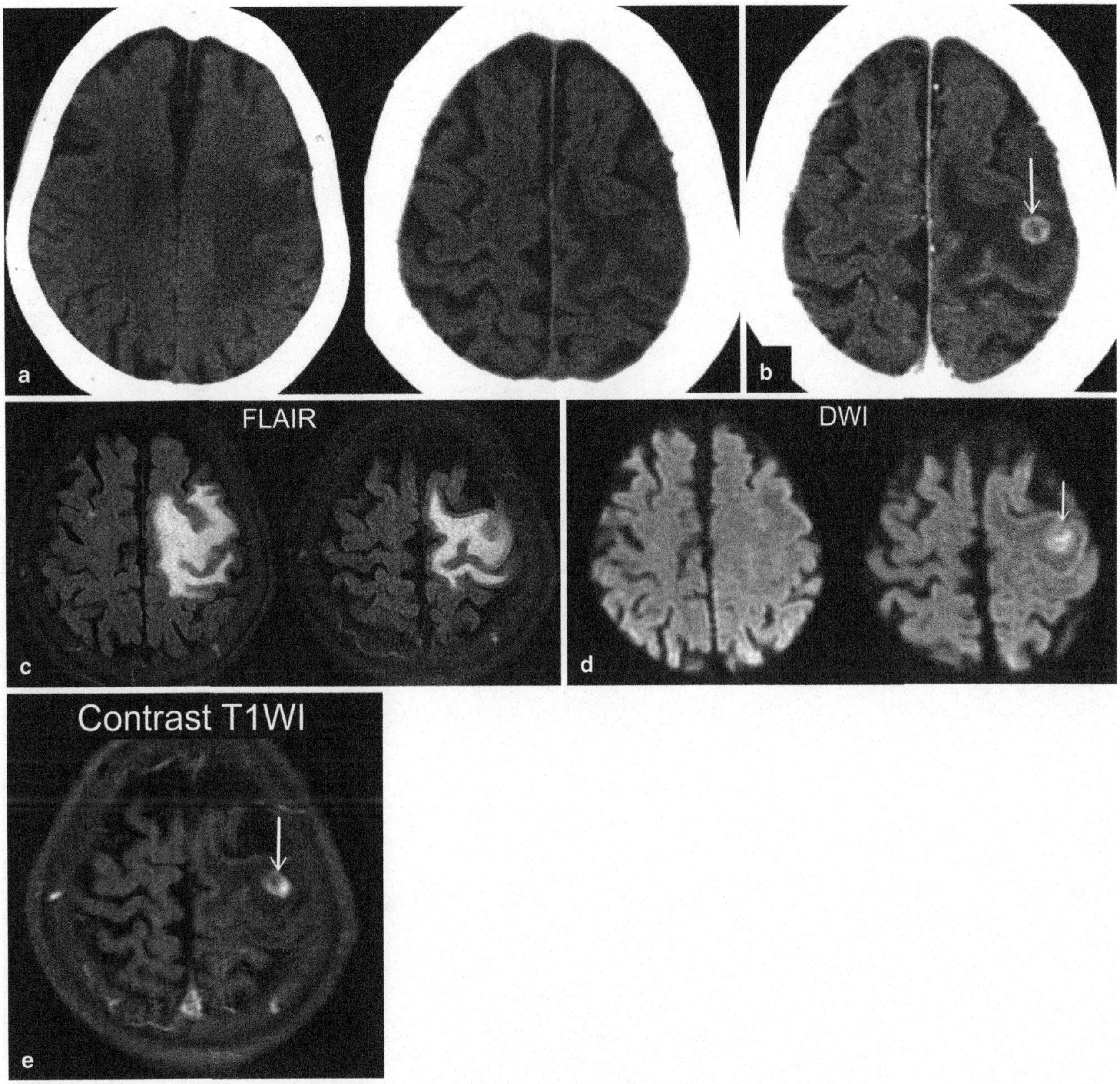

Fig. 2.30 F/96, WM edema presents a stroke symptom. The patient was diagnosed with a stroke based on right limb weakness and received a CT examination. (**a**) CT: an area of brain tissue edema in the left parietal lobe. Although it is in the MCA territory, it is very similar to MCA infarction edema. However, because the edema is mainly in white matter (WM), it forms palm-shaped. WM edema is vasogenic edema; we must perform contrast medium injection to identify a possible lesion within the edema. (**b**) Contrast-enhanced CT: A small lesion (arrow) within the edema area is enhanced out. (**c**, **d**) MRI: WM edema is hyperintensity (white) in FLAIR but lacks diffusion restriction; thus, no signal change is observed in DWI. The lesion itself, however, is slightly white (arrow) in DWI. (**e**) Contrast-enhanced T1WI: A lesion is enhanced out (arrow). This lesion is small and surrounded by significant WM edema, most commonly found in metastasis or brain abscess. This patient later failed to provide pathological proof to confirm that this is metastasis or brain abscess

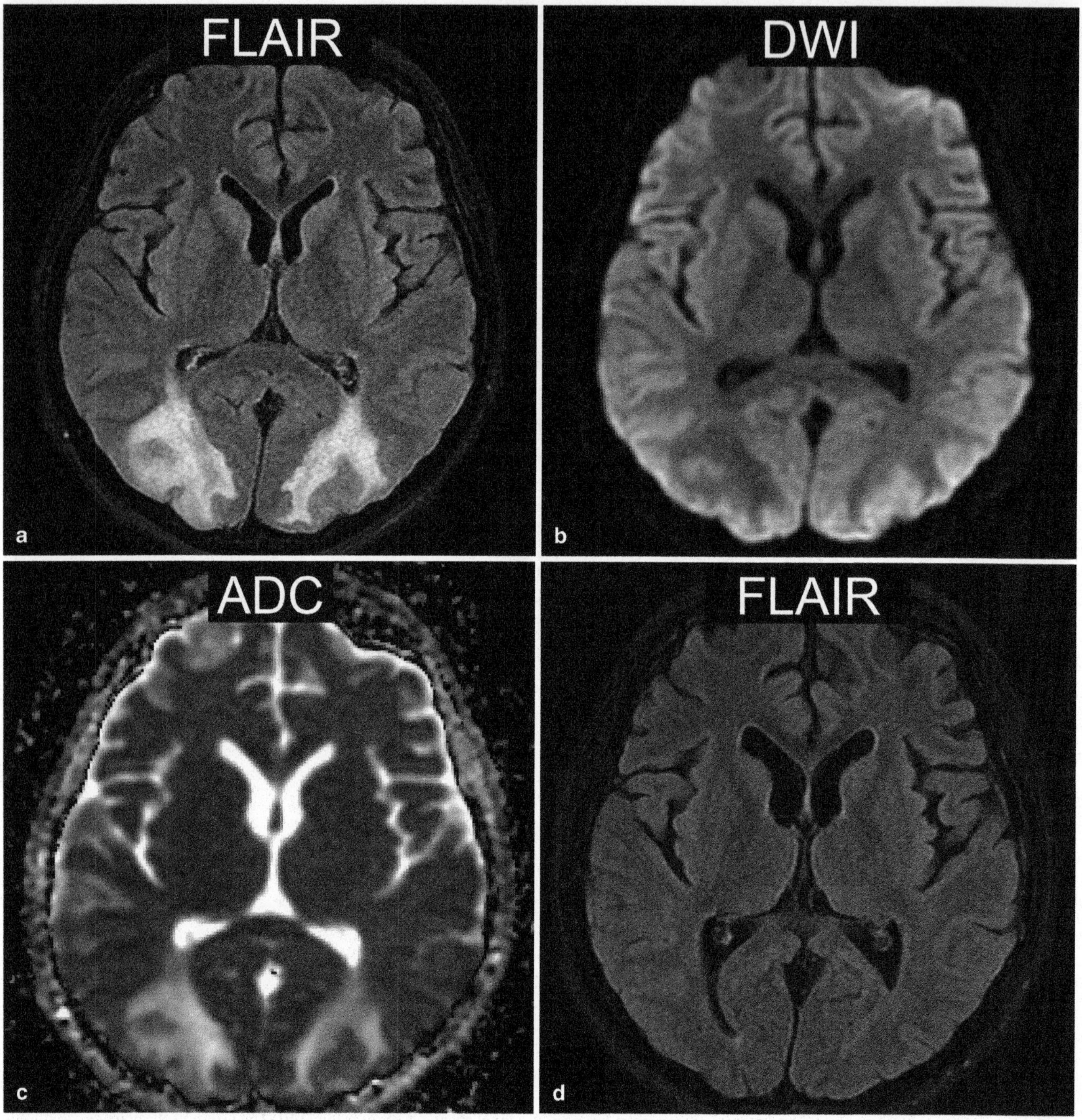

Fig. 2.31 F/15, PRES. This girl suffered a coma after persistent convulsion. (**a–c**) MRI: FLAIR showing symmetrical hyperintensity in the bilateral occipital lobes, no signal change in DWI, and hyperintensity in ADC. The findings indicate the absence of diffusion restriction and is vasogenic edema. According to the clinical course and MRI, this is possible PRES. (**d**) The patient recovered very well. Follow-up MRI after 10 months: FLAIR shows no sequelae. Note: Posterior reversible encephalopathy syndrome (PRES) is brain tissue edema caused by high blood pressure-induced BBB disruption, which causes vasogenic edema mainly in the occipital lobes. This case may feature persistent convulsions that cause transient hypertension, leading to PRES

2.8 Brain Atrophy

Brain atrophy identification is most sensitive in observation of a widened subarachnoid space around brain tissue, namely in the widening of the sulci, cisterns, fissures, and ventricles. Direct inspection of shrunken brain tissue volume, especially in comparison with normal contralateral brain tissues, clearly reveals brain atrophy.

2.8.1 Generalized Brain Atrophy

The causes are complex and include the following:

1. Generalized brain atrophy is more likely at aged people (Fig. 2.32), particularly in the frontal lobe.
2. If a patient has arteriosclerosis, brain atrophy occurs earlier and is more notable.
3. Chronic brain hypoxia.
4. The sequel of traumatic brain injury.
5. The sequel of meningitis (Fig. 7.5) and encephalitis.
6. Systemic lupus erythematosus.
7. Uremic encephalopathy.
8. Postradiation therapy.
9. Chronic alcoholism.

2.8.2 Focal Brain Atrophy

This is the sequel of focal brain injury. Observation of brain atrophy shows that surrounding sulci are widened, and nearby ventricles and cisterns are dilated, these features are usually accompanied by encephalomalacia and cavitary change.

The causes are as follows:

1. The sequel of cerebral contusion (Figs. 3.26 and 3.28).
2. Cerebral hemorrhage absorption (Fig. 2.36).
3. Old cerebral infarction region (Figs. 2.14 and 2.17).
4. Brain tissue atrophy near a big arteriovenous malformation.

2.8.3 Cerebral Hemiatrophy

Atrophy occurs on only one side of the brain and has the following causes:

1. Brain injury in children, in particular, the sequel of unilateral traumatic head injury, also known as the Dyke–Davidoff syndrome (Fig. 2.33) [6].
2. Sequel of unilateral intracranial major arterial infarction (Fig. 2.34).
3. Sturge-Weber syndrome with unilateral cerebral cortex hemangioma may associate with brain tissue atrophy.

2.8.4 Cerebellar Atrophy

1. Cerebellar atrophy occurs concurrently with cerebral atrophy. The causes are listed in the aforementioned generalized brain atrophy.
2. Cerebellar atrophy alone.
3. Combined brain stem atrophy:
   (a) Olivopontocerebellar degeneration (OPCD): in addition to cerebellar atrophy, it also associates with brain stem atrophy (Fig. 2.35).
   (b) Progressive supranuclear palsy: in addition to cerebellar atrophy, the midbrain is also atrophy.

In CT and MRI, cerebellar atrophy is observed through the widened cerebellar sulci, fourth ventricle, and CP angle cisterns.

2.8.5 Wallerian Degeneration

When the motor cortex or corona radiata of the corticospinal tract contains lesions, the remote structures of axons begin to demyelinate, and surrounding brain tissues undergo gliosis and atrophy. This process is called Wallerian degeneration and is most apparent in the brain stem.

In CT, only unilateral midbrain cerebral peduncle atrophy can be observed in most cases (Figs. 2.33 and 2.34). In MRI, atrophy of the pons and pyramid at lower positions can be observed. In T2WI and FLAIR, hyperintensity is observed at places through which the corticospinal tract passes before brain stem atrophy (Fig. 2.36).

When Wallerian degeneration is caused by subacute brain tissue injury, no brain stem atrophy be observed. However, remote regions through which axons pass begin to become demyelinated, and the MRI long TR images may show slight hyperintensity (Fig. 2.36). Therefore, signal changes can be observed in paths of the corticospinal tract, including the posterior limb of the internal capsule, cerebral peduncle of midbrain, pons, and pyramid of the medulla oblongata. Such signal changes represent early Wallerian degeneration.

The paramedian infarction of pons may cause a particular pattern of Wallerian degeneration, which can be observed in the pyramid of the medulla oblongata and bilateral middle cerebellar peduncles connecting the pons and cerebellum (Fig. 2.37) [7].

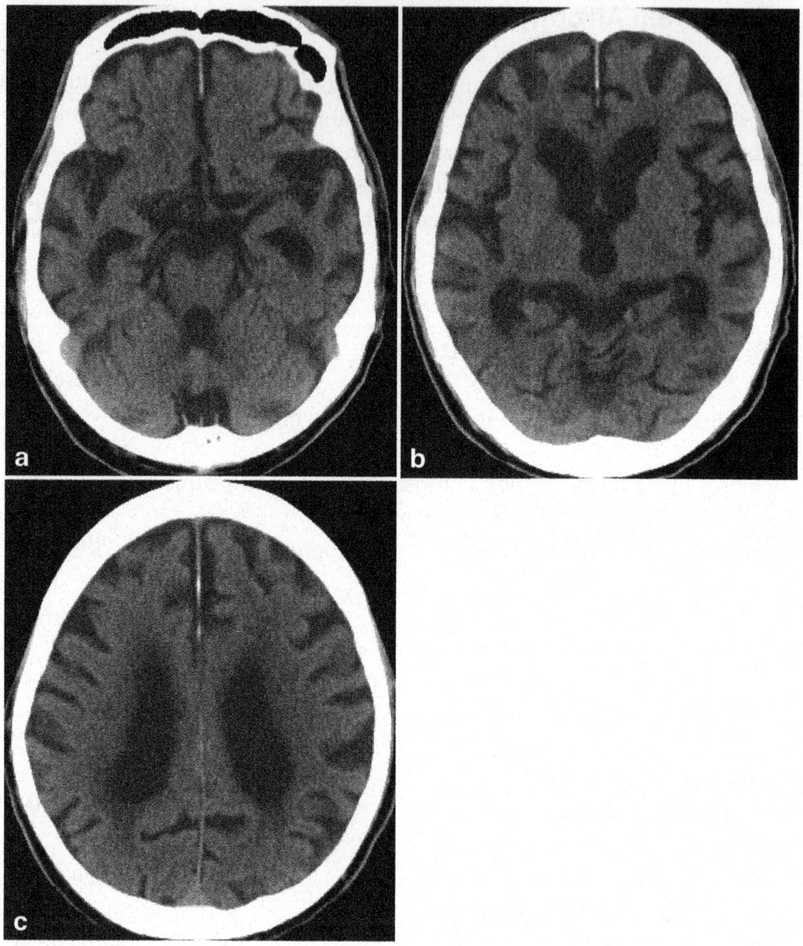

Fig. 2.32 M/87, Diffuse brain atrophy. CT: Brain tissue shows extensive atrophy because of age. The enlargement of all subarachnoid spaces, including ventricles, cisterns, fissures, and cortical sulci, indicates that the brain tissue is diffusely atrophic

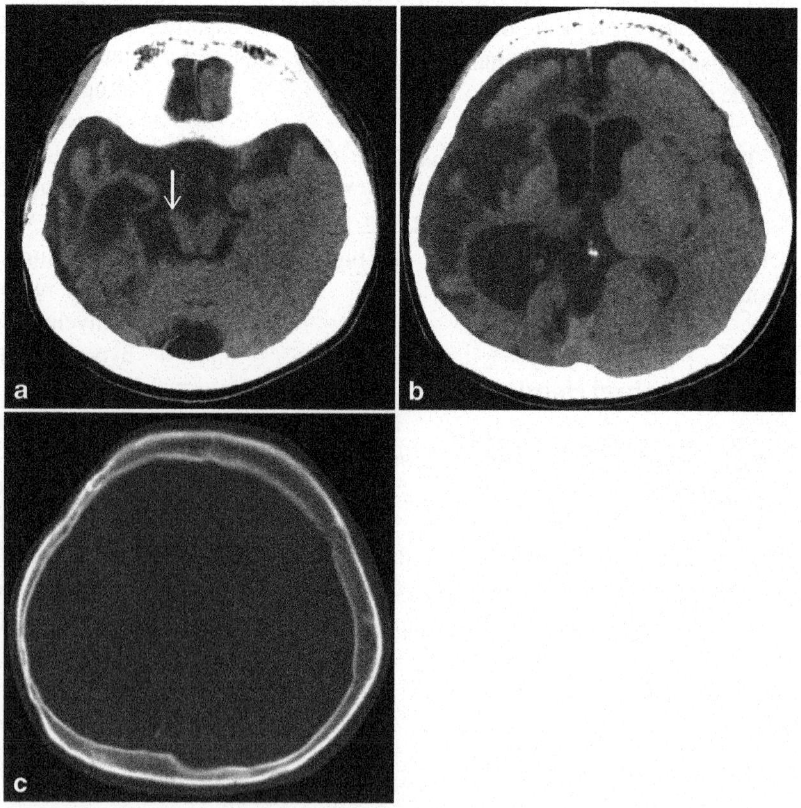

Fig. 2.33 M/20, Cerebral hemiatrophy. Seizure patients. The sequela of head injury in infancy. (**a**, **b**) CT: Severe atrophy of the right cerebral hemisphere; this is a sequela of head injury in infancy. There is atrophy of the right cerebral peduncle (arrow), indicating Wallerian degeneration. (**c**) CT, bone window: The right-side cranium is also thinning

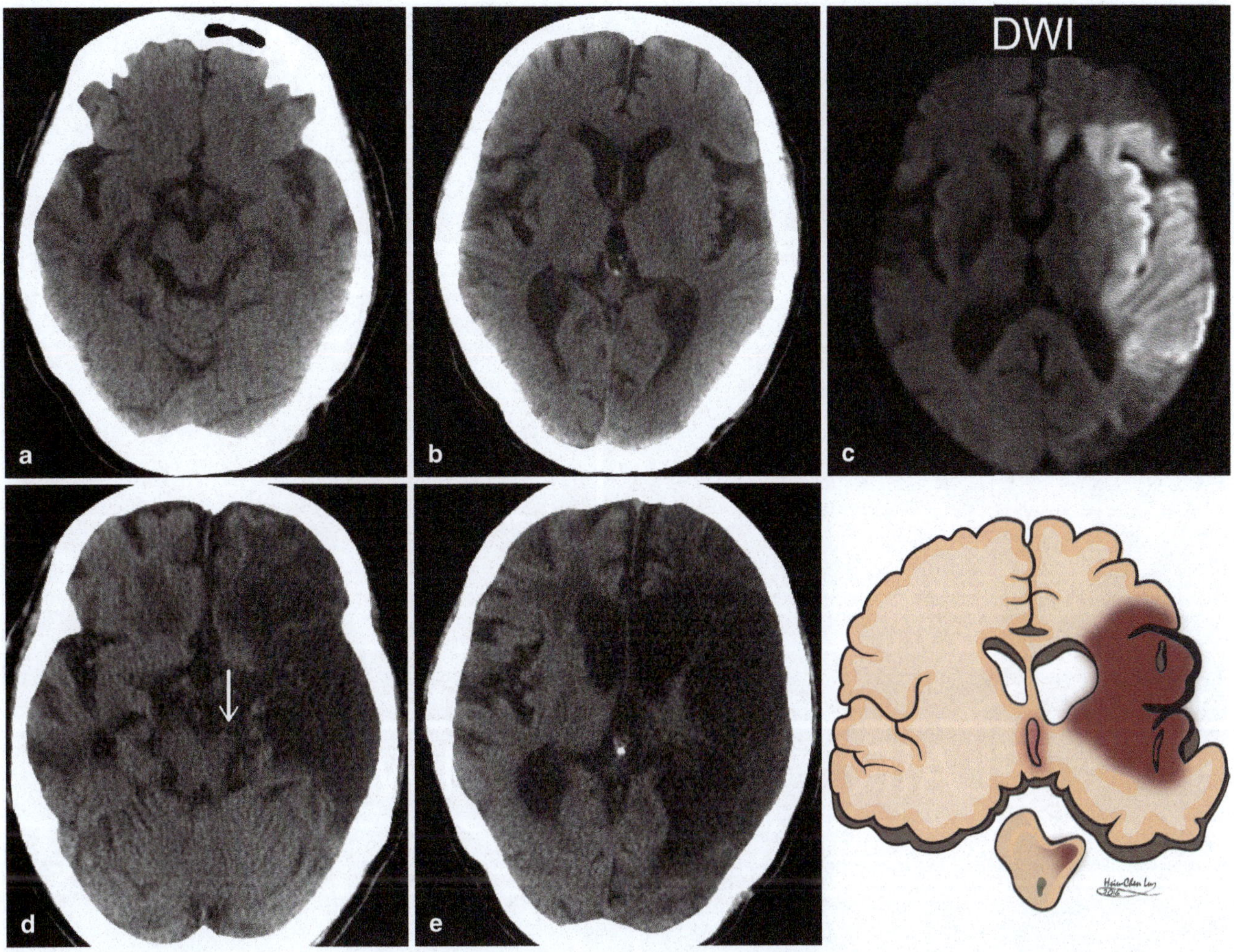

Fig. 2.34 F/85, Infarction causes cerebral hemiatrophy. (**a**, **b**) CT before stroke: diffuse brain atrophy due to age. The bilateral cerebral hemispheres, bilateral lateral ventricles, and bilateral cerebral peduncles are symmetrical. (**c**) MRI, DWI: Hyperintensity in the left MCA territory; this is acute infarction due to occlusion of left MCA. (**d**, **e**) Follow-up CT after 3 years: A large area of old brain tissue damage is present in the left cerebral hemisphere. This area shows hypodensity and reduces brain volume. The left lateral ventricle is enlarged, and the left cerebral peduncle is atrophied (arrow) because of Wallerian degeneration

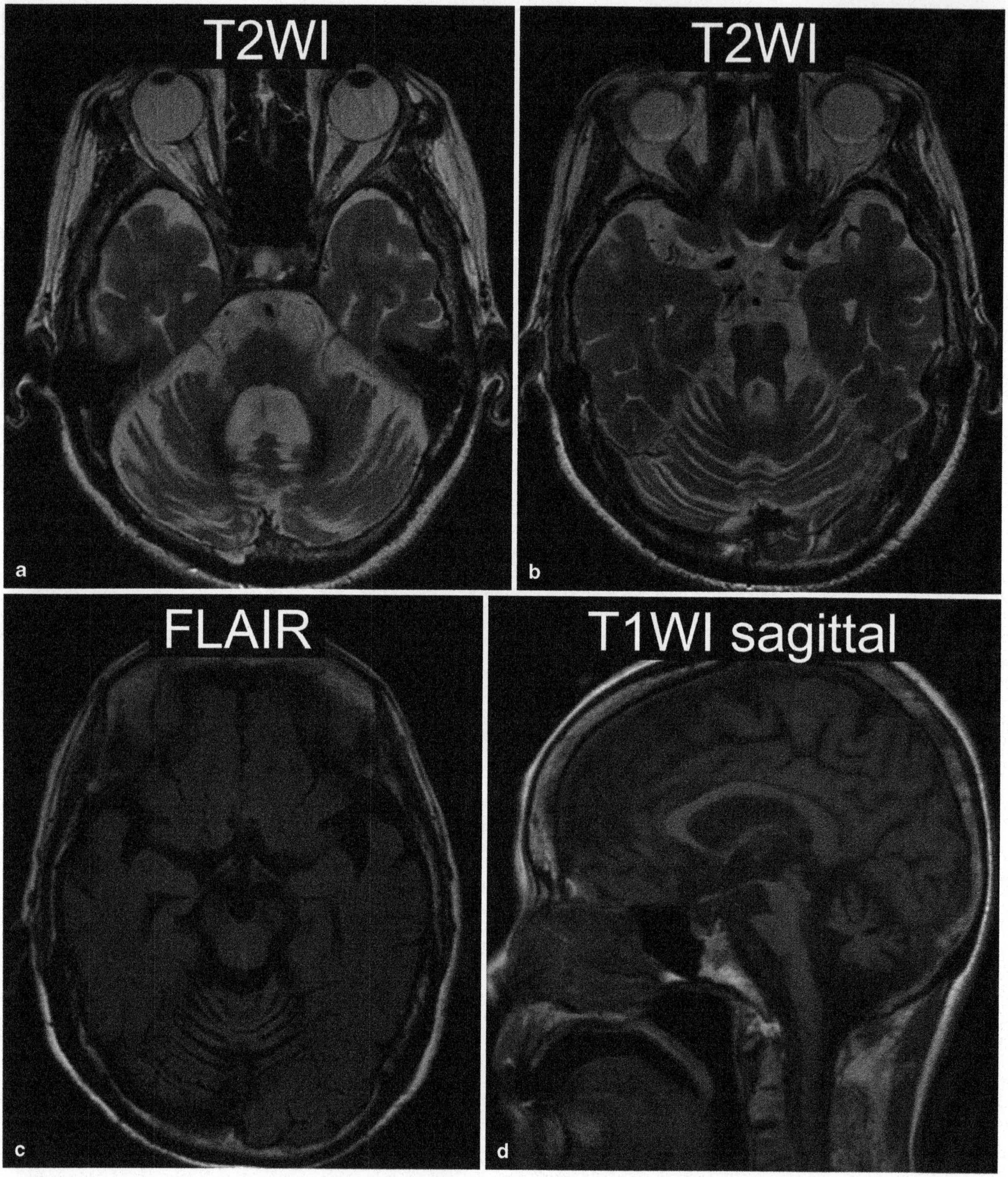

Fig. 2.35 F/66, OPCD (olivopontocerebellar degeneration). (**a–c**) MRI, T2WI, FLAIR: severe atrophy of the cerebellum and brainstem. The cerebellar sulci are very wide, and the fourth ventricle is dilated. (**d**) T1WI, sagittal: severe atrophy of cerebellum and brainstem. The subarachnoid spaces in the posterior fossa are wide

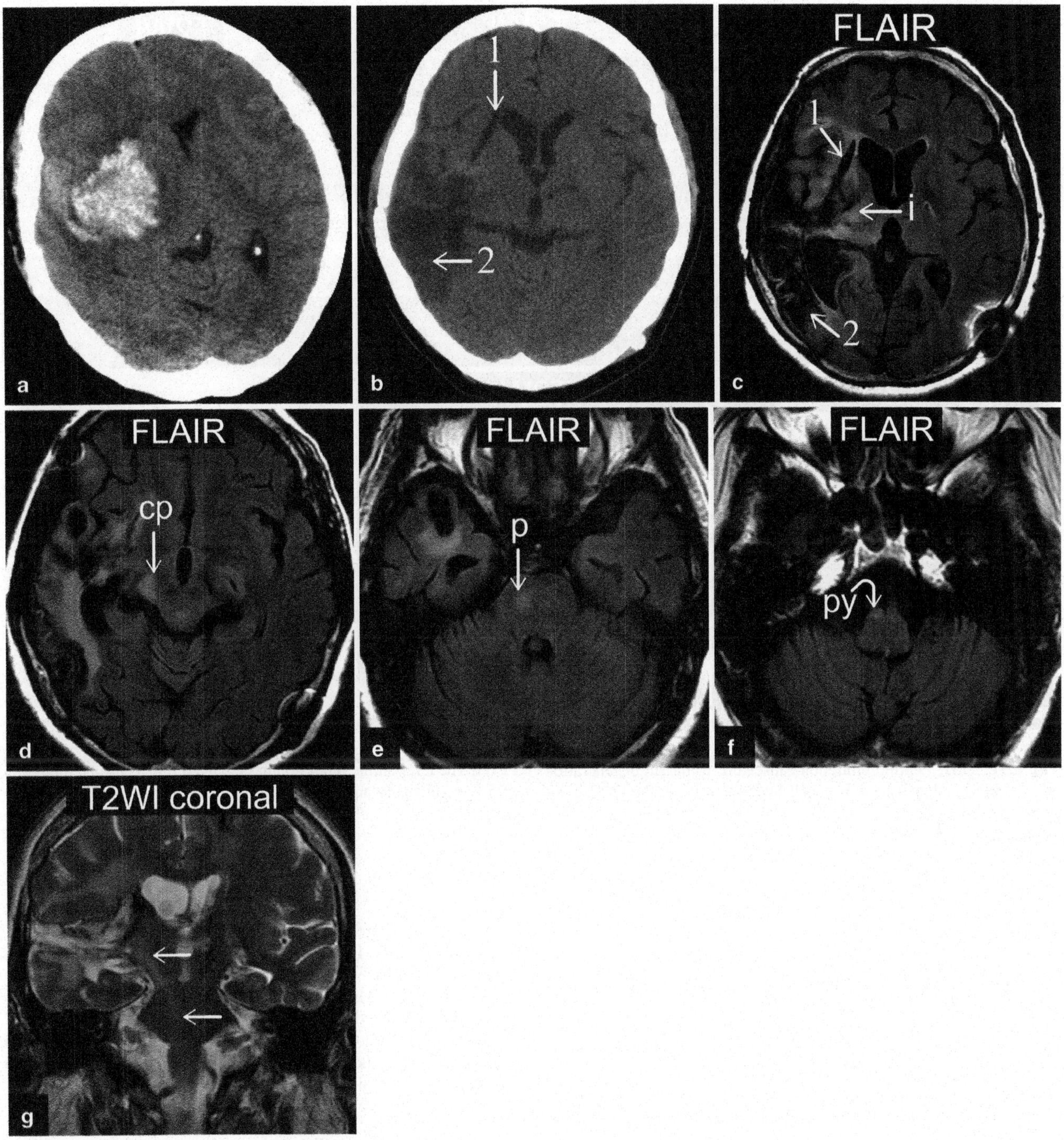

Fig. 2.36 F/58, ICH, and infarction cause Wallerian degeneration. (**a**) CT: Acute hematoma in the right putamen because of hypertension clinically presented left-side hemiplegia. (**b**) CT after 3 months: Right putamen hematoma had been absorbed, showing linear hypodensity (1). Another brain tissue edema (2) in the right temporal lobe caused by acute infarction. (**c–f**) MRI after half a year: An old ICH presents as a linear cavity (1) in the right putamen and an area of old infarction (2) in the right temporal lobe. Hyperintensity along the course of the right corticospinal tract, including the internal capsule (i), cerebral peduncle (cp), pons (p), and the pyramid (py) of the medulla oblongata. (**g**) T2WI, coronal section, clearly shows the hyperintensity along the course of the right corticospinal tract. Note, only the signal change is observed at this time, no tissue atrophy, such as cerebral peduncle atrophy, is observed yet

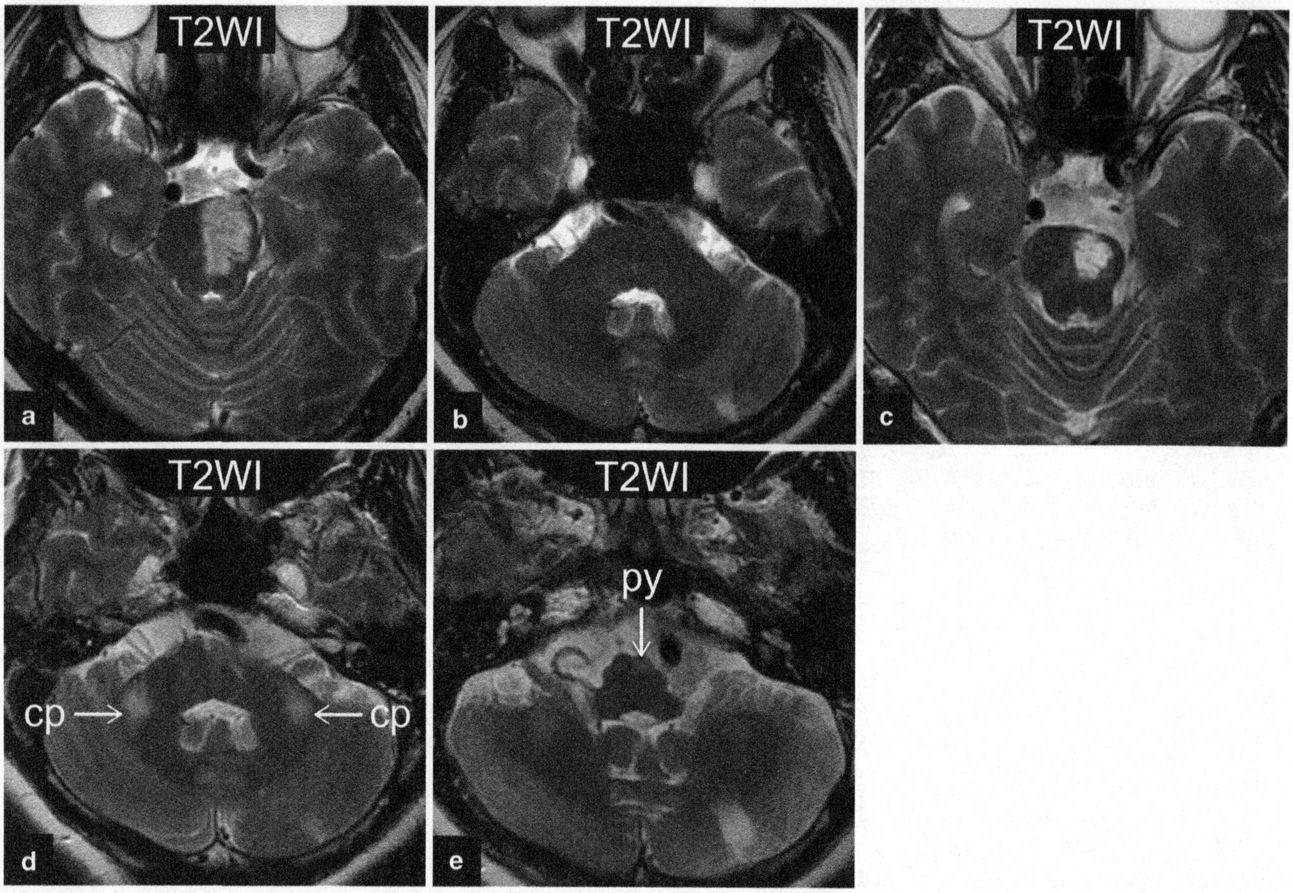

Fig. 2.37 F/57, Pontine infarction causes the Wallerian degeneration of cerebellar peduncles. (**a**, **b**) MRI: hyperintensity in the left side of pons. This is acute infarction edema; the bilateral middle cerebellar peduncles are normal at this time. (**c**–**e**) Follow-up MRI 8 months later, T2WI: The left pontine infarction has changed into a chronic infarction with hyperintensity and focal brain tissue atrophy. The hyperintensity of the pyramid (py) of the medulla oblongata and the bilateral middle cerebellar peduncles (cp) reflect Wallerian degeneration

References

1. Stuckey SL, et al. Hyperintensity in the subarachnoid space on FLAIR MRI. AJR. 2007;189:913–21.
2. Taoka T, et al. Sulcal hyperintensity on fluid-attenuated inversion recovery MR images in patients without apparent cerebrospinal fluid abnormality. AJR. 2001;176:519–24.
3. Verma A, et al. Magnetic resonance spectroscopy—revisiting the biochemical and molecular milieu of brain tumors. BBA Clin. 2016;5:170–8.
4. Ho ML, et al. Cerebral edema. AJR. 2012;199:W258–73.
5. Rosenberg GA. Ischemic brain edema. Prog Cardiovasc Dis. 1999;42:209–16.
6. Shen WC, et al. Magnetic resonance imaging of cerebral hemiatrophy. J Formos Med Assoc. 1993;92:995–1000.
7. Zhang ZY, et al. Clinical and radiological features of Wallerian degeneration of the middle cerebellar peduncles secondary to pontine infarction. Chin Med J. 2018;131:665–71.

Medical Imaging of Head Injury

3

Abstract

The imaging classification of head injury includes (1) extracerebral lesions: EDH, SDH, SDE, and chronic SDH; (2) intraparenchymal lesions: contusion edema and hemorrhage, contusion hematoma, contusion edema, and diffuse axonal injury (DAI); (3) traumatic SAH and IVH; (4) others: linear fracture, depressed fracture, and pneumocephalus; (5) extracranial lesions: facial bone fractures, paranasal sinuses bleedings, blow-out fracture of the orbital floor, and cervical spinal fracture or subluxation; and (6) sequelae of head injury: brain tissue encephalomalacia or porencephaly, focal or diffuse brain atrophy, and hydrocephalus. CT is the first diagnostic modality for head injury and can diagnose all the above conditions. MRI is an auxiliary tool for head injury. For DAI, MRI can detect microbleeding and deep brain tissue contusion edema, which CT may miss.

3.1 Imaging Classification of Head Injury

Brain and cranium damages caused by head trauma can be divided into several categories (Fig. 3.1).

3.1.1 Extracerebral Lesions

Acute epidural hematoma, EDH.
Acute subdural hematoma, SDH.
Subdural effusion, SDE.
Chronic subdural hematoma, ChrSDH.

3.1.2 Intracerebral (intraparenchymal) Lesions/Brain Contusion

Brain contusion edema.
Contusion edema and hemorrhage.
Traumatic intracerebral hematoma.
Diffuse axonal injury, DAI.

Traumatic subarachnoid hemorrhage, traumatic SAH.
Traumatic intraventricular hemorrhage, traumatic IVH.

3.1.3 Other Injuries

Bony fracture of the cranium.
 Linear fracture.
 Depression fracture.
Traumatic pneumocephalus.
Facial bones fracture, orbital fracture, skull base fracture.
Paranasal sinus bleeding.
Foreign bodies.

3.1.4 Sequela of Head Injury

Focal or diffuse brain atrophy.
Encephalomalacia or porencephaly.
Hydrocephalus.

3.2 Diagnostic Tools for Head Injury

Computed tomography (CT) is the most important diagnostic tool for acute head trauma, post-traumatic follow-up, and head injury sequelae [1, 2]. Owing to its rapidity, examination through CT can be completed under mild sedation even if the patient is unconscious and confused. Moreover, made possible by the advancement of CT instruments, the addition of coronal and sagittal reconstructions to axial sections is helpful in diagnosis.

X-ray: Traditional skull X-ray has been abandoned because it is meaningless given that it can only be used to examine skull fractures.

W.-C. Shen, *Diagnostic Neuroradiology*, https://doi.org/10.1007/978-981-15-4051-6_3

Magnetic resonance imaging (MRI) is unsuitable for the emergency examination of head traumas because it takes longer time to acquire. It cannot be performed when a patient is agitated or when oxygen or intubation is used. MRI is an auxiliary tool for CT. No apparent lesions appear on CT even though clinical symptoms are severe. For example, MRI is helpful in examining diffuse axonal injury (DAI). MRI can be utilized in visualizing brain tissue damage and brain hemorrhages, especially microbleeds. MRI is more precise than CT for small and chronic subdural hematomas (SDHs).

3.3 Several Basic Concepts for the Interpretation of Head Injury

1. **Coup or contrecoup:** Most intracranial hemorrhages and brain tissue contusions caused by head injuries occur in the same side as the traumas (Figs. 3.4, 3.5, 3.6, and 3.7). However, approximately 30% occur in another side (Figs. 3.4, 3.8, and 3.30). For example, a head injury may be in the right side with scalp swelling or cranial bone fracture, but the intracranial hemorrhage (EDH or SDH) and cerebral contusion are in the left side, or the injury may be on the posterior of the head, but bleeding and edema are in the frontal or temporal lobes.
2. **Delayed bleeding and cerebral edema:** Head trauma often has delayed bleeding (Figs. 3.29 and 3.30) and delayed cerebral edema (Fig. 3.15). Clinically, there is a lucid interval, where by a patient remains awake at the beginning of the trauma but gradually slips into unconsciousness after a few hours. Therefore, repeating a CT examination at any time in conjunction with clinical changes is necessary.
3. **Post-decompression hemorrhage**: Sometimes, new bleeding may begin after the surgical removal of a hematoma for decompression. Because a hematoma produces high pressure, so the other torn vessels are compressed and no bleeding. As the pressure reduces after surgical removal of the first hematoma, the other torn blood vessels begin to bleed and form a second hematoma (Figs. 3.31 and 3.43).
4. **Bone window setting and imaging reconstructions:** The bone window for the CT imaging of head trauma must be adjusted for the examination of the skull (Figs. 3.5, 3.6, 3.25, 3.29, 3.34, and 3.35) and the skull base in addition to the routine brain window. Meanwhile, facial bones, orbits, and paranasal sinuses must be checked (Figs. 3.25 and 3.39). Blow-out fractures at the floor of the orbital cavity are visible only through coronal reconstruction (Figs. 3.37 and 3.38). The entire cervical spine must be scrutinized for the prevention of missing cervical spine fractures or subluxation (Fig. 3.40). In addition to coronal and sagittal reconstruction, 3D image reconstruction can be added for the clarification of the diagnosis of fractures (Fig. 3.39).

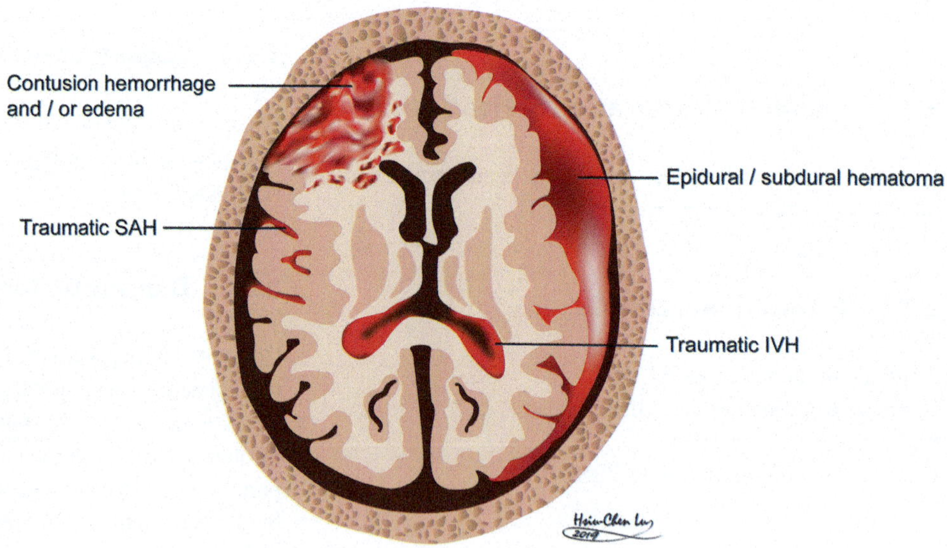

Fig. 3.1 The classification of head injury

3.4 Acute Epidural Hematoma (EDH)

The bleeding of the meningeal artery causes acute epidural hematomas (EDHs) during head trauma.

3.4.1 CT Shape

A typical EDH exhibits a biconvex shape on CT (the cranium and the outer edge of the hematoma form a biconvex shape together) or a fusiform shape with a high uniform density of hematoma (Figs. 3.2, 3.3, 3.4, 3.5 3.6, 3.26, and 3.28).

A dark-gray area that appears in the hematoma reflects the hematoma contains uncoagulated blood or continued arterial bleeding during CT scanning; this is called "swirl sign" (Figs. 3.3 and 3.4).

EDHs are usually located in the temporal and parietal regions and may step across the midline (e.g., falx) to the opposite side if located in the frontal region (Fig. 3.5). An EDH in the posterior fossa or occipital region may step across the tentorium (Fig. 3.6).

EDHs usually cause a strong mass effect. An excessively strong mass effect causes uncal and transtentorial herniations (Fig. 3.3). Therefore, emergency surgery is often needed to remove the EDH.

EDHs may occur alone or in association with brain contusion, cerebral edema, SAH, and intraventricular hemorrhage (IVH).

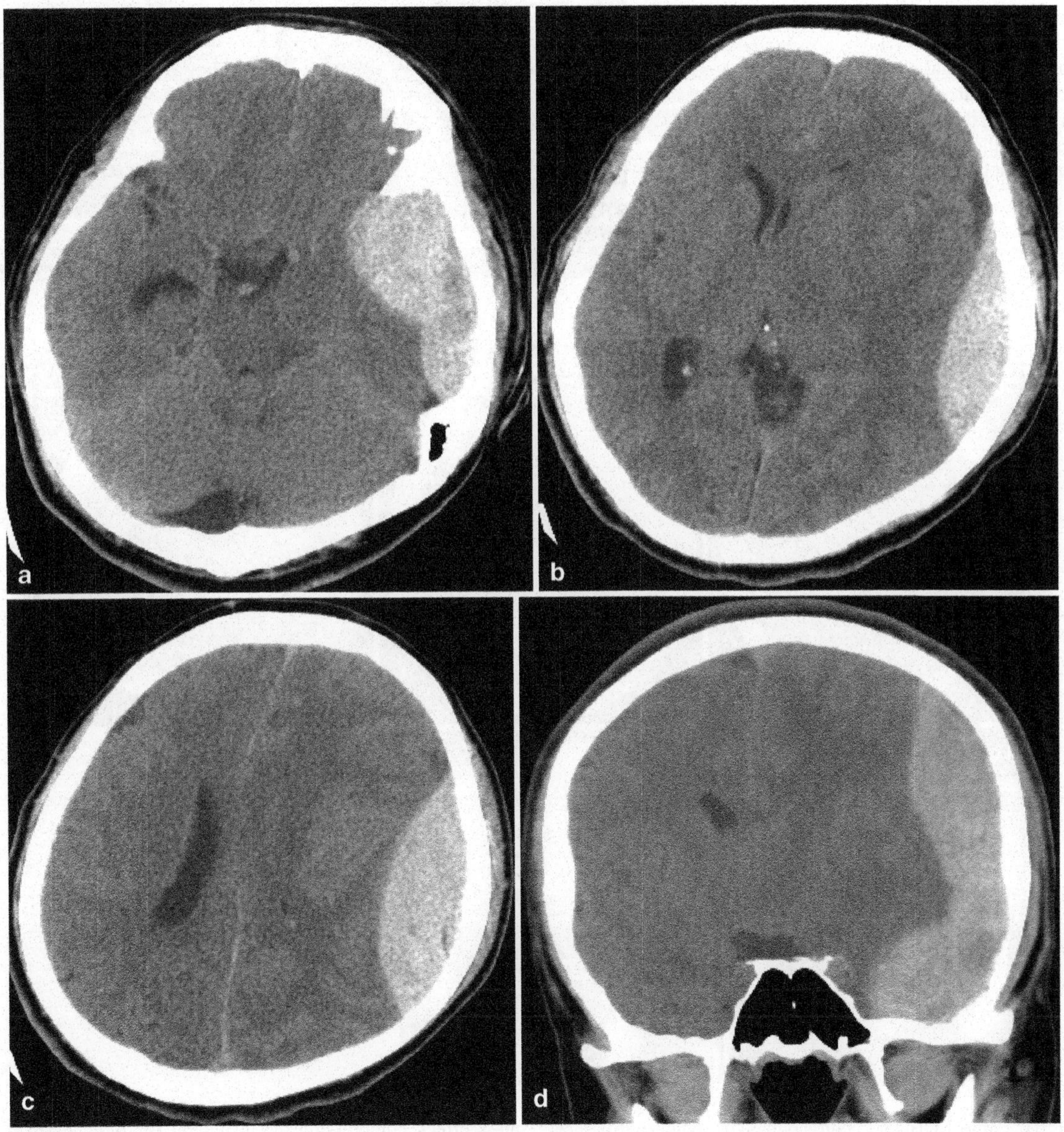

Fig. 3.2 M/26, Epidural hematoma (EDH). (**a–c**) CT, Axial section. (**d**) Coronal reconstruction. A large blood clot on the left cerebral surface, showing the fusiform shape and homogeneous hyperdensity, this is a typical EDH. The EDH causes a strong mass effect; the ipsilateral ventricle is severely compressed. The brain tissue appears normal, and no delayed bleeding or edema in the brain tissue after the surgical removal of EDH. The prognosis of this patient is excellent

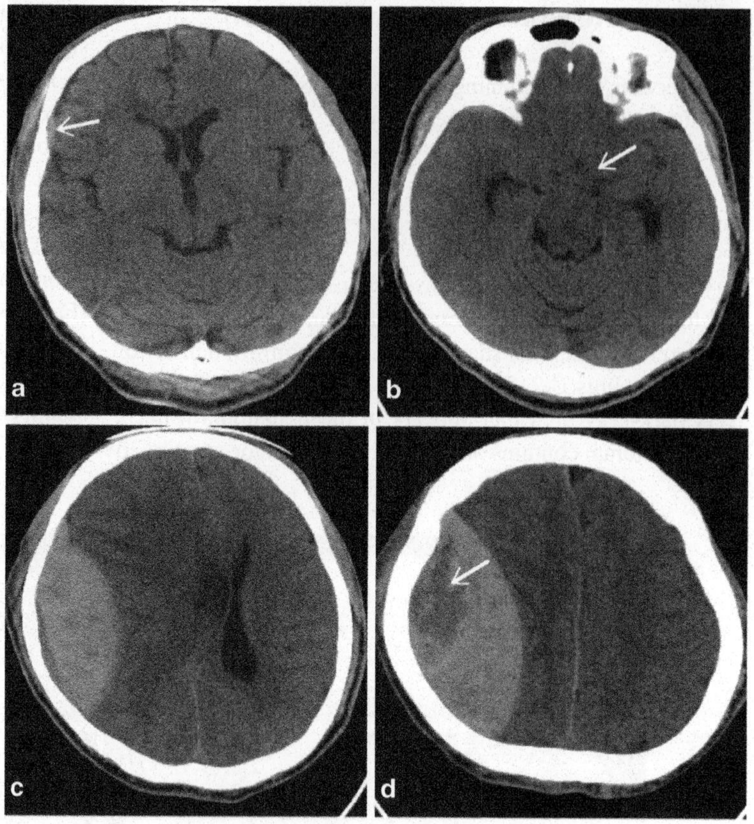

Fig. 3.3 M/49, Delayed bleeding. (**a**) Emergency CT was performed immediately after the head injury. Only a small EDH is observed (arrow). The patient was observed in the emergency unit. CT has performed again several hours later due to the deterioration of consciousness and abnormal respiration. (**b**–**d**) The CT was taken 5 h after the first CT. The small EDH has changed into a large fusiform hematoma, a typical EDH feature. A hypodense area (arrow in **d**) within this EDH, representing an uncoagulated blood clot, indicates that the hematoma was still bleeding actively. We call it "swirl sign." This hematoma causes a strong mass effect with uncal herniation based on the disappearance of the suprasellar cistern (arrow in **b**)

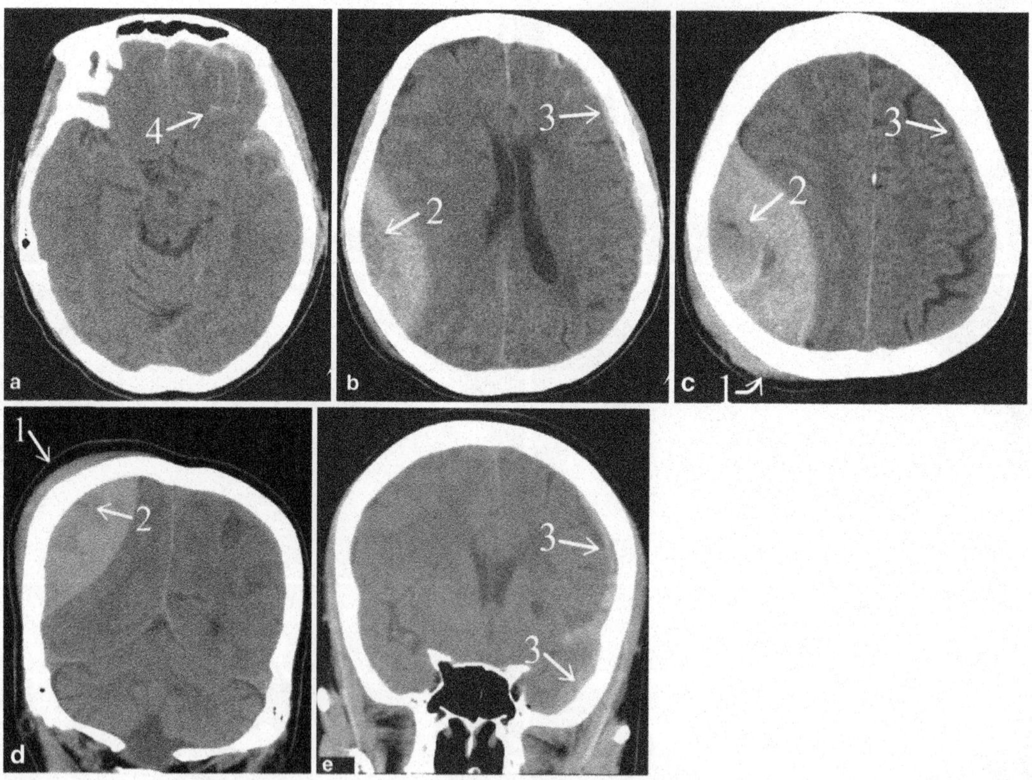

Fig. 3.4 F/63, Large EDH and contrecoup SDH, contusion hemorrhage. (**a**–**c**) CT, axial section. (**d**, **e**) Coronal reconstruction. The scalp swelling on the right parietal region is the impact position (1). A massive EDH on the same side. The hematoma in the EDH is not uniformly white and contains a hypodense area (2) which represents uncoagulated blood clot because of active bleeding (swirl sign). This EDH causes the mass effect, compressing the ipsilateral ventricle. A small crescentic hematoma, which is an SDH, is present in the contralateral frontal region (3). Linear hemorrhages in the left frontal lobe (4), which is the contusion hemorrhage in the brain tissue. The SDH (3) and contusion hemorrhage (4) are the contrecoup injuries

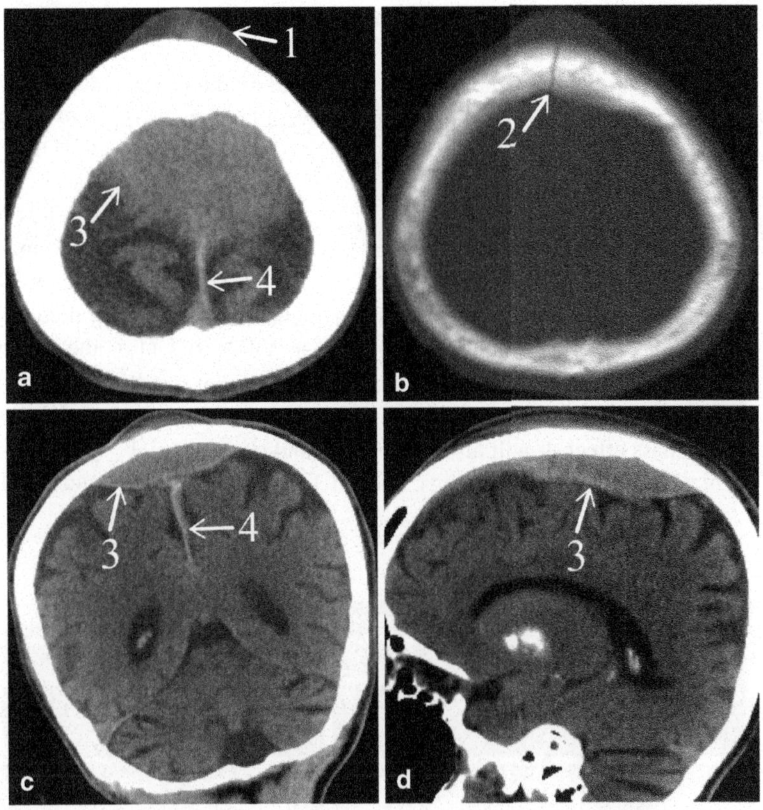

Fig. 3.5 M/45, Acute EDH across the falx. (**a**) CT, axial section. (**b**) Axial, bone window. (**c**) Coronal reconstruction. (**d**) Sagittal reconstruction. The scalp swelling on the head (1) is the impact position. The underlying skull has a linear fracture (2). There is a fusiform hematoma in the left and the right frontal regions, is an acute epidural hematoma (EDH) (3), this EDH across the falx (4). Only EDH can step across falx, subdural hematoma (SDH) cannot

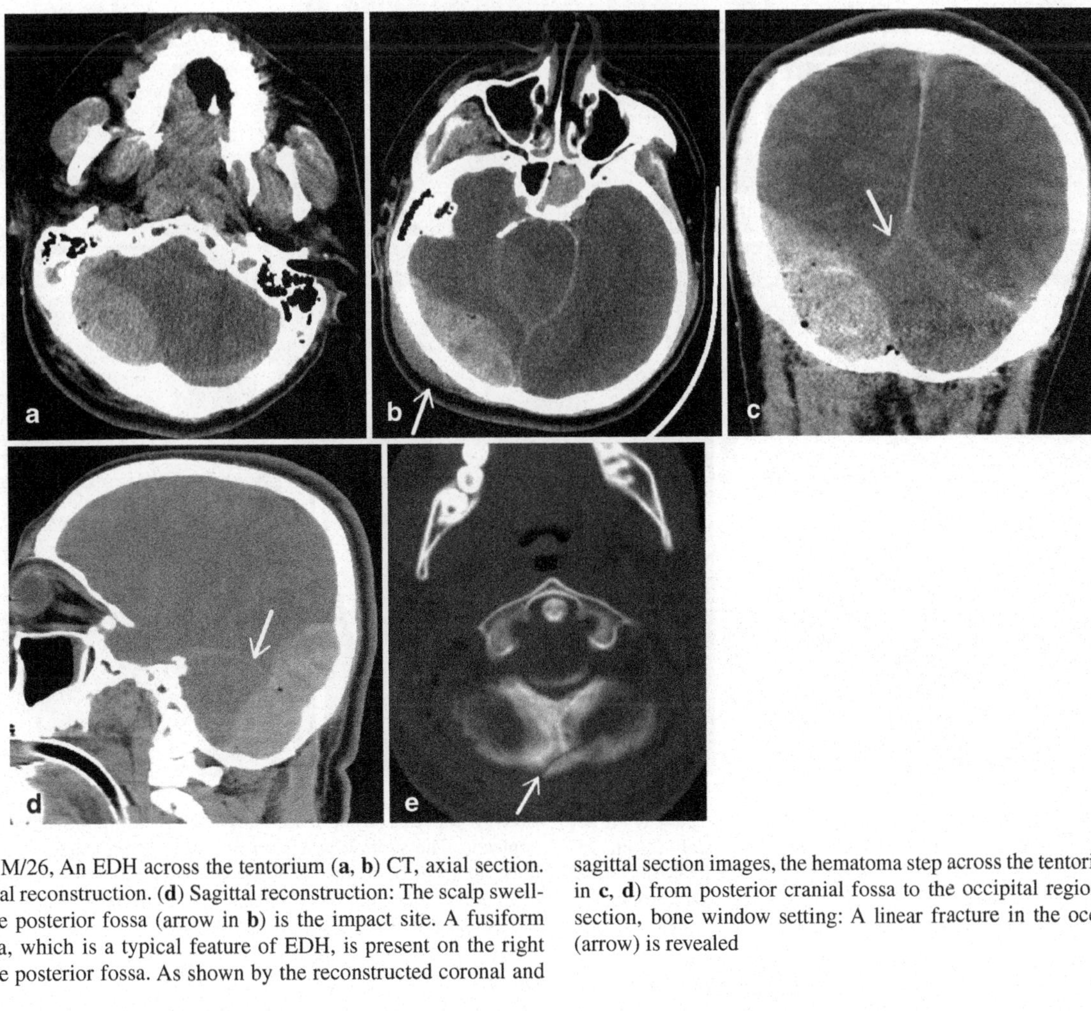

Fig. 3.6 M/26, An EDH across the tentorium (**a**, **b**) CT, axial section. (**c**) Coronal reconstruction. (**d**) Sagittal reconstruction: The scalp swelling on the posterior fossa (arrow in **b**) is the impact site. A fusiform hematoma, which is a typical feature of EDH, is present on the right side of the posterior fossa. As shown by the reconstructed coronal and sagittal section images, the hematoma step across the tentorium (arrows in **c**, **d**) from posterior cranial fossa to the occipital region. (**e**) Axial section, bone window setting: A linear fracture in the occipital bone (arrow) is revealed

3.5 Acute Subdural Hematoma (SDH)

Acute subdural hematomas (SDHs) are caused by the injury of the cerebral cortical artery or a cortical vein laceration in the dura mater by a head injury.

3.5.1 CT Shape

A typical acute SDH exhibits a high-density hematoma with a sickle or crescent shape (Figs 3.4, 3.7, 3.8, 3.9, 3.10 3.11, 3.15, 3.19, 3.20, 3.31, 3.41, 3.42, and 3.43). Given that it will penetrate back and forth, the SDH may be long and causes a strong mass effect. It will also cause uncal and transtentorial herniations in severe cases (Figs. 3.9 and 3.31).

Acute SDHs may extend into the subdural space along the tentorium (Figs. 3.9 and 3.10).In the CT axial section, the tentorial SDH is easily mistaken as an intracerebral hematoma (Fig. 3.10), so we need the coronal sections to clarify it is SDH. Occasionally, the SDH exists in the interhemispheric fissure (Fig. 3.11), or the SDH in frontal or parietal surface extends into the interhemispheric fissure (Fig. 3.43).

Some acute SDHs will mix with low-density fluid likely because blood clots have not yet coagulated, this is also called "swirl sign" (Fig. 3.8) or because of the laceration of the arachnoid membrane, therefore, CSF flows into the subdural space and mixes with blood clots (Fig. 3.9).

In some SHDs that remain untreated, blood clots may gradually evolve into subacute or chronic SDHs (Figs. 3.19 and 3.20) or even subdural effusions (SDEs).

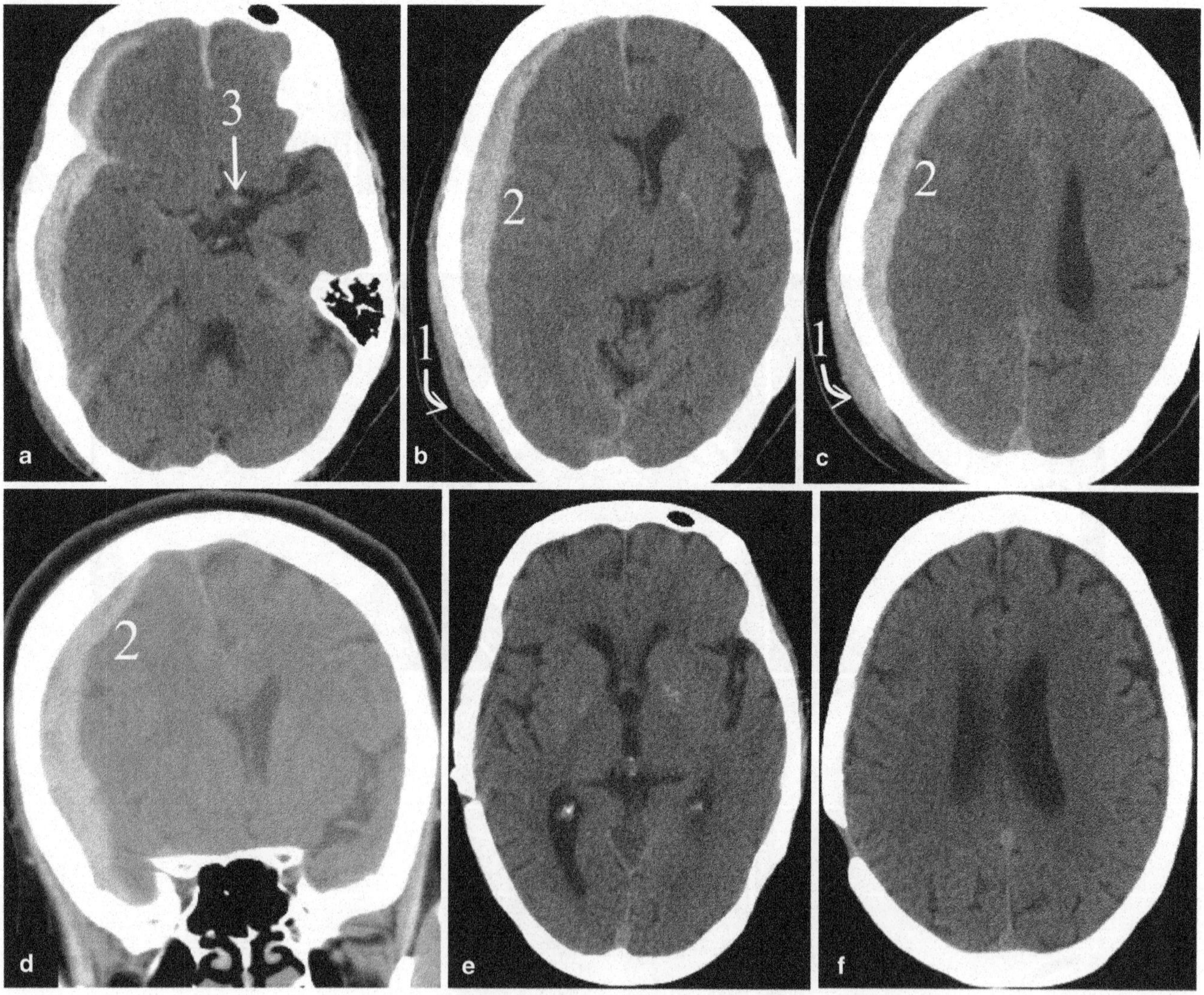

Fig. 3.7 F/72, Acute subdural hematoma (SDH). The patient hit her head when she slipped in the bathroom. (**a–c**) CT, axial section. (**d**) Coronal reconstruction: The swollen scalp in the right temporo-occipital region (1) is the impact position. A crescentic hematoma is present in the ipsilateral fronto-temporo-parietal region (2). It is a typical acute SDH. It causes a strong mass effect, compressing the ipsilateral lateral ventricle. The suprasellar cistern is not yet significantly deformed (3); thus, no uncal herniation is observed. (**e, f**) The mass effect has disappeared, and the lateral ventricle and sulci have returned to normal after the removal of the SDH by craniotomy

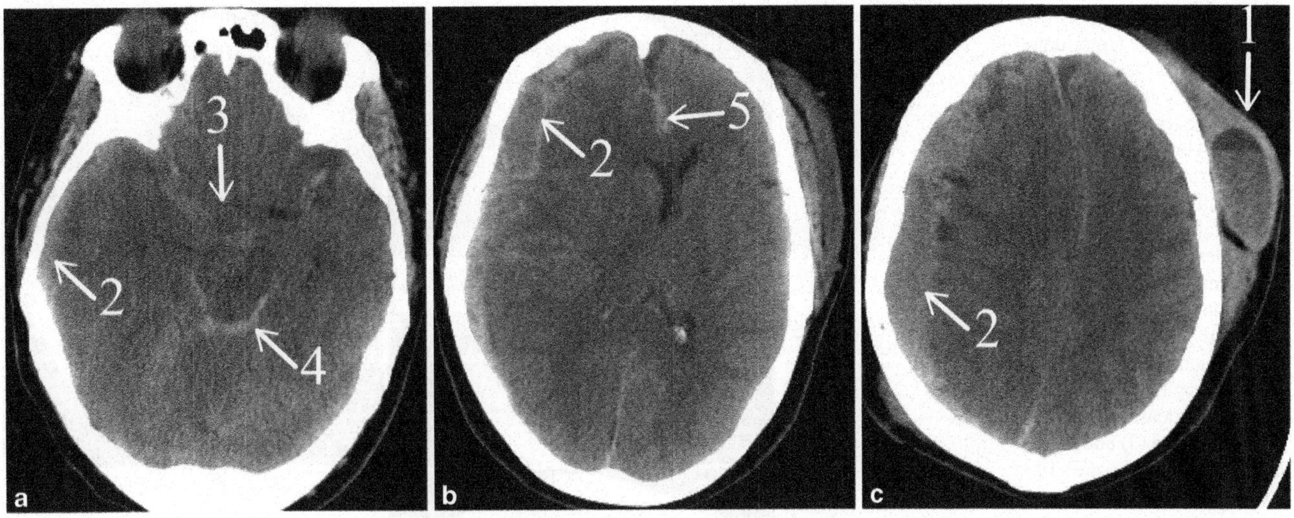

Fig. 3.8 F/75, Contrecoup SDH, SAH. Head injury caused by a car accident. (**a–c**) CT: The scalp on the left frontal region is severely swollen and has a large hematoma (1). SDH (2) is present on the right side. So, this is a contrecoup lesion. The SDH is not as hyperdense as a typical acute hematoma. This characteristic may reflect that the blood has not yet fully coagulated. Blood clots are present in the suprasellar cistern (3), quadrigeminal cistern (4), and interhemispheric fissure (5); these are traumatic SAH

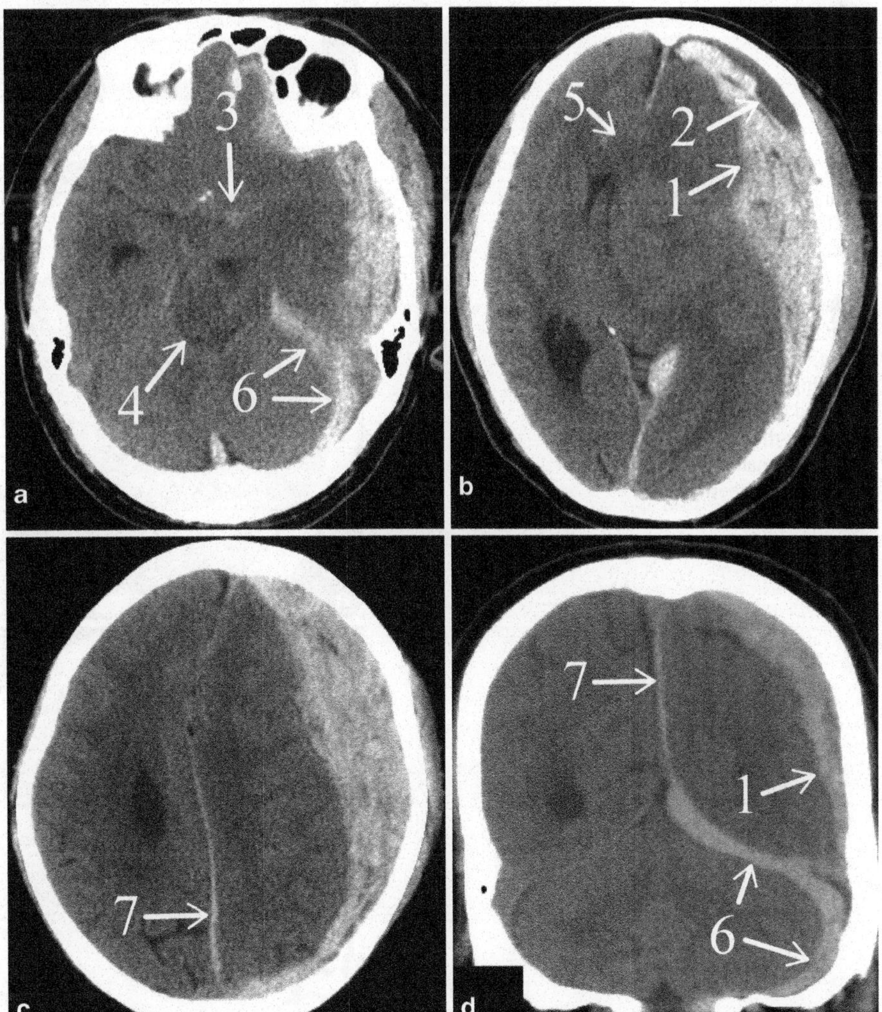

Fig. 3.9 M/75, A large SDH. (**a–c**) CT, axial sections. (**d**) Coronal reconstruction: A large SDH in the left cerebral surface (1). It contains fluid (2) possibly due to CSF leakage. The large SDH causes strong mass effect and the disappearance of the suprasellar cistern (3) and quadrigeminal cistern (4), reflecting uncal/transtentorial herniations. A subfalcine herniation (5) is also observed. Another SDH is present on the left side of the posterior fossa and extends to the infratentorial edge (6). The linear hyperdensity in the interhemispheric fissure (7) is a traumatic SAH

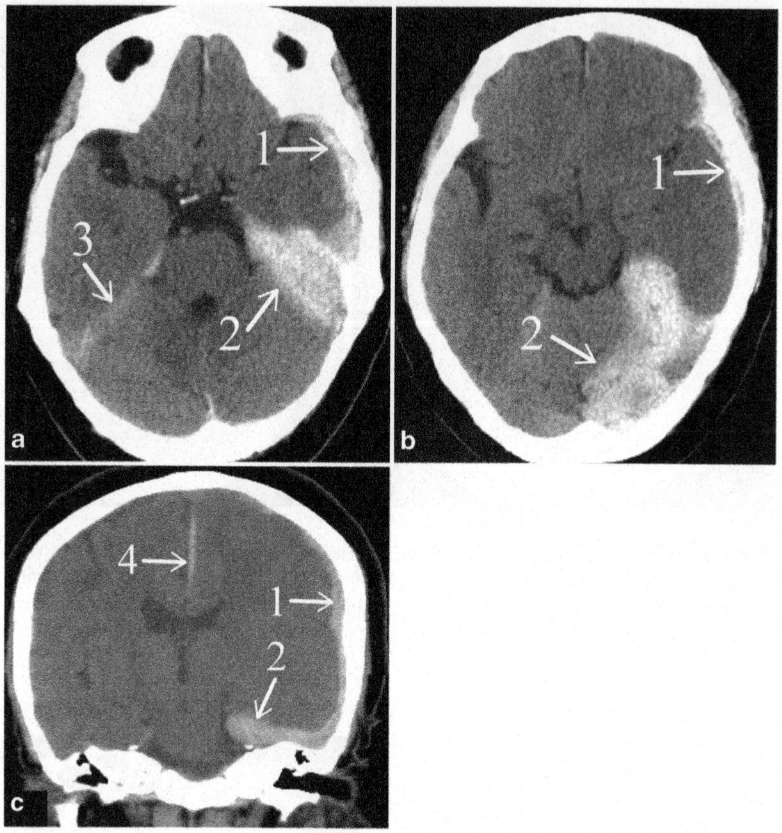

Fig. 3.10 F/51, An SDH extends along the tentorium. (**a**, **b**) CT, axial section. (**c**) Coronal reconstruction: An SDH in the left temporal region (1) extends back to the tentorial region (2). In the axial section (**a**, **b**), the SDH in the tentorial region resembles a big intracerebral hematoma (ICH). However, in the coronal reconstruction (**c**), apparently, it is an SDH (2) that is extended from the left temporal region (1). The linear hyperdensity in the right tentorium (3) and interhemispheric fissure (4) are traumatic SAH

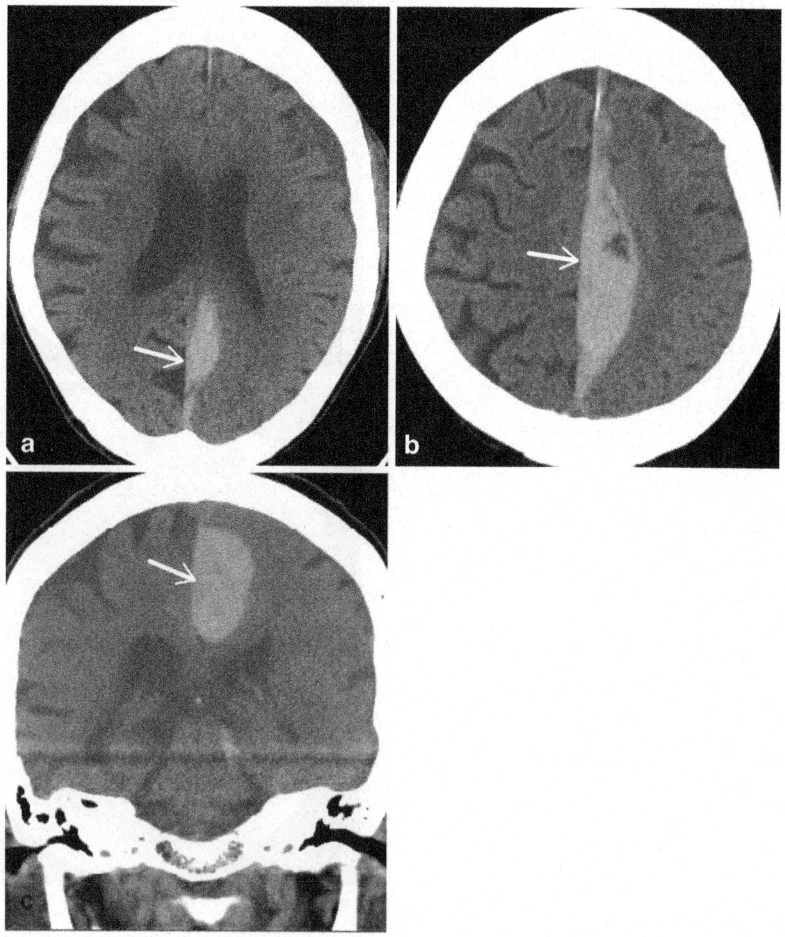

Fig. 3.11 F/80, SDH in the interhemispheric fissure. (**a**, **b**) CT, axial section. (**c**) Coronal reconstruction: Usually, if the blood clot appears as linear hyperdensity in the interhemispheric fissure, it is SAH, as in the above Figs. 3.9 and 3.10. If the blood clot (hematoma) is as wide as this patient, it is a subdural hematoma (SDH) in the interhemispheric fissure

3.6 Subdural Effusion (SDE)

SDEs have the following characteristics:

SDEs are formed gradually several days after trauma and are usually bilateral (Fig. 3.12, 3.13, 3.14, and 3.18). Or the acute SDH that remains untreated, the blood clots gradually evolve into SDE.

SDEs often occur among babies and the elderly.

SDEs are usually located outside the frontal and parietal lobes (Figs. 3.12, 3.13, 3.14, 3.18, and 3.21) and sometimes in the posterior fossa, the tentorial edge (Fig. 3.15), and interhemispheric fissure (Figs. 3.14 and 3.15).

Most SDEs will self-absorb and do not require surgical drainage. Surgical drainage is required for SDEs that increase in size or evolve gradually into chronic SDHs (Figs. 3.18 and 3.21).

VP shunt installation, craniotomy, and meningitis can also cause SDEs.

SDEs may rebleed from the membrane, in which subdural effusion mixes with hematoma (Fig. 3.13).

SDEs may form chronic subdural hematomas (CSDH) gradually (Figs. 3.18 and 3.21).

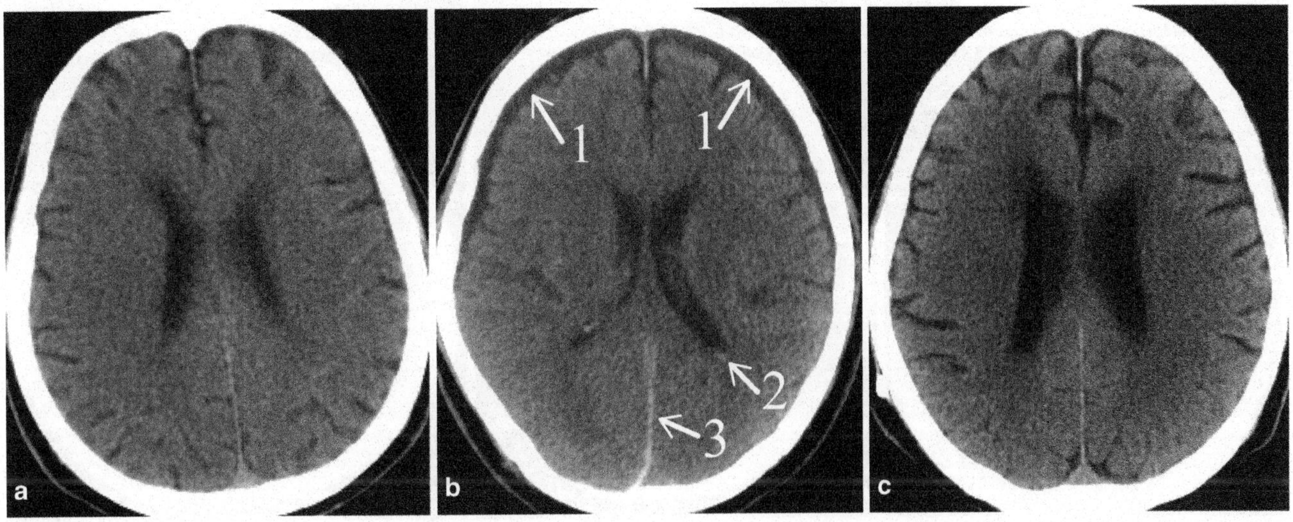

Fig. 3.12 F/68, Subdural effusion (SDE). The patient suffered a headache after head trauma. (**a**) CT on the day of head trauma: Only cortical atrophy is observed. (**b**) CT, fourth day: Given that the patient's headache intensified, CT was performed again after 4 days. SDEs (1) are present in the bilateral frontal regions. Trace IVH (2) in the left lateral ventricle and SAH in the interhemispheric fissure (3) are observed. (**c**) Follow-up CT, 4 months later: The patient's headache gradually improved after conservative treatment, and CT showed that the SDEs, SAH, IVH completely disappeared after 4 months

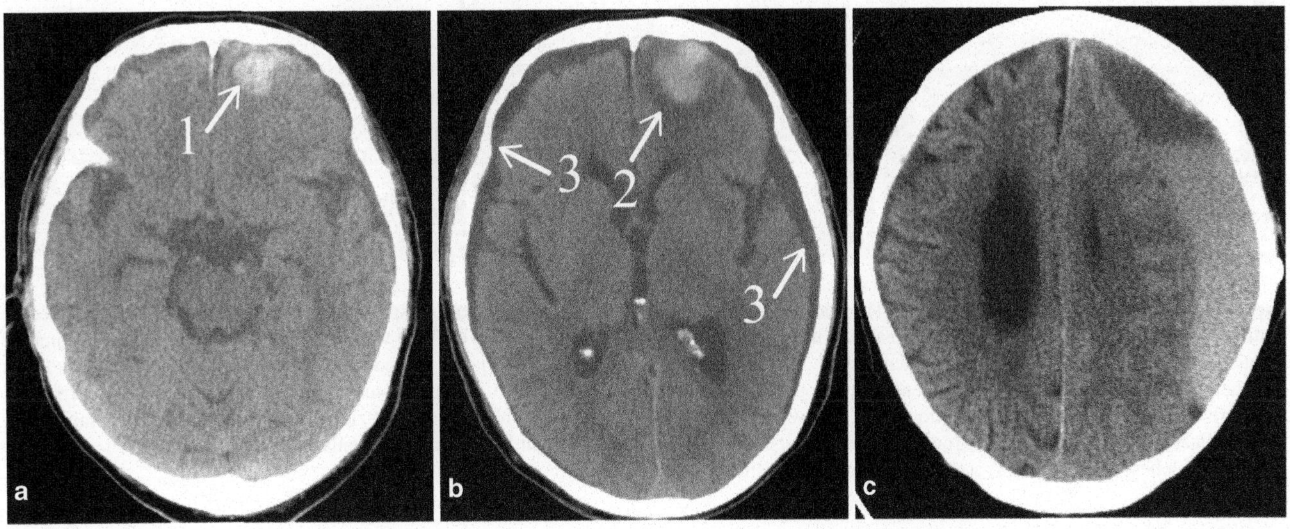

Fig. 3.13 M/87, Contusion hemorrhage, SDEs, and rebleeding with SDH. (**a**) An emergency CT after head trauma shows a brain contusion hematoma in the left frontal lobe (1). (**b**) One week later, the follow-up CT shows brain tissue edema around the contusion hematoma in the left frontal lobe (2) and bilateral SDEs (3). (**c**) After 3 months, the left SDE rebleeded to form a SDH with fluid blood level

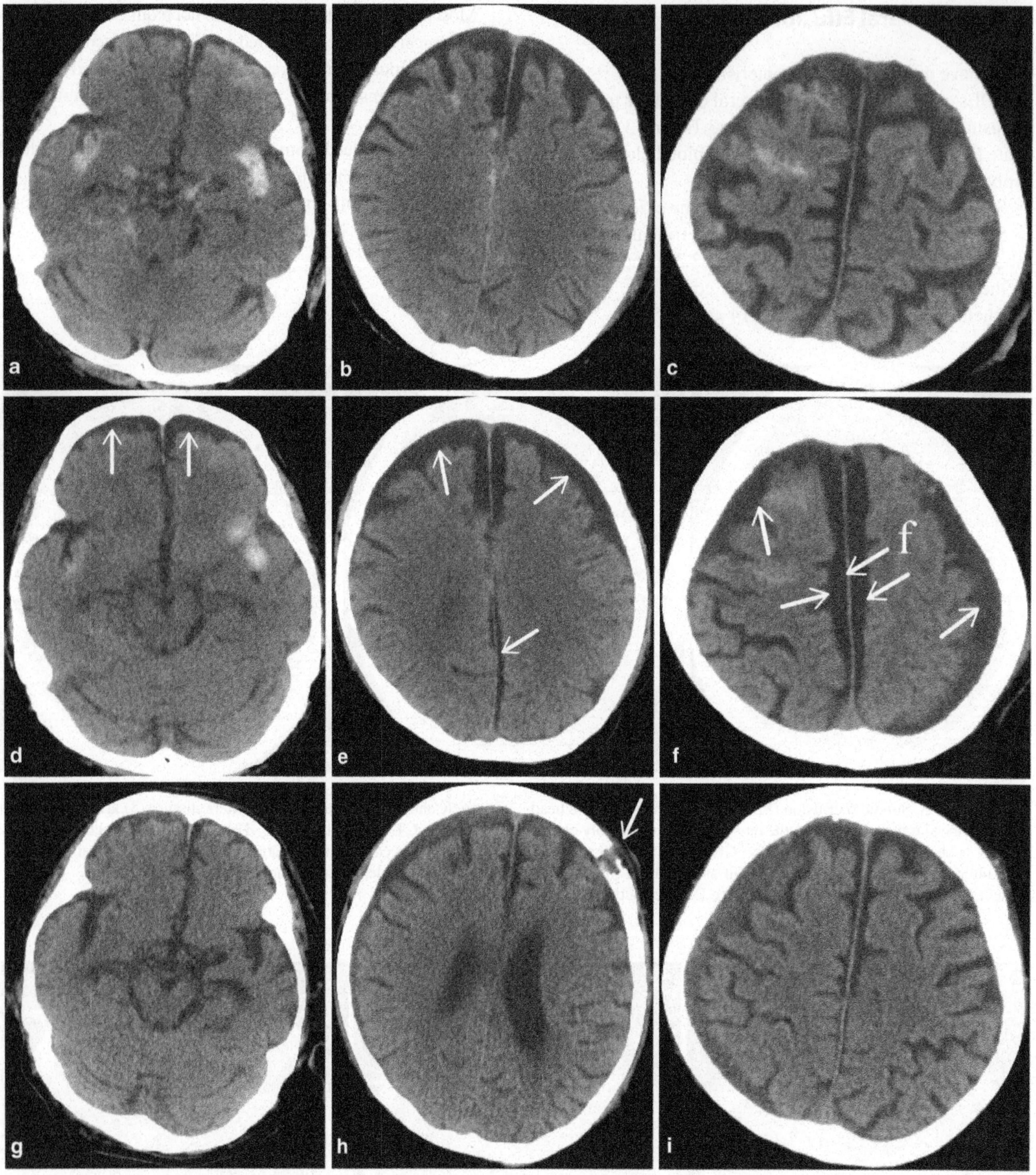

Fig. 3.14 M/65, Traumatic SAH, SDEs. The patient slipped and injured his head. (**a–c**) The emergency CT shows traumatic SAH in bilateral Sylvian fissures, suprasellar cistern, right ambient cistern, interhemispheric fissure, and sulci. Apparent brain atrophy, the cerebral sulci are wide. (**d–f**) One week later, follow-up CT shows that the SAH has drastically reduced, and SDEs (arrows) are present outside the bilateral frontal lobes. SDEs (arrows) are also present on both sides of the falx (**f**) in the interhemispheric fissure. Determining the presence or absence of SDE is difficult when the brain is atrophied, and the sulci are wide. The SDE is diagnosed in this patient because they had two CTs for comparison. (**g–i**) The surgeon did a burr hole in the left frontal bone (arrow) to drain the left-side SDE. The left SDE has disappeared, and the right SDE has slightly enlarged

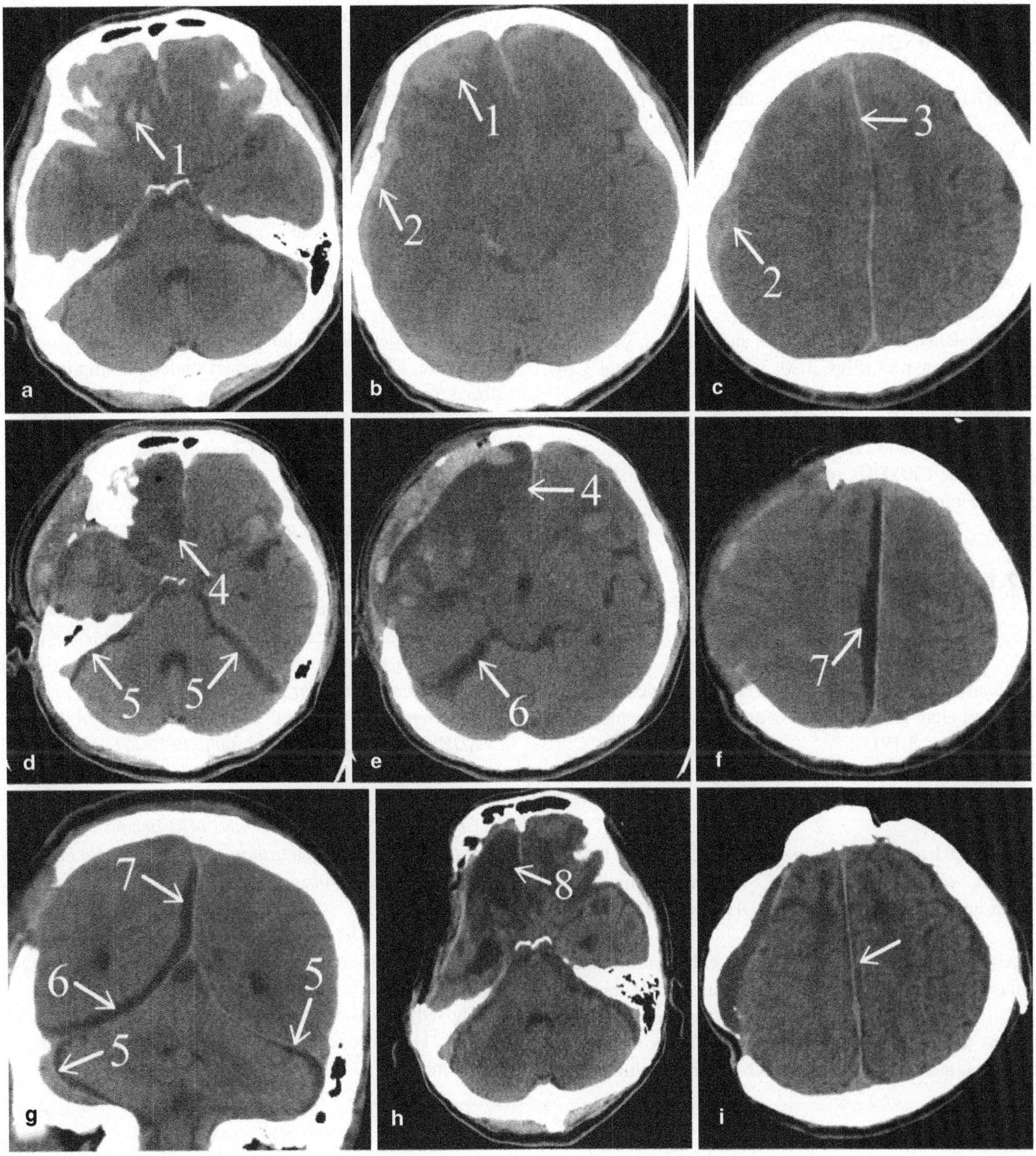

Fig. 3.15 M/67, Contusion hemorrhage, SDH, SAH, SDEs, and sequela. Head trauma caused by falling because of drunkenness. (**a–c**) Emergency CT: The right frontal lobe has contusion hemorrhage (1). Acute SDH in the right fronto-tempo-parietal region (2). The linear hyperdensity in the interhemispheric fissure is traumatic SAH (3). The patient underwent craniectomy, and part of the frontotemporal bone was removed to reduce intracranial pressure. (**d–f**) Follow-up CT on the 18th day showed a large area of contusion edema (4) in the right frontal lobe. Delayed SDEs are present in the bilateral CP angle cisterns (5), right tentorium upper edge (6), and interhemispheric fissure (7). (**g**) Coronal reconstruction. Clearly to see the SDEs. (**h, i**) CT took 2 years later: the right frontal contusion area has turned into encephalomalacia (8). The linear hyperdensity (arrow) in the interhemispheric fissure is the falx and no more SDE

3.7 Chronic Subdural Hematoma (ChrSDH)

ChrSDH is a common disease that mainly occurs in the elderly and is a type of head trauma (Figs. 3.17, 3.18, 3.19, 3.20, 3.21, 3.22, 3.23, and 3.24).

Most ChrSDHs are diagnosed using CT scans. Four kinds of densities are present in CT due to the different components of blood clots:

- Mild hyperdensity (Fig. 3.17),
- Isodensity (Fig. 3.18),
- Hypodensity (Figs. 3.19, 3.20, and 3.21),
- Mixed densities (Figs. 3.20, 3.21, 3.22, 3.23, and 3.24).

Some ChrSDHs will exhibit fluid blood levels (Fig. 3.23), whereby light blood flows on top, whereas dense blood clots sink. Some ChrSDHs rebleed and show the mixing of old and new blood clots (Fig. 3.23).

3.7.1 Etiology of ChrSDH [3]

Two mechanisms of ChrSDH pathogenesis (Fig. 3.16):

1. In an acute SDH that does not receive surgical treatment, blood clots gradually evolve and slowly become chronic SDH (Fig. 3.19).

   A minimal amount of acute SDH → CSF absorption occurs and gradually enlarges to form a ChrSDH (Fig. 3.20).
2. No SDH in head trauma → SDE develops a few days later → SDE slowly absorbs CSF → capsular microvascular hemorrhage creates a ChrSDH (Figs. 3.18 and 3.21).

Given that most ChrSDHs in the elderly are caused by minor head trauma, for example, walking into doors or walls or falling, head injury is easily overlooked because the conditions are mild. If CT is performed for the above minor head trauma, only a small blood clot in the brain parenchyma or subarachnoid space (Figs. 3.17 and 3.22) or a small SDH (Fig. 3.20) or SDE (Figs. 3.18 and 3.21) may be observed. A layer of the outer membrane (capsule) forms and envelopes SDHs or SDEs that do not absorb themselves, creating an area with an osmolality that is higher than that of the outer CSF and that gradually absorbs CSF. Besides, the microvessels of the capsule repeatedly bleed. Thus, the hematoma increases in size day by day. A mass effect is formed from 2 weeks to 2 months. This mass effect compresses the brain tissues, causing headaches, dizziness, unstable gait, and hemiparesis, which are highly similar to stroke symptoms. An elderly patient deteriorates as their intelligence declines or shows minor changes in personality. Therefore, CT or MRI performed under the impression of stroke or the degeneration of an elderly may reveal a ChrSDH (Fig. 3.23).

Therefore, four sources of ChrSDH exist:

1. *Apparent head trauma wherein small SDH is untreated. The doctor asked the patient and family if the patient had any symptoms back between 2 weeks and 2 months. CT and MRI revealed a ChrSDH (Figs. 3.19 and 3.20).*
2. *Apparent head trauma wherein CT shows small SDE. The doctor asked the patient and family if the patient had any symptoms back between 2 weeks and 2 months. CT and MRI discovered a ChrSDH (Figs. 3.18 and 3.21).*
3. *Apparent head trauma, but CT did not find SDH or SDE. The patient had symptoms back between 2 weeks and 2 months. ChrSDH was detected by CT and MRI (Figs. 3.17 and 3.22).*
4. *ChrSDH was found in CT and MRI because of the suspected stroke or degeneration of the elderly. No history of head trauma was observed (Fig. 3.23).*

If a young adolescent has ChrSDH, a congenital arachnoid cyst should be considered, given the slow bleeding of the capsule of an arachnoid cyst (Figs. 3.24 and 6.73).

ChrSDH can be drained through a burr hole surgery (Fig. 3.21). The operation is simple, and the prognosis is excellent.

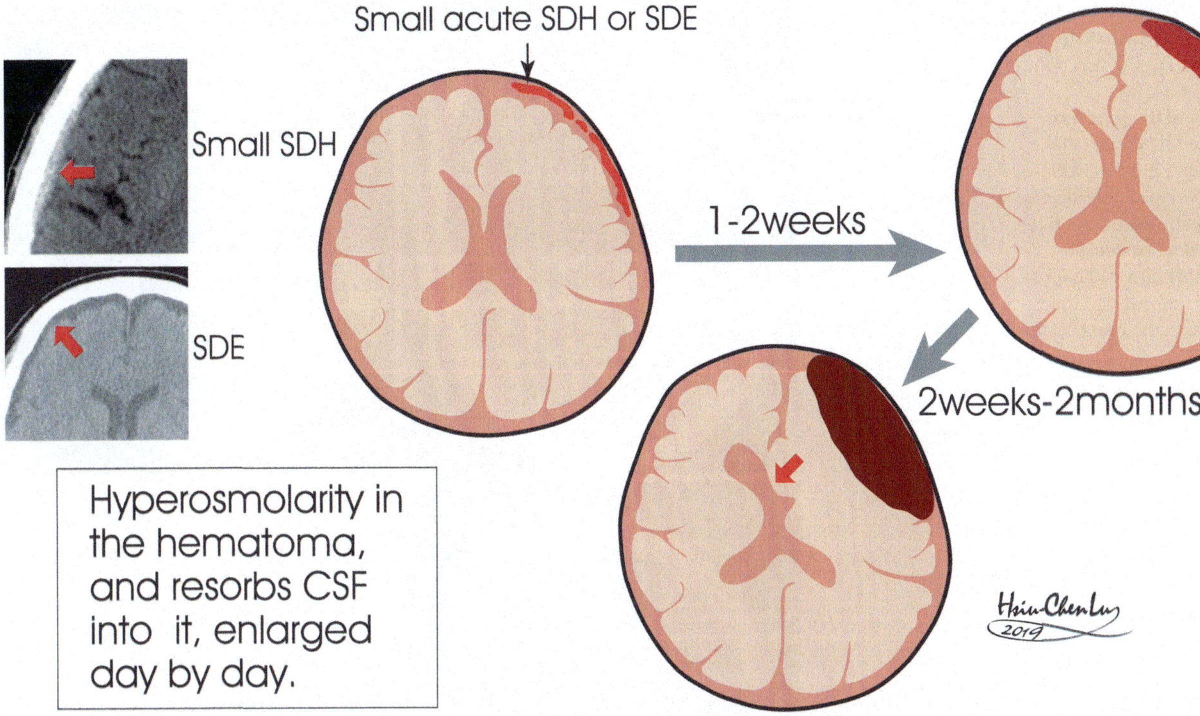

Fig. 3.16 Two mechanisms of chronic subdural hematoma (ChrSDH) pathogenesis: (1) Acute SDH → gradual evolution, development from acute to subacute, and then to chronic. Minimal amount of acute SDH → CSF absorption occurs and gradually enlarges to form a ChrSDH. (2) No SDH in head trauma → SDE develops a few days later → SDE slowly absorbs CSF → capsular microvascular hemorrhage creates a ChrSDH

Fig. 3.17 M/68, Chronic subdural hematoma (ChrSDH), initial CT lacked SDH or SDE. (**a**) CT: CT on the day of head trauma. The right frontal lobe has a small contusion hemorrhage (arrow). No SDH or SDE is noted. (**b**, **c**) CT: After 2 months, the patient developed headache, dizziness, and left-limb weakness. He was sent to the emergency department for CT. CT showed a large and mild hyperdense ChrSDH, which causes a mass effect and compresses the brain cortex

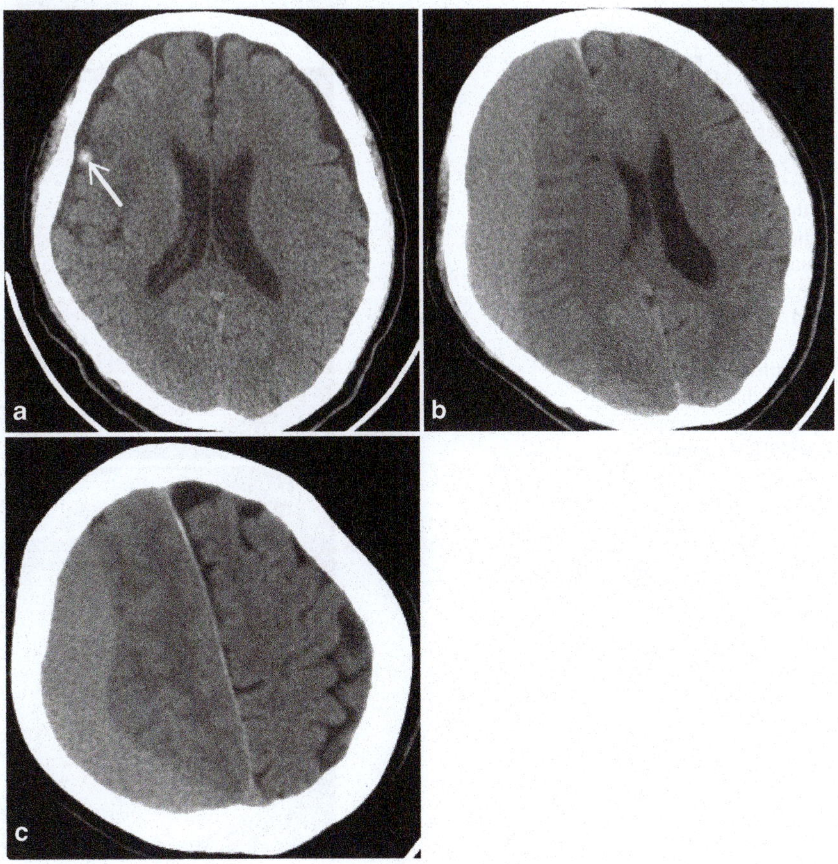

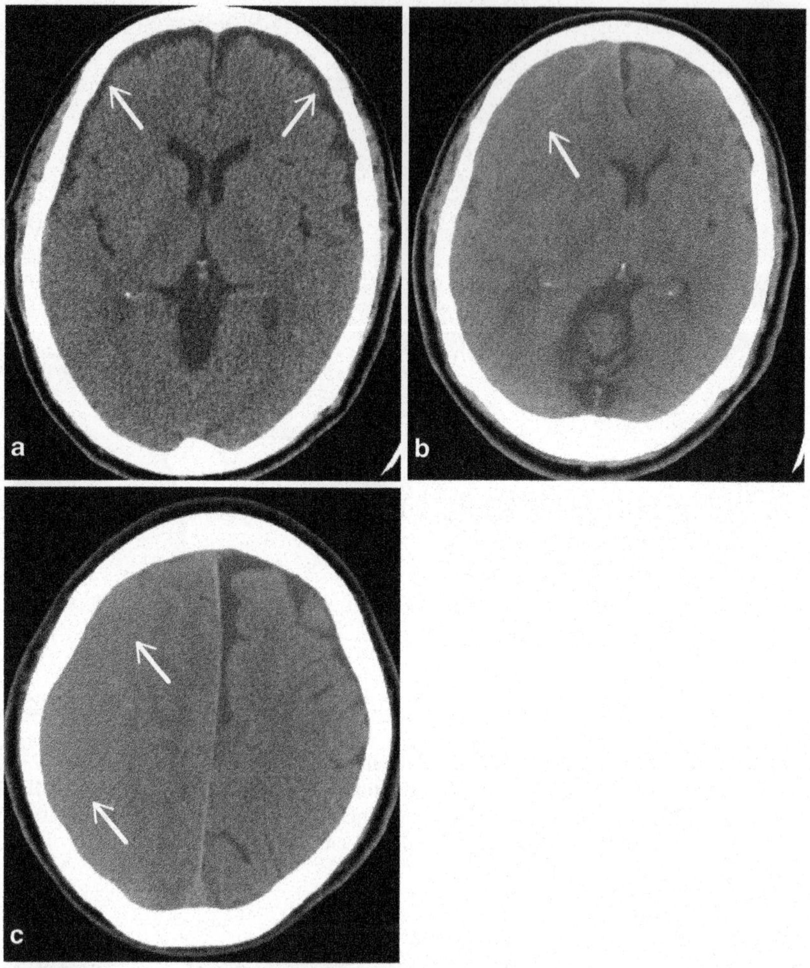

Fig. 3.18 M/68, SDEs, and chronic SDH. The patient fell on his head. (**a**) CT was done 2 days after the fall, CT shows thin SDEs (arrows) outside the bilateral frontal lobes. After 2 months, the patient developed a headache and left-limb weakness. (**b**, **c**) CT showed an isodense chronic SDH (arrows) over the right frontoparietal lobes, it compresses the brain cortex

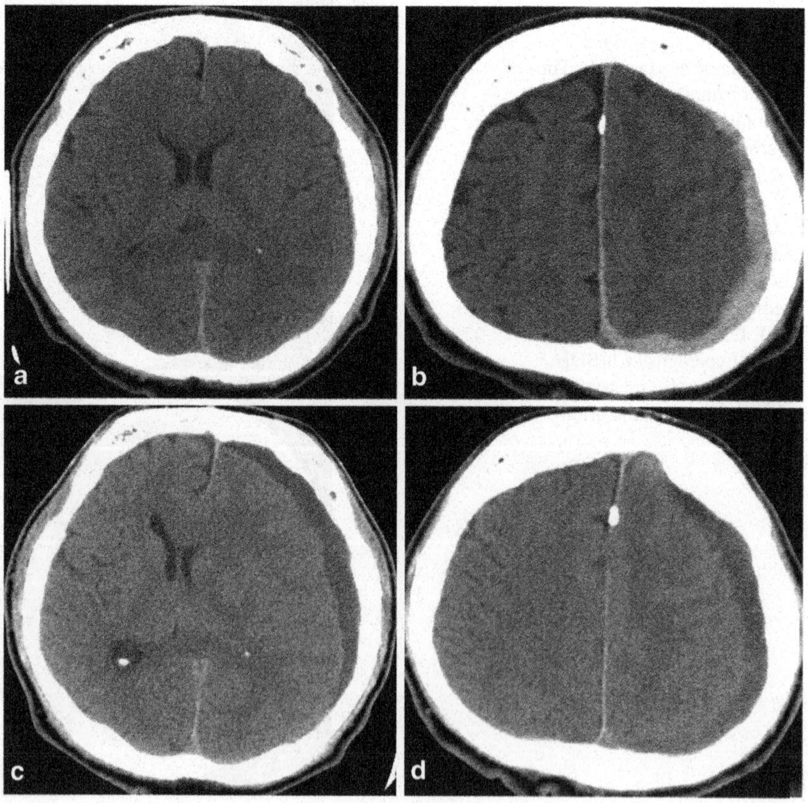

Fig. 3.19 M/47, Acute SDH evolved into chronic SDH. (**a**, **b**) Emergency CT after head injury: An acute crescent shape hyperdense hematoma in the left frontoparietal region was identified as an acute subdural hematoma. Surgery was not performed. (**c**, **d**) The patient experienced a persistent headache for 2 months. Follow-up CT showed that the SDH has changed into a hypodense ChrSDH, it compresses the brain cortex and the left lateral ventricle

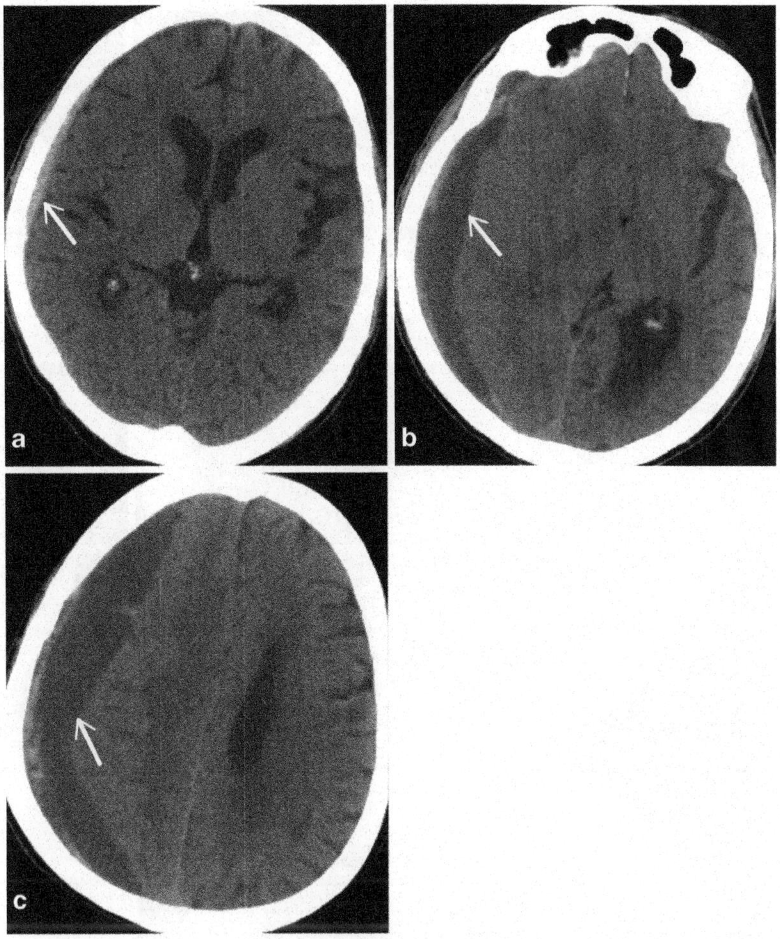

Fig. 3.20 M/77, Acute SDH developed into ChrSDH. (**a**) CT for head trauma: A thin layer of SDH (arrow) on the right side. The family decided not to operate and opted for observation because the hematoma was small. After a month, the patient gradually became weak on the left side of his body and experienced headache, dizziness, and unstable gait. (**b**, **c**) Follow-up CT: The SDH has evolved into a large ChrSDH (arrow) that contains hypodense and some hyperdense blood clots. It causes a strong mass effect, and compresses the brain cortex and right lateral ventricle

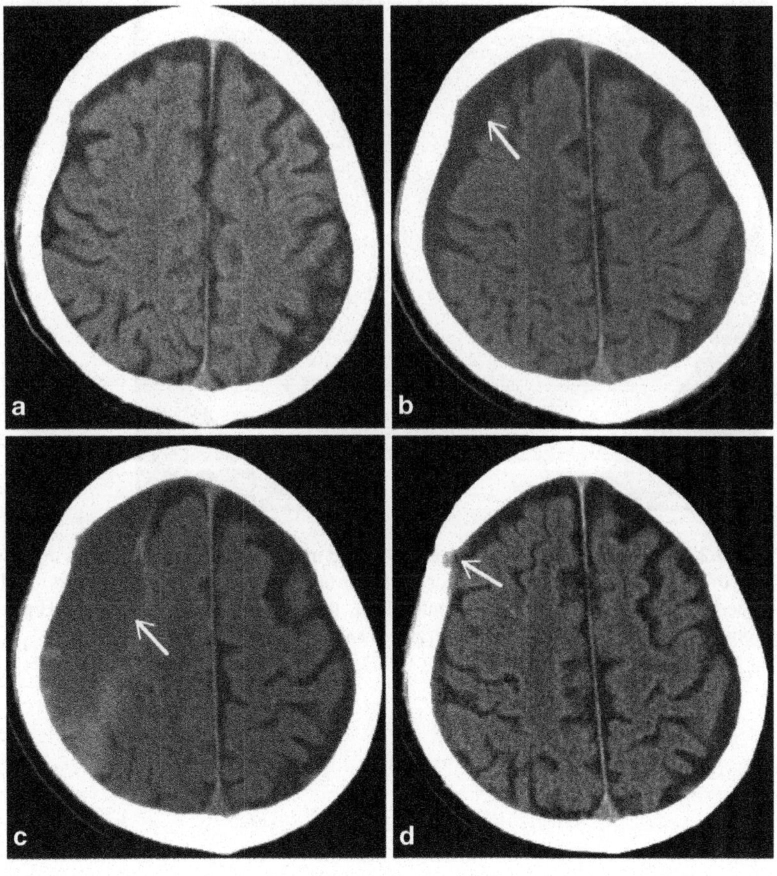

Fig. 3.21 M/74, SDE developed into ChrSDH. (**a**) CT: On the day of head trauma, CT only showed brain atrophy and sulcal widening. (**b**) Follow-up CT after 5 days: SDE in the Rt. frontal region (arrow), it slightly compresses the brain cortex. SDE usually develops after a few days of head injury, especially in the elderly. After 2 months, the patient gradually felt left-limb weakness and complained of headaches, dizziness. Follow-up CT was performed. (**c**) Follow-up CT: The SDE gradually formed a chronic SDH (arrow) containing hypodense and hyperdense blood clots. It severely compresses the brain cortex. The patient received surgery, the neurosurgeon made a burr hole and drained out all the oil-like chronic blood clot. (**d**) Follow-up CT: A burr hole (arrow) in the right frontal bone. No residual subdural hematoma

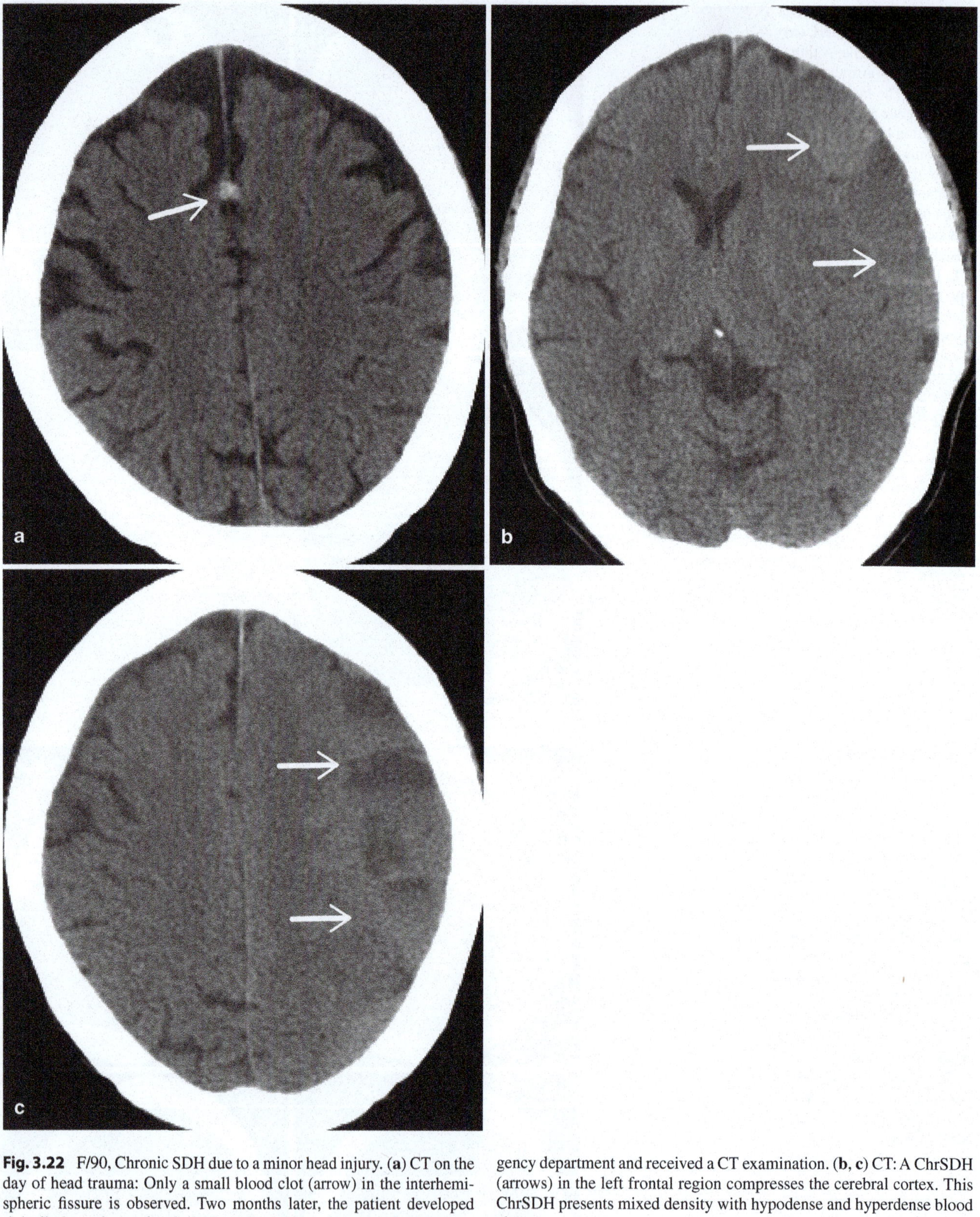

Fig. 3.22 F/90, Chronic SDH due to a minor head injury. (**a**) CT on the day of head trauma: Only a small blood clot (arrow) in the interhemispheric fissure is observed. Two months later, the patient developed right-limb weakness, headache, and dizziness and was sent to the emergency department and received a CT examination. (**b**, **c**) CT: A ChrSDH (arrows) in the left frontal region compresses the cerebral cortex. This ChrSDH presents mixed density with hypodense and hyperdense blood clots

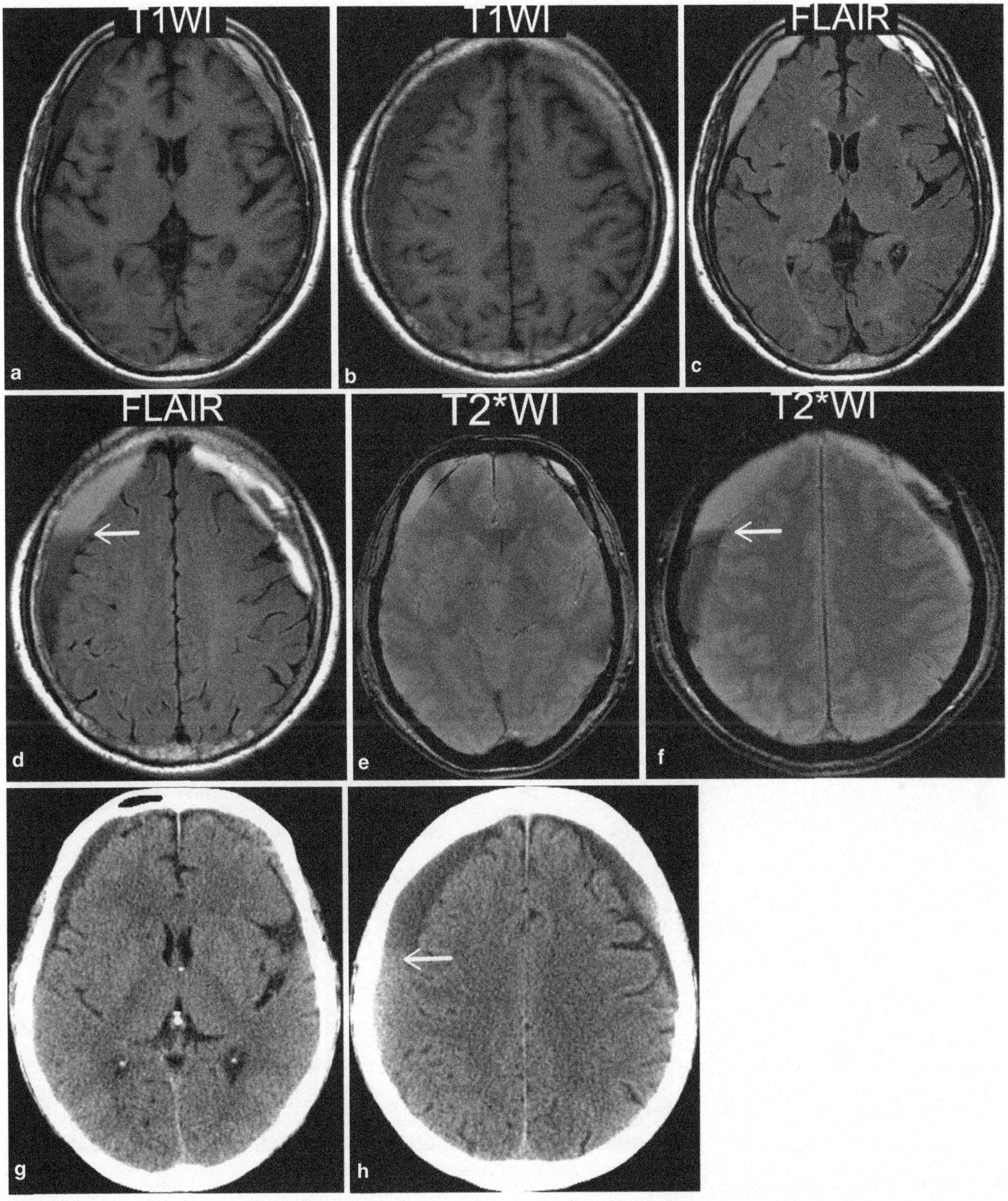

Fig. 3.23 M/76, Bilateral chronic SDHs. The patient was suspected of having a stroke due to headaches, dizziness, and weakness of both limbs. MRI examination was arranged. (**a–f**) MRI: MRI shows SDHs on the bilateral frontal regions. The signal intensities of the SDHs are nonuniform, in FLAIR and T2*WI, fluid-blood level (arrows) is noted. (**g**, **h**) CT was conducted on the same day: CT shows that these are hypodense ChrSDHs with rebleeding. The right SDH forms a fluid-blood level (arrow)

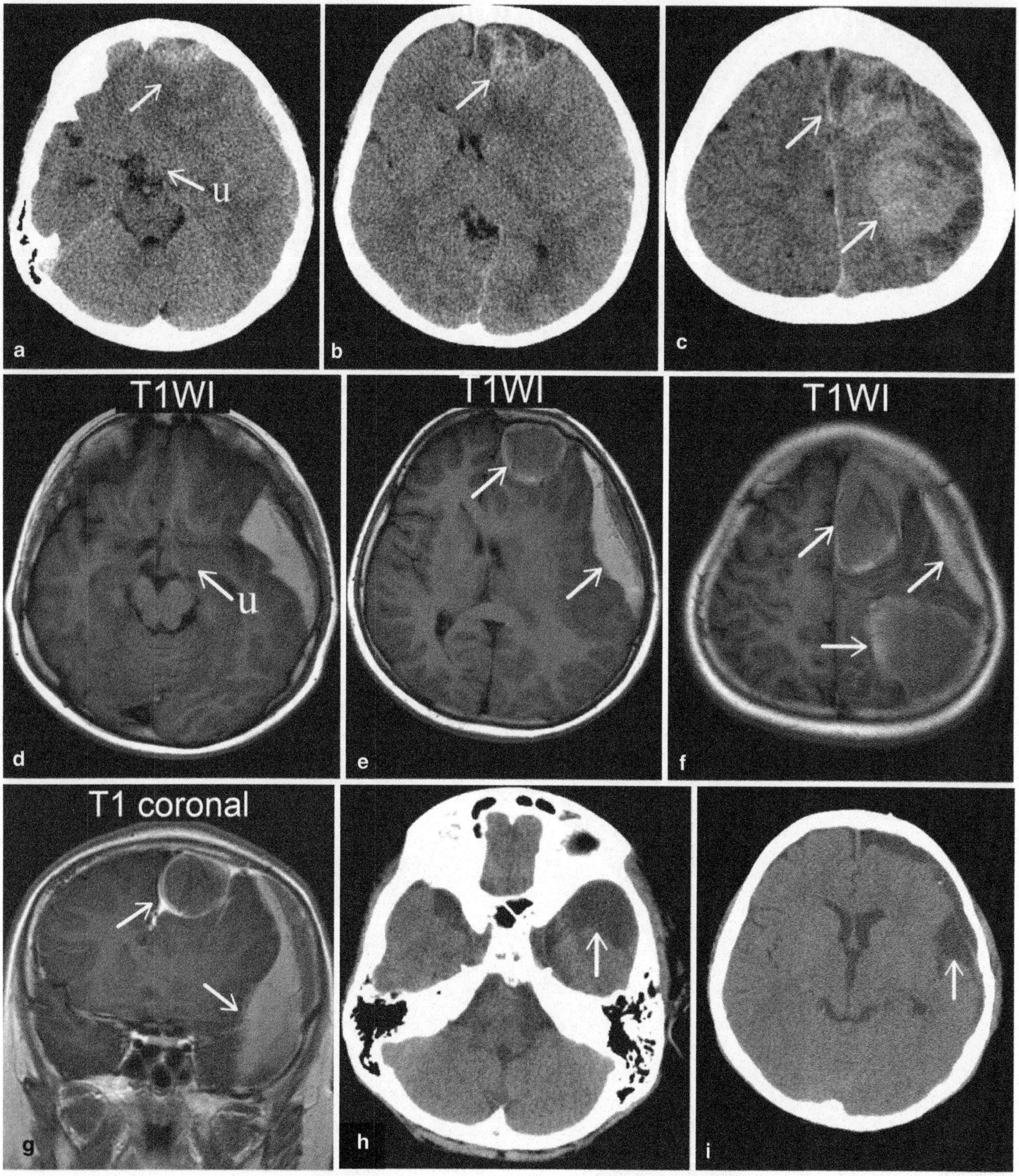

Fig. 3.24 M/10, Arachnoid cyst caused ChrSDH. This boy suffered severe headaches and nausea, vomiting for 3 days. (**a–c**) Emergency CT: Reveals inhomogeneous density in the frontal lobe with strong mass effect causing uncal herniation (u). Determining the lesion on these CT images is difficult; thus, MRI was performed after CT. (**d–g**) MRI T1WI: The lesion is identified as a lobulated ChrSDH (arrows), and it causes a strong mass effect with uncal herniation (u). The neurosurgeons drained the ChrSDH, and an arachnoid cyst in the left middle cranial fossa was found. (**h, i**) Postoperative CT: The left middle cranial fossa has an arachnoid cyst (arrows). The ChrSDH disappeared with some residual SDE in the left frontal region

3.8 Brain Contusion

The injuries are in the brain tissue caused by external forces. Brain contusions have several types.

Brain edema combined with hemorrhages (contusion edema and hemorrhages): This is the most common type of brain contusion. It features irregular cerebral edema and punctate or small hematomas in the area of impact injury. Some only have one area of contusion (Fig. 3.28), and some have several areas of contusion (Figs. 3.26, 3.27, 3.29, 3.30, and 3.31).

Local brain edema: Less common than other types (Figs. 3.15 and 3.26).

Focal contusion hematoma: No association with cerebral edema, which may be caused by the rupture of a single vessel in the brain (Figs. 3.13, 3.29, 3.30, 3.32, 3.42, and 3.43).

Diffuse brain edema: A large area or even the entire cerebral hemisphere has extensive brain edema. The pathological mechanism is unclear. Some diffuse brain edemas may be caused by the traumatic occlusion of large blood vessels and induce cerebral hypoxia and edema (Fig. 3.25).

Diffuse axonal injury: Diffuse axonal injury (DAI), also known as shearing injury, should be suspected if the clinical symptoms of a patient are severe, especially if the patient is in a coma and CT is negative or only reveal minimal findings (Figs. 3.32 and 3.33) that do not correspond to the clinical signs. Following are the CT and MRI findings for DAI, MRI has a higher diagnostic rate than CT for DAI (Fig. 3.33).

CT: A spotted hemorrhage or small area of brain edema is present, particularly in the deep locations of the brain (Fig. 3.32), such as the corpus callosum, basal ganglia, brainstem, and gray–white matter junction. In some cases, only trace SAH and IVH are seen in CT (Fig. 3.33).

MRI: T1WI, similar to CT, reveals small blood clots in the above areas. FLAIR and T2WI are highly sensitive and can visualize small lesions with the high signal that represents cerebral edema or hemorrhage. The minor deep brain tissue edema in DAI may show hyperintensity on DWI (Fig. 3.33), thus reflecting that the edema is cytotoxic edema. T2*WI or SWI is a necessary pulse sequence that can detect deep hemorrhages in the brain and increase the diagnostic rate of DAI.

Several concepts for reading brain contusions:

1. Some cerebral contusion hemorrhages and cerebral edemas are not found through urgent CT, or only mild injury is diagnosed, but delayed hemorrhage and edema will be observed (Figs. 3.29 and 3.30). Therefore, CT should be conducted when the patient's clinical symptoms change.
2. A brain contusion is often combined with SDH (Figs. 3.4, 3.15, 3.25, 3.42, and 3.43), EDH (Figs. 3.4, 3.26, and 3.28), SAH (Figs. 3.25, 3.29, 3.30, and 3.42), or IVH (Figs. 3.29 and 3.32).
3. Brain contusion hemorrhage co-occurs with EDH or SDH. The EDH or SDH has stronger mass effects, so the contusion hemorrhage is suppressed and has less bleeding. When the EDH or SDH is surgically removed, intracranial pressure decreases, and cerebral contusion hemorrhage expands. This phenomenon is called postdecompression hemorrhage (Figs. 3.31 and 3.43).

After a long period in the brain contusion area, blood clots are absorbed gradually and evolve into encephalomalacia (Figs. 3.26 and 3.28) or even undergo cavitary change (Fig. 3.43), which may cause epilepsy. A severe brain contusion is an important cause of intellectual damage or even results in a vegetative state.

3.9 Traumatic SAH, IVH

Traumatic subarachnoid hemorrhage (traumatic SAH) (Figs. 3.8, 3.9, 3.10, 3.12, 3.14, 3.15, 3.25, 3.28, 3.29, 3.30, 3.33, 3.35, 3.42, 3.43, and 3.44) and traumatic intraventricular hemorrhage (traumatic IVH) (Figs. 3.12, 3.29, and 3.32) are common in head injury. They may occur along, but more often associate with SDH, EDH, and brain contusion. Some DAI cases, CT only see traumatic SAH and IVH, but cannot detect microbleed or small deep brain tissue edema (Fig. 3.33).

In CT, traumatic SAH is commonly seen in the sulci of cerebral hemispheres, the fissures (such as Sylvian fissure and interhemispheric fissure), the cisterns (such as suprasellar cistern and quadrigeminal cistern), and the tentorial edge. CT is sensitive to the diagnosis of SAH and IVH. In the adult, the SAH in the interhemispheric fissure is easily confused with falx calcification (Fig. 3.30). The SAH in the tentorium edge or interhemispheric fissure is not easy to distinguish from SDH (Fig. 3.43). Generally speaking, the linear hyperdensity is SAH (Figs. 3.25, 3.29, and 3.30); the wider blood clot is SDH (Figs. 3.9, 3.10, 3.11, and 3.43). Coronal reconstruction can help distinguish SAH and SDH.

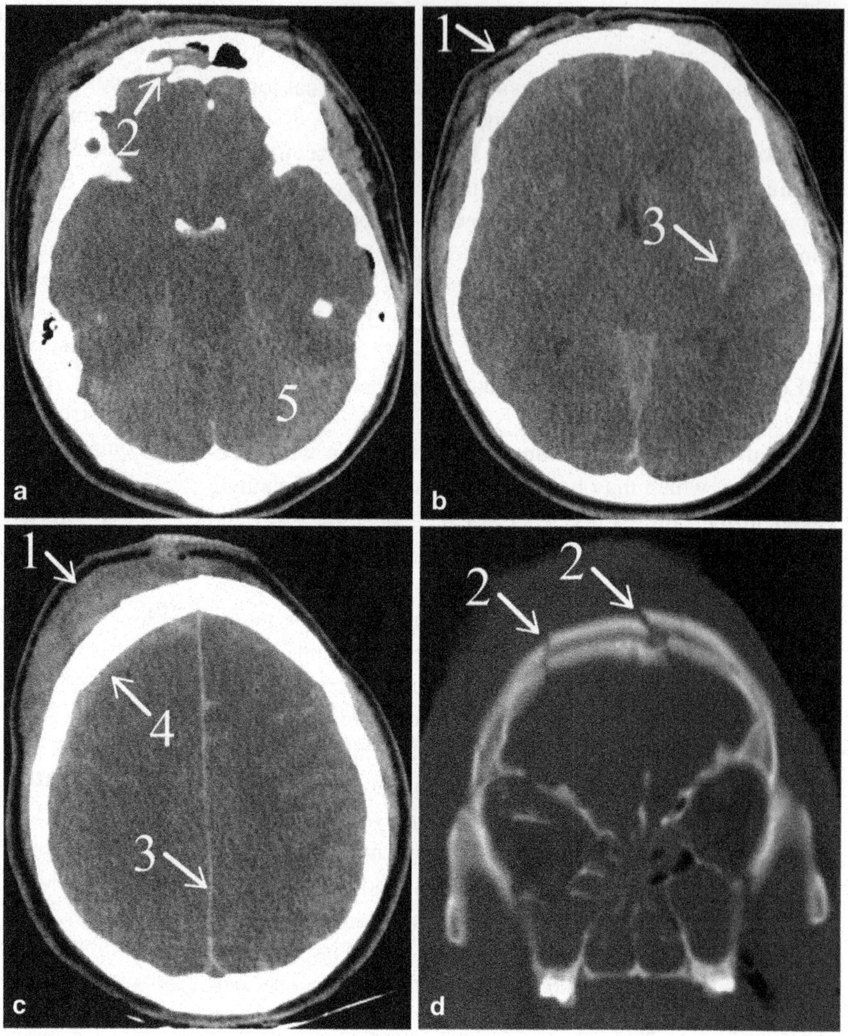

Fig. 3.25 M/16, Cranial bony fracture, diffuse brain tissue edema. This boy encountered a car accident that caused severe head trauma and coma. (**a**–**c**) CT: A very swollen scalp (1), fractures in the skull (2), SAH (3) in the Sylvian fissure and interhemispheric fissure, and small SDH (4). Diffuse brain tissue edema in the bilateral cerebral hemispheres showing slight gray-dark, the disappearance of the cisterns and sulci, and the compression of the bilateral ventricles. These characteristics indicate extensive brain edema. Only the cerebellar density is normal (5) and appears in gray-white. It is called the "white cerebellar sign." (**d**) Coronal reconstruction, bone window: Multiple skull fractures (2) can be seen, and the paranasal sinuses are full of blood clots. CT cannot determine whether the diffuse brain edema is caused by brain contusion or cerebral hypoxia caused by respiratory arrest

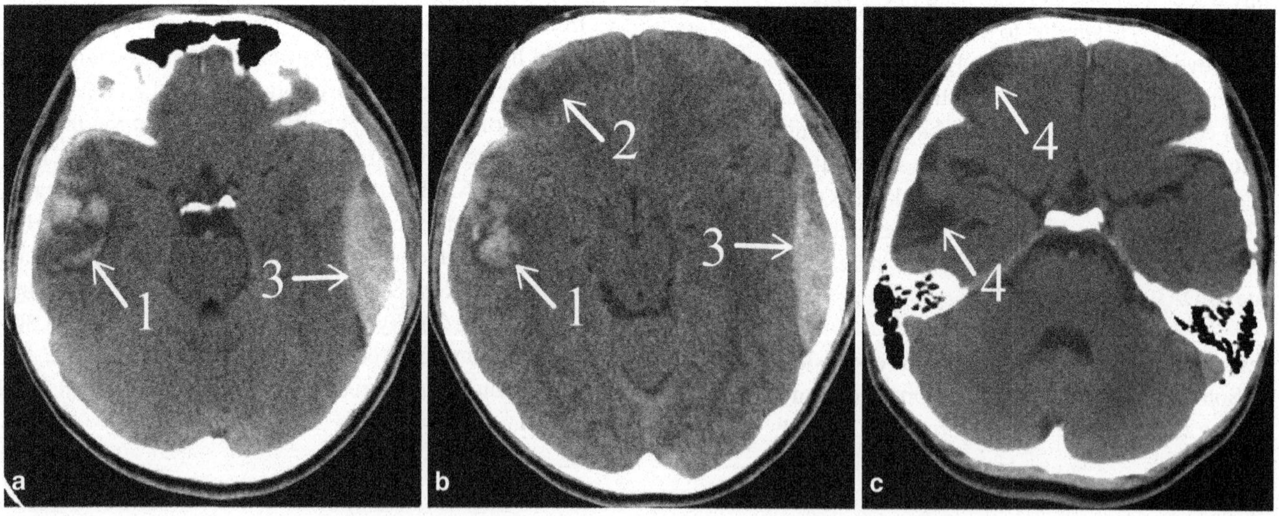

Fig. 3.26 M/42, Contusion hemorrhage, edema, EDH, and encephalomalacias. (**a**, **b**) Emergency CT: Contusion hemorrhage mixed with edema (1) in the right temporal lobe. Another small contusion edema (2) in the right frontal lobe. An EDH (3) in the left temporal region. The patient began to exhibit epileptic symptoms several months after the surgical removal of EDH. (**c**) CT after 11 months: The previous contusion areas have turned into encephalomalacias (4) in the right temporal lobe and frontal lobe. The old brain tissue lesion in the temporal lobe is the cause of epilepsy

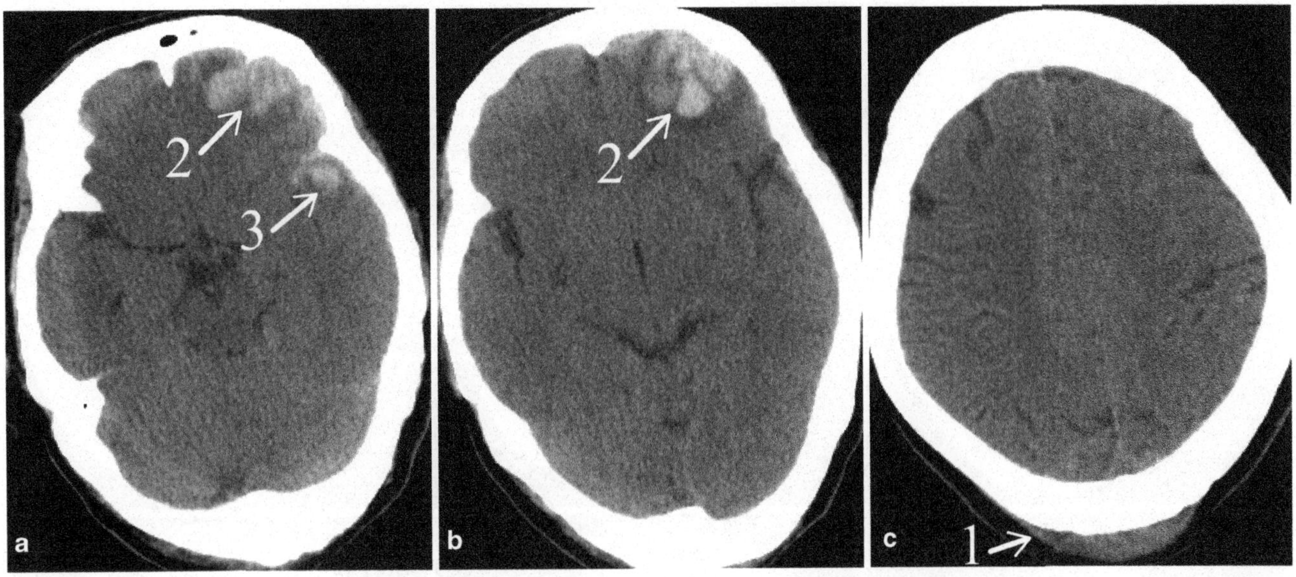

Fig. 3.27 F/60, Contrecoup contusion hemorrhages. The posterior of the head hit the ground due to a fall. (**a**–**c**) CT: Scalp swelling on the rear of the head (1) is the impact site. An area of brain contusion is present in the left frontal lobe (2), that is, blood clot plus brain tissue edema. A small contusion hemorrhage is also present in the left temporal lobe (3). The hit is on the posterior of the head, and the contusion hemorrhages are in the frontal and temporal lobes. Thus, this is a contrecoup injury

Fig. 3.28 F/59, Contusion hemorrhages, SAH, and EDH. Head trauma caused by a car accident. (**a**–**c**) CT: Left scalp swelling (1). The right temporal lobe has a typical brain contusion (2), which is irregular bleeding plus brain tissue edema. The linear hemorrhages in the sulci of the right frontal lobe are traumatic SAH (3). Both of these are contrecoup injuries. The fusiform hematoma in the left temporal region is EDH (4). The patient started to experience epilepsy symptoms a year after. (D) Follow-up CT after 1 year: An area of encephalomalacia (5) in the right temporal lobe of the previous contusion area. The expansion of the temporal horn (6) of the right lateral ventricle represents the atrophy of the surrounding brain tissue. This old injury in the temporal lobe is the cause of epilepsy

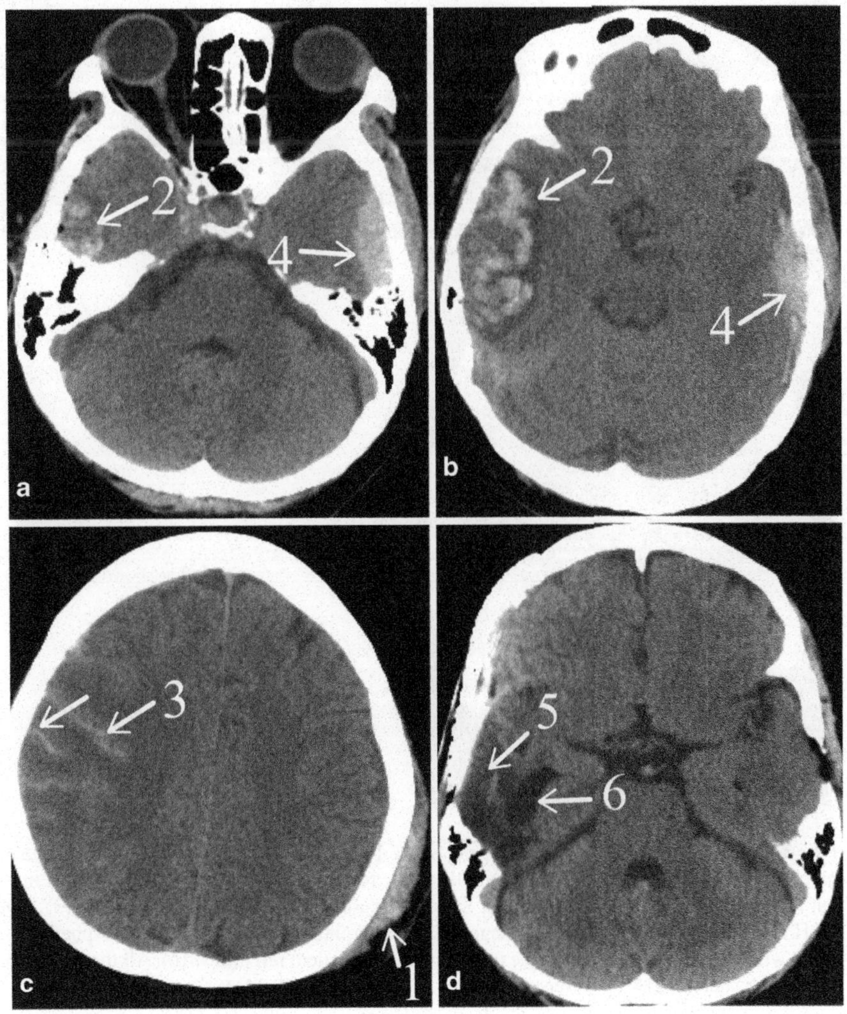

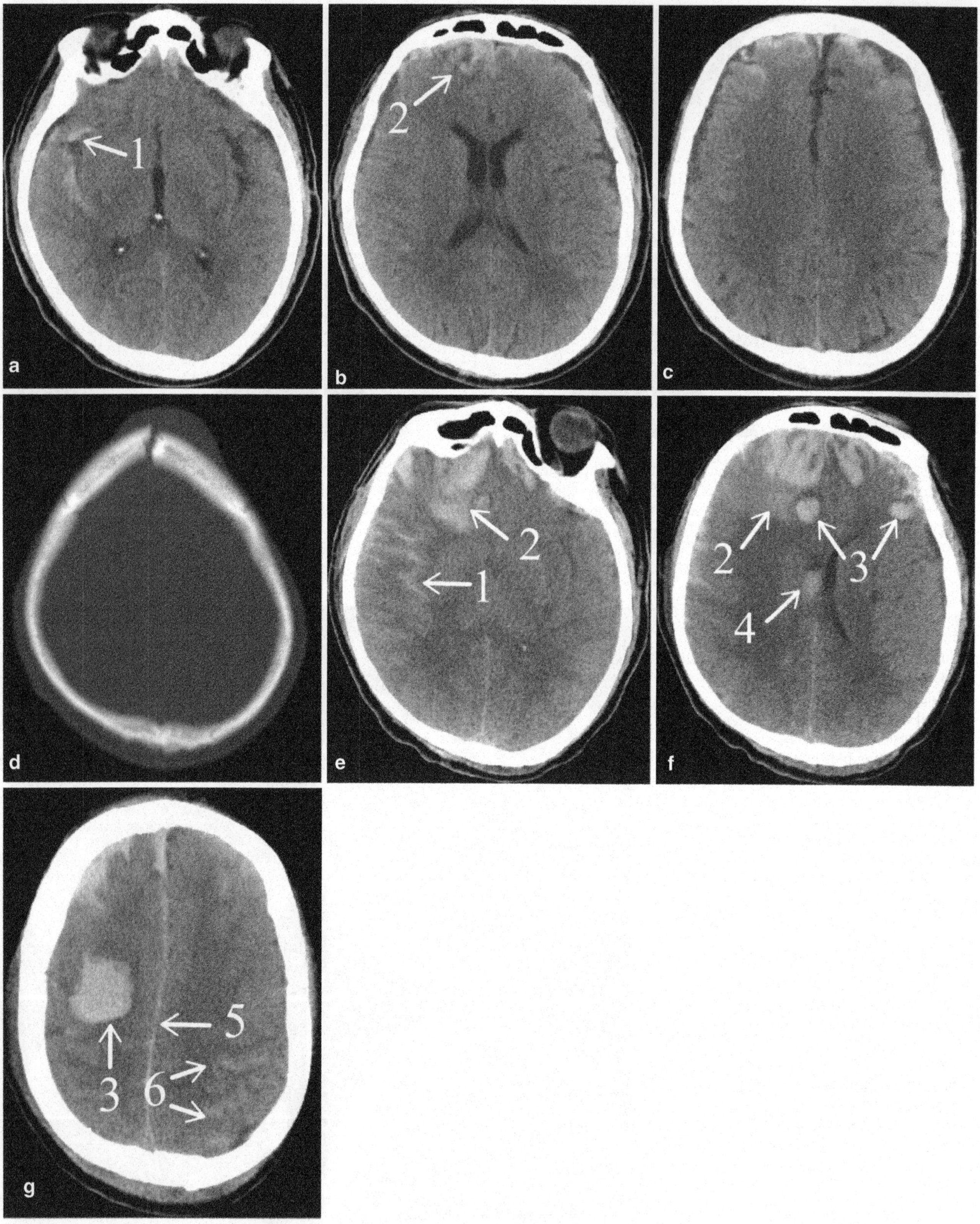

Fig. 3.29 M/72, Contusion hemorrhages, SAH, IVH, and delayed hemorrhages. The head injury caused by fall and the patient was awake but restless. (**a–c**) Emergency CT: Right Sylvian fissure has traumatic SAH (1) and small contusion hemorrhages (2) in the frontal lobes. (**d**) Bone window: A linear fracture in the frontal bone. The patient fell into a coma 4 h later. (**e–g**) CT was repeated after 4 h from the first CT: More SAH in the right Sylvian fissure (1) and increasingly severe contusion hemorrhages in the frontal lobes (2). Other new ICHs in the bilateral frontal lobes (3). Some IVH in the right lateral ventricle (4). SAH in the interhemispheric fissure (5) and SAH in the sulci of the left parietal lobe (6). All the above are delayed hemorrhages

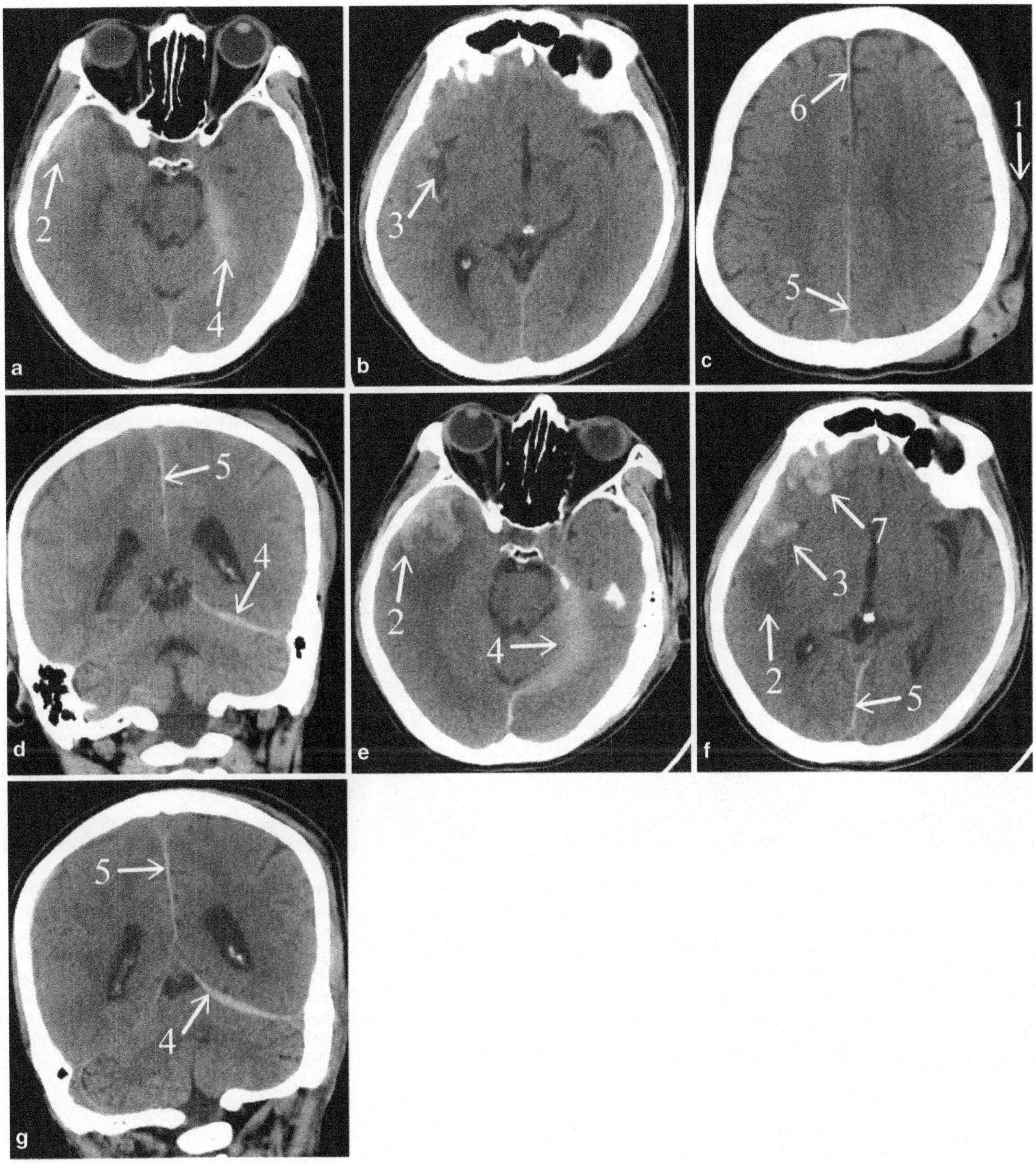

Fig. 3.30 M/56, Traumatic SAH, and delayed contusion hemorrhages. (**a–c**) Emergency CT, axial section, and (**d**) coronal reconstruction: Scalp swelling and subcutaneous hemorrhage on the left side (1) represent the location where the head was hit. A small contrecoup contusion hemorrhage (2) in the right temporal lobe and a small amount of SAH (3) in the right Sylvian fissure are observed. A blood clot on the left tentorial edge (4) seems similar to an ICH because it appears wide but emerges as linear in the coronal reconstruction; hence, it is SAH or SDH. A white line present in the interhemispheric fissure represents SAH (5) and is common in head trauma but cannot be confused with falx calcification (6). Follow-up CT 5 days later. (**e, f**) CT, axial section (**g**) coronal reconstruction: The range of contusion hematoma in the right temporal lobe extends, combines with cerebral edema (2) and causes a mass effect. The nearby Sylvian fissure is compressed and disappears (3). A new hematoma (7) in the right frontal lobe is a delayed hemorrhage. Increasing hematoma on the left tentorium (4). The axial section seems to have widened similar to ICH but appears as linear in the coronal reconstruction; thus, it is SAH or SDH not ICH. The white line in the interhemispheric fissure represents SAH (5)

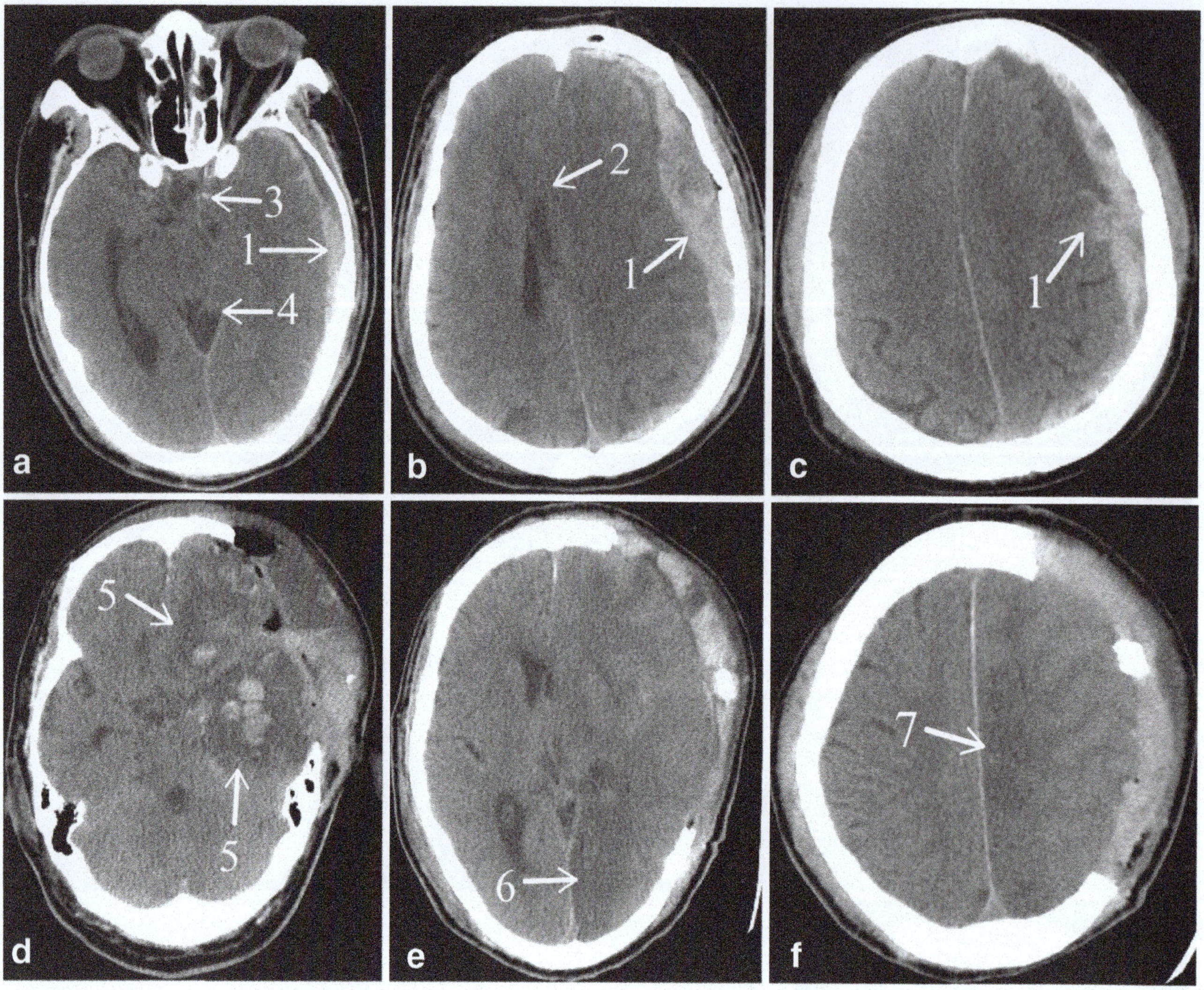

Fig. 3.31 M/63, SDH, delayed contusion hemorrhage and edema, and infarction edema. Head injury caused by a car accident. (**a–c**) Urgent CT: A large acute subdural hematoma (SDH) (1) in the left cerebral surface, producing a powerful mass effect. The flattening of the ipsilateral ventricle and the shifting of the midline to the right represent subfalcine herniation (2). The disappearance of the suprasellar cistern (3) and quadrigeminal cistern (4) represent uncal/transtentorial herniations. Craniectomy was performed to remove the SDH and remove part of the cranial table to reduce intracranial pressure. (**d–f**) CT after 2 days reveals the presence of two areas of brain tissue edemas and hemorrhages (5) in the left frontal lobe and temporal lobe. These are typical delayed contusion edemas and hemorrhages. Brain tissue edema is observed in the left occipital lobe (6), this edema is the cerebral infarction edema of the left posterior cerebral artery (PCA) caused by uncal/transtentorial herniations and cannot be confused with contusion edema. There is also a long strip of cerebral edema (7) in the left frontoparietal lobes, which is the left anterior cerebral artery (ACA) infarction caused by subfalcine herniation

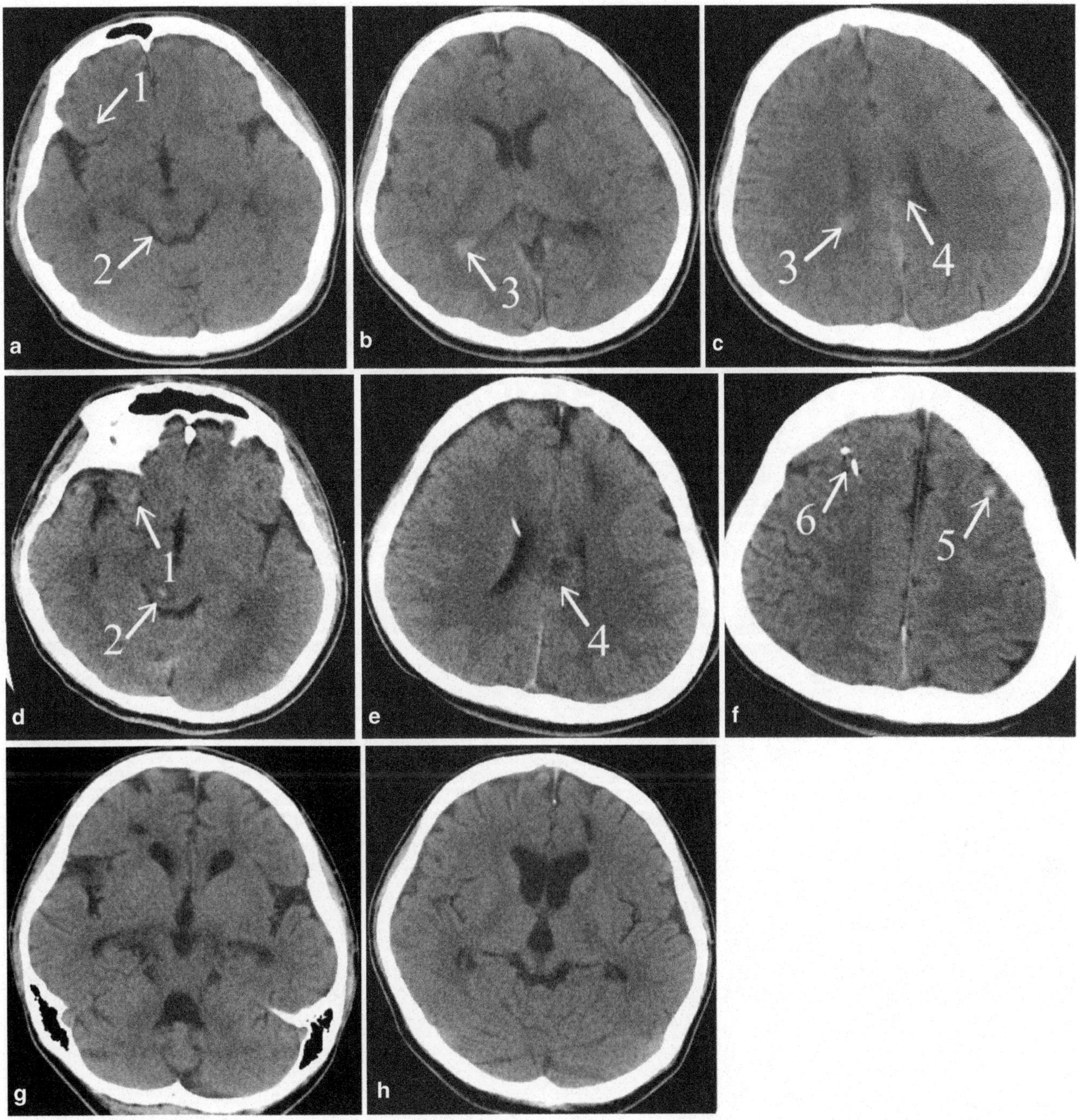

Fig. 3.32 M/19, Diffuse axonal injury, DAI. The head injury caused by a traffic accident. The patient was riding a motorcycle when he hit a car. The patient was in a coma. (**a–c**) Emergency CT: Only some tiny hematomas in the right frontal lobe (1) and midbrain (2). IVH (3) in the right lateral ventricle. A small hematoma in the corpus callosum (4). The above CT images seem cannot explain the coma. (**d–f**) Continued coma, fourth-day CT: Hemorrhage and edema with increased visibility in the right frontal lobe and midbrain. The left frontal lobe also has a small hematoma (5). An intracranial pressure monitoring device (6) in the right frontal lobe. The patient subsequently remained in a semi-vegetative state. (**g, h**) Follow-up CT after 7 months: dilated ventricles and widened cerebral cortex sulci, indicating diffuse brain atrophy. Therefore, the head injury incurred 7 months ago was DAI

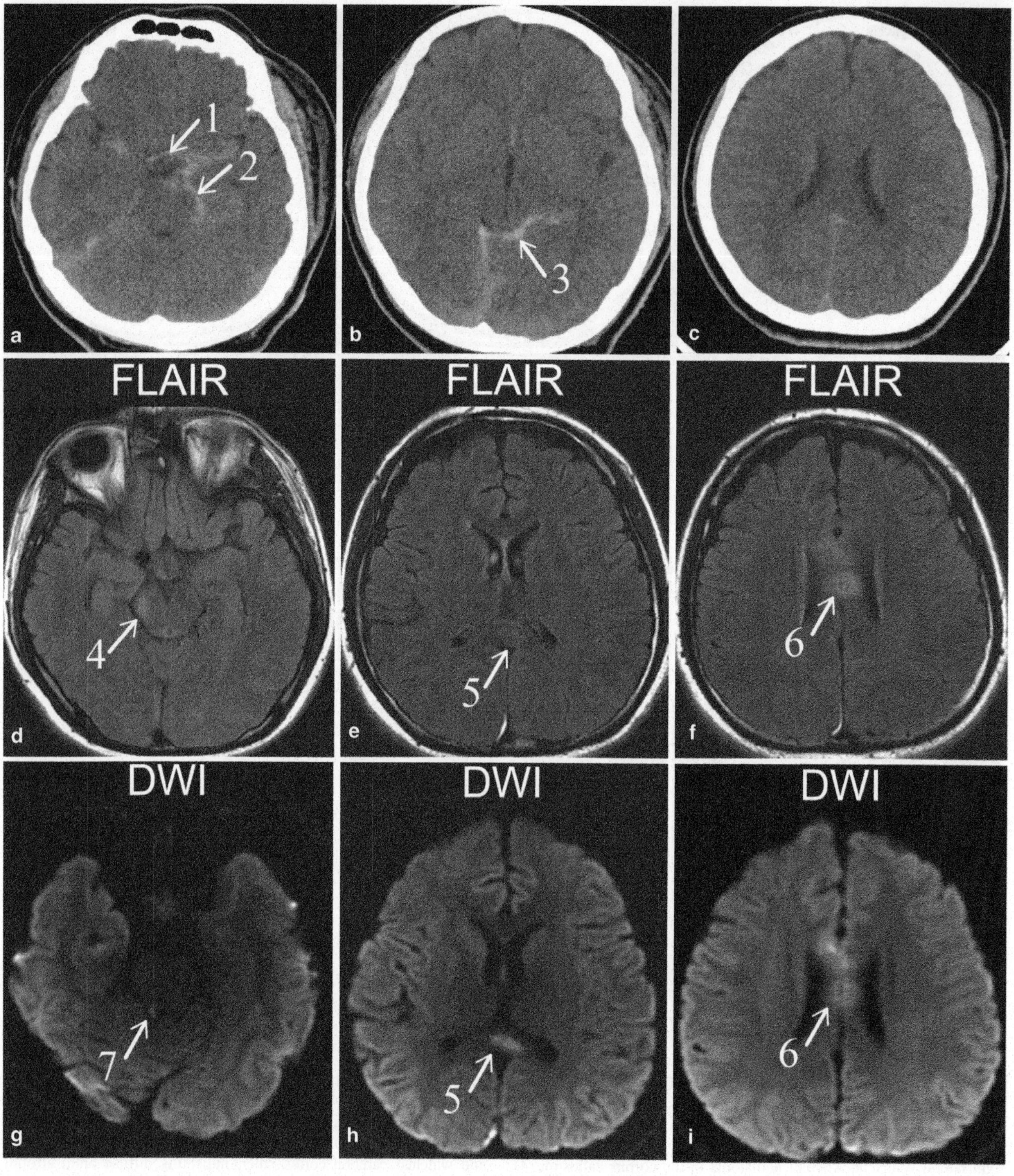

Fig. 3.33 M/20, Diffuse axonal injury, DAI. The head injury caused by a motorcycle hitting a car; the patient was in a coma. (**a–c**) Emergency CT: Traumatic SAH in the suprasellar cistern (1), peripontine cistern (2), and quadrigeminal cistern (3). Continued comatose state. MRI was performed on the 11th day. (**d–f**) MRI, FLAIR: Hyperintense lesions in the right side of the midbrain (4), the splenium (5), and body (6) of the corpus callosum represent contusion edemas. (**g–i**) DWI: Hyperintense lesions in the right colliculus of the midbrain (7), the splenium (5), and body (6) of the corpus callosum represent cytotoxic edema in these areas. T2*WI did not detect small hemorrhages in the brain tissue (not shown). From the MRI findings and clinical presentation of coma, this patient had a typical DAI

3.10 Other Injuries

3.10.1 Cranial and other fractures

3.10.1.1 Linear Fracture

The CT of head trauma is best routinely adjusted to the bone window for the examination of the skull and the skull base for the prevention of missing linear fractures (Figs. 3.5, 3.6, 3.25, and 3.35). Although clinically linear fractures do not need to be treated.

3.10.1.2 Depressed Fracture

Depressed fractures seen through routine CT must be surgically removed of the bone fragments that trapped in the brain (Fig. 3.34). The bone window must be adjusted for more clearly to show the bone fragments and distinguish with the surrounding hematomas.

3.10.1.3 Other Fractures

In addition to skull fractures, the facial bones (Fig. 3.39), orbits (Figs. 3.37 and 3.38), or the entire cervical spine (Fig. 3.40) must be scrutinized for fractures. Coronal and sagittal reconstruction images are vital at this point.

3.10.2 Traumatic Pneumocephalus

3.10.2.1 Sources of Air

Gases in the paranasal sinus or the mastoid are raised after the skull base fracture (Fig. 3.35).

The gases enter the intracranial CSF spaces directly after a skull fracture.

These gases may be concentrated in the subdural space but diffuse quickly along the CSF in the intracranial subarachnoid space (Fig. 3.36).

3.10.3 Foreign Bodies

CT can detect bullets, shrapnel fragments, blades, and other items left in the brain and skull. The metal objects may produce radial artifacts on CT (Fig. 3.41).

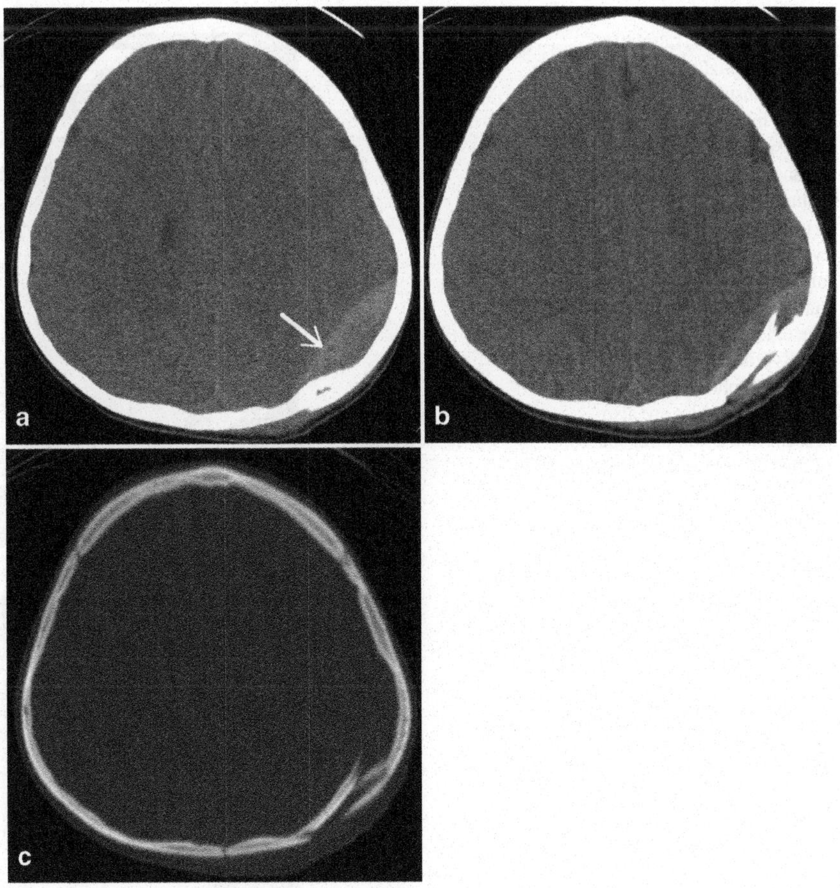

Fig. 3.34 M/31, Depressed fracture, and EDH. Head trauma caused by falling from a height. (**a**, **b**) CT, axial section. (**c**) Bone window setting: A depressed fracture in the left parietal bone and a fusiform hematoma under the fracture indicates EDH (arrow)

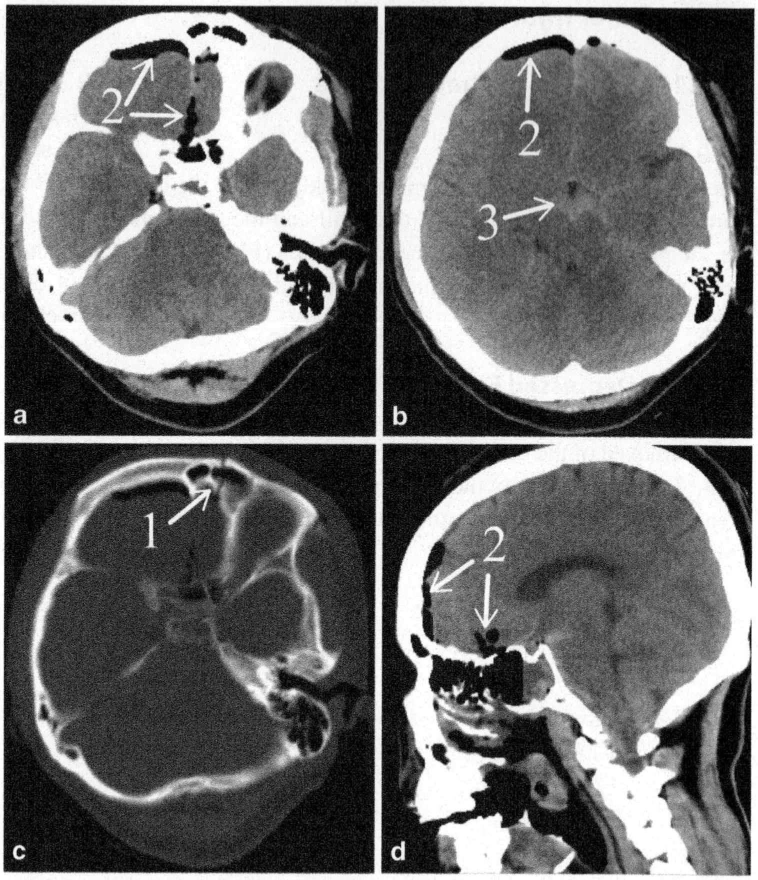

Fig. 3.35 F/39, Traumatic pneumocephalus, SAH. An impact on the frontal area resulted in head trauma. (**a**, **b**) CT, axial section, (**c**) Bone window, (**d**) Sagittal reconstruction: A linear fracture (1) in the left frontal bone is seen in the bone window setting; the fracture passes through the underlying frontal sinus. Thus, air may enter the intracranial spaces and cause pneumocephalus. Airs in the subdural space of anterior cranial fossa (2), and SAH in the suprasellar cistern (3) are observed

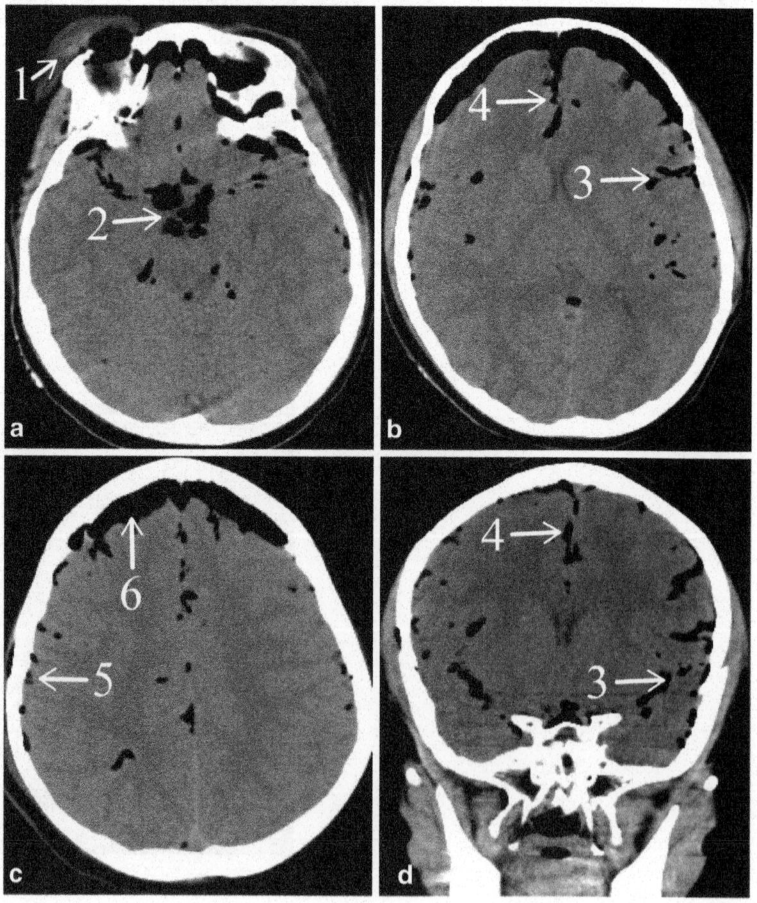

Fig. 3.36 F/6, Traumatic pneumocephalus. The head injury caused by a small truck falling into a valley. (**a**–**c**) CT, axial section. (**d**) Coronal reconstruction: CT shows the right eye swelling (1), the air is present under the skin of eyelid, and considerable amounts of intracranial air, mainly in the subarachnoid space, i.e., suprasellar cistern (2), Sylvian fissure (3), interhemispheric fissure (4), and sulci (5). Airs are also present in the subdural spaces of the bilateral frontal regions (6). The CT findings are indicating severe traumatic pneumocephalus

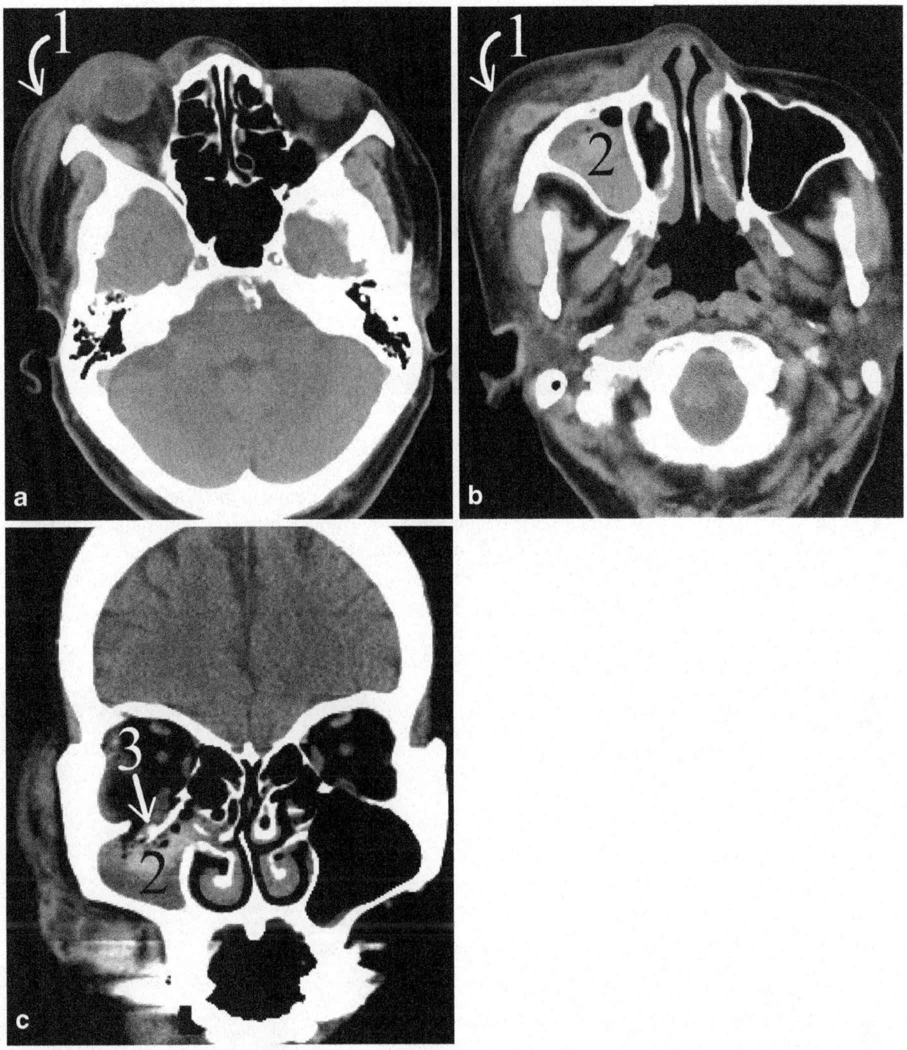

Fig. 3.37 F/69, Blow-out fracture, paranasal sinus bleeding. A patient with Parkinson's disease fell and hit his right cheek and eyelids. (**a**, **b**) CT, axial section, and (**c**) Coronal reconstruction: Subcutaneous swelling and hemorrhage on the right orbit and cheek (1). A blood clot in the right maxillary sinus (2). The coronal reconstruction shows a depressed fracture in the right orbital floor; this is a typical blow-out fracture (3)

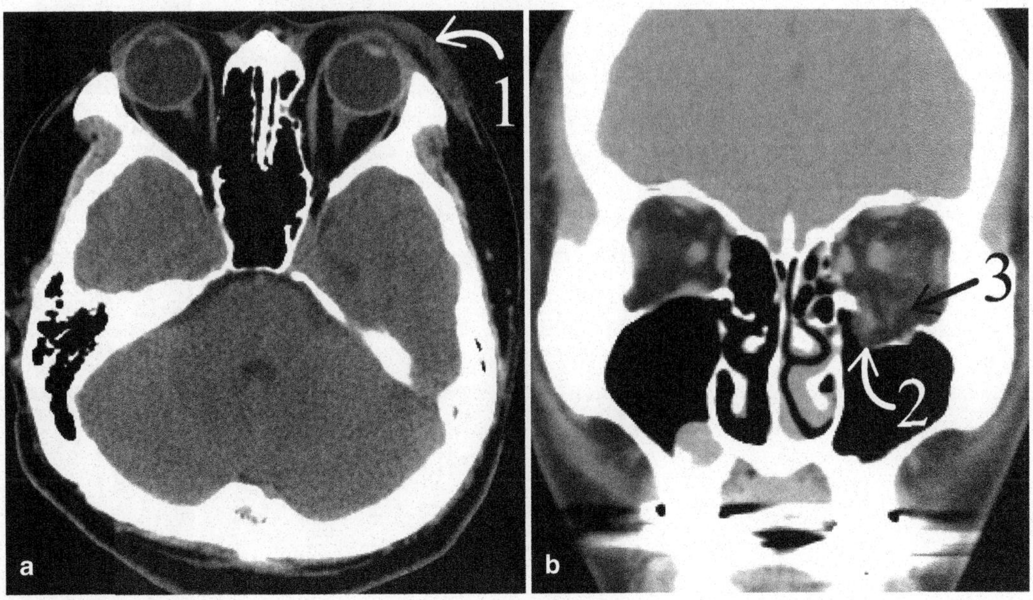

Fig. 3.38 M/27, Blow-out fracture of the orbit. The left eye was hit by a baseball. (**a**) CT, axial section, and (**b**) Coronal reconstruction: The left eyelid skin is swollen due to the impact (1). A depressed fracture (2) in the orbital floor; this is a typical blow-out fracture. The fatty tissue in the orbital cavity collapses with a depressed fracture (3). Fat may sometimes fall into the maxillary sinus

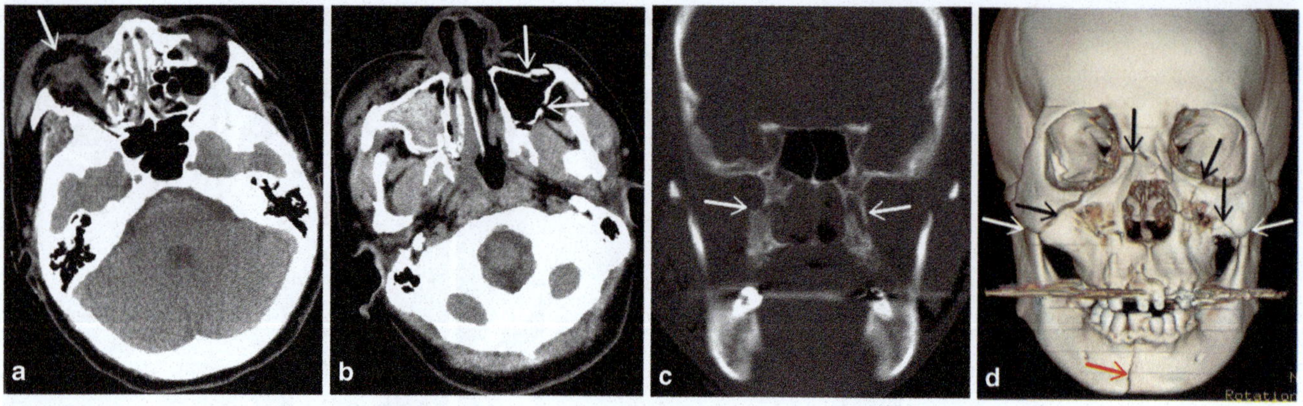

Fig. 3.39 F/38, Le Fort II facial bone fractures. Facial injury caused by a traffic accident. (**a**) CT, axial section: Right eye swelling and subcutaneous emphysema (arrow). (**b**) Axial section: Fractures are present in the bilateral maxillary sinuses (arrows). A blood clot in the right maxillary sinus. (**c**) Coronal reconstruction and bone window: Fractures in the bilateral pterygoid plates (arrows). (**d**) 3D reconstruction: This is Le Fort II facial bone fracture (transverse fractures passing through bilateral zygomatic arches, maxillary sinuses wall, orbital floors, and nasofrontal suture). Another linear fracture (red arrow) is present in the mandible symphysis

Fig. 3.40 M/20, Cervical spine fracture. A traffic accident caused a loss of consciousness and inconsistent breathing. Thus, an endotracheal tube was inserted. (**a**) CT, axial section, and (**b**) sagittal reconstruction. (**c**) Sagittal reconstruction and bone window: No apparent injury in the brain is observed. Given that the examination range includes the cervical spine, a fracture and posteriorly displacement of the C7 vertebral body (arrows) are noted. (**d**) MRI, T2WI, sagittal: Shows that the fracture fragment slightly compresses the spinal cord. No edema or bleeding in the spinal cord is observed

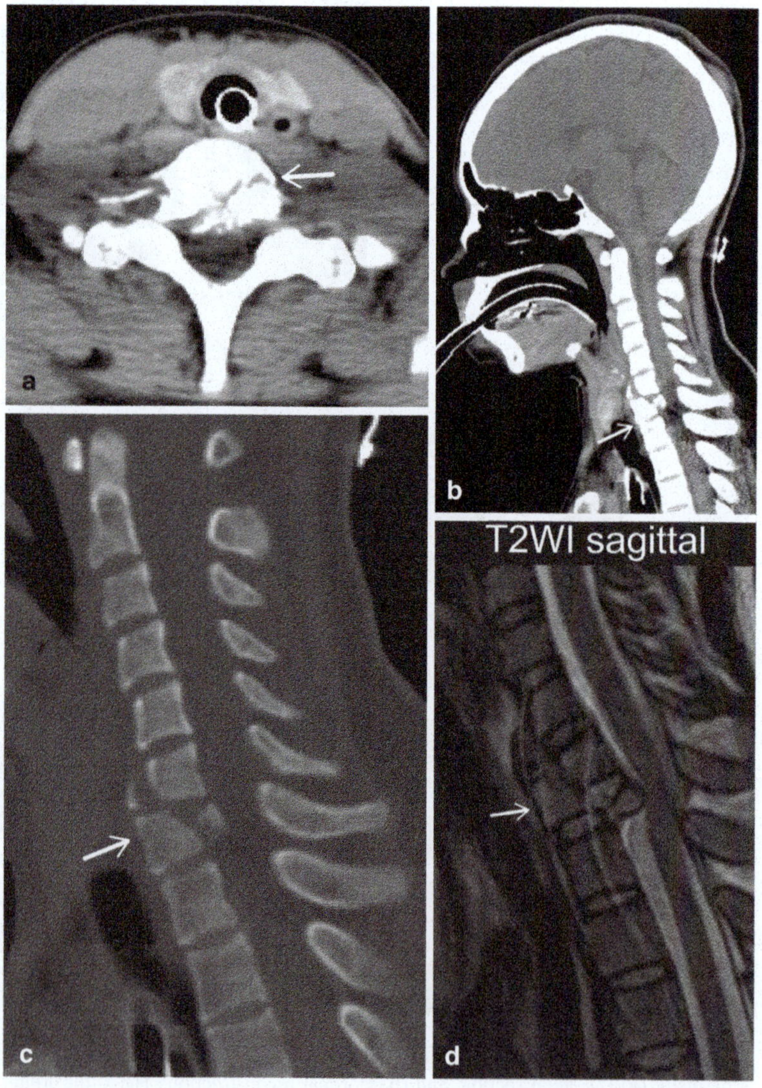

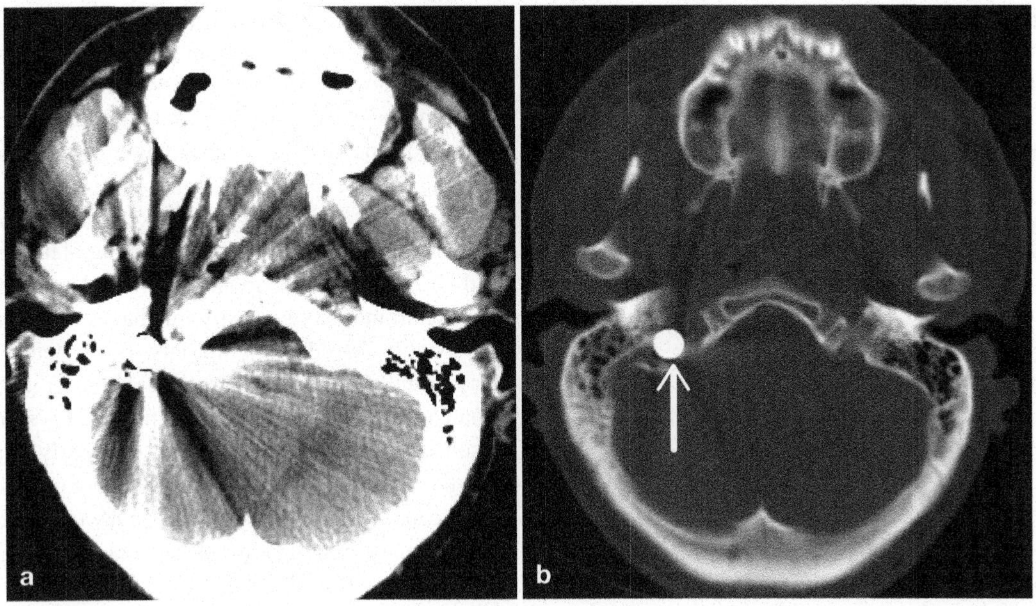

Fig. 3.41 M/23, Gunshot injury. (**a**) CT, axial section: A bullet is stuck in the right mastoid. The bullet produces a potent radiation artifact because it is metal. (**b**) Bone winding setting: Adjusting the bone window to remove the radiation artifact. The bullet (arrow) is clearly visible

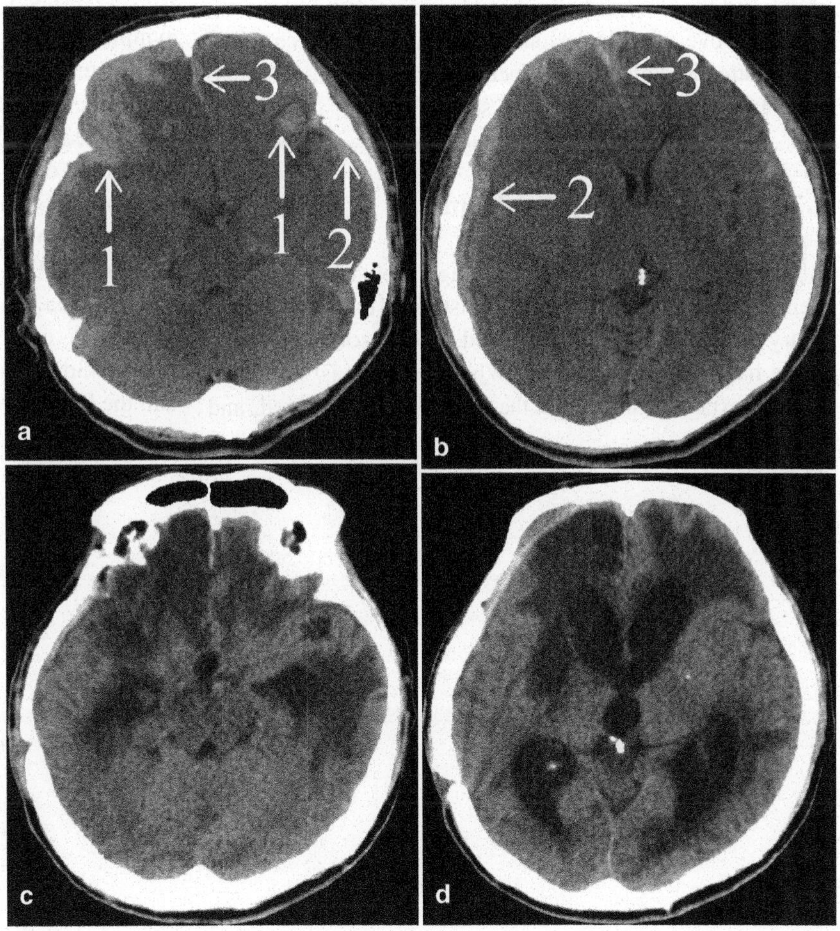

Fig. 3.42 M/67, Sequela of head injury. (**a, b**) CT: Severe head injury, contusion hemorrhages in the bilateral frontal lobes (1) and SDH (2) and SAH (3). (C, D) Follow-up CT 3 months later: Encephalomalacias in the bilateral frontal lobes are the sequela lesions of brain contusion. The dilatation of the ventricles indicates hydrocephalus; it is caused by traumatic SAH

3.11 Sequelae of Head Injury

3.11.1 Diffuse Brain Atrophy

The whole brain will atrophy gradually in severe brain contusion. The gradual dilatation of the sulci and ventricles seen on follow-up CT or MRI indicate brain tissue atrophy (Figs. 3.32 and 3.44).

3.11.2 Hydrocephalus

Patients who have SAH or IVH will gradually develop communicating hydrocephalus because of poor CSF circulation (Fig. 3.42).

3.11.3 Encephalomalacia or Cavitary Change

The brain contusion area will gradually become necrotic, and the brain tissue will soften (encephalomalacia; Figs. 3.15, 3.26, 3.28, and 3.42) or exhibit cavitary changes (Fig. 3.43). The density is reduced to gray-dark, the brain tissue is atrophied, and the surrounding subarachnoid space widens.

The above sequela lesion is the most crucial cause of post-traumatic epilepsy, intellectual degeneration, personality changes, and even vegetative state.

3.12 Shaken Baby Syndrome

Infants less than 7 or 8 months of age should be held with their necks supported so that the twisting of the neck and the injury of the head can be prevented. The reason is that their necks have not yet hardened. When the neck is shaken in some unexpected situations, the brain can be damaged, and intracranial hemorrhage and cerebral edema may occur. Given the absence of apparent external head trauma, this injury is known as a shaken baby syndrome. Most cases of this syndrome are caused by child abuse [4]. In some cases, the syndrome may be caused by unintentional excessive shaking by parents or caretakers.

The early symptoms of shaken baby syndrome may include vomiting, restlessness, crying, lethargy, paleness, and seizures without apparent external trauma. Therefore, this syndrome may be easily misdiagnosed as meningitis or encephalitis based on symptoms. Early detection with CT may reveal only a few subarachnoid hemorrhages (SAHs) or small SDHs. It is difficult to diagnose and is sometimes mistaken for slight head trauma. Improper early treatment often causes severe cerebral palsy and other neurological sequelae.

The series of CT and MRI changes in shaken baby syndrome can be divided into five phases.

Phase 1 occurs 1–2 days after the appearance of symptoms. CT detects only thin-layer SDH, SAH (Figs. 3.43a, b and 3.44a, b), and SDE, but no apparent cerebral edema.

Phase 2 occurs 2–7 days after symptom onset. CT detects unilateral (sometimes with contralateral frontal lobe) or bilateral cerebral edema in the cerebral hemispheres (Fig. 3.44c). SDH and SAH persist. At this time, the patient's symptoms have worsened and even developed into a coma.

Phase 3 occurs on days 7–20 after symptom onset. CT or MRI reveals hemorrhagic infarction in the original area of cerebral edema (Fig. 3.44d, e).

Phase 4 occurs 20 days to 5 months after symptom onset. A chronic SDH appears, and the necrosis begins in the above cerebral edema and infarct area.

Phase 5: For more than 5 months, the SDH disappears, but the area of brain damage may develop atrophy. If it occurs on one side, it appears as cerebral hemiatrophy (Fig. 3.43d); if it occurs on both sides, the ventricles expand, and the brain parenchyma becomes thin.

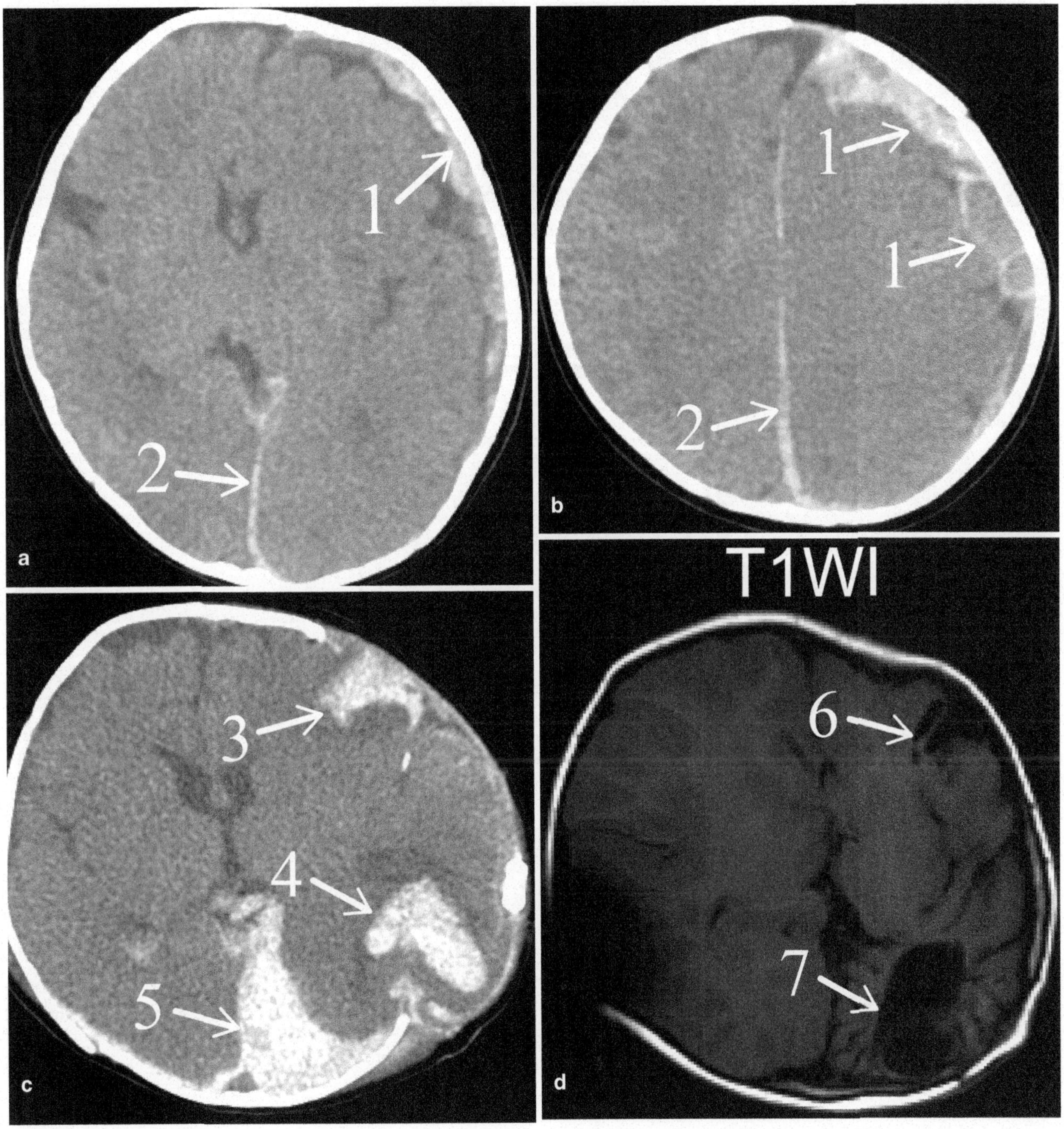

Fig. 3.43 M/3 months, shaken baby syndrome. This infant was possibly a victim of child abuse. (**a**, **b**) Emergency CT: An acute SDH in the left cerebral surface (1) and SDH in the interhemispheric fissure (2). An emergency craniectomy was performed to remove the SDH and remove part of the cranial table, allowing brain tissue to herniate out and relieve high intracranial pressure. (**c**) CT, 5 days later: New intracerebral hematomas (ICH) in the left frontal lobe (3) and parietal lobe (4). A big SDH in the posterior of the interhemispheric fissure (5). The ICH and SDH are delayed hemorrhages. (**d**) MRI, 1 year later, T1WI: Left-side cerebral hemiatrophy and porencephalic cysts in the frontal lobe (6) and parietal lobe (7) are the sequela of previous ICHs

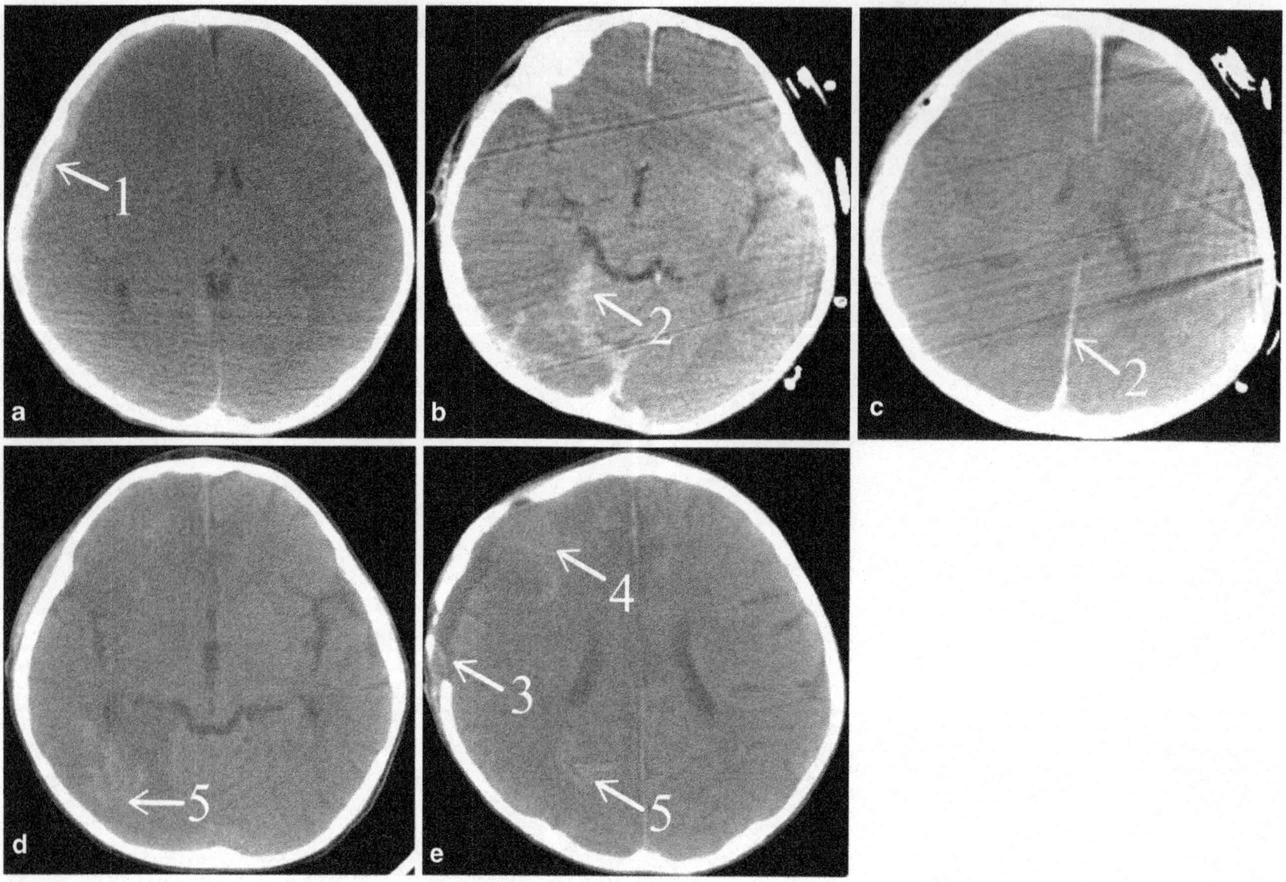

Fig. 3.44 M/14 months, shaken baby syndrome. A possible victim of child abuse. (**a**) Emergency CT: An acute SDH in the right frontal region (1). (**b**, **c**) CT on the fourth day: Diffuse brain tissue edema in the right cerebral hemisphere and SAH in the tentorium and interhemispheric fissure (2). (**d**, **e**) CT on the tenth-day postcraniectomy: Part of the right frontal bone was removed (3) to relieve intracranial pressure. Diffuse brain tissue edema is present and mixes with hemorrhages (4, 5) in the right cerebral hemisphere. This is a kind of hemorrhagic transformation in infarction brain tissue. The right cerebral hemisphere is expected to shrink gradually

References

1. Davis PC. Head trauma. AJNR Am J Neuroradiol. 2007;28:1619–21.
2. Provenzale JM. Imaging of traumatic brain injury: a review of the recent medical literature. AJR Am J Roentgenol. 2010;194:16–9.
3. Park SH, et al. Chronic subdural hematoma preceded by traumatic subdural hygroma. J Clin Neurosci. 2008;15:868–72.
4. Hsieh KL, et al. Revisiting neuroimaging of abusive head trauma in infants and young children. AJR Am J Roentgenol. 2015;204:944–52.

Medical Imaging of Cerebral Hemorrhagic Stroke

4

Abstract

Two types of hemorrhagic stroke include intracerebral (intraparenchymal) hemorrhage (ICH) and subarachnoid hemorrhage (SAH). The acute ICH shows hyperdensity on CT and can easily be diagnosed. In the subacute stage, the density of hematoma gradually decreases, and the brain edema around the hematoma becomes obvious. In the chronic stage, a linear cavity in the original ICH location is observed and associated with peripheral brain tissue atrophy. MRI is an auxiliary tool for diagnosing ICH. The evolution of ICH is complicated in MRI, and it is divided into five stages. ICH is most often caused by hypertension, and the locations are in deep areas, such as the putamen, thalamus, brainstem, and cerebellum. Lobar hemorrhage is primarily caused by amyloid angiopathy, AVM, and tumor bleeding. For the diagnosis of ICH, plain CT is usually sufficient. In young stroke and lobar hemorrhage, contrast-enhanced CT plus CTA and even DSA can be performed to find a vascular anomaly or others. Most spontaneous SAH is caused by the rupture (leakage) of an aneurysm. Most aneurysms are located in the circle of Willis. CTA can detect most of the aneurysms. In addition to SAH, 30% of aneurysm rupture may combine ICH. The ICH provides a valuable clue to surmise the location of aneurysms, such as if an ICH is in the frontal lobe or septum pellucidum, the aneurysm is in the ACoA; an ICH in the mesial temporal lobe, the aneurysm is in the ICA/PCoA; and a hematoma in Sylvian fissure, the aneurysm is in the bifurcation of MCA.

Cerebral Stroke

A stroke, also known as a cerebrovascular accident (CVA), occurs (1) when an intracerebral hemorrhage forming a hematoma which compresses the brain tissue, or (2) occlusion of the intracerebral artery, causes brain tissue ischemia, supplied by the affected blood vessel, resulting in edema of the brain tissue. Each of these conditions produces symptoms related to the area of the brain be involved, such as limb weakness, facial numbness or paralysis, dysphonia, dysphagia, blurred vision, headaches, dizziness, vomiting, and consciousness disturbance, severe cases can result in coma and even death. Following the acute phase, many patients are left with long-term disabilities.

There are two major types of stroke:

1. Hemorrhagic stroke, which is divided into (Fig. 4.1) the following:
   (a) Intracerebral hemorrhage (ICH) or intraparenchymal hemorrhage (IPH)
   (b) Subarachnoid hemorrhage (SAH)
2. Ischemic stroke (see Chap. 5), which is divided into the following:
   (a) Embolism.
   (b) Thrombosis.
   (c) Systemic hypoperfusion.

4.1 The Evolution of ICH in CT and MRI

CT and MRI are often repeatedly performed at any time during the acute, subacute, and chronic phases of a hemorrhagic stroke if clinically indicated. During each of these phases, due to the continuous resolution of the intracerebral hematoma (ICH), the CT and MRI images continuously change, and these changes need to be understood to read these images properly (see Table 4.1).

The hemorrhagic stroke generally requires an urgent CT because the acute hematoma appears white (hyperdense) in the CT, and has an attenuation value of 70–90 HU, making it is easy to recognize. In most cases of intracranial hemorrhage caused by stroke or head trauma, the CT image is made after the patient has been at the hospital for 3 or 4 h, and this is when the acute hematoma appears white, providing the most explicit image (Fig. 4.2).

But in cases where the patient is already in the hospital or the injury takes place near the hospital, it might be possible to do the

W.-C. Shen, *Diagnostic Neuroradiology*, https://doi.org/10.1007/978-981-15-4051-6_4

CT within 1 or 2 h, during the hyperacute hematoma phase, at that time the hematoma may not have coagulated or may have just solidified, so its density will not be very white, is gray, and the attenuation value will be 40–50 Hu (Figs. 4.2 and 4.3).

Hematomas that have not been surgically removed gradually resolve, and as they resolve, their color in the CT and MRI continually changes. In the CT, the hematoma is initially white (hyperdense) and gradually fades, and peripheral brain edema becomes increasingly apparent (Figs. 4.4 and 4.5), making the mass effect stronger.

The MRI provides a highly detailed view of the changing composition of the hematoma, which has been divided by researchers [1, 2] into five stages. Table 4.1 shows the changes of CT and MRI images in the five stages:

1. **Hyperacute hematoma**: Less than 12 h from onset; composed of oxyhemoglobin. Appears gray less than 2 h (Figs. 4.2, 4.3 and 4.34), or white more than 2 h in CT. For head injury and hemorrhagic stroke, urgent CT is the first examination modality, CT often performs within several hours after the onset of symptoms, so always present white (Figs. 4.2–4.30), only rare cases have the opportunity to do CT examination less than 2 h, and the hematoma shows gray (Figs. 4.2 and 4.3). In MRI, there is an isointense on T1WI and hyperintense on T2WI, FLAIR. However, it is rarely possible to make an MRI at such an early stage.
2. **Acute hematoma**: 12 h–2 days, composed of deoxyhemoglobin. Appears white in CT (Figs. 4.2–4.30); in MRI, T1WI is gray; T2WI, FLAIR, and T2*WI are dark (Figs. 4.6, 4.23, 4.24, and 4.25).
3. **Early subacute hematoma**: 2 days–2 weeks, composed mainly of methemoglobin (intracellular). Still appears white in CT, gradually turning white at T1WI, still dark at T2WI, FLAIR, and T2*WI (Figs. 4.6 and 4.7).
4. **Late subacute hematoma**: 2 weeks–2 months, composed mainly of methemoglobin (extracellular). The hematoma gradually becomes dark gray in CT, or a little grayish white only in the middle, easily mistaken for brain edema (Figs. 4.4, 4.8, and 4.9). This is the best time for an MRI because the entire hematoma contains methemoglobin; when all of the pulse sequences are white, the surrounding edema gradually disappears. T2*WI is also white, and the adjacent hemosiderin deposition is dark (Figs. 4.7, 4.8, 4.9, and 4.10).
5. **Chronic hematoma**: 2 months and later, composed mainly of hemichromes (ferritin/hemosiderin). After the blood clot is entirely resolved, it gradually becomes a linear cavity, and the surrounding brain tissue gradually atrophies. In the CT can be seen the linear cavities, some long and slender, and some somewhat wider (Figs. 4.4, 4.5, 4.6, 4.11, and 4.12). At T2WI in the MRI can be seen the water in the linear cavity, which appears white; at T2*WI, the edge hemosiderin deposition is dark (Figs. 4.6, 4.7, and 4.10).

If the stroke results in long-term paralysis, it will cause Wallerian degeneration, which is most easily seen in the brainstem (Fig. 4.12) (see also Chap. 2; Fig. 2.34).

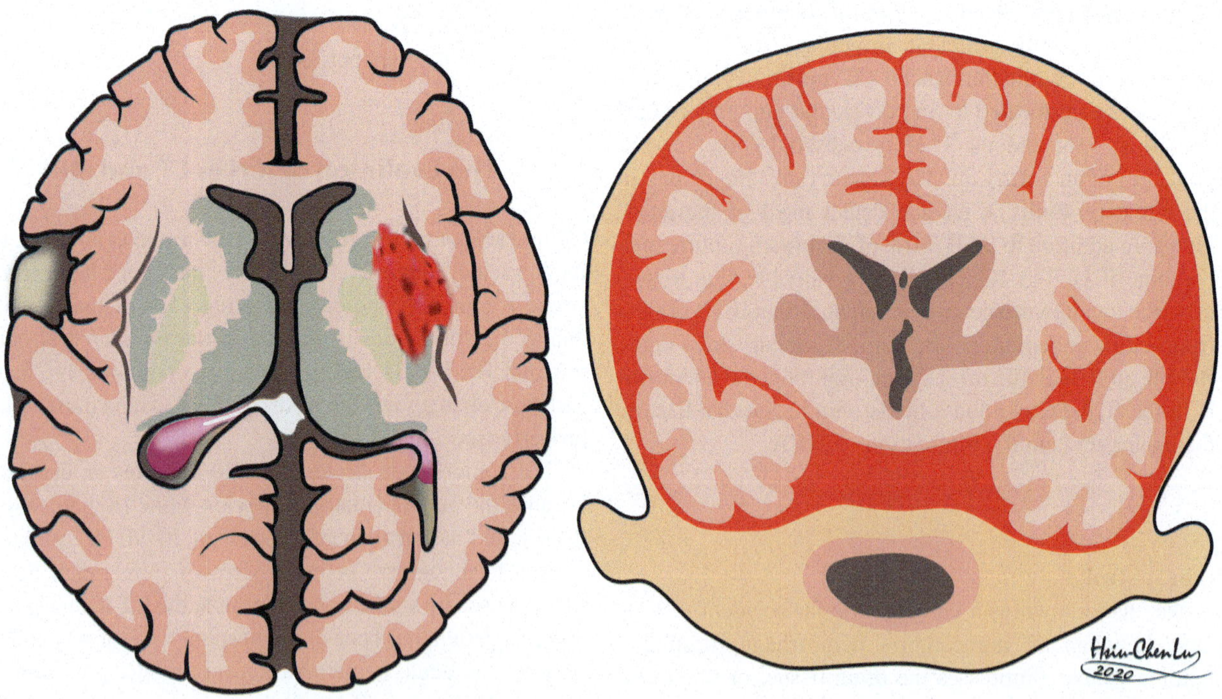

Fig. 4.1 Two types of hemorrhagic stroke: (1) ICH: Intracerebral hematoma (ICH), a parenchymal hemorrhage in the brain tissue. (2) SAH: Subarachnoid hemorrhage (SAH), hemorrhage in the subarachnoid spaces, such as suprasellar cistern, Sylvian fissures, interhemispheric fissure, sulci; mixes with the cerebrospinal fluid (CSF); no hematoma is formed

Table 4.1 Evolution of intracerebral hematoma (ICH) and changes in CT and MRI images

Timing	CT	MRI
Hyper-acute Less than 12 h. The blood clot is not yet solidified (less than 2 h) or just solidify (over 2 h)	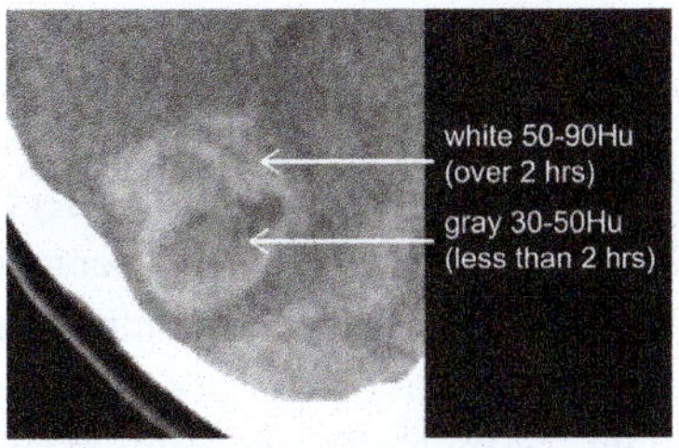 	Very few opportunities to do MRI Hematoma contains oxyhemoglobin T1WI: isointensity T2WI/FLAIR, DWI: bright T2*WI: variable
Acute 12 h–2 days 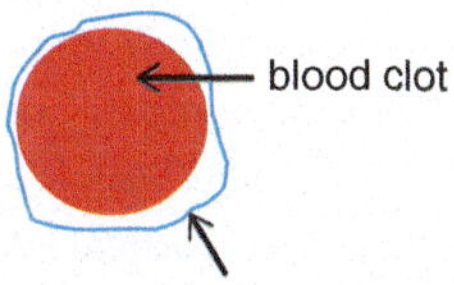 some peripheral edema	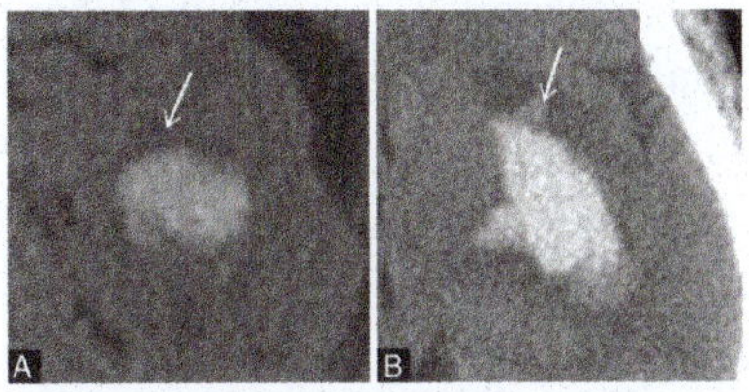 ICH, white 70~90Hu some peripheral edema	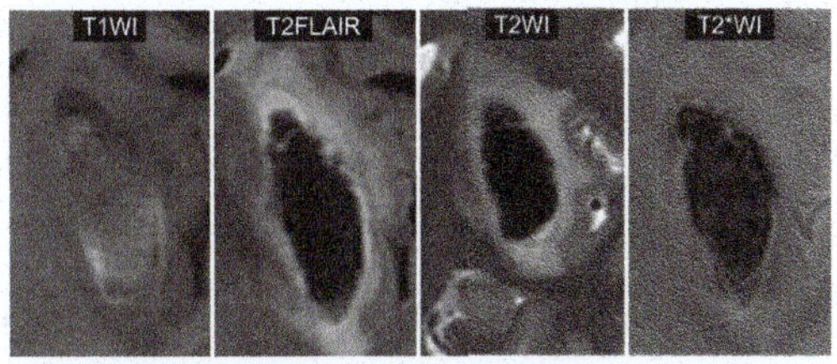 Hematoma contains deoxyhemoglobin T1 gray; long TR dark, peripheral edema is obvious. T2*WI dark.
Early subacute 2 days~2 weeks more peripheral edema 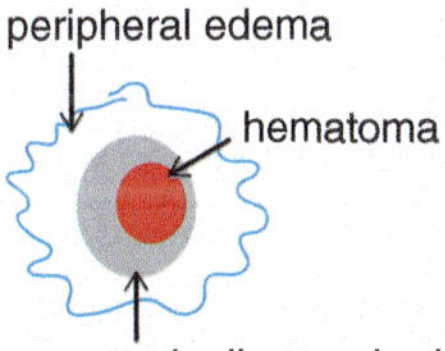 hematoma gradually resorbed	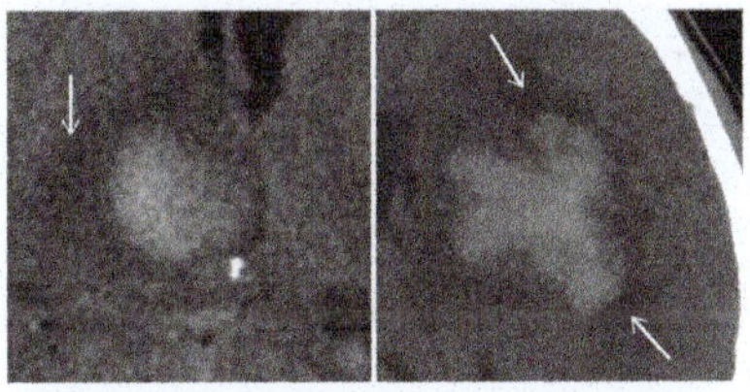 Hematoma white, gradually shinking more obvious peripheral edema (gray)	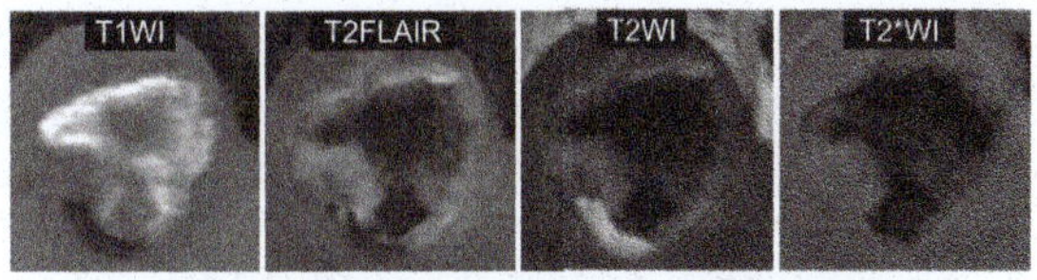 Hematoma contains methemoglobin (intracellular), T1 gray; long TR dark, more peripheral edema, T2*WI dark.
Late subacute 2 weeks~2 months 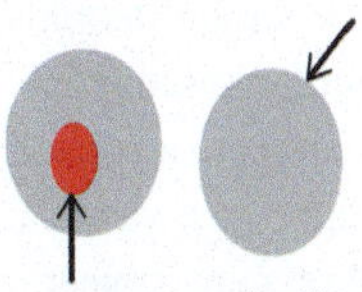 The hematoma gradually shrinks no more peripheral edema	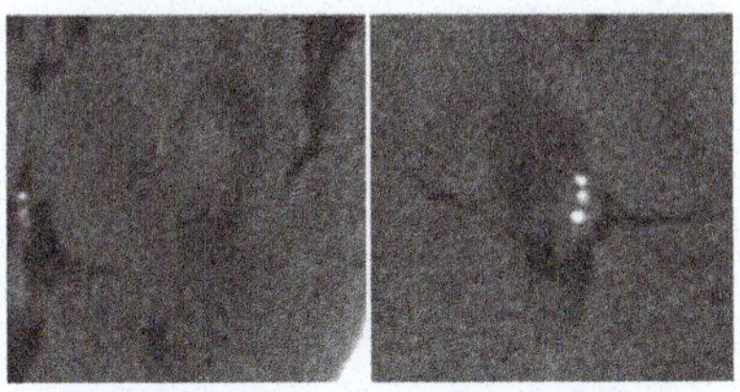 residual white in middle / hematoma totally gray	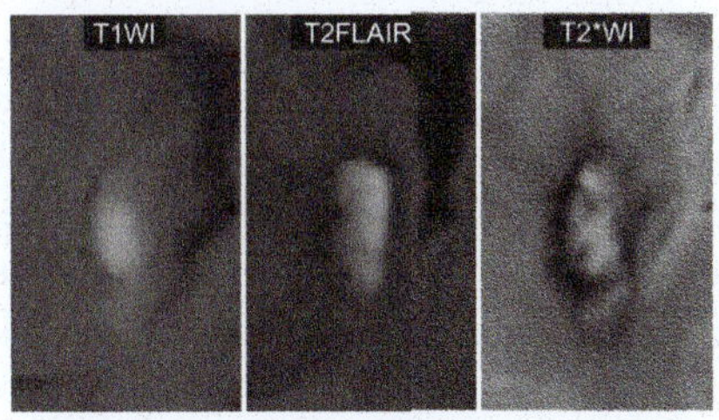 hematoma contains methemoglobin (extracellular), white in every pulse sequence. T2*WI: peripheral hemosiderin deposition, dark.
Chronic 2 months~years 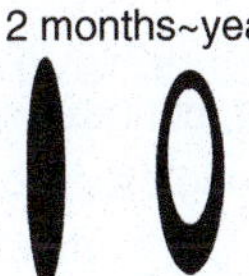 linear cavity / linear cavity fluid and peripheral hemosiderin	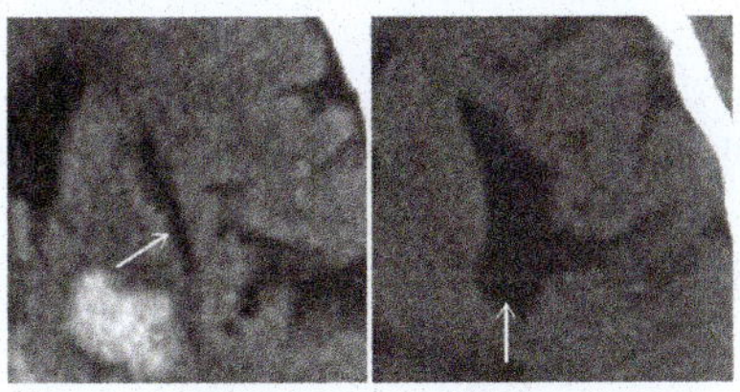 CT: linear cavity, dark	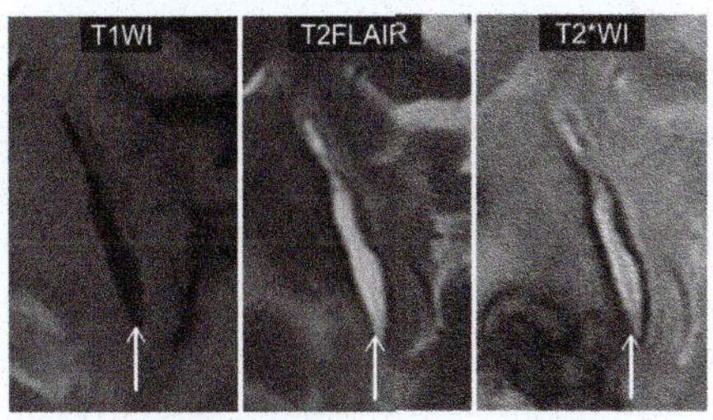 T1: linear cavity, dark T2 WI, T2*WI: fluid, white, rim: hemosiderin, dark

4.2 Neuroimaging of Intracerebral Hemorrhage (ICH)

The causes of intracerebral hemorrhagic (ICH) stroke are as follows:

1. Hypertensive hemorrhagic stroke, the most common (Figs. 4.2 and 4.4–4.23)
2. Amyloid angiopathy (Figs. 4.24 and 4.25)
3. Vascular diseases, such as AVM (Figs. 4.26–4.30), aneurysm (Figs. 4.3, 4.32, and 4.33), venous malformation, and hemangioma (Fig. 4.34)
4. Tumor bleeding (Figs. 4.35 and 4.36)
5. Diseases with hemorrhagic tendency, e.g., leukemia (Fig. 4.37), liver dysfunction, taking an anticoagulant.

4.2.1 Hypertensive Hemorrhagic Stroke

This is the most common type of hemorrhagic stroke and usually occurs in hypertensive patients over the age of 50, but can also occur in the 30s or 40s if high blood pressure is not properly controlled. Most cases occur in winter, but some also occur during late fall or early spring, when there are rapid temperature changes. In strokes caused by high blood pressure, the bleeding usually occurs at the following locations, in order of likelihood:

Putamen (Figs. 4.2, 4.5, 4.6, 4.10–4.15, and 4.18)
Thalamus (Figs. 4.4, 4.6, and 4.16, 4.17, and 4.18)
Pons of the brainstem (Figs. 4.7, 4.8, and 4.19)
Cerebellum (Fig. 4.20)
Lobar hemorrhage (Figs. 4.9 and 4.22)
Caudate nucleus (Fig. 4.21)
Midbrain and medulla oblongata of the brainstem (Fig. 4.23)

When a hematoma occurs in the thalamus or caudate nucleus, both of which are very close to the ventricles, it can easily break into the ventricles, causing intraventricular hemorrhage (IVH) (Figs. 4.6, 4.16, 4.17, and 4.21). When the hemorrhage occurs in the putamen, cerebral cortex, or cerebellum, although it is far from the ventricles, if the hematoma is large, it also can rupture into the ventricles and causes IVH (Figs. 4.14 and 4.20). Besides, these ICHs may directly flow into the subarachnoid space, causing secondary SAH (Fig. 4.12), or IVH followed by a CSF circulation resulting in secondary SAH.

The size of ICH induced by hypertension is usually determined at the moment of vessel ruptures. The ICH immediately compresses the ruptured small blood vessel, and this stops the bleeding. However, it occasionally happens that soon afterward, the hematoma becomes larger, which is a rebleeding (Figs. 4.13 and 4.17), rather than continuous bleeding.

Sometimes the ICH caused by high hypertension is small (Figs. 4.5, 4.11, 4.13, and 4.17); sometimes, a large amount of bleeding forms a large hematoma (Figs. 4.13 and 4.14), creating a strong mass effect. This is not necessarily related to how the rise of blood pressure.

4.2.2 Cerebral Amyloid Angiopathy

Amyloid angiopathy refers to the deposition of ß-amyloid in the cerebral cortex, leptomeninges, or arteriolar wall. This arterial lesion is common in Alzheimer's disease and is also seen in elderly people who have no neurological symptoms. Amyloid angiopathy is one of the causes of hemorrhagic stroke. When the bleeding occurs in the cerebral cortex or subcortex, it is called a lobar hemorrhage. Most occur in the frontal, parietal, occipital, and temporal lobes, and occasionally in the cerebellum and corpus callosum, rebleeding is typical (Fig. 4.24). This phenomenon is different from hypertensive hemorrhage, in which the bleeding typically occurs in the basal ganglia, thalamus, cerebellum, and brainstem.

CT can be used to diagnose a cortical or subcortical hemorrhage (Fig. 4.24). In addition to the bleeding seen in the CT, the MRI can detect asymptomatic microbleeds on T2*WI and SWI (Figs. 4.24 and 4.25). Since amyloid angiopathy is also a type of small vessel disease, CT and MRI can detect leukoaraiosis in patient with amyloid angiopathy (see Chap. 5 for details).

4.2.3 Vascular Disease

Vascular disease includes the following:

Arteriovenous malformation (AVM) (Figs. 4.26–4.30)
Aneurysm (Figs. 4.3, 4.32, and 4.33)
Venous malformation
Hemangiomas (such as cavernous hemangioma) (Fig. 4.34)

Any of the above vascular diseases may rupture and bleed, causing a stroke; most strokes amongst younger people fall into this category. Bleeding caused by vascular disease has a high chance of rebleeding in a short time. Therefore, it is usually necessary to perform surgery or embolization of the vascular anomaly as soon as possible after bleeding to prevent rebleeding.

4.2.4 Arteriovenous Malformation (AVM)

AVM is the leading cause of stroke amongst young people (Figs. 4.26–4.30). Most AVMs are congenital, but rarely rupture during childhood; most ruptures occur in adolescence and young adulthood as a result of excessive tension, excitement, or fatigue.

AVMs can produce symptoms without rupturing. Some AVMs rob most of the blood supply, causing the surrounding brain tissue to atrophy and producing the symptoms of a seizure; others may only cause headaches and dizziness (Fig. 4.31).

CT: An AVM that has not been ruptured has a slightly higher density in the CT than the brain tissue, and sometimes calcification is seen (Fig. 4.31). Injection of the contrast medium greatly enhances the image, making it possible to see blood vessels that are twisted and thickened, resembling an earthworm, this is called "bag of worms sign"; in the surrounding area can be seen the thickened supply arteries and drainage veins (Figs. 4.28, 4.29, and 4.31).

When AVM causes an intracerebral hemorrhage, the hematoma is seen in the CT. After the contrast medium is injected, it is possible to see abnormal blood vessels in or nearby the hematoma (Figs. 4.26, 4.27, 4.28, and 4.29), suggesting that AVM caused this hematoma. After composing the 3D CTA, CTA can clearly show the "bag of worms sign" (Figs. 4.28 and 4.31), but no further information for the diagnosis of AVM.

MRI: MRI can see the AVM itself, even a very small AVM. MR angiography is also helpful for AVM diagnosis.

Digital subtraction angiography (DSA): Traditional cerebral angiography is used to confirm the diagnosis, and DSA can clearly show the feeding arteries and drainage veins. The DSA is required especially for evaluating whether or not to adopt embolization treatment (Figs. 4.26, 4.29, and 4.31).

4.2.5 Tumor Bleeding

Intracerebral tumors such as malignant metastatic tumors (Fig. 4.35) and glioblastoma (Fig. 4.36) are susceptible to bleeding, and may be accompanied by symptoms similar to those of a stroke; they are clinically considered to be a CVA, and thus require a CT.

As mentioned above (Sect. 4.1), during the acute phase of ICH caused by hypertension, the edema in the peripheral area is minimal, and it is not until the hematoma is absorbed 8–30 days after the onset that the surrounding brain tissue edema appears extensively (Figs. 4.4 and 4.5). Therefore, when clinical signs indicate that an acute stroke has just occurred, but brain tissue edema appears around the ICH in the CT, especially if it is white matter edema, it should be highly suspected that there is a tumor hidden in the hematoma.

If tumor bleeding is suspected, the contrast medium can be injected intravenously; if the white hematoma becomes whiter, this indicates that there is a tumor in the ICH (Fig. 4.35).

4.2.6 Patients Prone to Bleeding

Patients who have a bleeding tendency are also prone to hemorrhagic stroke. The diseases with bleeding tendencies include hemophilia, leukemia (Fig. 4.37), SLE, uremia, and liver cirrhosis. The cerebral hemorrhage caused by these diseases can occur anywhere in the brain, and often several occur at the same time (multiple hemorrhages).

4.2.7 Diagnosis of Brain Tissue ICH

- **CT**: For hemorrhagic stroke, CT is the first and most important diagnostic tool because a new intracerebral hematoma (ICH) is white in the CT, making it easy to identify. Moreover, for hypertensive ICH, CT is enough to make a diagnosis; no further tests are required [3].
- **MRI**: For acute bleeding, MRI is not an ideal diagnostic tool because (1) in comparison to CT, although the MRI is as sensitive as CT to detect the acute ICH, in different pulse sequences, the signs are more complicated and challenging to interpret. (2) An MRI usually takes about 20 minutes. Since in the acute phase of hemorrhagic stroke, the patient is usually confused and irritable and may need to be intubated with an endotracheal tube, the MRI is not suitable for an emergency examination. However, in the late subacute phase, ICHs are difficult to see in a CT but can be seen in an MRI because at this time, the ICH contains methemoglobin, which is white (hyperintense) in each pulse sequences of MRI [3].
- **Cerebral angiography**

  Cerebral angiography can be divided into three types:
  1. CT angiography (CTA)
  2. MR angiography (MRA)
  3. Digital subtraction angiography (DSA)

  CTA is the first-line diagnostic tool, especially for patients with ICH and SAH. To determine if the cause is AVM or an aneurysm, CTA is usually the first test to carry out. If the CTA provides a precise diagnosis, then it may not be necessary to perform DSA prior to surgery; but when considering whether to perform an embolization treatment, the DSA will be required. The DSA provides the best results, but it is an invasive test. MRA is only suitable for conscious patients.
- **Indication of angiography**

  In the vast majority of hemorrhagic strokes, CT is sufficient, but angiography should be considered in the following three conditions:
  1. All types of stroke in young adults (young stroke):

     Young hemorrhagic stroke is usually the result of AVM (Figs. 3.26, 3.27, 3.28, 3.29, and 3.30) or some other vascular disease, so following the CT diagnosis of a cerebral hemorrhage, it is necessary to do a CTA, or even a DSA immediately.

     Here "young adult" means under the age of 30. After ruling out definite hypertension and other common causes of bleeding, such as head trauma, leukemia, and drug abuse, all non-traumatic intracerebral hemorrhages should be regarded as young stroke.

     Patients in their 30s and 40s who do not suffer from such predisposing conditions such as hypertension, DM, and uremia also fall into this category. After using CT to diagnose the intracerebral hemorrhage, a CTA should be made, and it may also be necessary to do a DSA to look for vascular disease.

Angiography is ineffective on some diseases, known as VMOTA (vascular malformation occult to angiography), including cryptal AVM (Fig. 4.30), thrombosed AVM, and cavernous hemangioma (Fig. 4.34).

2. Unusual locations of intracerebral hemorrhage:

   For people over the age of 40, if the location of bleeding is not any of those typical for hypertensive hemorrhagic stroke (i.e., basal ganglion, brainstem, deep layer of cerebrum/cerebellum), angiography should be considered. Conditions with a fairly complex etiology include aneurysm, AVM, tumor hemorrhage, moyamoya disease, and other vascular anomalies.

   For lobar hemorrhage, before the DSA is considered, when the hemorrhage is detected in plain CT, the contrast medium can be injected, sometimes the abnormal blood vessels are enhanced (Figs. 4.26, 4.27, 4.28, 4.29 and 4.33), which is helpful to diagnosis.

3. For both primary and spontaneous SAH, more than 85% of all cases are caused by the rupture of an aneurysm, so angiography must be used to check for an aneurysm, which can be surgically removed or endovascular embolized to avoid rebleeding (more details in Sect. 4.3).

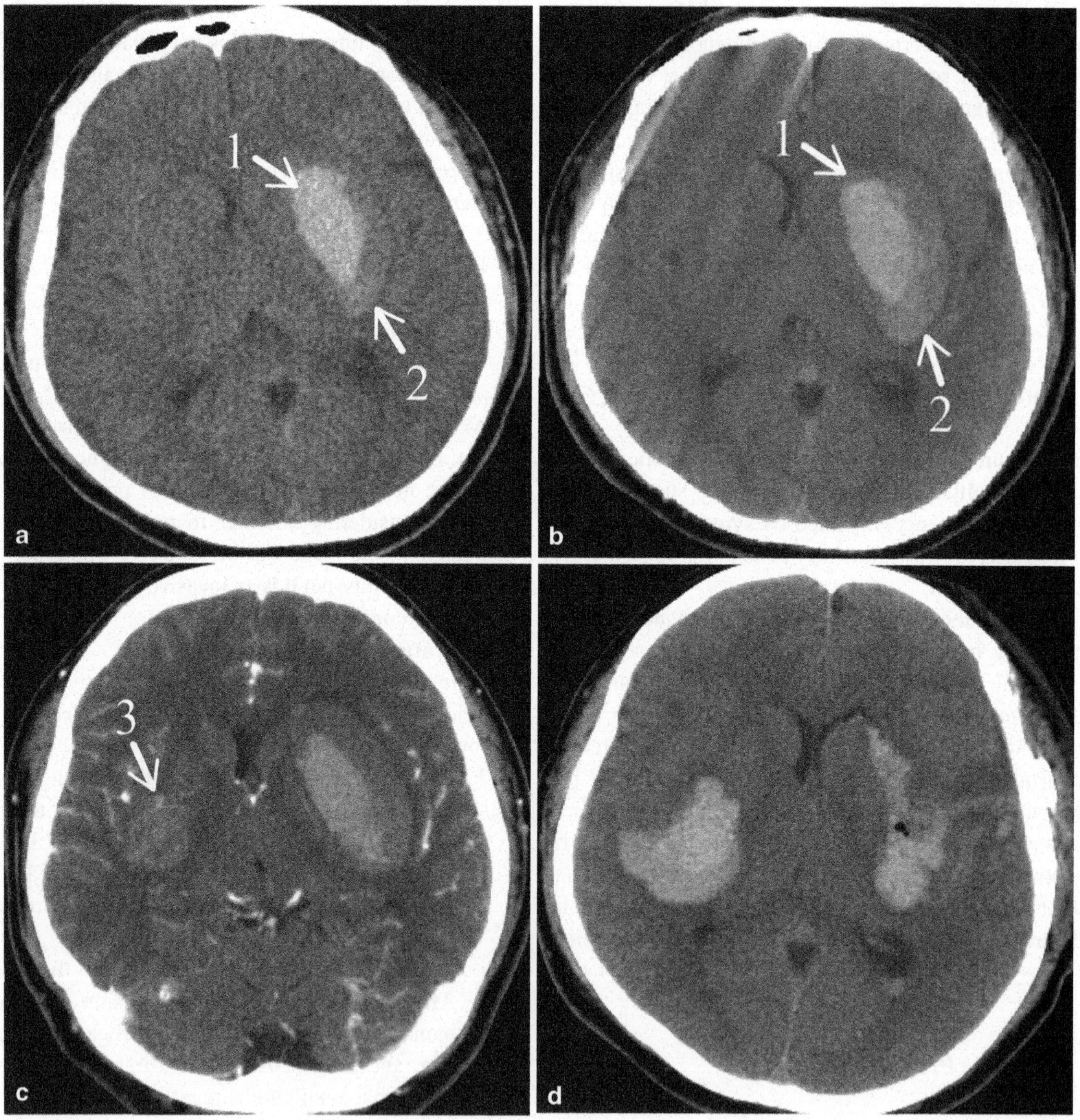

Fig. 4.2 M/29, Young hypertensive stroke, repeat cerebral hemorrhage in a short time. This patient suffered a sudden onset of confusion and right-sided hemiplegia. (**a**) CT: A hematoma in the left putamen; the middle part of hematoma is white (1), 80–90 Hu. The peripheral portion is gray (2), 40–50 Hu, which may indicate secondary bleeding. Because this was a young stroke, CT was done again, and the contrast medium was injected to look for possible AVM or other vascular diseases. (**b**) CT, separated by 1.5 h: The hematoma in left putamen still showed two densities; the periphery is gray, and the density increased to 45–60 Hu (2). (**c**) CT, after injection of contrast medium, separated by just a few minutes. It was surprising to find an acute hemorrhage in the contralateral putamen (3); density is 40–50 Hu. Then, the patient underwent a left hematoma drainage procedure. (**d**) CT, 2 days later: The left putamen still had residual blood clots after drainage surgery, and the hematoma in the right putamen became white with a density of 80–90 Hu

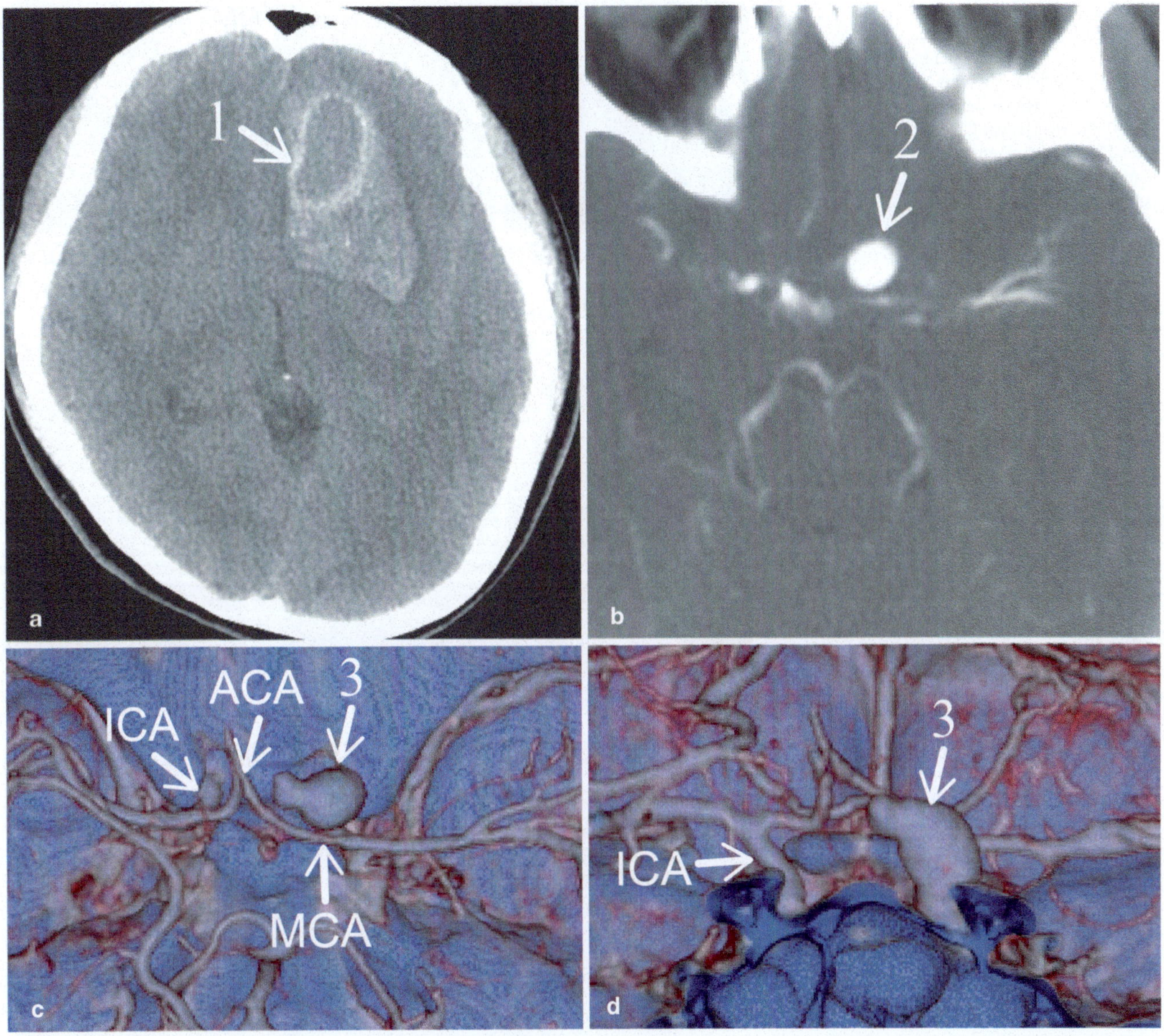

Fig. 4.3 F/36, A large aneurysm causes an intracerebral hemorrhage. A healthy young woman had a sudden severe headache. (**a**) CT: A hyperacute intracerebral hematoma (ICH) in the left frontal lobe. It is not very white; the average density is 50 Hu. A darker part (1) in the hematoma, which means there is bleeding; this is an uncoagulated blood clot, the average density is only 40 Hu. (**b**) Source image of CTA: A spherical structure (2) in which contrast medium accumulation, a large aneurysm is suspected. (**c**, **d**) CTA confirms that this is a large aneurysm (3) that arises from the left internal carotid artery (ICA)

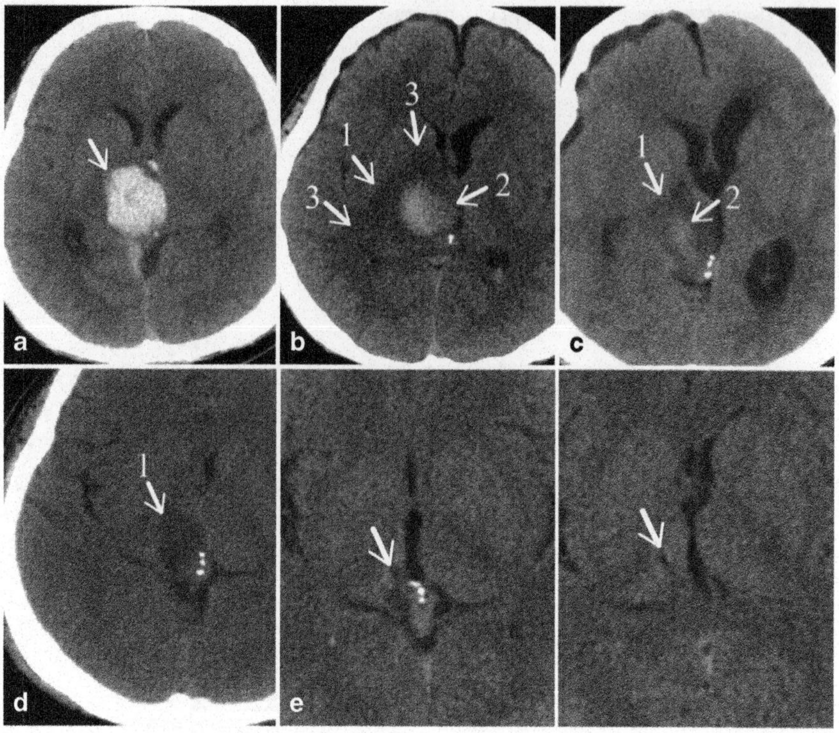

Fig. 4.4 M/54, Hypertension causing thalamus hemorrhage. (**a**) CT: An acute hematoma in the right thalamus, showing uniform white (hyperdense), 70–90 Hu. (**b**) Repeat CT after 17 days: The hematoma is in absorption, gradually becoming gray-dark (1) on the periphery, white (2) in the middle, and brain tissue edema around (3). (**c**) CT 1 month later: The hematoma is dark gray (1), the center remains gray (2), and the peripheral brain tissue edema has disappeared. (**d**) CT 2 months later: The whole hematoma is dark gray (hypodense), so it is easily mistaken for brain edema. (**e**) CT 3 years later: A linear cavity in the original bleeding area (arrow)

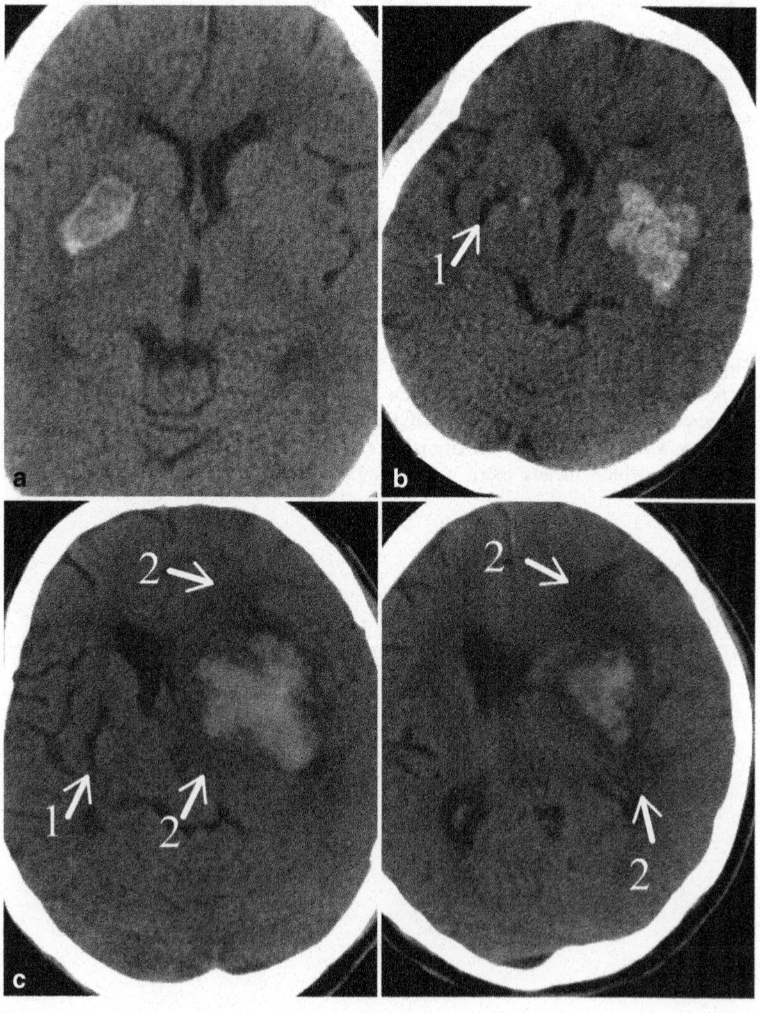

Fig. 4.5 F/44, Hypertension causing two separate putamen hemorrhages. (**a**) CT: The first stroke, right putamen hemorrhage; CT shows hyperdensity. Because the hematoma was small, conservative treatment was adopted. (**b**) Another stroke after 2 years; CT shows left-side putamen hemorrhage, the hematoma is more massive than the last time. A linear cavity (1) in right putamen; this is a sequela lesion of previous ICH. (**c**) On day 8, the patient's right limb more weakened, and she began to lose consciousness. CT: The hematoma is in absorption, with severe peripheral white matter edema (2), making the mass effect stronger, and causing the left ventricle to be more severely compressed. After CT, the neurosurgeon did an endoscopic surgery to remove the hematoma

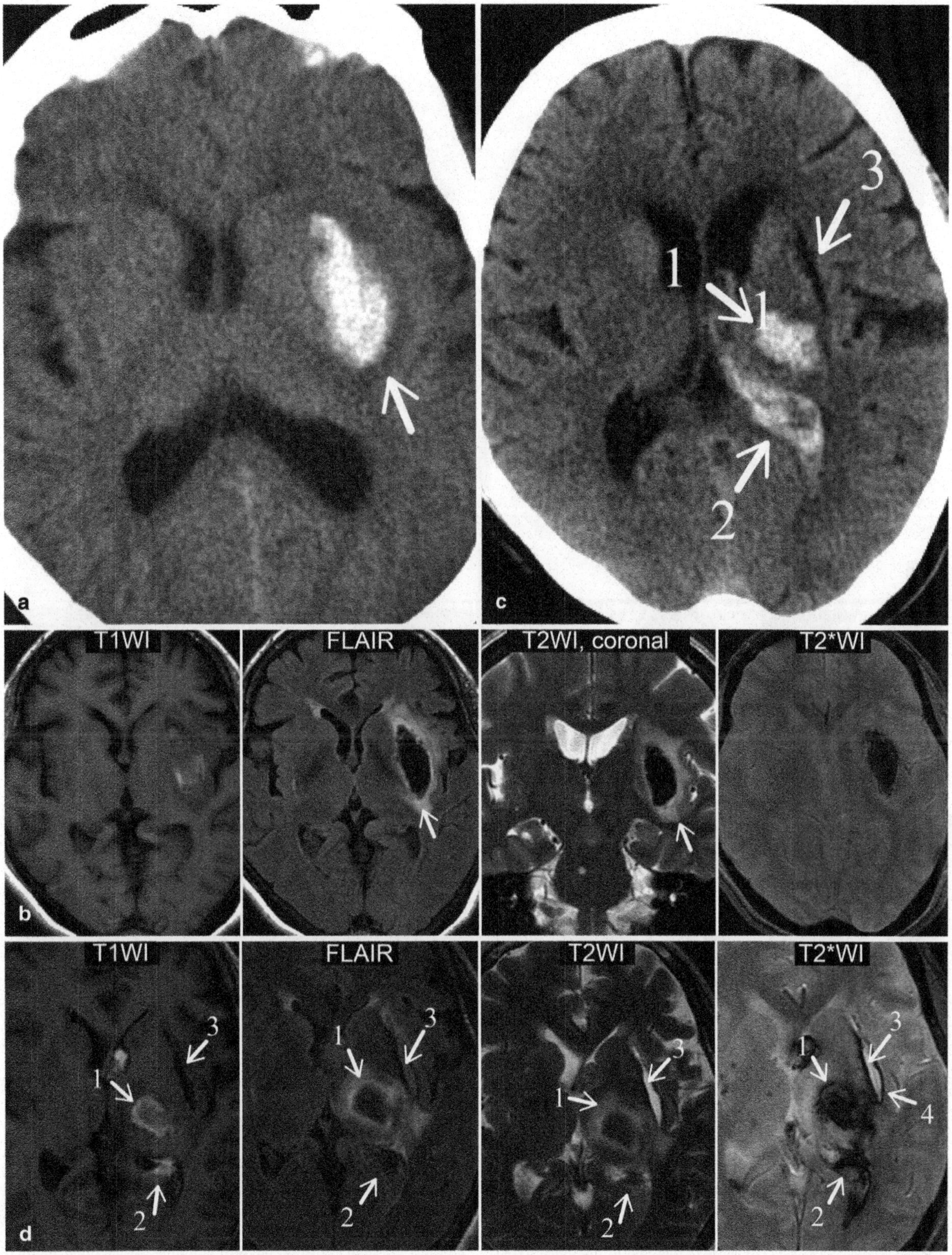

Fig. 4.6 F/52, Hypertensive putamen hemorrhage, and thalamic hemorrhage. Sudden onset of right-sided hemiplegia and dysphonia. (**a**) CT: An acute hematoma in left putamen shows homogeneous hyperdensity. (**b**) MRI on the second day: The hematoma appears isointense on T1WI, and hypointensity on FLAIR, T2WI, and T2*WI; the hematoma contains deoxyhemoglobin at this time. (**c**) Two years later, another stroke. CT shows an acute hematoma in the left thalamus (1), which has ruptured into the left lateral ventricle (2). The linear cavitary lesion in left putamen (3) is a sequela of previous ICH. (**d**) Eight days later, MRI was performed: The hematoma appears hyperintense on T1WI (1) and hypointense on T2WI, FLAIR, and T2*WI. The peripheral brain tissue edema is apparent. At this time, the hematoma is in the early subacute stage, which contains intracellular methemoglobin. The sequela lesion in left putamen mainly contains fluid, showing hyperintensity (3), and with rim hemosiderin deposition (4). Still, some residual IVH (2)

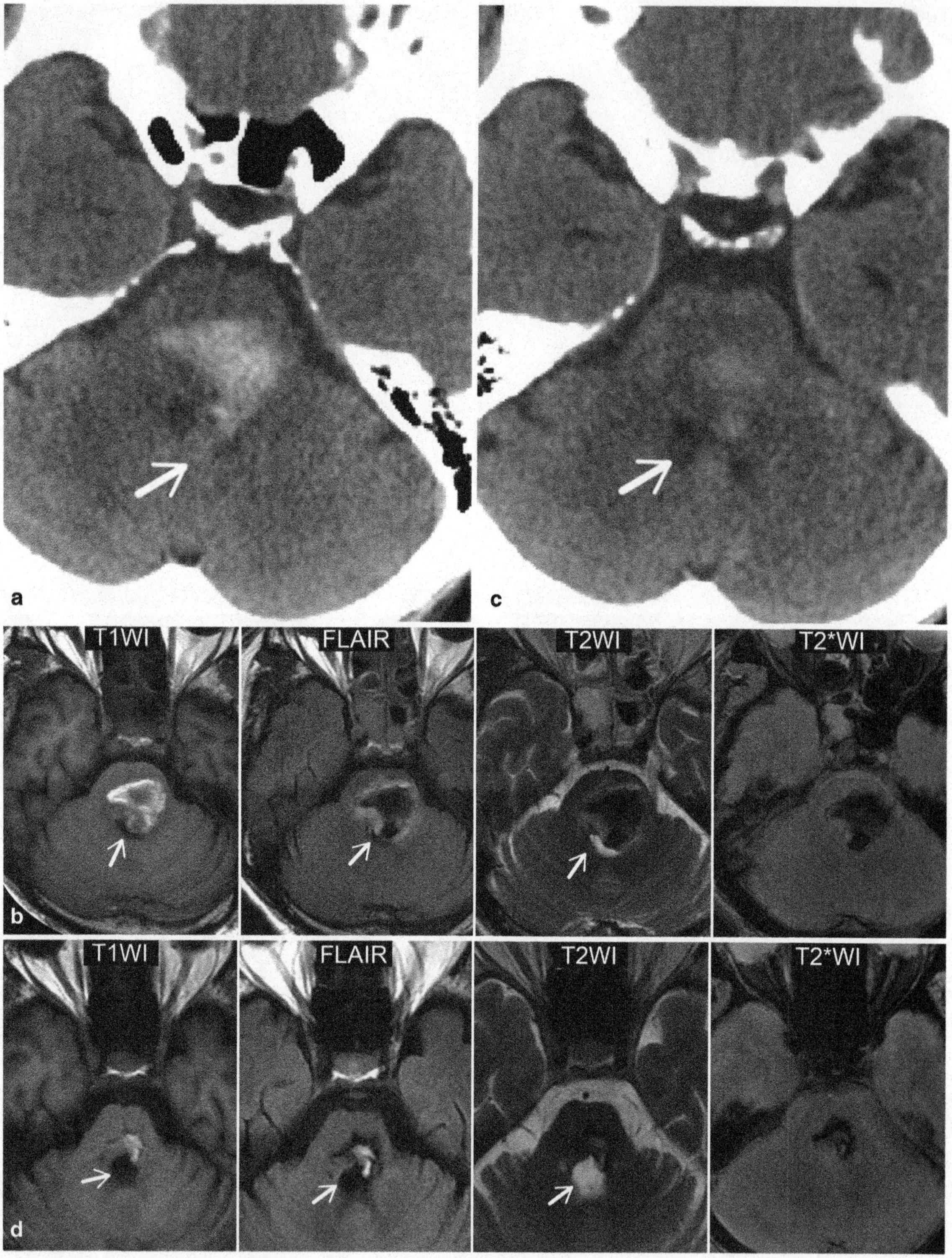

Fig. 4.7 M/52, Pontine hemorrhage caused by hypertension. Sudden loss of consciousness. (**a**) CT: An acute hematoma in the pons, hyperdense. (**b**) MRI was done on the fifth day; the hematoma is in the early subacute stage. At this time, T1WI is white (hyperintense), and dark (hypointense) on FLAIR, T2WI, and T2*WI, because the hematoma contains intracellular methemoglobin. A small circle of edema surrounds the hematoma; the edema is white (hyperintense) on T2WI and FLAIR. (**c**) CT on 16th day: The hematoma is gradually absorbed; the middle is gray, and the rest is darker. (**d**) MRI after 2 months: The blood clot has gradually shrunk, but still contains extracellular methemoglobin, which is white (hyperintense) on all pulse sequences. The periphery of the hematoma contains hemosiderin at this time, so it is dark on FLAIR, T2WI, and T2*WI, and there is no more edema around the hematoma. (**e**) Note: In (**a**), (**b**), and (**c**) the hematoma has a mass effect, the fourth ventricle (arrows) is compressed, and in (**d**), the hematoma shrunk, and the fourth ventricle (arrows) is slightly enlarged

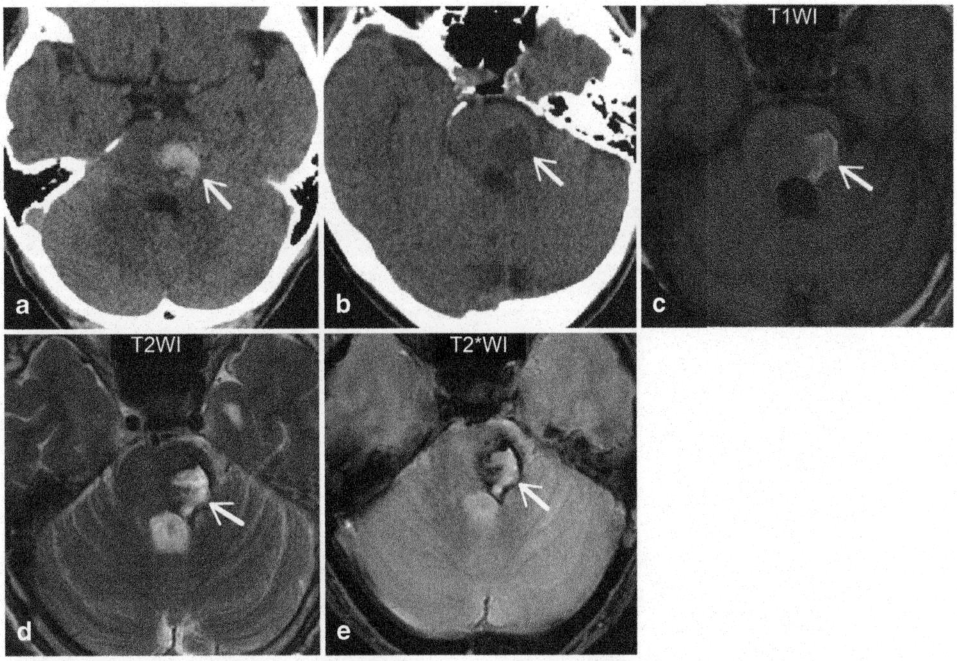

Fig. 4.8 F/61, Pontine hemorrhage caused by hypertension. (**a**) CT: an acute hematoma in the left side of pons (arrow). (**b**) CT, one and a half months later: The hematoma is in the late subacute stage, appearing hypodense (dark gray) (arrow), which is easily misconstrued as brain tissue edema. (**c**) MRI in T1WI, (**d**) T2WI, and (**e**) T2*WI: The hematoma shows hyperintensity in all pulse sequences (arrows), because the hematoma is in late subacute stage, containing extracellular methemoglobin. In T2WI and T2*WI, there is hemosiderin deposition in the periphery of the hematoma, showing rim hypointensity

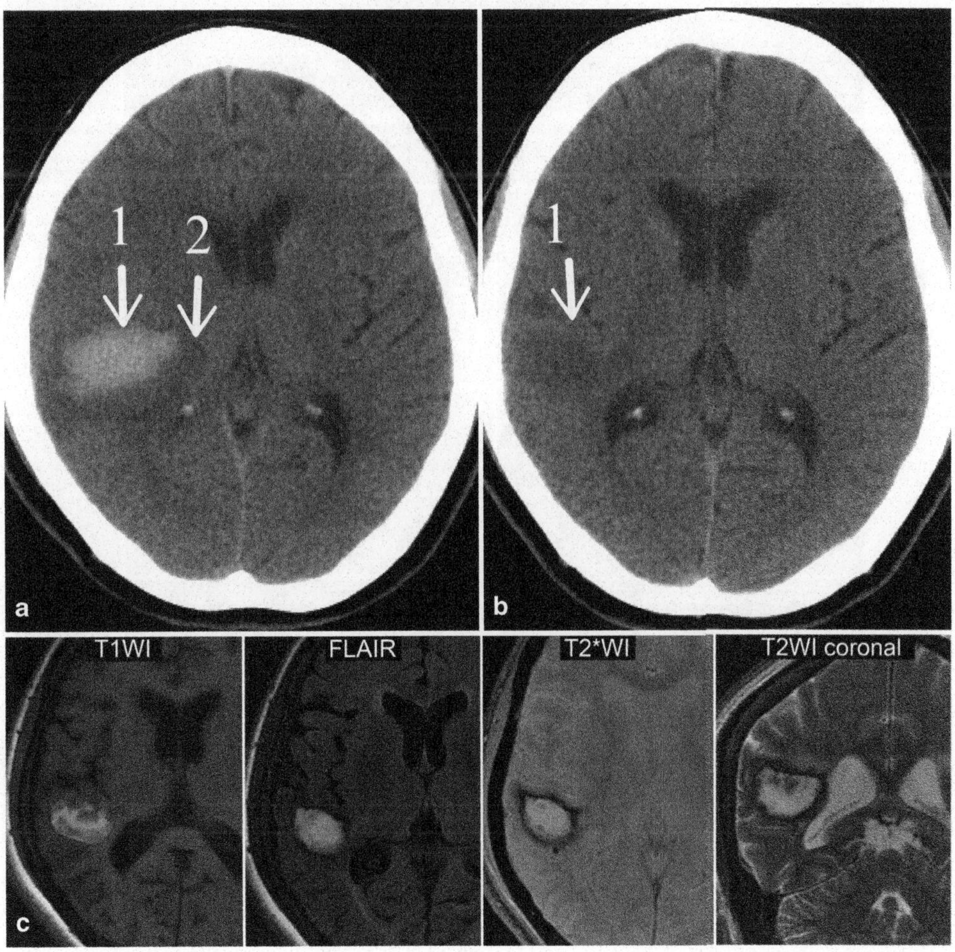

Fig. 4.9 F/52, Lobar hematoma due to hypertension. (**a**) CT, 7 days after stroke: A hematoma in the right temporal lobe (1); the hematoma is hyperdense (white), and there is peripheral brain tissue edema (2) because the hematoma is in resorption. (**b**) CT, 2 months later: The entire hematoma appears as mild hypodense (1), and is very similar to brain tissue edema. (**c**) MRI on the same day as CT: The hematoma is in late subacute stage, contains extracellular methemoglobin, showing hyperintensity in all pulse sequences, including T1WI, T2WI, FLAIR, and T2*WI. There is peripheral hemosiderin deposition showing hypointensity in T2WI and T2*WI

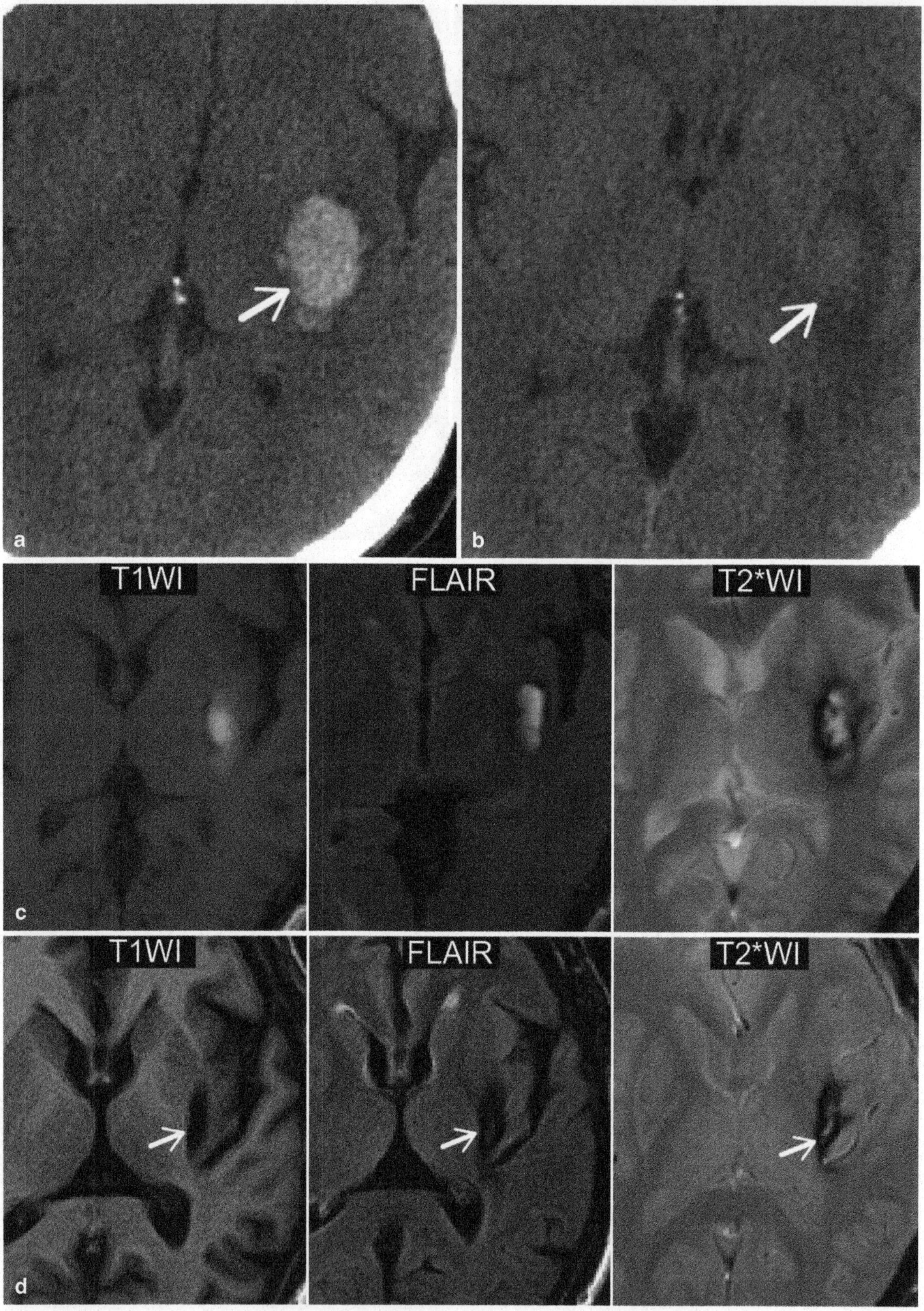

Fig. 4.10 M/59, Putaminal hemorrhage caused by hypertension. Sudden onset of right hemiparesis. (**a**) CT: An acute hematoma in left putamen appears as homogeneous hyperdensity (white). The mass effect is minimal, so no surgery was performed. (**b**) CT, 27 days later: The hematoma is in the late subacute stage, has changed to mild hypodense (gray-dark) (arrow), and is mixed with mild hyperdensity in the middle (gray). (**c**) MRI, 40th day: The hematoma is in the late subacute stage, showing hyperintensity (white) in T1WI, FLAIR, and T2*WI, and mainly contains extracellular methemoglobin. In T2*WI, the periphery of the hematoma is dark because of hemosiderin deposition. (**d**) MRI, a half year later: Chronic stage of the hematoma appears as a linear cavity in T1WI, and also dark in FLAIR and T2*WI because of hemosiderin deposition

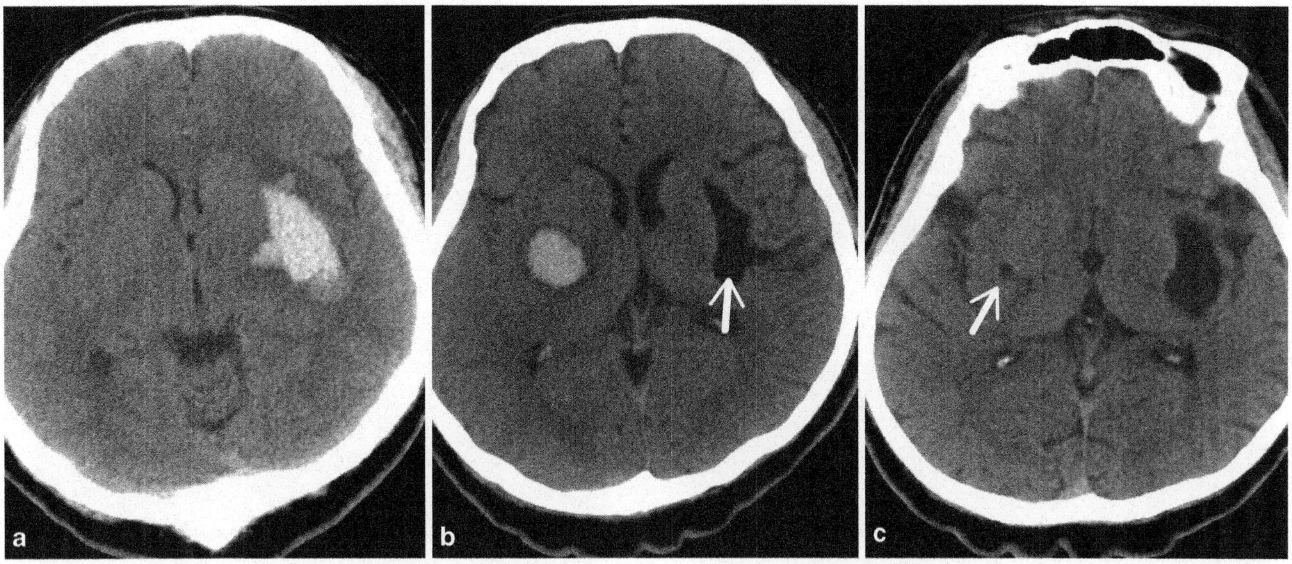

Fig. 4.11 M/49, Two putaminal hemorrhages due to hypertension. (**a**) CT: An acute hematoma in left putamen, appearing as homogeneous hyperdense (white); conservative treatment. (**b**) Six years later, another stroke occurred; CT shows a small acute hematoma in the right putamen. The previous left putaminal hematoma changed into a linear cavity (arrow); the cavity is broader because it may be connected to the sulcus, allowing the CSF to enter and exit. (**c**) One year later, follow-up CT: The right putaminal hematoma has changed into a small cavity

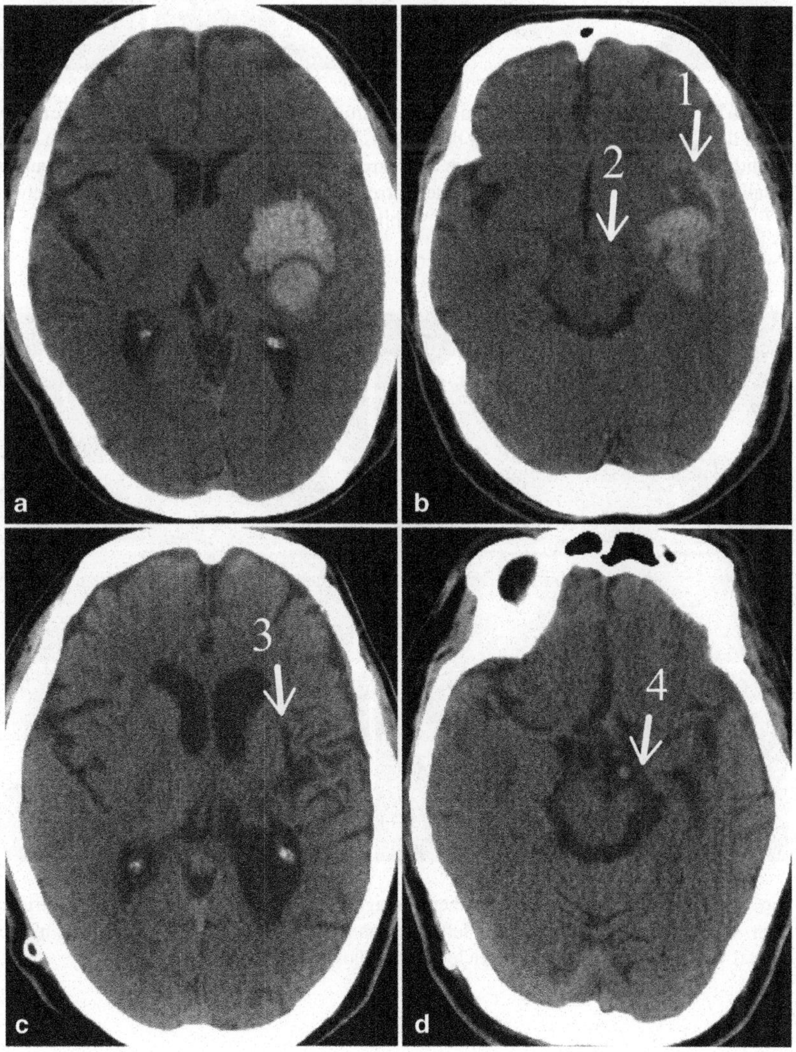

Fig. 4.12 M/56, Hypertensive putaminal hemorrhage, causing Wallerian degeneration. (**a, b**) CT: An acute hematoma in left putamen; the hematoma ruptured into the left Sylvian fissure (1). At this time, the bilateral cerebral peduncles of the midbrain are symmetrical (2), and the left lateral ventricle is smaller than the right lateral ventricle because it is compressed by the putaminal hematoma. This patient had persistent right-side hemiplegia after this stroke. (**c, d**) CT 6 years later: The previous putaminal hematoma has changed into a linear cavity (3) with peripheral brain tissue atrophy causing dilatation of left lateral ventricle. Significant atrophy of left cerebral peduncle of the midbrain (4) due to Wallerian degeneration

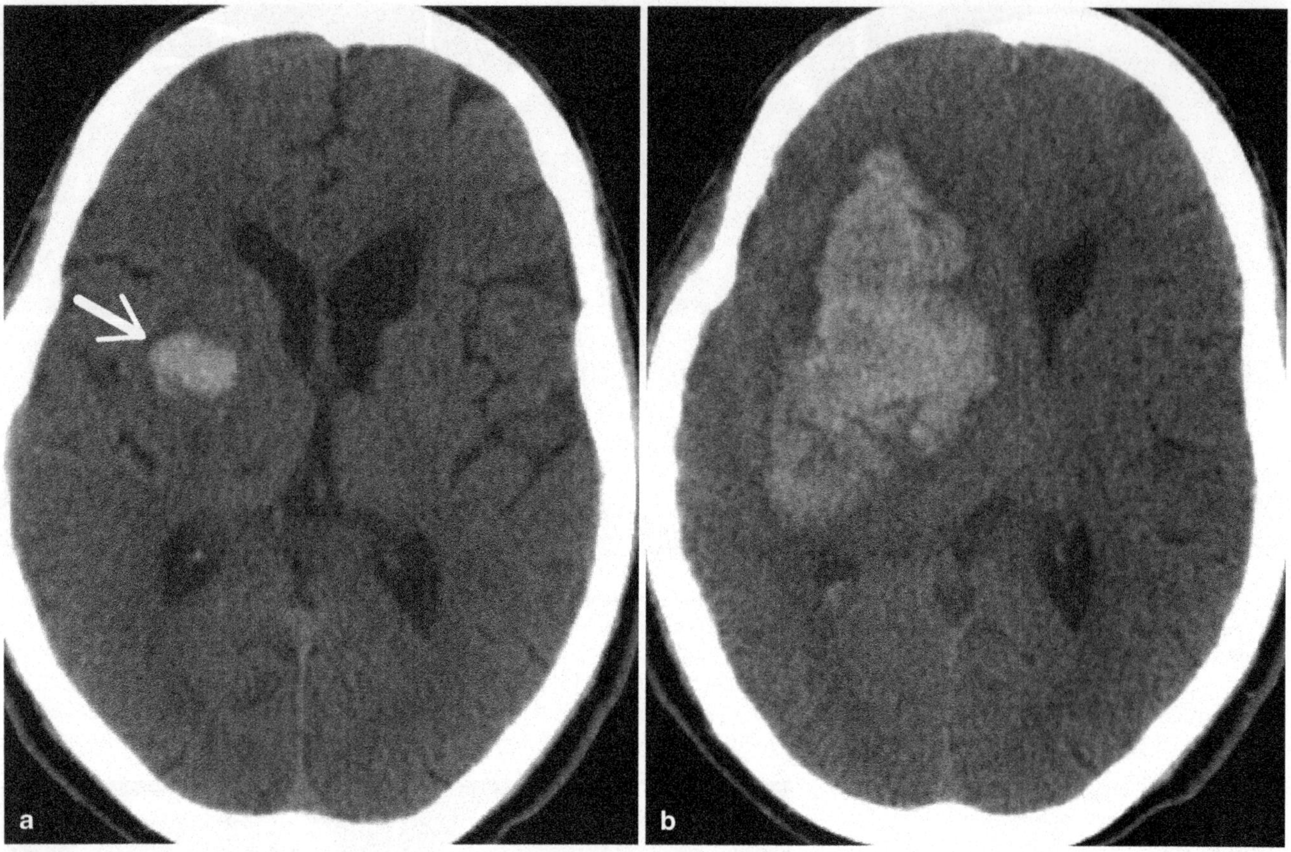

Fig. 4.13 M/59, Hypertensive hemorrhagic stroke, rebleeding in a short time. The patient suddenly felt that his left limbs were numb and slightly weak. CT performed about 4 h after stroke. (**a**) CT: showing a small acute hematoma in the right putamen (arrow). (**b**) Two hours after CT, the patient's left side was suddenly wholly paralyzed, along with loss of consciousness. When another urgent CT was performed, it was found that the putaminal hematoma had become very large. Note that this is putamen rebleeding due to hypertension, instead of continuous bleeding between secondary CT

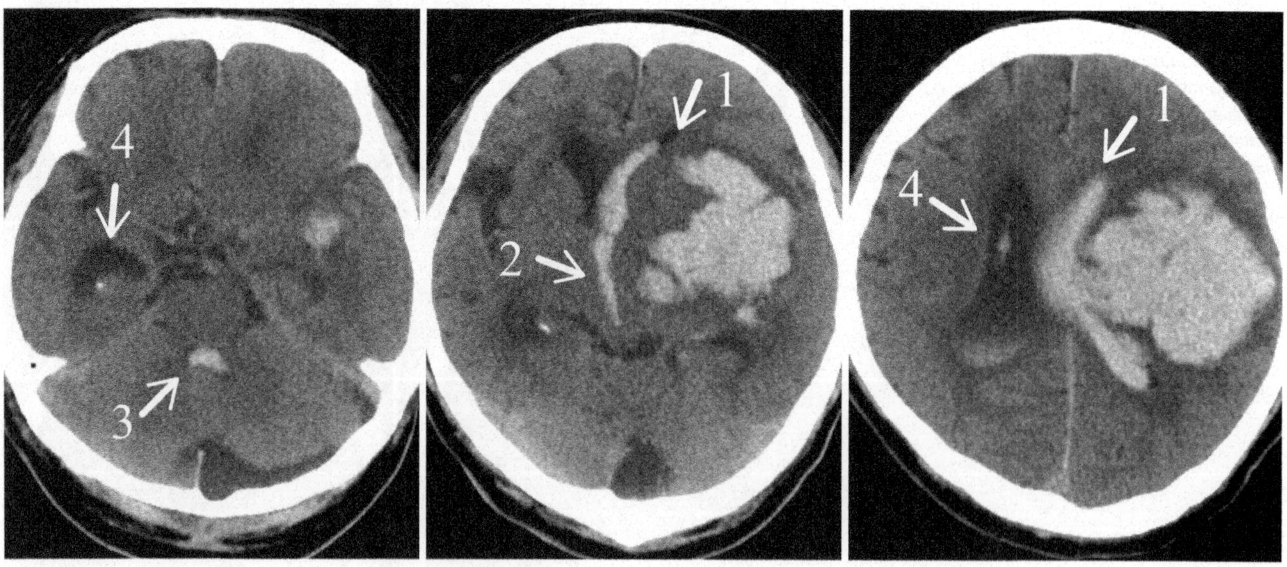

Fig. 4.14 M/50, Putaminal massive hemorrhage caused by hypertension. CT: A big acute hematoma in left putamen ruptures into the left lateral ventricle (1) and third ventricle (2), and flowing down into the fourth ventricle (3). The contralateral lateral ventricle is dilated (4), representing hydrocephalus

Fig. 4.15 F/83, Fall with scalp swelling after stroke. This older woman was found to have fallen; her scalp was swollen and bleeding, so CT was done with head trauma. (**a**) CT, axial; (**b**) CT, coronal: A big acute hematoma in left putamen; the left lateral ventricle is compressed and shrunken (arrow). Although there is a severe swelling of the scalp (s) caused by head trauma, this putaminal hemorrhage cannot be caused by the head trauma, so it can be surmised that she first had a stroke accompanied by limb weakness, causing her to fall, resulting in head trauma

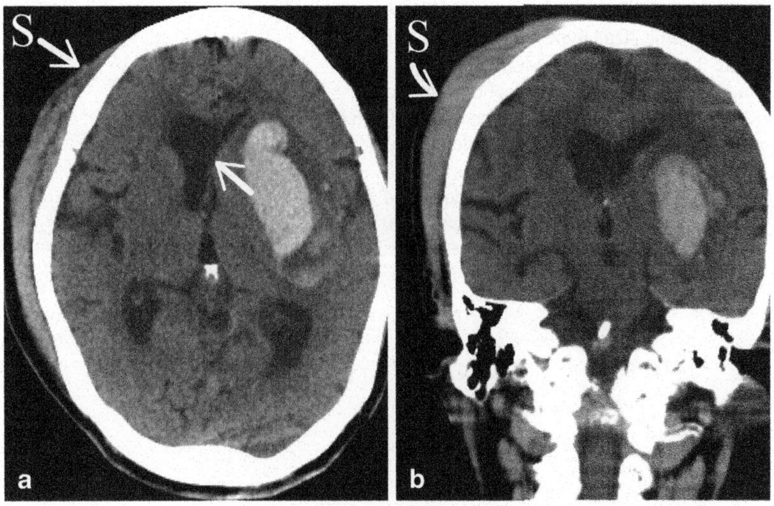

Fig. 4.16 F/88, Thalamic hemorrhage, caused by hypertension. CT: An acute hematoma in left thalamus (1), which has ruptured into the third ventricle (2). There are calcifications in the bilateral globus pallidus (3) and the pineal gland (4); all are physiological calcifications, not to be mistaken as hematomas

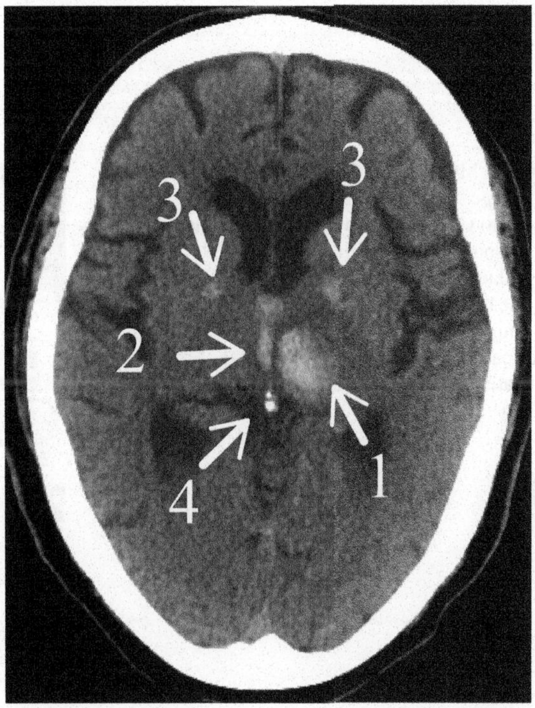

Fig. 4.17 M/65, Repeat thalamic hemorrhages. A hypertension patient suddenly felt numbness of the right face and right hand. (**a**) CT: A small acute hematoma in left thalamus (1); this is a typical hypertensive hemorrhage. Two old lacunar infarctions are seen in the bilateral putamen (2). After 5 h, the patient suddenly suffered right-sided hemiplegia and unconsciousness. (**b**) CT: the left thalamic hematoma enlarged (3) and ruptured into the lateral ventricle (4). This is a repeat hemorrhage caused by hypertension

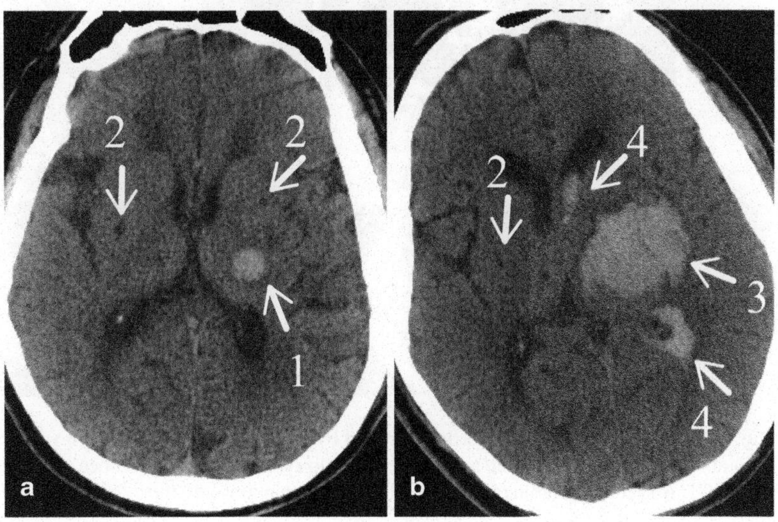

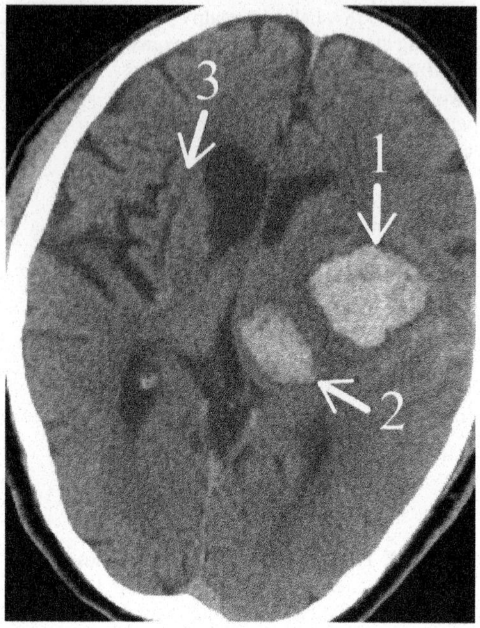

Fig. 4.18 M/60, Putamen, thalamus bleeding at the same time. This hypertension patient had a stroke 3 years ago, caused left hemiplegia. This time he suffered a sudden onset of right-sided hemiplegia. CT: Two acute hematomas in the left putamen (1) and thalamus (2), which are typical hypertensive hemorrhages. There is a linear cavity (3) in the right putamen, a sequela of a previous hematoma (the stroke 3 years ago)

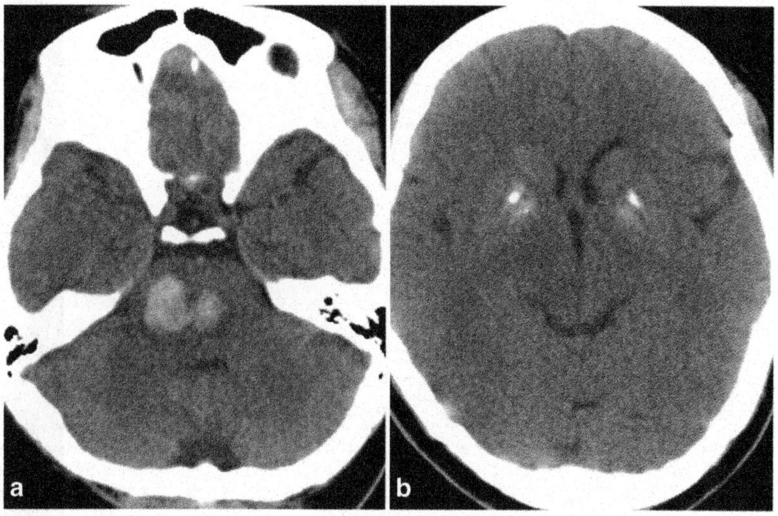

Fig. 4.19 M/41, Hypertensive pontine hemorrhage. Sudden coma in a hypertensive patient. (**a**) CT: Two acute hematomas in the pons. A spontaneous pontine hemorrhage is always due to hypertension; there is usually only one hematoma, but this patient has two. (**b**) Symmetrical calcifications in the bilateral globus pallidus, which are physiological calcifications, and should not be mistaken for bleeding

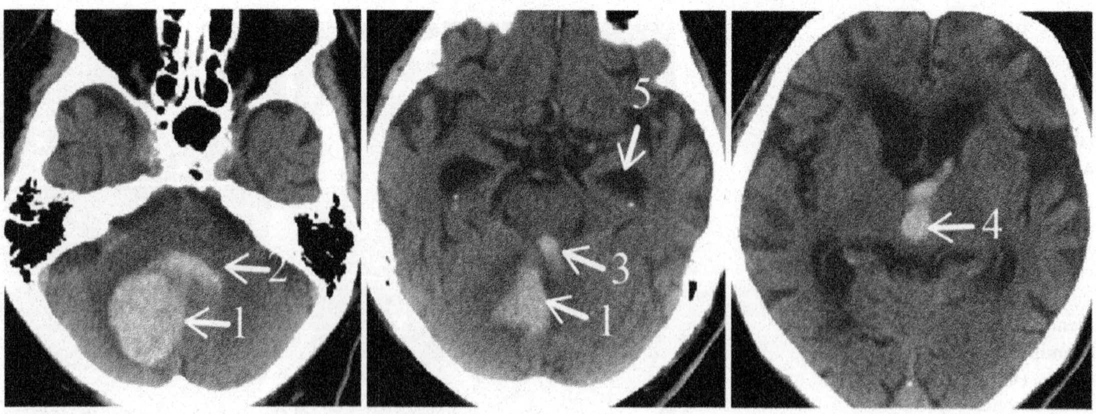

Fig. 4.20 M/85, Cerebellar hemorrhage caused by hypertension. The patient waked up in the morning and felt severely dizzy, nauseous, and weak. CT: An acute hematoma in right cerebellum (1), ruptures into the fourth ventricle (2), flowing up into the third ventricle (4) via the aqueduct (3), causing hydrocephalus. Dilatation of the bilateral temporal horns (5), indicating hydrocephalus

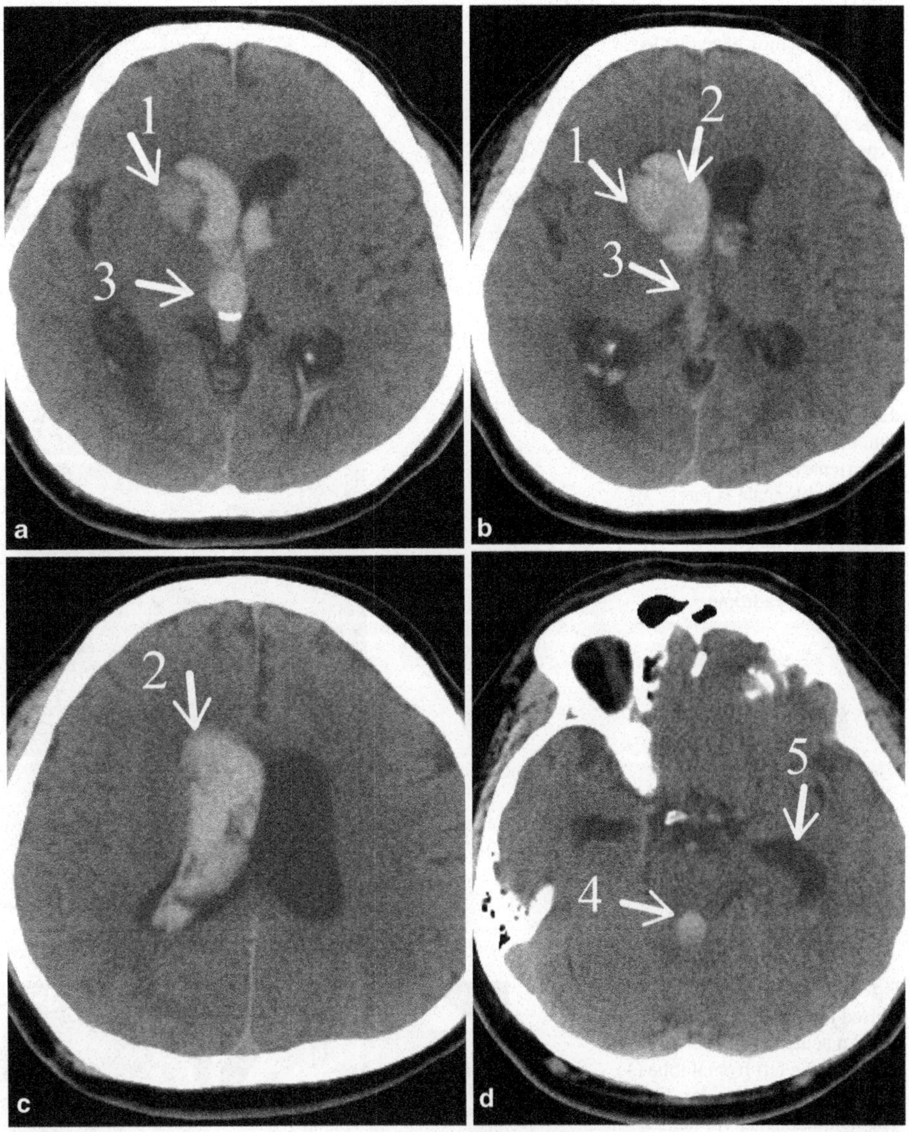

Fig. 4.21 M/35, Caudate nucleus hemorrhage due to hypertension. (**a–d**) CT: An acute hematoma in the right caudate nucleus (1), ruptured into the right lateral ventricle (2) and third ventricle (3), and flowing down into the aqueduct (4). Dilatation of bilateral temporal horns (5), indicating hydrocephalus

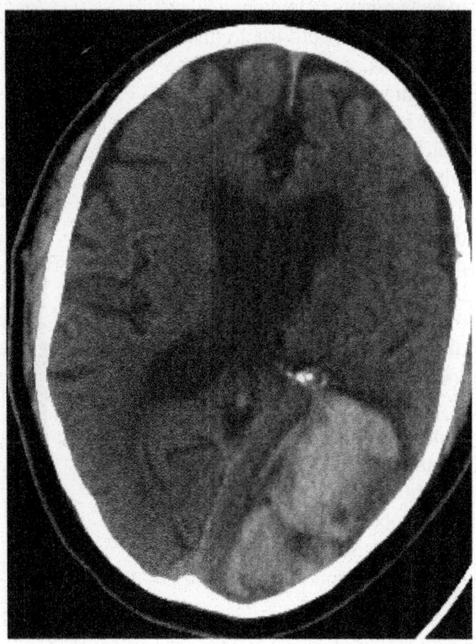

Fig. 4.22 M/86, Lobar hemorrhage caused by hypertension. Sudden onset of blurred vision, headache, and right limb weakness. Hemorrhagic stroke was suspected. CT: Big acute hematoma in the subcortex of the left occipital lobe due to hypertension. Hypertension causing this kind of lobar hemorrhage is relatively rare

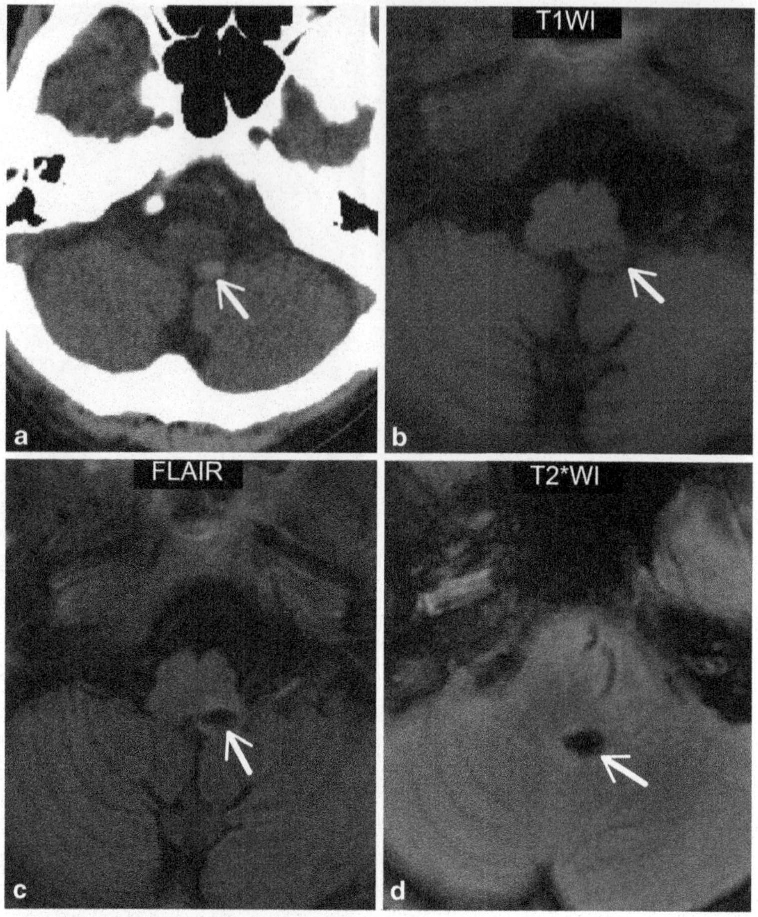

Fig. 4.23 M/55, Medulla oblongata hemorrhage due to hypertension. A hypertensive patient with dizziness and unsteady gait. (**a**) CT: A small hyperdense lesion in the left inferior cerebellar peduncle of the medulla oblongata, suggesting an acute hematoma. (**b–d**) MRI was immediately performed: This lesion is isointense at T1WI and not easily recognized. It appears hypointense in FLAIR and T2*WI, so this is definitely an acute hematoma containing deoxyhemoglobin. Hypertensive hemorrhage in medulla oblongata is rare. Hemorrhage or infarction in the inferior cerebellar peduncle may cause Wallenberg syndrome

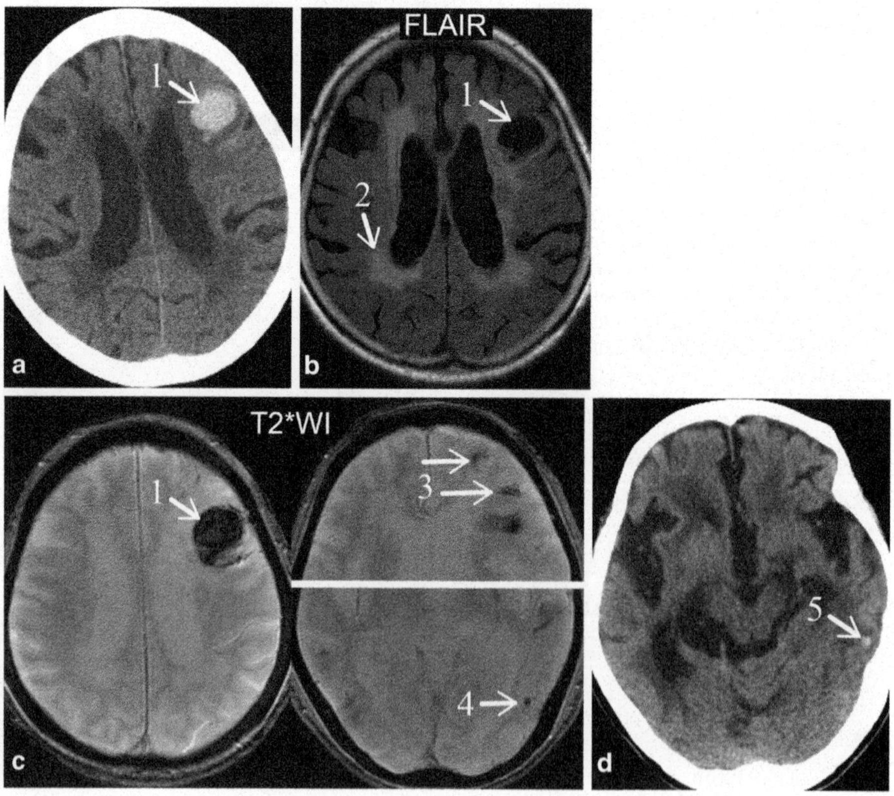

Fig. 4.24 F/86, Lobar hemorrhage caused by amyloid angiopathy. (**a**) CT: An acute hematoma in the cortex of the left frontal lobe (1). (**b**) MRI on the same day, FLAIR: The hematoma is hypointense (dark) (1). The periventricular hyperintensity is leukoaraiosis (2). (**c**) T2*WI: In addition to this acute hematoma, which appears hypointense (1), there are also two other small hypointense lesions, which are possibly old hematomas with hemosiderin deposition (3). There is another microbleed (4) in the left parietal lobe. Surgery was performed to remove the acute hematoma, and pathology confirmed that amyloid angiopathy is the cause of this acute hematoma. (**d**) A follow-up CT was performed 2 years later, revealing a small hemorrhage in the cortex of the left temporal lobe (5). For the elderly patient who has repeat hemorrhages in the lobar cortex, amyloid angiopathy should be suspected, rather than hypertension

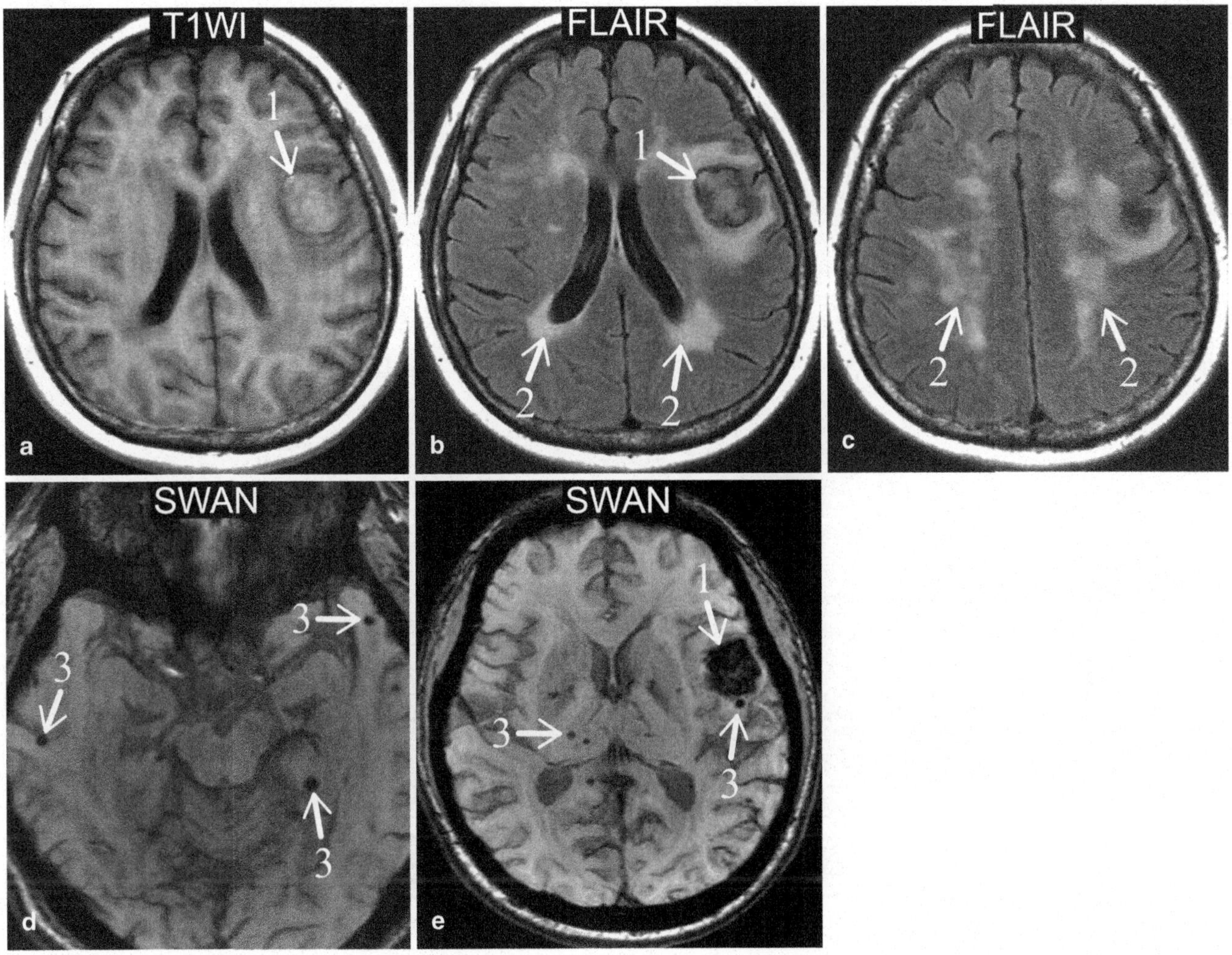

Fig. 4.25 F/50, Amyloid angiopathy causing lobar hemorrhage and microbleeds. The patient suddenly had weakness in the right limbs, and MRI was performed on the second day. (**a**) T1WI: A small acute intracerebral hematoma (ICH) (1) in the cortex of the left frontal lobe, showing isointense on T1WI. (**b**) FLAIR: The ICH (1) showing hypointense in FLAIR, and with peripheral brain tissue edema. There is periventricular hyperintensity (PVH) (2); the PVH is a kind of leukoaraiosis. (**c**) FLAIR, there are subcortical white matter hyperintensities (2) in the bilateral centrum semiovale; these are also leukoaraiosis. (**d, e**) SWAN: The ICH is showing hypointensity (1). In addition to this lobar hematoma, there are many microbleeds (3); some are in the lobar cortex, some in the thalamus. After surgical removal of the lobar ICH, the pathology confirmed amyloid angiopathy. According to reference, the microbleeds in the lobar cortex are also caused by amyloid angiopathy

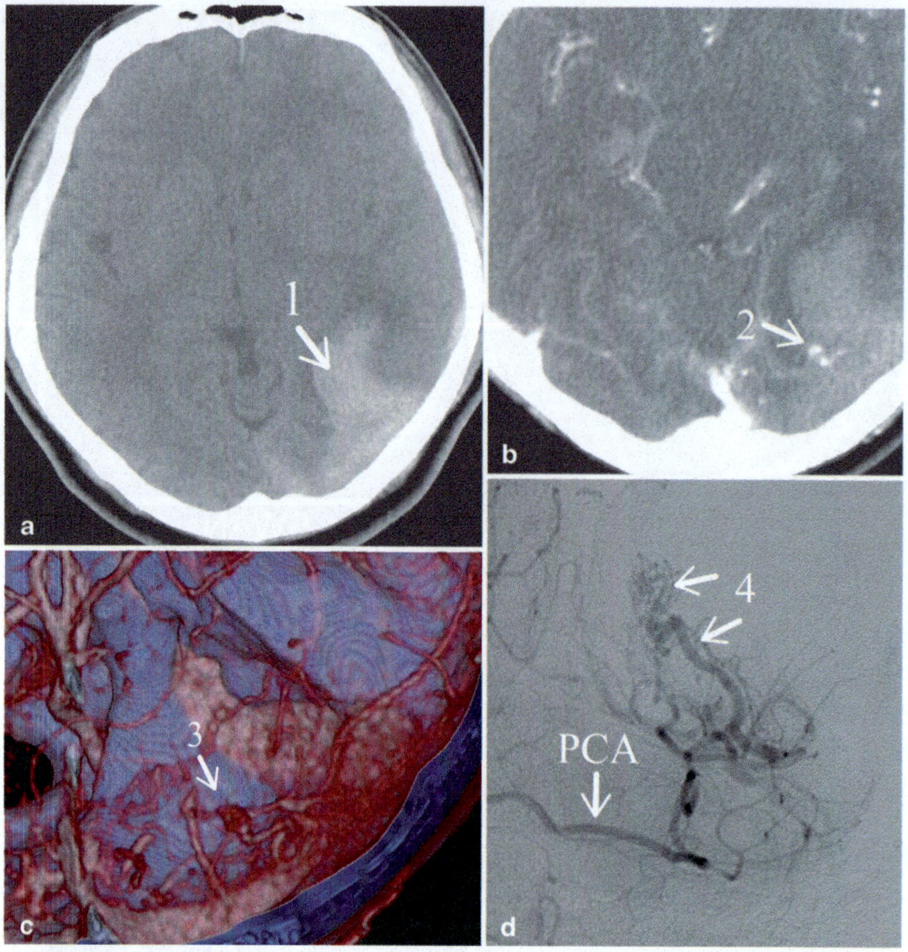

Fig. 4.26 M/27, AVM bleeding. The patient suffered a sudden severe headache. (**a**) CT: An acute intracerebral hematoma (ICH) (1) in the left occipital lobe. (**b**) CTA source image: Some slightly dilated small blood vessels (2) can be seen, suspected to be AVM. (**c**) CTA: There are abnormally dilated vessels (3) in the ICH, suspected to be AVM (3). (**d**) DSA: confirms this is a small AVM (4) supplied by the PCA

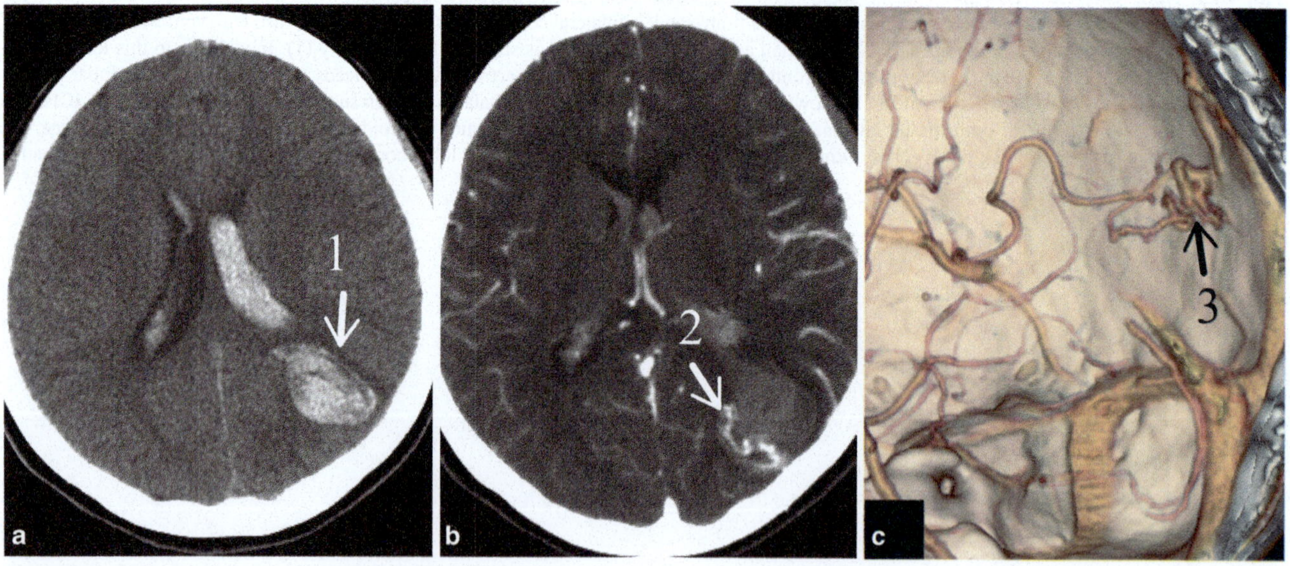

Fig. 4.27 F/15, AVM bleeding. The patient suddenly suffered a severe headache, vomiting. (**a**) CT: An acute intracerebral hematoma (ICH) (1) in left parieto-occipital lobes and ruptures into the lateral ventricles. (**b**) CTA, source image: Visible abnormal blood vessels (2) in the ICH; since this is a young stroke, it is likely AVM. (**c**) CTA: There are abnormally dilated vessels in the ICH, suspected to be AVM (3). Because the ICH is in a superficial position, so, without further angiography study, the neurosurgeon directly did craniotomy to remove the ICH and the AVM

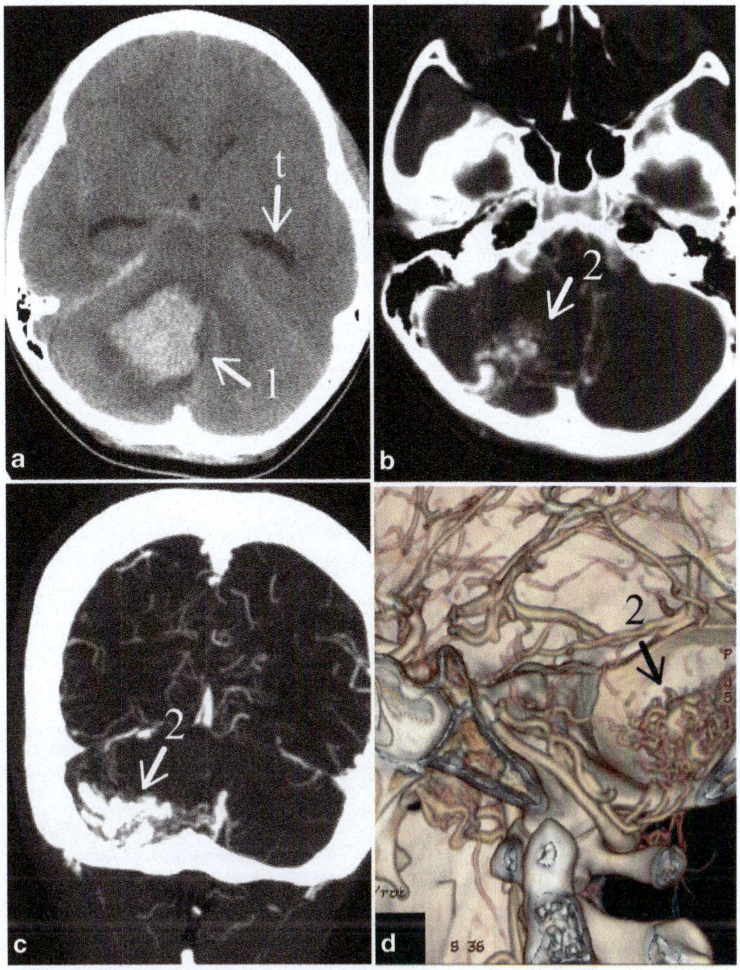

Fig. 4.28 F/15, A big AVM caused cerebellar hemorrhage. The patient suddenly suffered severe headache, vomiting, and then went into a coma. (**a**) CT: An acute hematoma (1) in the right cerebellum, which compresses the fourth ventricle and the aqueduct, causing obstructive hydrocephalus. The bilateral temporal horns (t) are dilated, representing hydrocephalus. (**b, c**) Source images of CTA: Axial (**b**) and coronal views (**c**) show a cluster of irregularly expanding blood vessels (2), presenting the so-called bag of worms sign, which is a large AVM. (**d**) CTA: A cluster of abnormal vascularity (2), this is also a "bag of worms sign," which is AVM. Due to the urgent situation, the neurosurgeon did not require DSA and did craniotomy directly to remove the cerebellar hematoma and the huge AVM

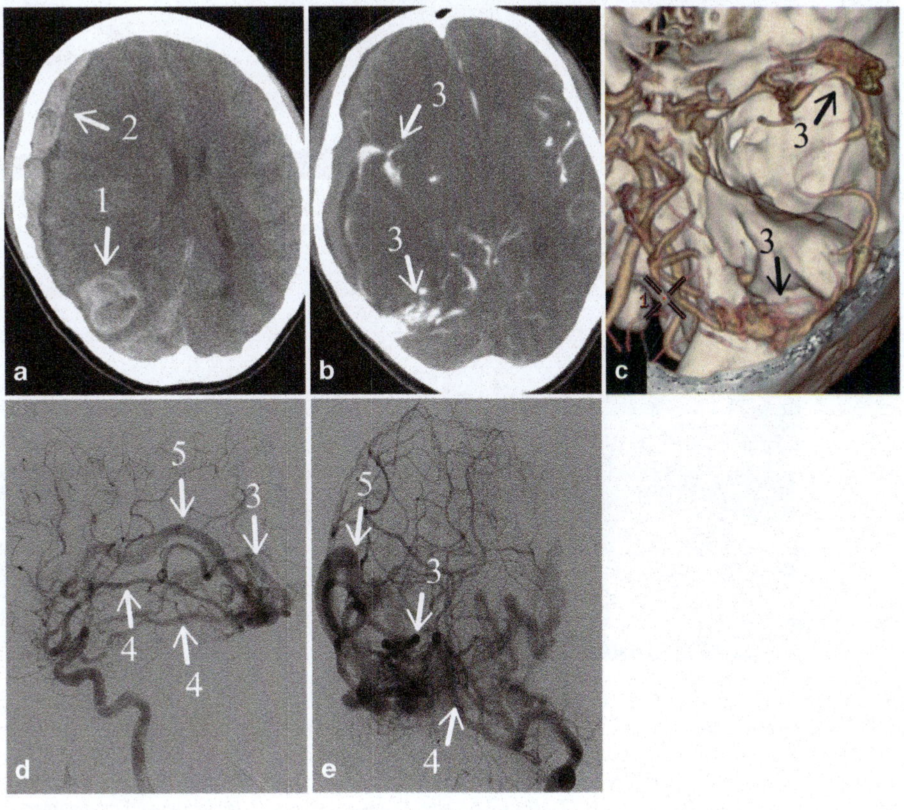

Fig. 4.29 F/17, A big AVM caused ICH and SDH. The patient suffered a sudden and severe headache and left-sided hemiparesis. (**a**) CT: An intracerebral hematoma (ICH) (1) in the right occipital lobe, and subdural hematoma (SDH) (2) outside the right cerebral hemisphere. (**b**) CTA source image: Abnormally dilated vessels (3), one is nearby the ICH, suspected to be AVM. (**c**) CTA: The same findings as to the above source image. (**d, e**) DSA, sagittal (**d**), and AP (**e**) views: A big AVM (3) in the right occipital lobe, the supplied arteries (4) and the drainage veins (5) have become very large

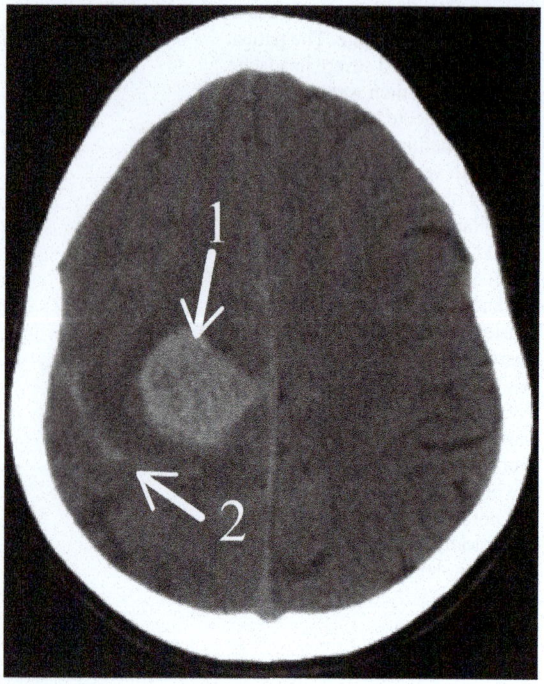

Fig. 4.30 F/29, VMOTA. A healthy lady, with sudden onset of severe headache and left limb weakness. CT: An acute hematoma (1) in the right parietal lobe, and with SAH in the peripheral sulci (2). Because this is a young stroke, digital subtraction angiography (DSA) was done, but no abnormal vascularity was detected (not shown). The patient had surgery to remove this hematoma. The pathologist found small arteriovenous malformation (AVM) in the hematoma microscopically. This kind of small vascular anomaly cannot be detected by angiography, which is called a VMOTA (vascular anomaly occult to angiography)

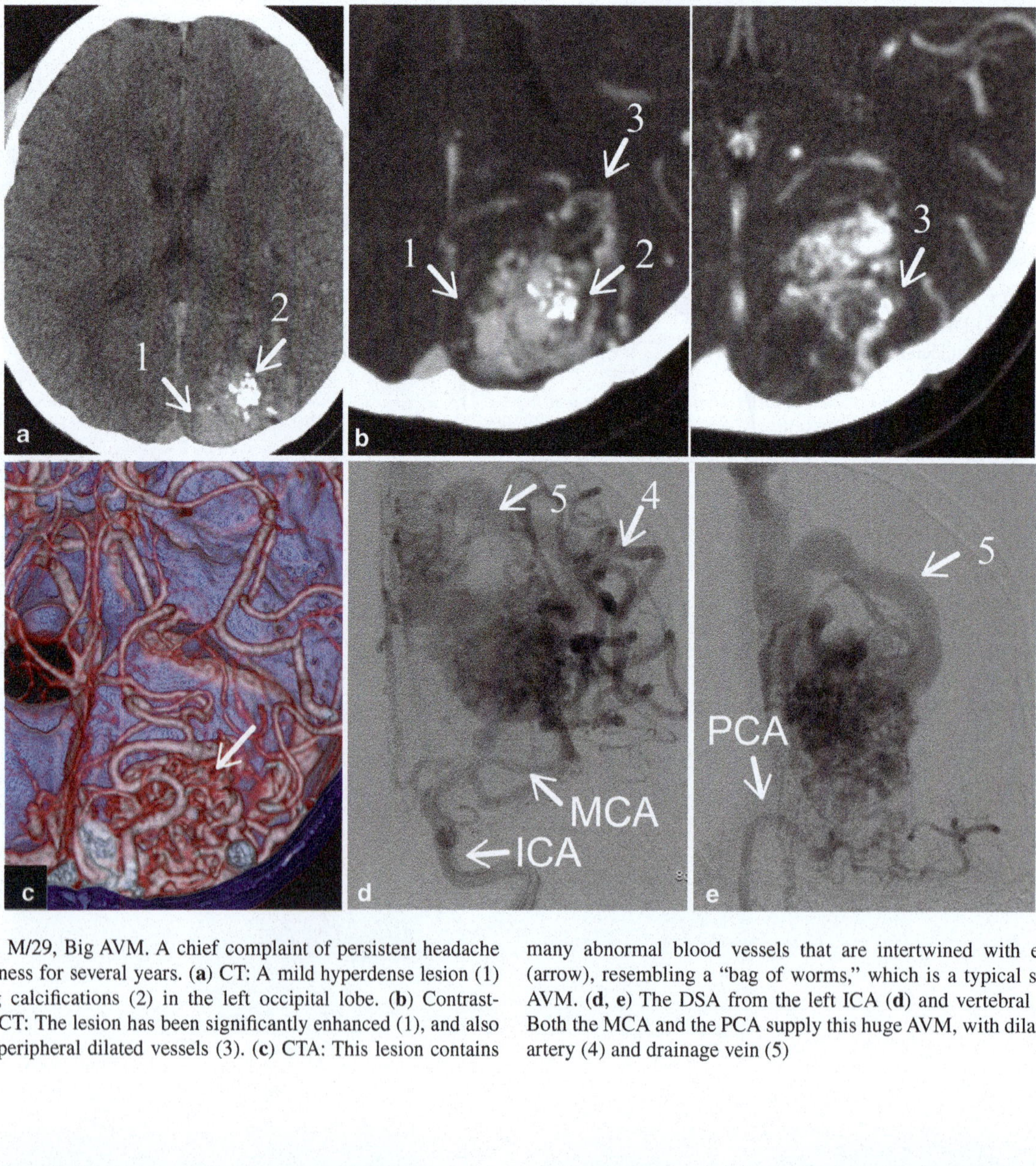

Fig. 4.31 M/29, Big AVM. A chief complaint of persistent headache with dizziness for several years. (**a**) CT: A mild hyperdense lesion (1) containing calcifications (2) in the left occipital lobe. (**b**) Contrast-enhanced CT: The lesion has been significantly enhanced (1), and also revealing peripheral dilated vessels (3). (**c**) CTA: This lesion contains many abnormal blood vessels that are intertwined with each other (arrow), resembling a "bag of worms," which is a typical sign for an AVM. (**d, e**) The DSA from the left ICA (**d**) and vertebral artery (**e**): Both the MCA and the PCA supply this huge AVM, with dilated supply artery (4) and drainage vein (5)

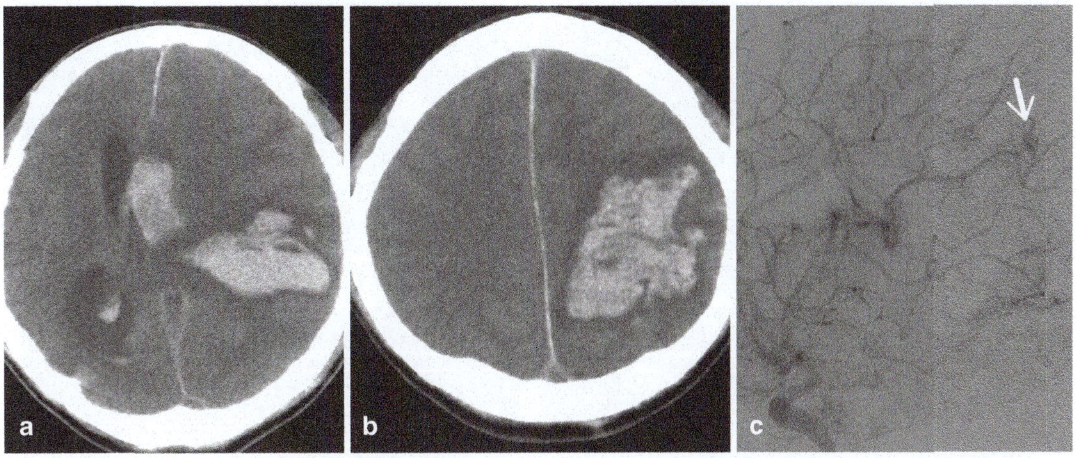

Fig. 4.32 M/49, Intracerebral hematoma due to rupture of a mycotic (infectious) aneurysm. A heart disease patient, sudden onset of right-sided hemiplegia, and coma. (**a**, **b**) CT: A big acute intracerebral hematoma (ICH) in the left frontal lobe and ruptures into the ventricles. This is an unusual location for an ICH and requires angiography to determine whether there is a vascular lesion? (**c**) DSA: An aneurysm (arrow) in the distal portion of the left middle cerebral artery (MCA). An aneurysm formed in the distal of the main intracranial artery, a mycotic aneurysm should be considered. It turned out that this patient has infectious endocarditis and has septicemia, and *Staphylococcus aureus* is cultured in blood. So, this aneurysm is a mycotic aneurysm arising from bacterial infection of the arterial wall

Fig. 4.33 F/83, Intracerebral hematoma caused by rupture of an aneurysm. Sudden and severe headache. (**a**, **b**) CT: A big acute intracerebral hematoma (ICH) in the corpus callosum. (**c**) Source image of CTA: An abnormally dilated vascularity within the ICH, which is suspected to be an aneurysm (arrow). (**d**) CTA: Confirms that this is an aneurysm (arrow) of the right anterior cerebral artery (ACA)

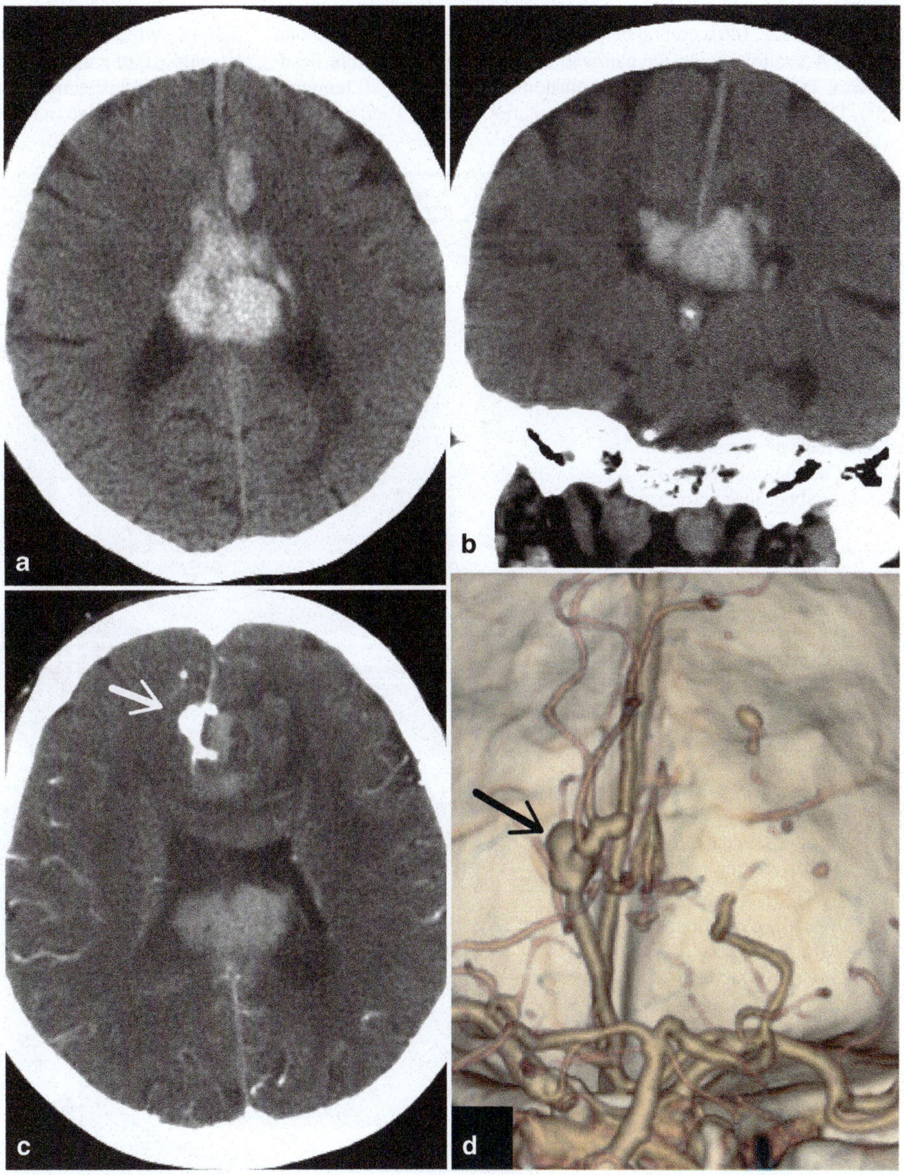

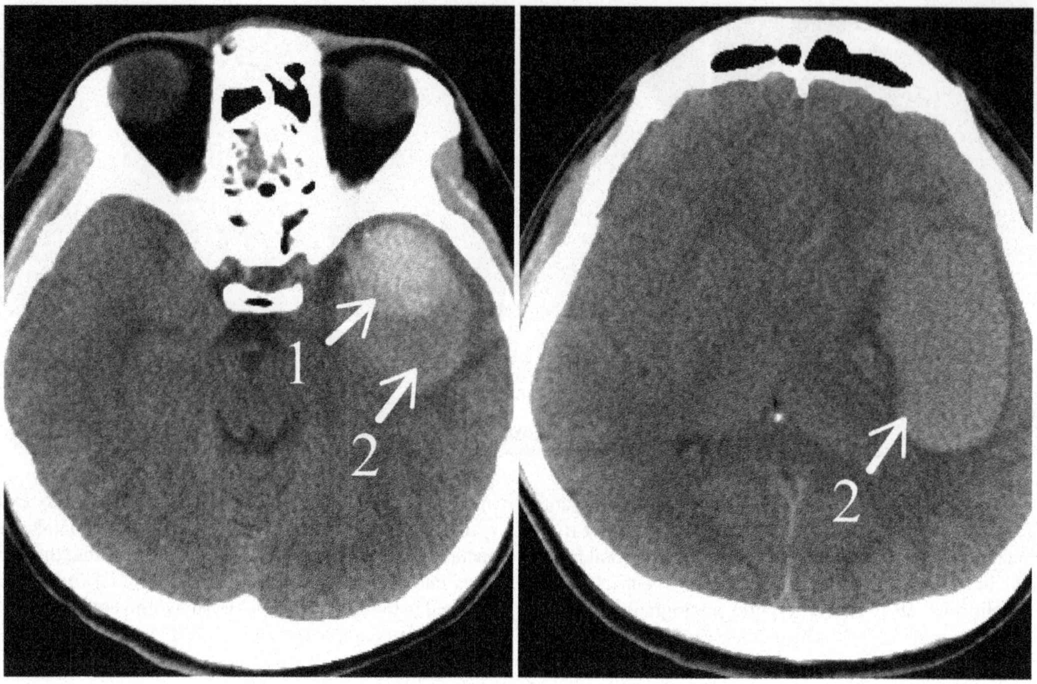

Fig. 4.34 F/22, Intracerebral hematoma caused by a cavernous hemangioma. A healthy young woman who suddenly suffered severe headaches. CT: An acute intracerebral hematoma (ICH) in the left temporal lobe. The blood clot has two different densities, white (1) and relatively gray (2), which may indicate two episodes of bleeding in a short time. No angiography was performed. After surgical removal of this ICH; the pathological inspection revealed that the cause of the bleeding was a cavernous hemangioma

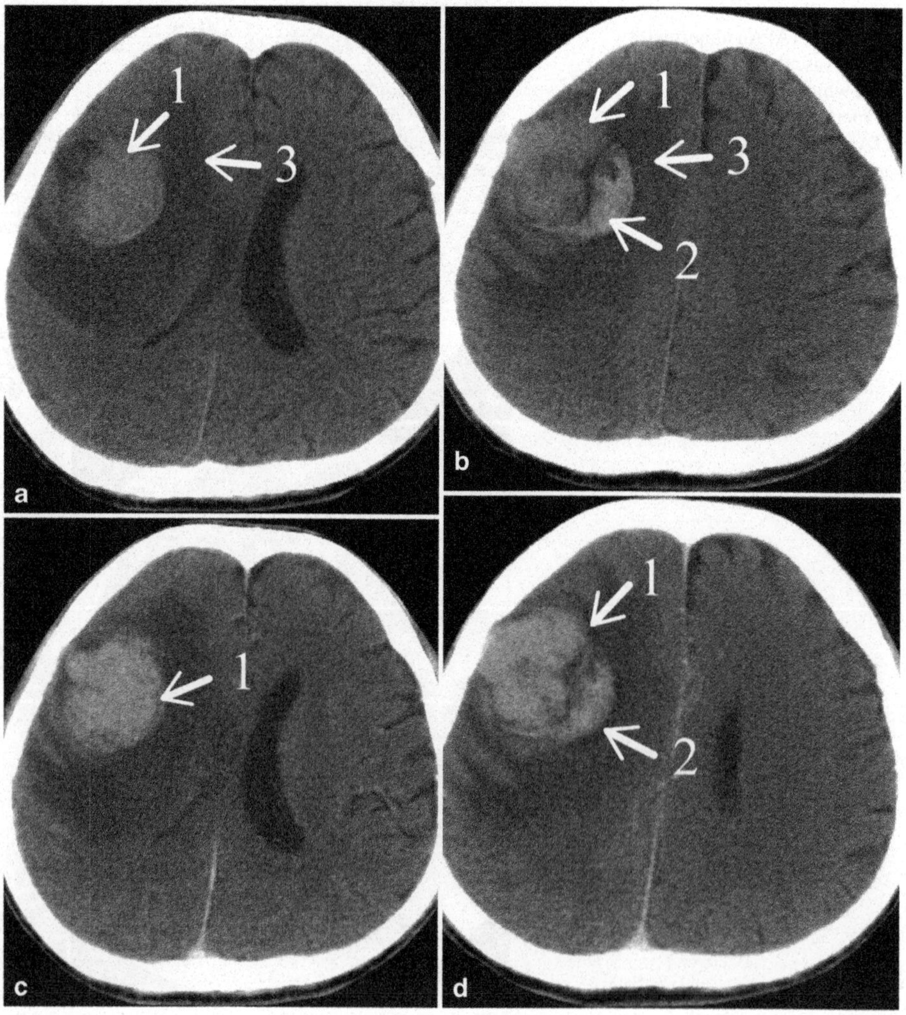

Fig. 4.35 M/54, Tumor bleeding. A patient with gastric cancer, sudden onset of left limb weakness, and severe headache. (**a**, **b**) CT: A large intracerebral hematoma (ICH) in the right frontal lobe (1, 2), accompanied by significant peripheral white matter edema (3). A new ICH should have no peripheral edema, so tumor bleeding is considered because before bleeding, a tumor always has peripheral brain tissue edema. (**c**, **d**) Contrast-enhanced CT: The ICH is enhanced and becomes whiter. A close comparison of (**b**) and (**d**) reveals that in (**b**), the ICH has two parts, which are gray (1) and white (2). After the contrast medium is injected, the two parts become all white. Therefore, the gray part (1) is enhanced to show a tumor plus bleeding, and the white part (2) is a pure hematoma. Surgical removal of the hematoma and pathology proved to be a metastatic tumor from gastric cancer, and with tumor bleeding

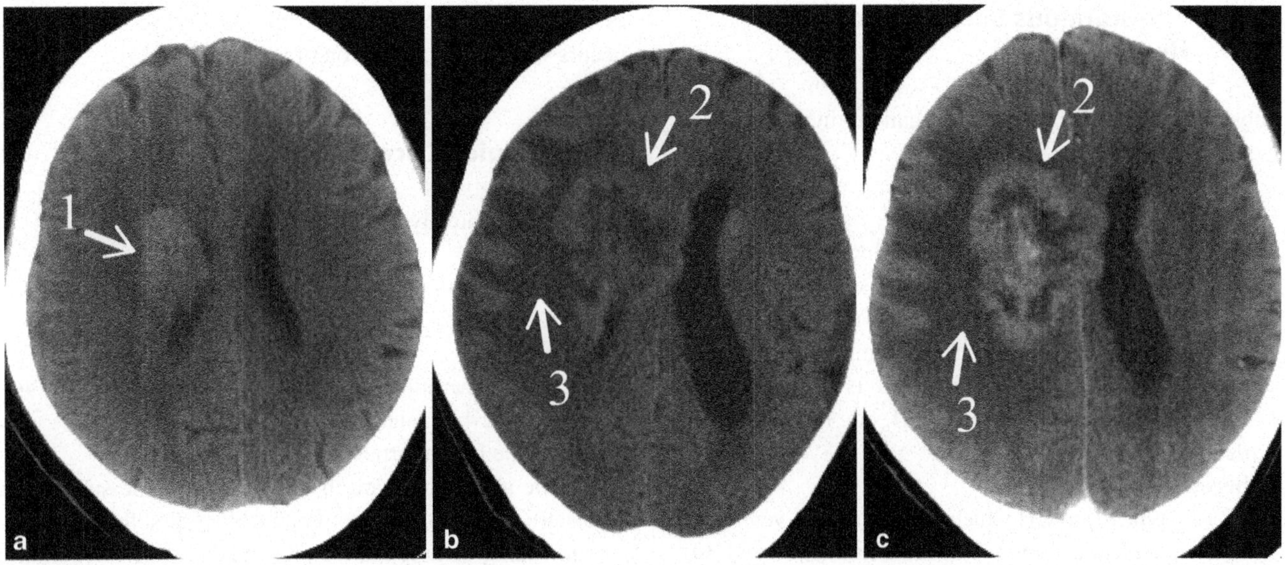

Fig. 4.36 F/78, Tumor bleeding. (**a**) The patient underwent CT for headache: A hematoma in the right caudate nucleus (1) beside the right lateral ventricle. Because the hematoma was not significant, no active interventional therapy was performed. After half a year, the patient felt more severe headaches and left-sided hemiparesis, and another CT was performed. (**b**) Plain CT: A tumor in the location of the previous bleeding site (2), with a large area of peripheral white matter edema (3). (**c**) Contrast-enhanced CT: The tumor is enhanced with irregular central necrosis (2), which is like a glioblastoma. Finally, surgery and pathology proved that this tumor is glioblastoma. So, the first CT showed that a hematoma in the right caudate nucleus was a tumor bleeding of this glioblastoma

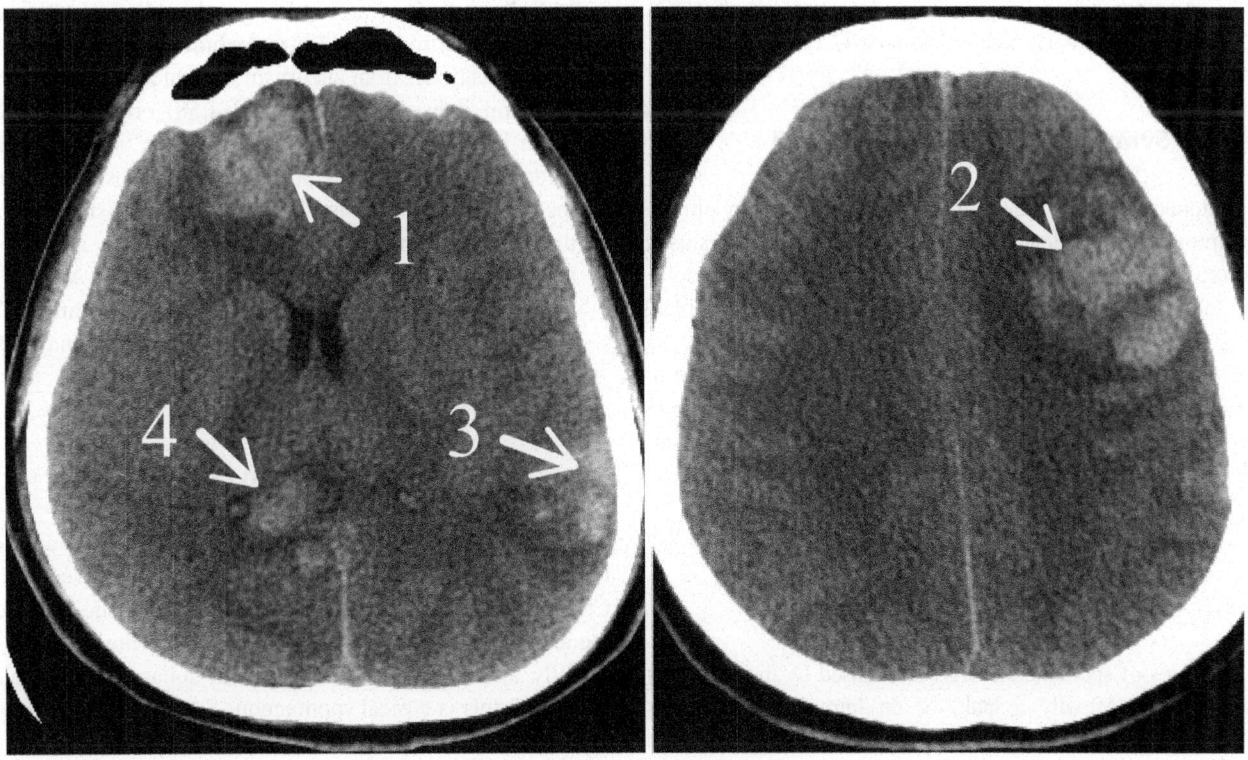

Fig. 4.37 M/38, Intracerebral hemorrhages caused by leukemia. A patient with acute myeloblastic leukemia (AML), who suffered a sudden onset of a seizure and coma. CT: Multiple intracerebral hematomas (ICHs) in the right frontal lobe (1), left frontal lobe (2), left parietal lobe (3), and the splenium of the corpus callosum (4)

4.3 Spontaneous Subarachnoid Hemorrhage

Subarachnoid hemorrhage (SAH) can be divided into three types:

1. **Traumatic SAH:**
   This type of SAH is usually located in the sulci, Sylvian fissures, interhemispheric fissure, or on the tentorial edge; it sometimes occurs in the suprasellar cistern and quadrigeminal cistern. Traumatic SAH results in noticeable scalp swelling and is often combined with brain contusion, EDH, SDH, etc. (see Chap. 3 for details)
2. **Secondary SAH:**
   This type is an ICH which breaks into the ventricles or other subarachnoid spaces (SAS) (Figs. 4.12 and 4.30).
3. **Spontaneous SAH or primary SAH:**
   This type of SAH occurs spontaneously, without head trauma, and without ICH. Especially when there is a large volume of bleeding in the suprasellar cistern, it may spread to other SASs; it often combined with IVH. This type of hemorrhagic stroke will be further discussed later in this section (Figs. 4.39–4.60, 4.62, 4.64, and 4.66).
   Another primary intraventricular hemorrhage (IVH) (Fig. 4.68) is also a type of primary SAH, which is rare.

4.3.1 Symptoms of Spontaneous SAH

Spontaneous SAH is a kind of stroke. The main clinical symptoms are sudden severe headache, dizziness, nausea, vomiting, consciousness decline, neck stiffness, photophobia, and other meningeal signs; thus, when mild, it appears very similar to meningitis. In severe cases of SAH, the patient may fall into a coma or even die. Since there are no typical stroke symptoms, which are familiar to the public, such as hemiparesis, limb weakness, mouth drooping, and facial numbness, it is likely to be neglected. Most people are unfamiliar with this kind of stroke.

4.3.2 Etiology of Spontaneous SAH

Most cases of spontaneous SAH are caused by the formation and rupture (actually a leak) of an intracranial aneurysm (Figs. 4.39–4.59, 4.62, 4.64, 4.65, and 4.66) [4]. A few cases are caused by AVM (Fig. 4.68). There is also a rare type of spontaneous SAH caused by bleeding in the sulcus rather than in the basal cisterns; this type is mainly caused by vasculitis [4].

In about 15–20% of SAH cases, it is not possible to locate the site of the bleeding (Fig. 4.60); this may indicate a case of intracranial arteriosclerosis; in which case the bleeding occurs without the formation of an aneurysm [5].

4.3.3 Typical Locations of Aneurysm

Aneurysms typically occur in these locations (Fig. 4.38):

1. Anterior communicating artery (ACoA) (Figs. 4.39–4.45, 4.65, and 4.66).
2. Where the posterior communicating artery (PCoA) enters the internal carotid artery (ICA)—ICA/PCoA (Figs. 4.46–4.50, 4.62, 4.63, and 4.65).
3. Tip of the basilar artery (Figs. 4.56 and 4.64).
   The above three are in the vicinity of the suprasellar cistern, so when they rupture, the blood first flows into the suprasellar cistern and then spreads into the surrounding SAS.
4. Bifurcation of the middle cerebral artery (MCA) (Figs. 4.45, 4.52, 4.53, 4.54, and 4.55).
   The aneurysm at this location is exactly inside the Sylvian fissure. When the rupture and hemorrhage occur, the Sylvian fissure contains most blood, and the blood permeates other SAS, sometimes even forms hematoma in Sylvian fissure, or breaks into the adjacent temporal lobe, thus forming ICH (intracerebral hematoma).
5. Other locations: If an aneurysm is located in the bilateral vertebral artery (Figs. 4.57 and 4.58) or basilar artery when bleeding occurs, the SAH is most obvious at the foramen magnum of the posterior cranial fossa, and then the blood spreads upward to the suprasellar cistern. As for the ICA, in addition to the ICA/PCoA, it may also occur at other locations (Figs. 4.3, 4.51, and 4.67). Any locations of ACA (Fig. 4.33), MCA (Fig. 4.55), and PCA (Fig. 4.59), especially at the proximal segment, may have the aneurysm to form.

4.3.4 Patterns of Aneurysm Bleeding

As described above, most aneurysms occur in the arteries located at the skull base. These arteries are immersed in the CSF and have not yet entered into the brain tissue, so when the aneurysm ruptures and bleeds, the blood flows into CSF directly and soon spreads along with subarachnoid spaces with CSF, this is typical spontaneous SAH.

Simple SAH accounts for about 70% of aneurysm hemorrhages, and about 25% are combined with ICH (Figs. 4.41, 4.42, 4.43, 4.44, 4.48, 4.50, and 4.54); i.e., when the aneurysm ruptures, the blood flows into the brain tissue to form an ICH. Only about 5% have ICH but no SAH (Figs. 4.3 and 4.66).

If the aneurysm formed in the artery in brain parenchyma is ruptured, it is most likely to be ICH (Figs. 4.32 and 4.33), instead of SAH. These aneurysms relatively far in the artery are usually considered as infected (mycotic) aneurysm (Fig. 4.32); endovascular infections should be checked, especially the patients with septicemia and endocarditis.

4.3.5 How to Find an Aneurysm?

Before the advent of CTA, after using CT to diagnose spontaneous SAH, it was necessary to do traditional angiography (DSA) to search for an aneurysm, which is an invasive procedure since it requires catheterization of an artery. The CTA image quality of multislice CT is good, and different angles are available. Hence, most aneurysms can be diagnosed by the mere use of CTA. For the very few cases that cannot be confirmed by CTA, the DSA is required for validating aneurysm (Fig. 4.55). In the cases the CTA fails to find aneurysm, there is little chance of finding it even using DSA [5]. In less than 10% of the SAH cases, no location of the bleeding point is seen by angiography (Fig. 4.60) [6].

Besides, the source images before the 3D CTA is composed should be read carefully. Sometimes the aneurysm (Figs. 4.44, 4.49, 4.51, 4.54, 4.56, 4.57, 4.59, 4.64, and 4.66) or AVM (Fig. 4.68) can be seen clearly in the source image or contrast-enhanced CT.

4.3.6 Aneurysm Bleeding and Rebleeding

As mentioned in the second section (Sect. 4.2.1), once an ICH forms, it immediately begins to press on the ruptured small blood vessels, stopping the bleeding. The SAH induced by aneurysm rupture is also mostly stopped immediately. This explains that some people have extensive bleeding, while others only bleed in small amounts. Also, the amount of bleeding is not necessarily related to the size of the aneurysm; sometimes, a large aneurysm has only a small amount of bleeding, and sometimes a small aneurysm has a large SAH. However, in SAH there is no hematoma to compress the aneurysm rupture, so there may still be some leakage in a short period of time (Fig. 4.43); as a result, there is a high chance of re-rupture and rebleeding within hours or days, and maybe even more severe (Fig. 4.50) [7].

An aneurysm does not really "rupture"; since the aneurysm only makes a fissure, it would be more precise to say it "leaks." Moreover, after rupturing and bleeding, the aneurysm remains, so if it is not quickly dealt with by surgical clamping or embolization, there is a high chance of this aneurysm re-rupturing and rebleeding within a few days or even within a few hours. Thus, once spontaneous SAH has been diagnosed using CT, it is necessary to immediately find the aneurysm and treat it to prevent rebleeding.

4.3.7 Using the Bleeding Pattern Seen in CT to Surmise the Location of the Aneurysm

Since most aneurysms occur in the SAS at the skull base, when they rupture, they tend to take the form of a SAH. SAHs are easy to see in CT and most are evenly distributed. Yet it is difficult to determine the location of an aneurysm by CT images alone; it is usually necessary to search using CTA. However, when some aneurysms bleed, in addition to producing a SAH, they also infiltrate the brain tissue to form an ICH (also see Sect. 4.3.4). When an SAH is combined with an ICH, the position of the aneurysm can be surmised from the CT image. For example:

1. If an SAH is combined with an ICH in the frontal lobe, or with a hematoma in the septum pellucidum, it can be surmised that the aneurysm is in the ACoA (Figs. 4.41, 4.42, 4.43, 4.44 and 4.66).
2. If an SAH is combined with an ICH inside the medial aspect of the temporal lobe, it can be surmised that the aneurysm is in ICA/PCoA (Figs. 4.48 and 4.50).
3. If an SAH is combined with a hematoma in the Sylvian fissure, or there is an ICH in the outer aspect of the temporal lobe, it can be surmised that the aneurysm is located in the MCA bifurcation (Figs. 4.52, 4.53, 4.54, and 4.55).
4. Elsewhere, if the foramen magnum or even the first or second section of the cervical vertebra has remarkable SAHs, it can be surmised that the aneurysm is located in the vertebral artery (Figs. 4.57 and 4.58).

4.3.8 SAH Complications

The most significant risk in SAH is that all the large arteries immersed in the SAS containing blood will cause a vasospasm, which in turn causes ischemic edema, which is a type of ischemic infarction. This kind of vasospasm varies from person to person; some are mild (Fig. 4.46), and some are quite severe or even fatal (Fig. 4.60), thus presenting a significant challenge for neurosurgeons treating SAH patients.

Another complication of SAH is communicating hydrocephalus. SAH has slight hydrocephalus in the acute phase; because the CSF becomes filled with blood, its circulation is impeded, resulting in a rapid onset of hydrocephalus. Later, even while the SAH is gradually shrinking, what cannot be seen in the CT, but the SAS may be becoming more adhesive, which impedes circulation of the CSF, and causing communicating hydrocephalus. This may require the neurosurgeon to install a VP shunt to facilitate long-term drainage.

A rarely seen complication of SAH is when, following bleeding, hemosiderin undergoes superficial siderosis in the brain tissue, especially in the cerebellum and brainstem (Fig. 4.58). After several years, it causes cerebellar atrophy, which results in balance disorders, gait instability, tinnitus, hearing loss, and other sequelae [8].

4.3.9 Minor SAH

When an aneurysm ruptures, there is not necessarily much bleeding with obvious SAH, sometimes the amount of SAH is minimal (Figs. 4.62, 4.64, and 4.66), in which case patient suffers a severe headache. When doing the CT, if the SAH is very small, it sometimes gets overlooked, and may even be misdiagnosed as a severe cold or meningitis.

When reading the CT, a slight dilatation of the bilateral temporal horns (Figs. 4.65 and 4.66) indicates mild hydrocephalus, which is often caused by meningitis. In this situation, it is necessary to look for any trace of SAH carefully; if SAH or aneurysm is present (Fig. 4.65), meningitis can be ruled out.

When a slight SAH is found, it is vital to do a CTA and search for an aneurysm as soon as possible and do embolization or surgical clipping to prevent further bleeding (Figs. 4.62, 4.64, and 4.66).

4.3.10 Unruptured Aneurysm:

Once an aneurysm has formed, how long does it take to rupture? It is uncertain (Fig. 4.49). When an aneurysm is tiny, it is unlikely to cause symptoms by compressing the adjacent structures (Figs. 4.61 and 4.63); it is usually only after rupturing and bleeding that symptoms are produced, prompting a medical examination leading to the discovery of an aneurysm. An aneurysm located at ICA/PCoA may compress the oculomotor nerve below it, producing ptosis or diplopia (Figs. 4.61 and 4.63). When an MRI is performed based on such symptoms, there is a chance to find the aneurysm using MRA before it ruptures.

When making an MRI examination of the brain, MRA is considered a routine procedure. This is especially true with the increasing prevalence in recent years of regular health examinations which include MRI and MRA, often resulting in the accidental discovery of an aneurysm. Do the unruptured aneurysms need management? According to a cohort research, the authors found the natural course of unruptured aneurysms varies according to the size, location and shape of the aneurysm. The aneurysms are larger than 5–7 mm, located in the ACoA, ICA and with irregular shape (Fig. 4.63) are associated with an increased risk of rupture [9]. Figure 4.67 is an example to perform a prophylactic embolization for an incidentally detected aneurysm to prevent rupture.

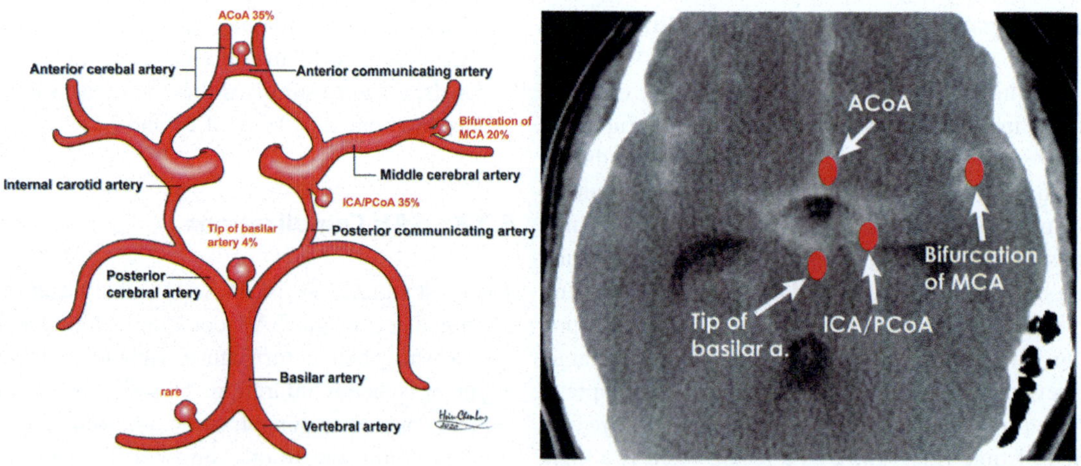

Fig. 4.38 The most common locations of aneurysms: (1) Anterior communication artery (ACoA). (2) Internal carotid artery/posterior communication artery (ICA/PCoA). (3) Tip of the basilar artery. (4) Bifurcation of the middle cerebral artery (MCA). (5) Other locations: Vertebral and basilar arteries, ICA, ACA, MCA, PCA. For the above locations, the aneurysms in the ACoA, ICA/PCoA, and the tip of the basilar artery are just around the suprasellar cistern, so the bleeding first flows into this cistern, and then spreads to other subarachnoid spaces (SAS). The aneurysm of the bifurcation of MCA is in the Sylvian fissure, so it first flows into this fissure and then spreads to the suprasellar cistern and other SASs

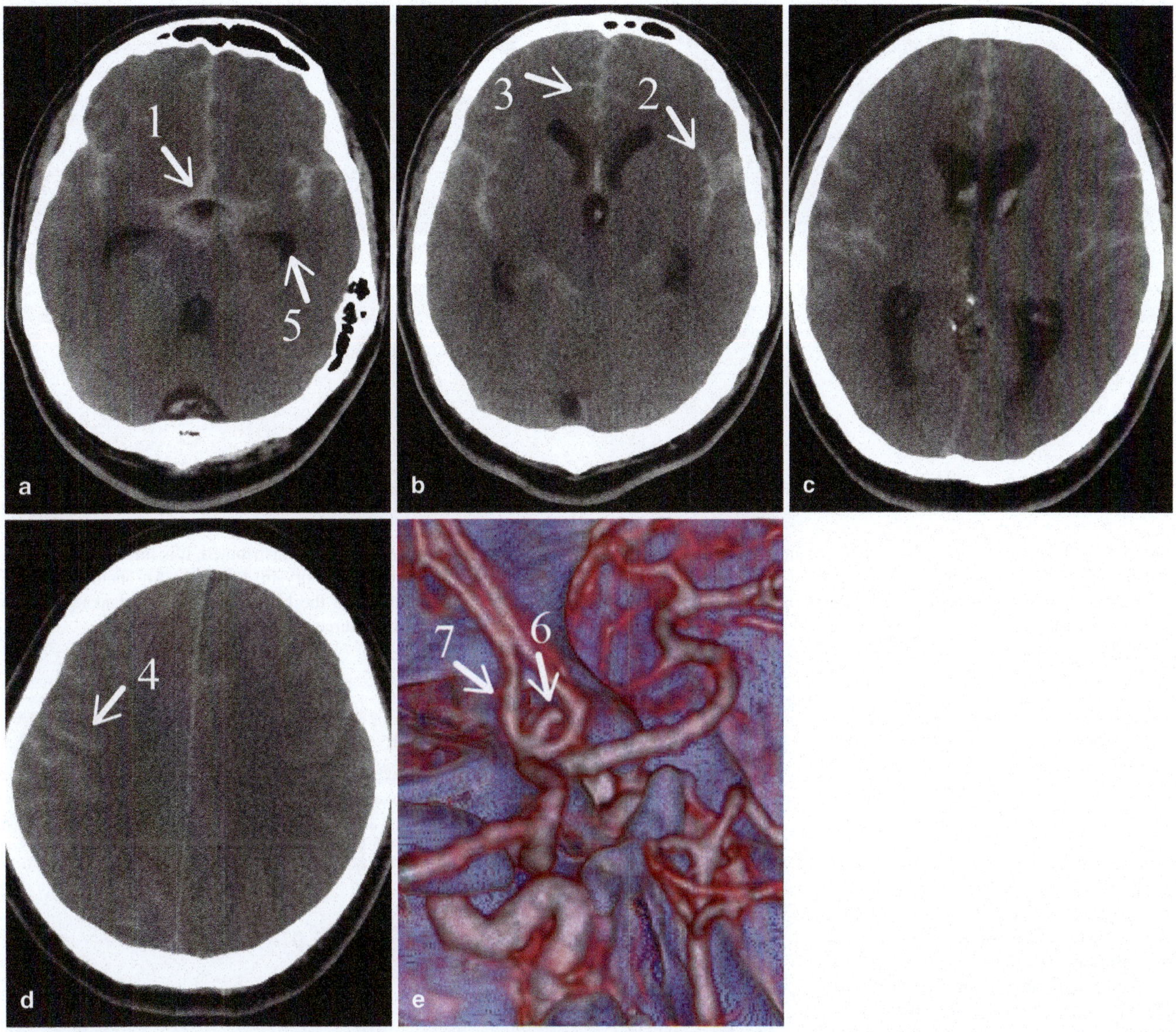

Fig. 4.39 M/38, SAH caused by rupture (leakage) of an ACoA aneurysm. The patient suffered a sudden onset of severe headache and then decreasing consciousness. (**a–d**) Blood clots in the suprasellar cistern (1), bilateral Sylvian fissures (2), interhemispheric fissure (3), and sulci (4); this is a typical pattern of spontaneous SAH. Mild dilatation of the bilateral temporal horns (5), indicating mild hydrocephalus. Because the SAH is evenly distributed, it is impossible to determine the precise position of the aneurysm. (**e**) CTA: An aneurysm (6) in the ACoA, which is between the bilateral ACAs (7). This aneurysm is the bleeder which has ruptured and causes diffuse SAH. Note that an aneurysm does not really "rupture"; since the aneurysm only makes a fissure, it would be more precise to say it "leaks." Thus a "ruptured" aneurysm continues to exist and keeps its original shape and has a high tendency of rebleeding in a short-time interval

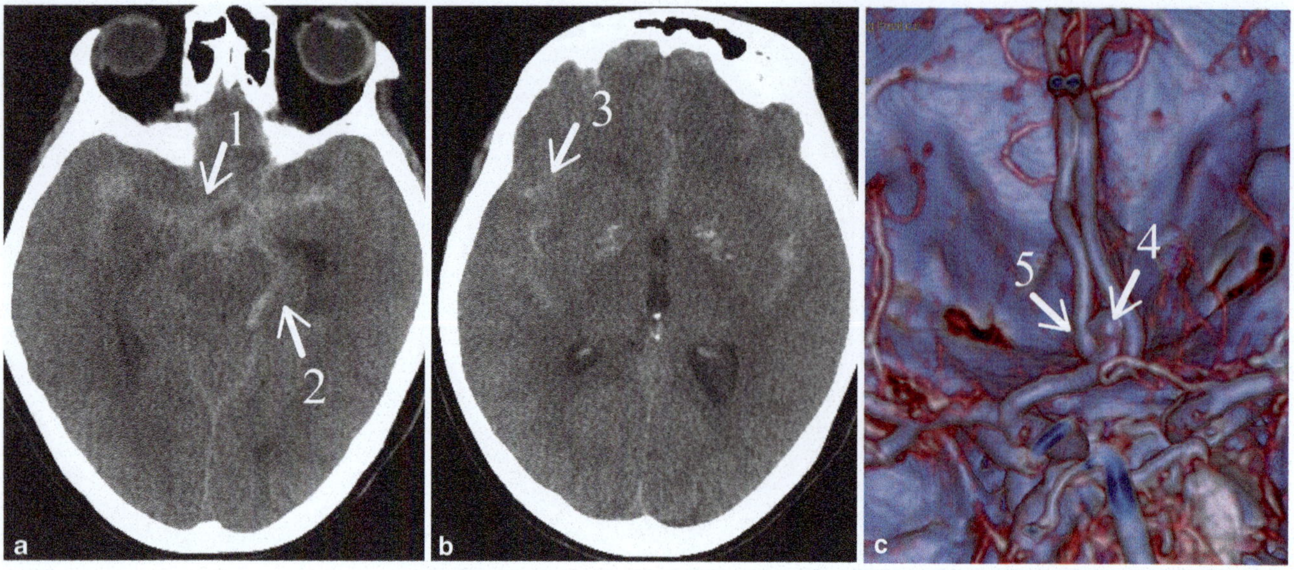

Fig. 4.40 M/59, SAH caused by leakage of an ACoA aneurysm. The patient suffered a sudden onset of severe headache. (**a, b**) CT: Blood clots in the suprasellar cistern (1), ambient cistern (2), and bilateral Sylvian fissures (3); this is spontaneous subarachnoid hemorrhage (SAH). Because the SAH is evenly distributed, it is impossible to speculate on the position of the aneurysm. (**c**) CTA: An aneurysm in the ACoA (4), which is between the bilateral ACAs (5); leakage of this aneurysm is the bleeding source of this diffuse SAH

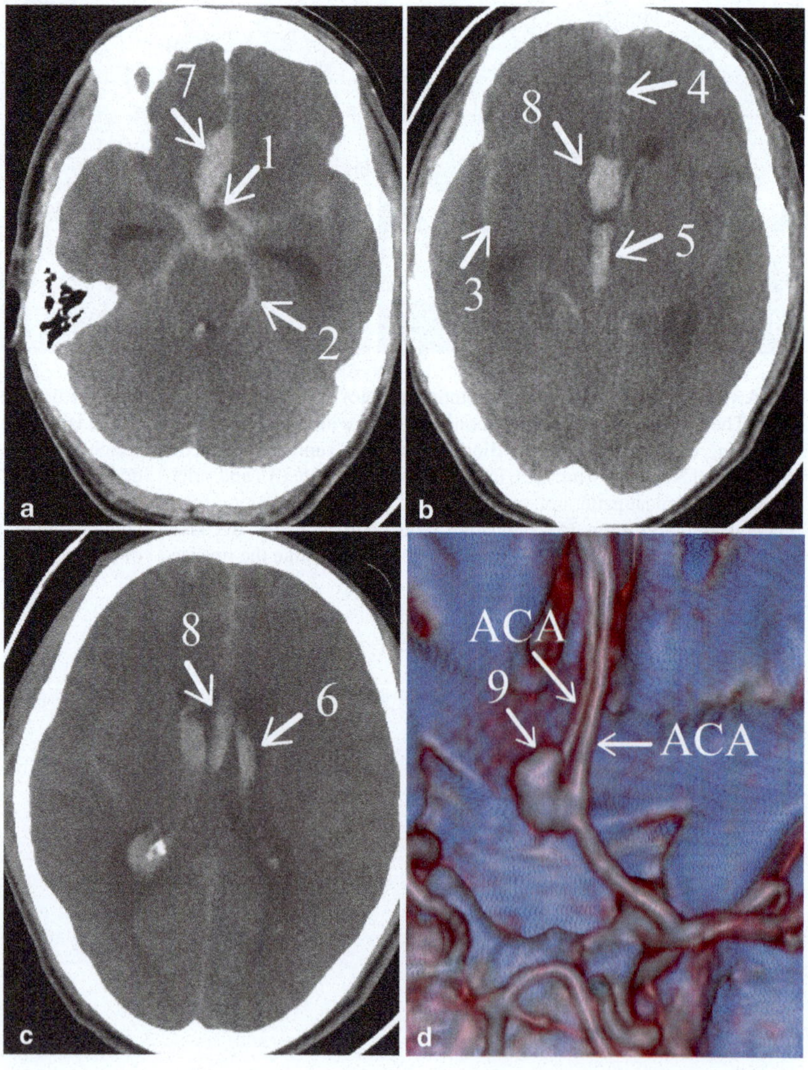

Fig. 4.41 F/49, An aneurysm in ACoA caused SAH and ICH. (**a–c**) CT: SAH in the suprasellar cistern (1), ambient cistern (2), Sylvian fissures (3), and interhemispheric fissure (4). Also, intraventricular hemorrhage (IVH) in the third ventricle (5) and bilateral lateral ventricles (6). Dilatation of temporal horns of bilateral ventricles, reflecting mild hydrocephalus. An intracerebral hematoma (ICH) (7) in the right frontal lobe, and a hematoma in the septum pellucidum (8) between the bilateral lateral ventricles. These two hematomas provide an important clue to predicting an aneurysm in the ACoA, which causes the above hemorrhages. (**d**) CTA: CTA confirms an aneurysm in the ACoA (9); this is the bleeding source of the above SAH, IVH, and ICHs

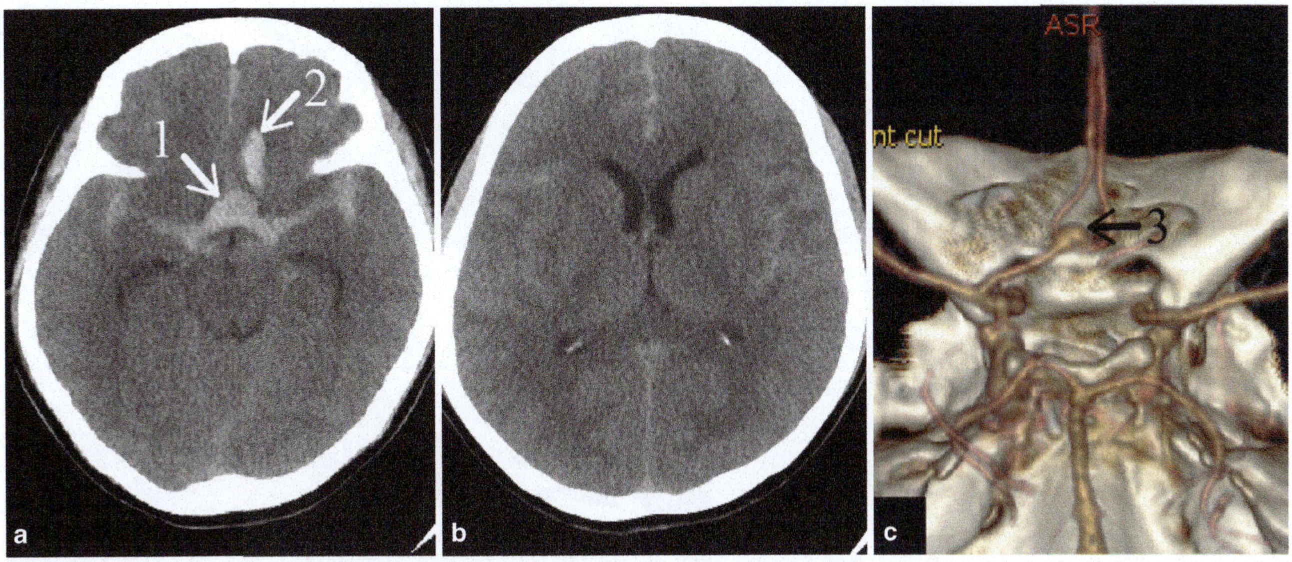

Fig. 4.42 F/47, ACoA aneurysm causing SAH and ICH. (**a**, **b**) CT: In addition to SAH in the suprasellar cistern (1), a small intracerebral hematoma (ICH) in the left frontal lobe (2), this ICH provides an important clue to speculate an aneurysm in the ACoA. Slightly dilatation of temporal horns of bilateral lateral ventricles, indicating mild hydrocephalus. (**c**) CTA: A small aneurysm (3) in the ACoA. The SAH and ICH are due to rupture (leakage) of this aneurysm

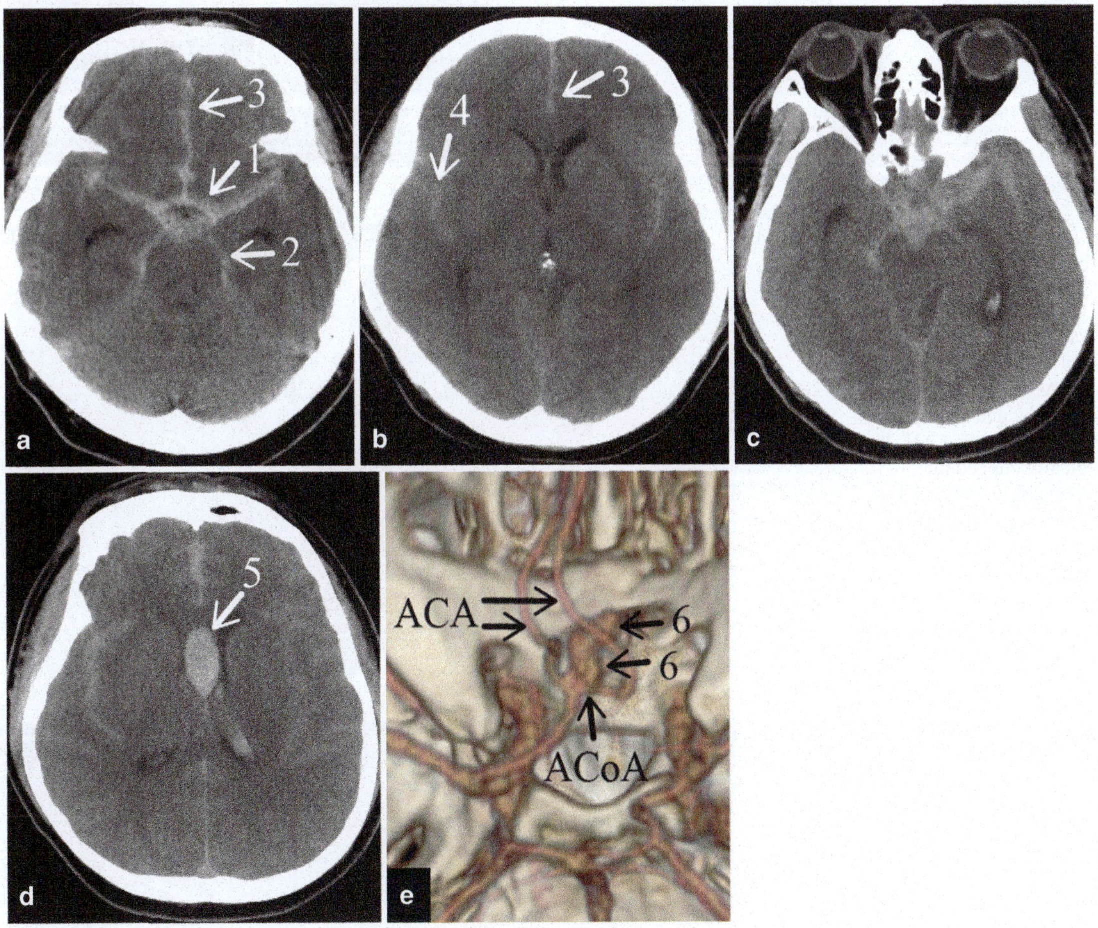

Fig. 4.43 M/50, ACoA aneurysm causing SAH and ICH. The patient suffered a severe headache and was referred by a regional hospital. (**a**, **b**) CT of the original hospital: SAH spread into the suprasellar cistern (1), peripontine cistern (2), interhemispheric fissure (3), and Sylvian fissures (4); with such SAH appearance, it is not possible to determine the location of the aneurysm. (**c**, **d**) The patient had a more severe headache and drowsiness when this repeat CT was made 3 h later: This CT shows a slight increase in the SAH and a new hematoma in the septum pellucidum (5), suggesting that the source of bleeding may be an aneurysm located in ACoA. (**e**) CTA: Confirms an aneurysm (6) in the ACoA

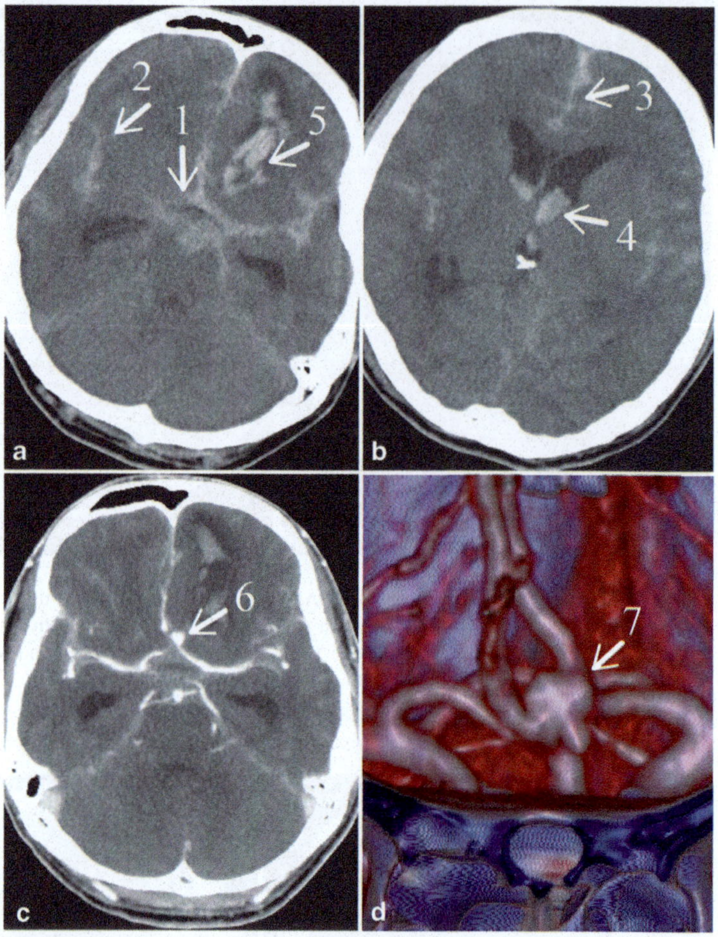

Fig. 4.44 M/47, ACoA aneurysm causing SAH and ICH. (**a**, **b**) CT: SAH in the suprasellar cistern (1), Sylvian fissures (2), and interhemispheric fissure (3); also, IVH in the bilateral lateral ventricles (4). An irregular hematoma (5) in the left frontal lobe (5); this hematoma suggests that the bleeding source is an aneurysm in the ACoA. (**c**) Source image of CTA: A suspected aneurysm in the ACoA (6). (**d**) CTA: Confirms an aneurysm (7) in the ACoA

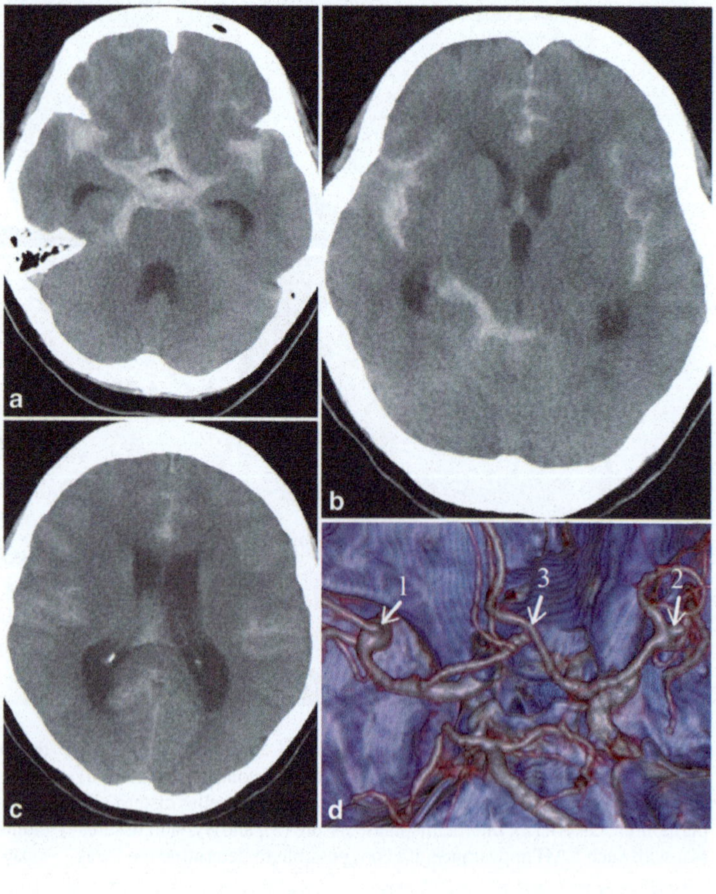

Fig. 4.45 F/59, Multiple aneurysms. (**a**–**c**) CT: A large amount of SAH, without any clues for surmising the location of the aneurysm. (**d**) CTA: three aneurysms, two are in the bifurcations of bilateral MCAs (1, 2), and one in the ACoA (3). The CTA cannot determine which aneurysm is the bleeding source of this SAH. The surgeon surgically clipped the aneurysms in the right MCA and ACoA and found that the SAH was caused by leakage of the aneurysm (1) in the right MCA bifurcation

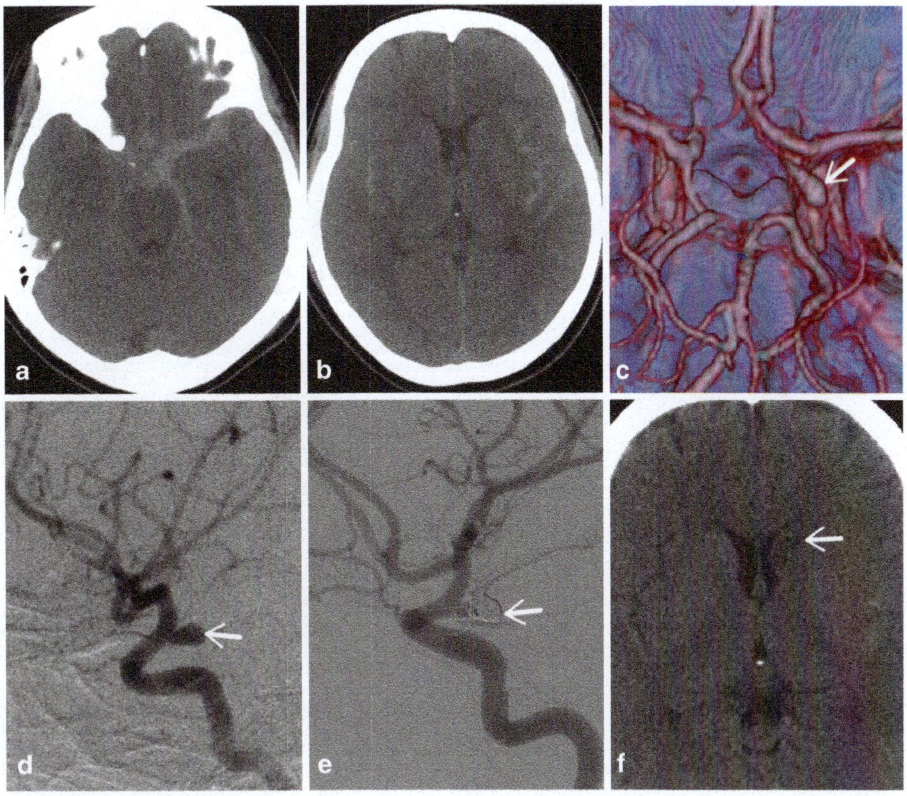

Fig. 4.46 F/42, SAH caused the vessel spasm. (**a, b**) CT: SAH in the suprasellar cistern and Sylvian fissures. (**c**) CTA: An aneurysm (arrow) at the left ICA/PCoA; this is the bleeding source. (**d, e**) Neuroradiologists did a DSA to confirm this aneurysm (arrow in **d**) and embolized this aneurysm with coils (arrow in **e**). (**f**) CT 1 week later: The left caudate nucleus has brain edema (arrow), which is an ischemic infarction; may be caused by vasospasm; this is a complication of SAH

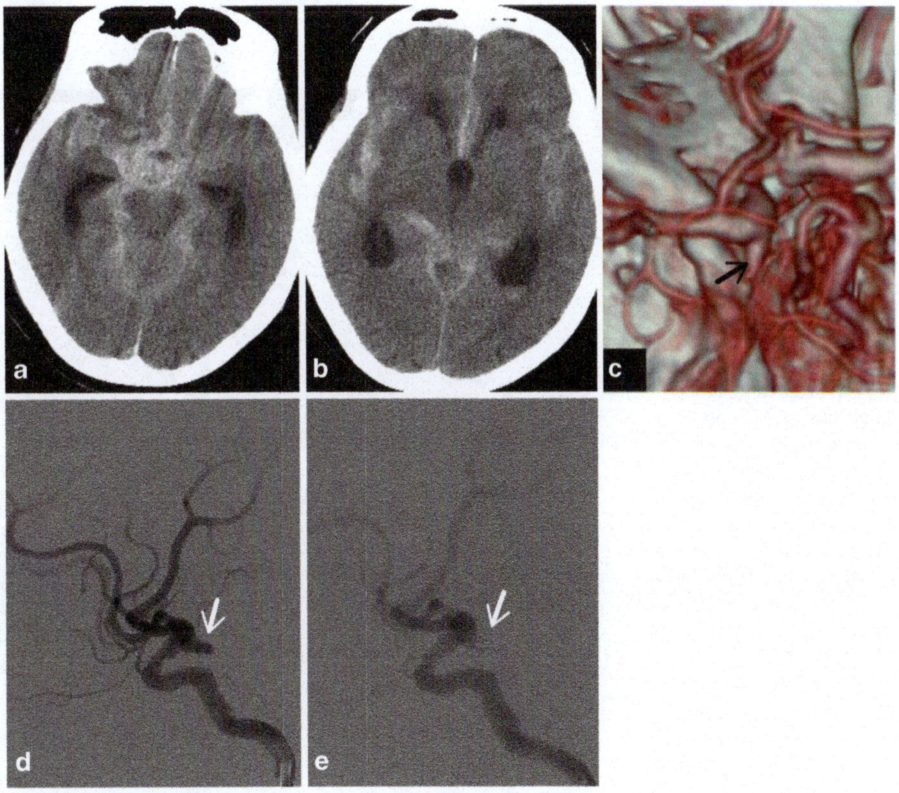

Fig. 4.47 F/86, SAH caused by an ICA/PCoA aneurysm. (**a, b**) The amount of SAH is large and evenly distributed, making it impossible to locate the aneurysm. The temporal horns of the bilateral lateral ventricles are slightly dilated, representing mild hydrocephalus. (**c**) CTA: Turned to several angles, revealing a suspected long-shape aneurysm (arrow) in the right ICA/PCoA. (**d, e**) The neuroradiologist performed a DSA and confirmed that this is an aneurysm (arrow in **d**) located in the right ICA/PCoA, and embolized this aneurysm with coils (arrow in **e**)

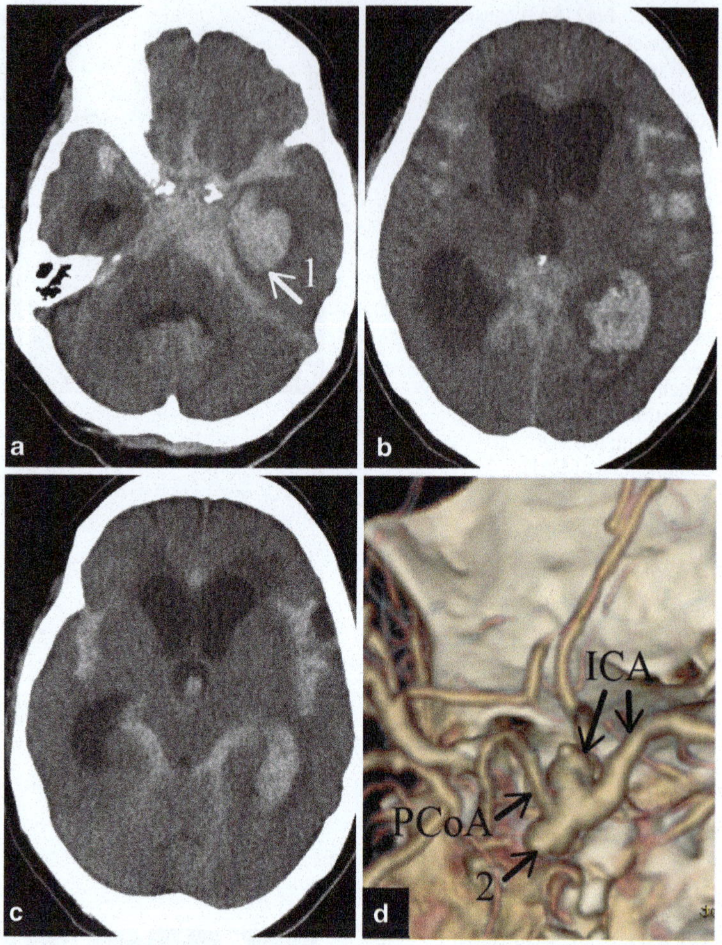

Fig. 4.48 F/72, An aneurysm in ICA/PCoA causing SAH and ICH. The patient suffered a severe headache and then fell into a coma. (**a**–**c**) CT: A large amount of SAH and IVH with hydrocephalus. An intracerebral hematoma (1) in the left temporal lobe; this ICH suggests that the bleeding point should be an aneurysm in the left ICA/PCoA. (**d**) CTA: Confirms a big aneurysm (2) in the left ICA/PCoA

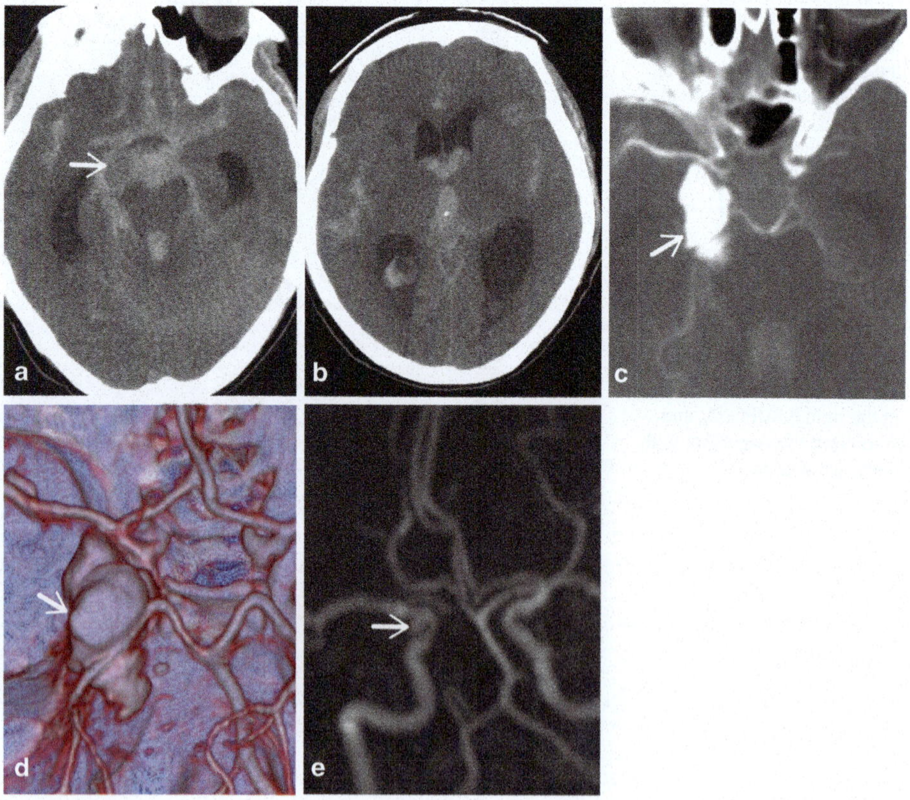

Fig. 4.49 F/77, A small aneurysm that has enlarged and ruptured. The patient suddenly had a severe headache and went into a coma. (**a**, **b**) CT: A large amount of SAH and mild hydrocephalus. A small spherical filling defect (arrow) in the suprasellar cistern is suspected to be an aneurysm. (**c**) CTA source image: A large amount of contrast medium flows out of the artery and collects (arrow); this is a giant aneurysm. (**d**) CTA: Confirms that this is a giant aneurysm (arrow). (**e**) Reviewed the medical history, it is found that an MRI was performed at another hospital 20 days ago. The MRA showed a small aneurysm (arrow) on the right ICA/PCoA. In summary, a small aneurysm will become larger and even rupture, so it must be treated as soon as possible

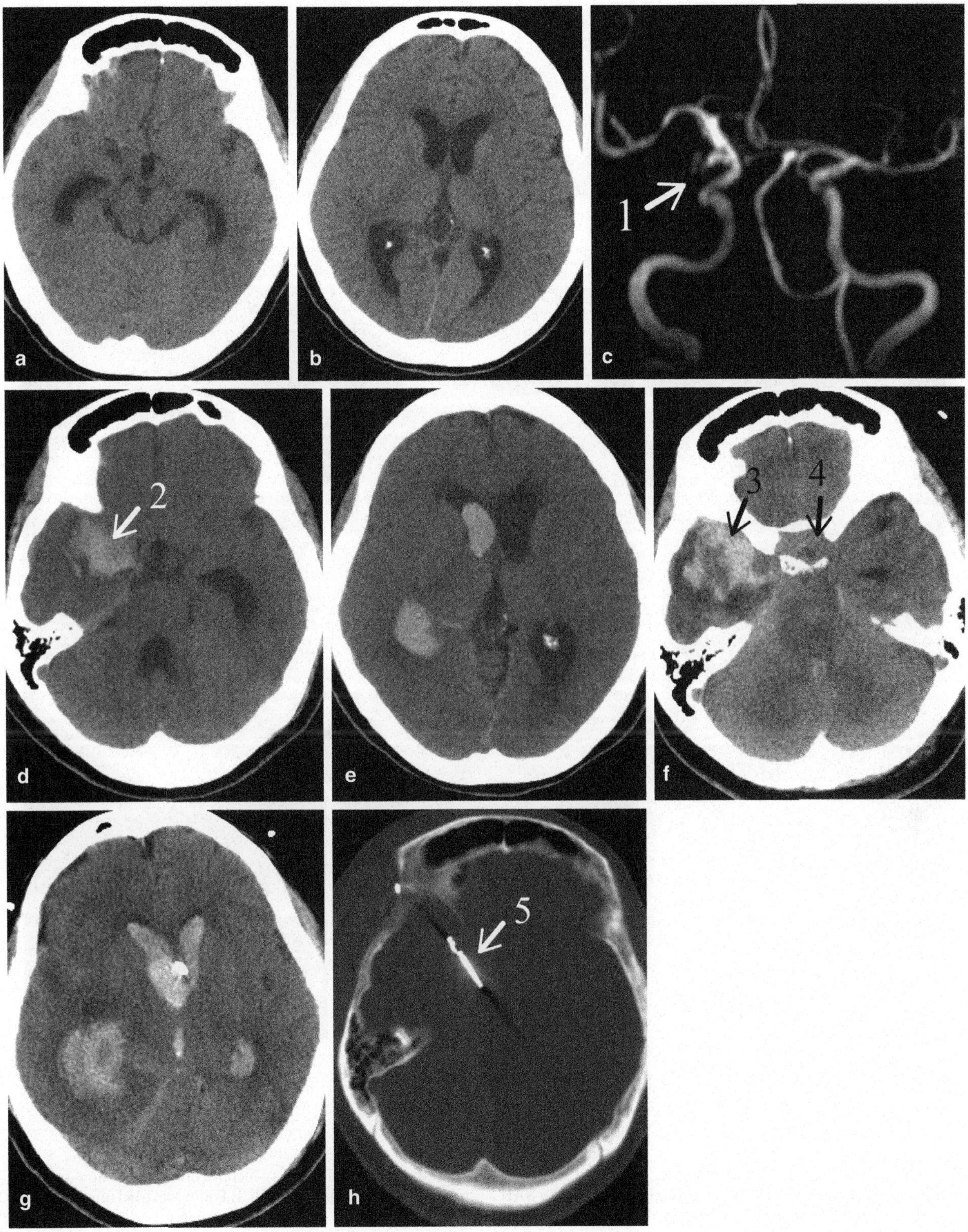

Fig. 4.50 F/59, An ICA/PCoA aneurysm caused repeat bleeding. (**a**, **b**) CT: Mild hydrocephalus, which may be caused by SAH or meningitis. (**c**) MRA: Shows an aneurysm (1) in the right ICA/PCoA, but no treatment was done. One month later, the patient had a severe headache again. (**d**, **e**) CT: Shows an intracerebral hematoma (ICH) (2) in the right temporal lobe and IVH in the right lateral ventricle. Two days later, the headache was more severe. (**f**, **g**) Repeat CT: Shows more bleeding. The ICH in the right temporal lobe is more extensive (3), with some SAH in the suprasellar cistern (4), and more IVH. This is the aneurysm in the right ICA/PCoA causing repeat bleeding. The neurosurgeon performed surgery to clip this aneurysm for preventing further bleeding. (**h**) CT, post-surgery, bone window: A surgical clip (5) is used to clamp this aneurysm

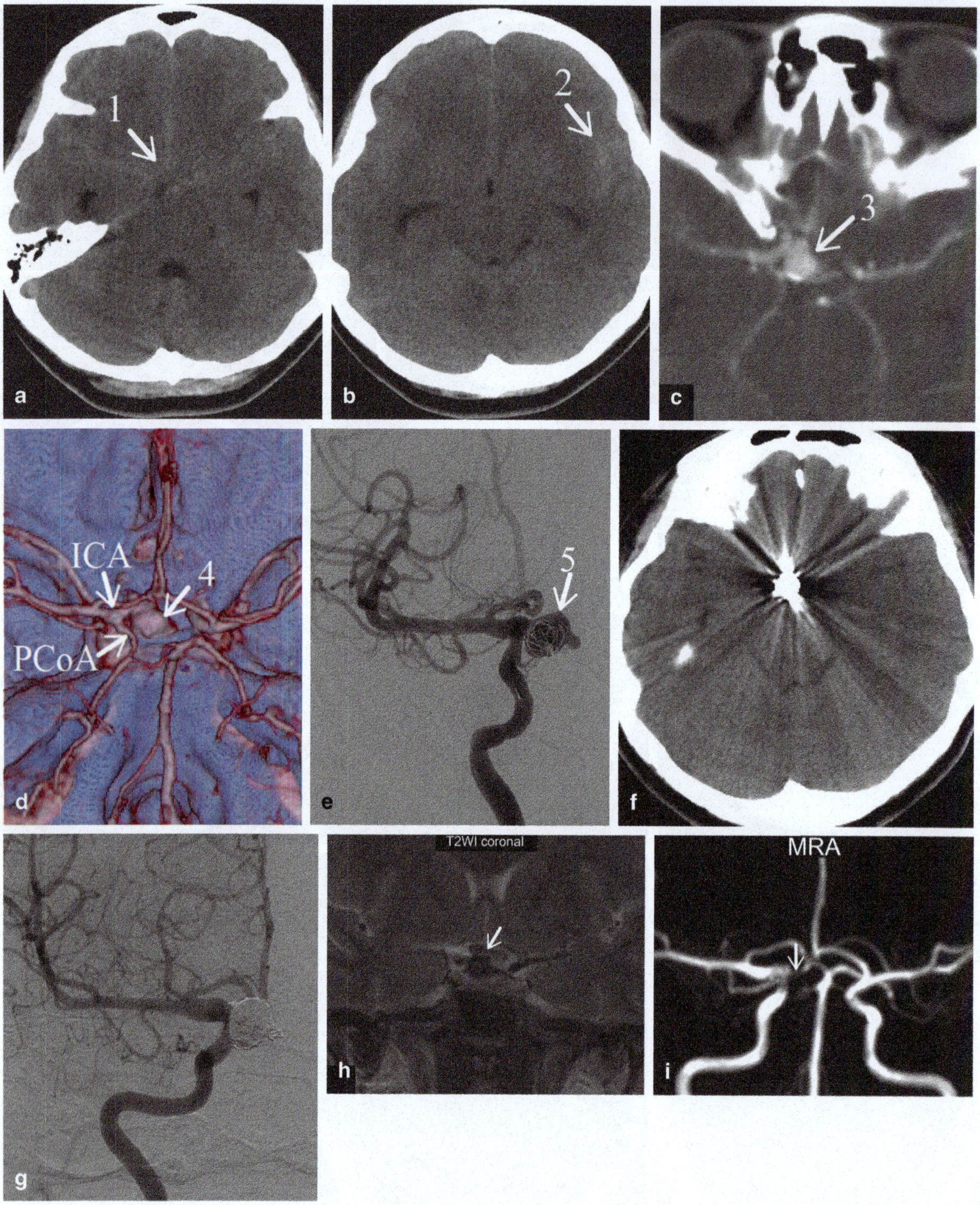

Fig. 4.51 F/38, An ICA aneurysm caused SAH. The patient suffered a severe headache, but consciousness was normal. (**a, b**) CT: Some SAH in the suprasellar cistern (1) and Sylvian fissure (2), with mild hydrocephalus. (**c**) CTA source image: There is an accumulation of contrast medium besides the right ICA, which may be an aneurysm (3). (**d**) CTA: Confirms that it is a large aneurysm (4), which is derived from the supraclinoid portion of the right ICA. (**e**) The neuroradiologist embolized this aneurysm with coils (5). (**f**) CT scan 1 week after embolization: The coils are producing strong metal artifacts. (**g**) Follow-up DSA: The coils are filling the aneurysm. (**h, i**) Follow-up MRI after 5 months: The coils are still in the original aneurysm position (arrow in **h**), but no artifact was produced. MRA shows that aneurysm has disappeared (arrow in **i**). Comment: The coils used to embolize aneurysm are metal, and may thus produce metallic artifacts in CT, but they are magnetically resistant, so a patient with coil embolization can safely undergo an MRI examination

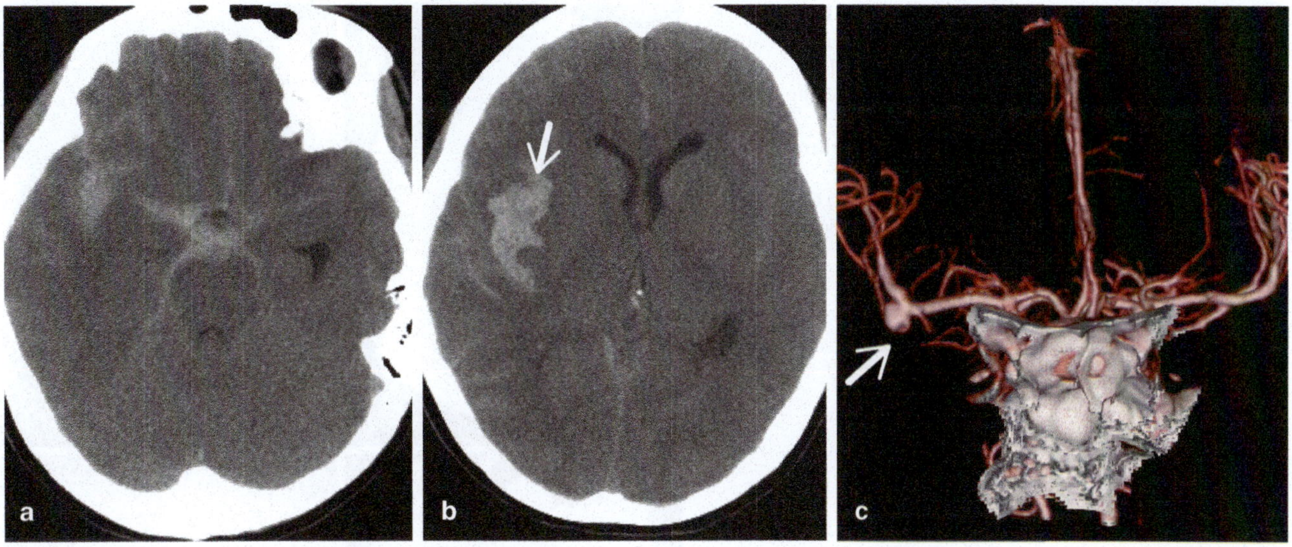

Fig. 4.52 F/35, An MCA bifurcation aneurysm caused SAH. (**a**, **b**) CT: SAH in the suprasellar cistern and large blood clot in the right-side Sylvian fissure (arrow), suggesting that the aneurysm should be in the right MCA bifurcation. (**c**) CTA confirms an aneurysm (arrow) in the right MCA bifurcation; this is the bleeding source of SAH

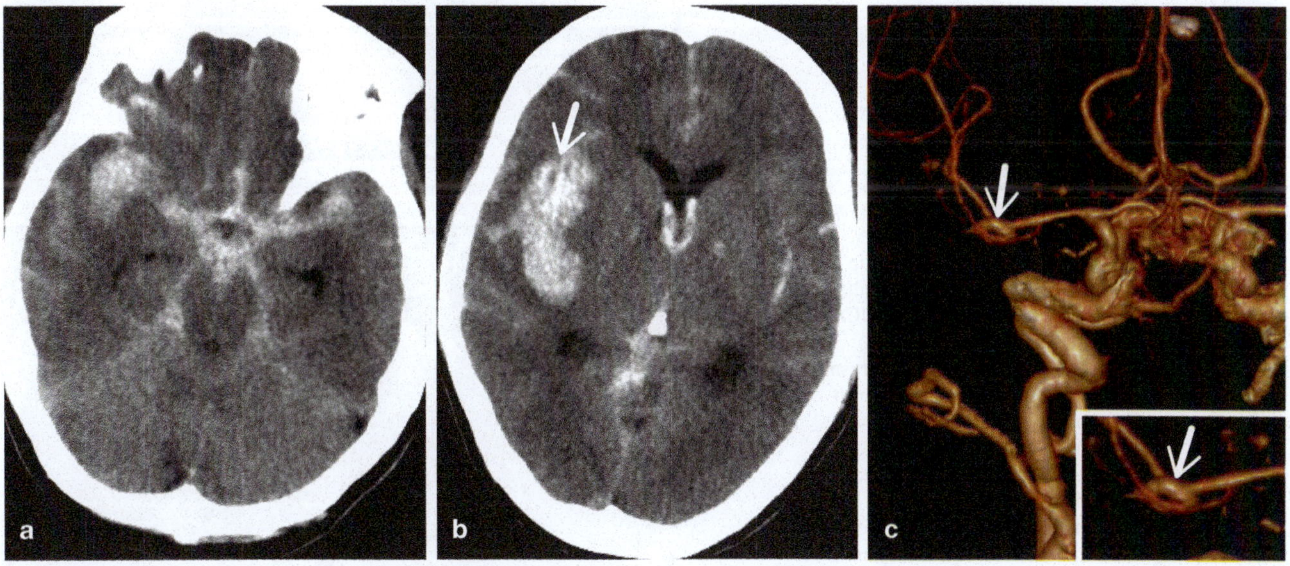

Fig. 4.53 F/53, SAH caused by an MCA bifurcation aneurysm. (**a**, **b**) CT: Large amount of SAH, and an especially large blood clot in the right Sylvian fissure (arrow), suggesting an aneurysm in the right MCA bifurcation. (**c**) CTA: Confirms an aneurysm (arrow) in the right MCA bifurcation to be the bleeding source of SAH. The bottom right box is the magnified view of this aneurysm

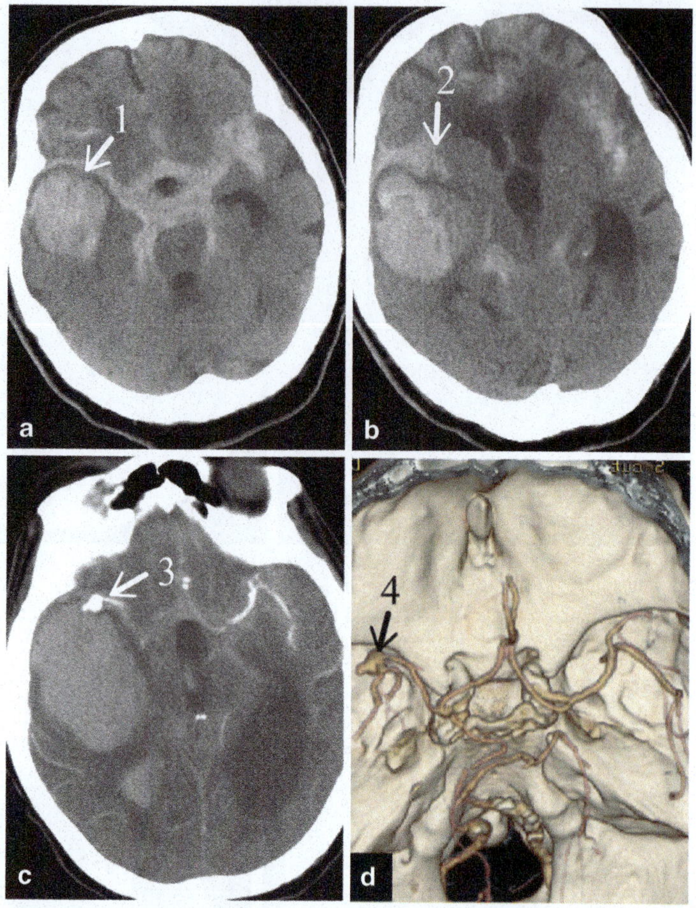

Fig. 4.54 F/81, MCA aneurysm causing SAH. (**a**, **b**) CT: Large amount of SAH, an intracerebral hematoma (ICH) (1) in the right temporal lobe, and more SAH in the right Sylvian fissure (2), suggesting that the bleeding point is an aneurysm in right MCA bifurcation. (**c**) Source image of CTA: We can see a small pocket where the contrast medium has collected (3) in the MCA bifurcation; this pocket is possibly an aneurysm. (**d**) CTA confirms that this is an aneurysm (4) in the bifurcation of right MCA; this is the bleeding point

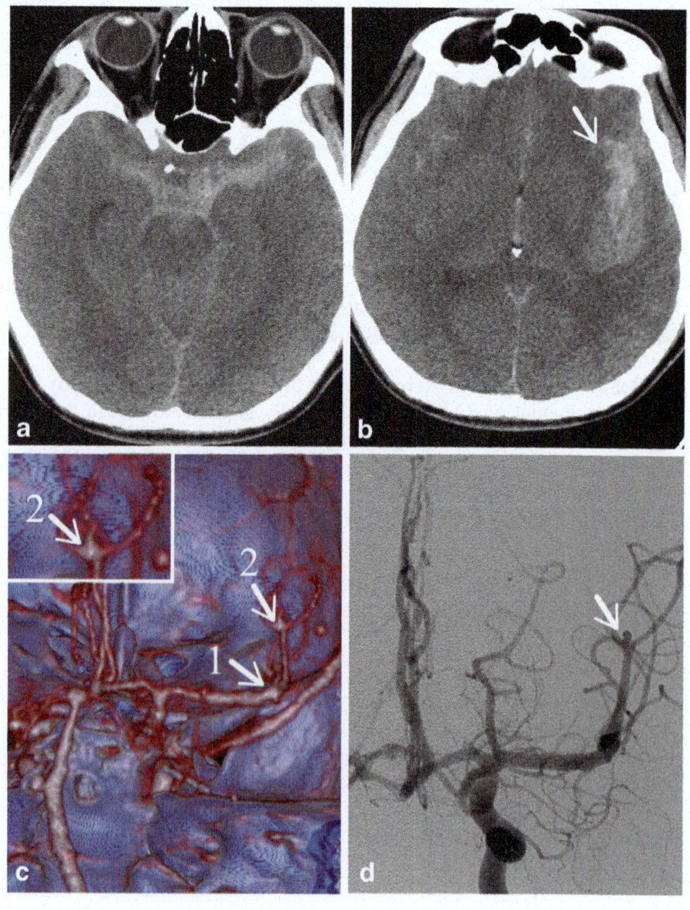

Fig. 4.55 M/42, An aneurysm in distal of MCA, causing SAH. (**a**, **b**) CT: SAH, large blood clot in left Sylvian fissure (arrow), suggesting that the bleeding point is an aneurysm in the bifurcation of left MCA. (**c**) CTA: However, no aneurysm is found in the MCA bifurcation (1); instead, a suspected aneurysm (2) is found in the distal portion of an MCA branch (left upper box is the magnified view of this aneurysm), necessitating a DSA to confirm this finding. (**d**) DSA: Angiogram reveals that this normal anatomic variation, a bifurcation in a branch of MCA, has an aneurysm (arrow). The neurosurgeon did craniotomy and confirmed that this aneurysm was the bleeding point of this SAH

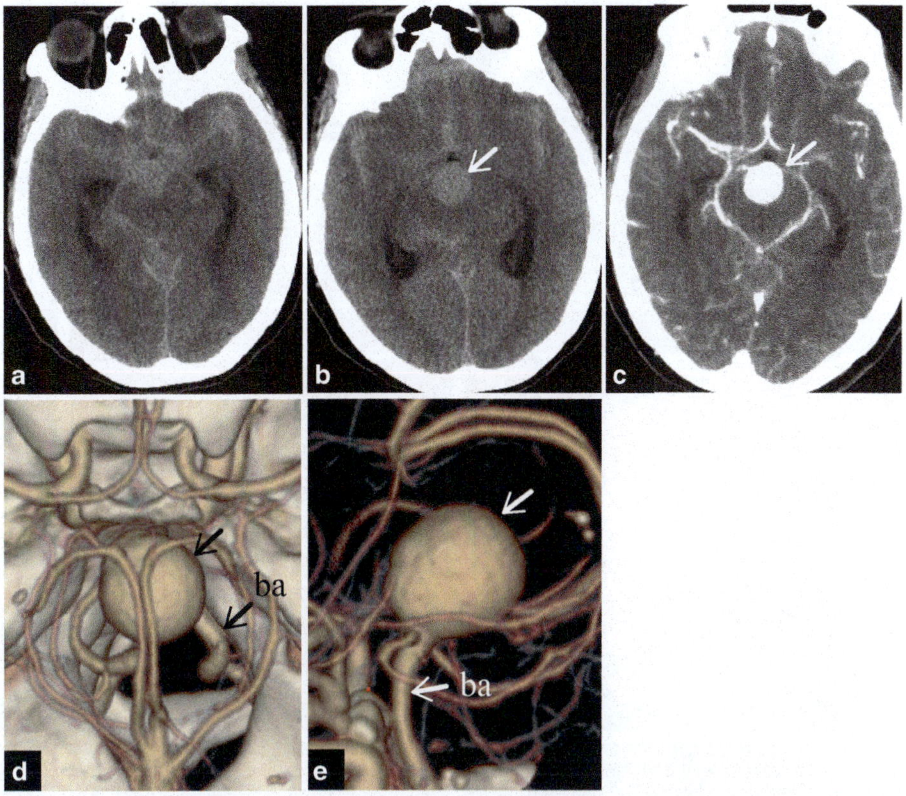

Fig. 4.56 F/58, A basilar artery tip aneurysm caused SAH. (**a, b**) CT: SAH and a round-shape blood clot (arrow) in the interpeduncular fossa, which is suspected to be an aneurysm. (**c**) Source image of CTA: Contrast medium is accumulated in this round area (arrow), suggesting a big aneurysm. (**d, e**) CTA confirms that this is a big aneurysm (arrow) in the tip of the basilar artery (ba)

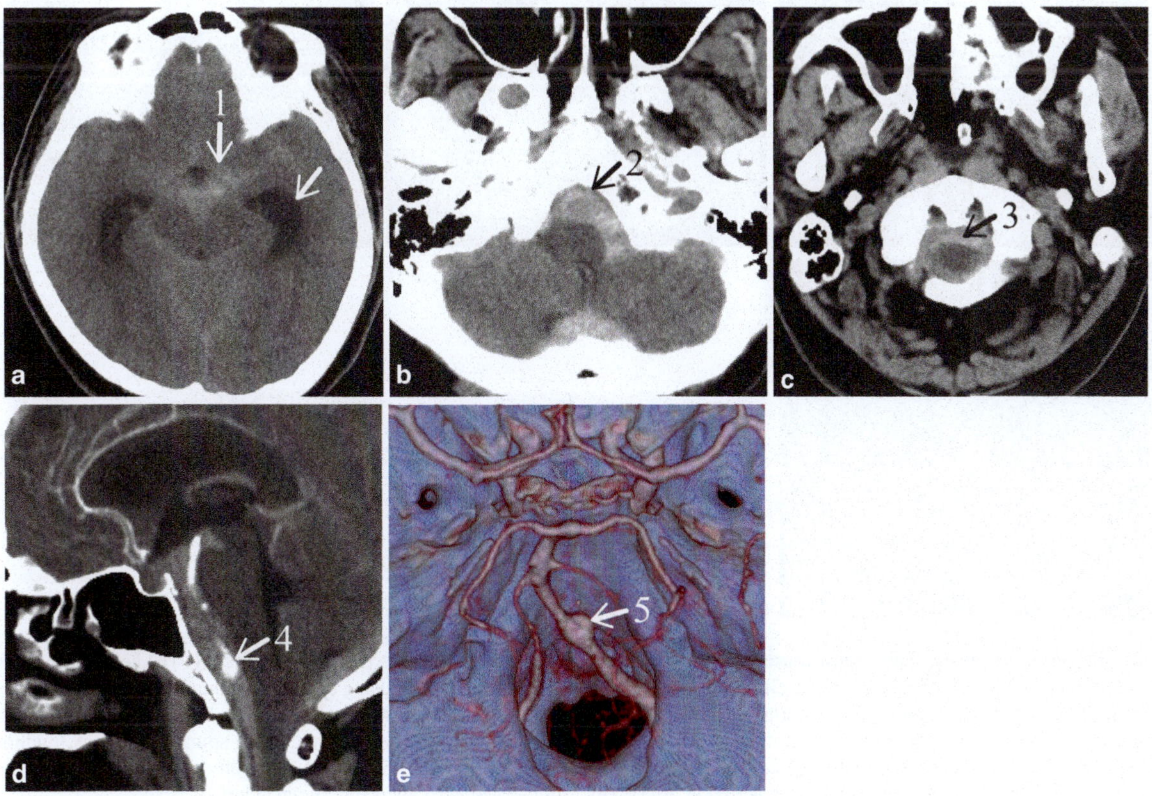

Fig. 4.57 M/49, A vertebral artery aneurysm caused SAH. (**a–c**) CT: SAH in the suprasellar cistern (1), dilatation of bilateral temporal horns (arrow), indicating hydrocephalus. In the posterior fossa, SAH is especially evident in the foramen magnum (2) adjacent to the medulla oblongata; the SAH has even reached the spinal canal at the C1-2 level (3). This type of SAH suggests an aneurysm in a very low location of an artery. (**d**) Source image of CTA, sagittal section: A small pocket contains contrast medium (4), resembling an aneurysm. (**e**) CTA confirms this is an aneurysm in the left vertebral artery (5); this is the bleeding source of this SAH

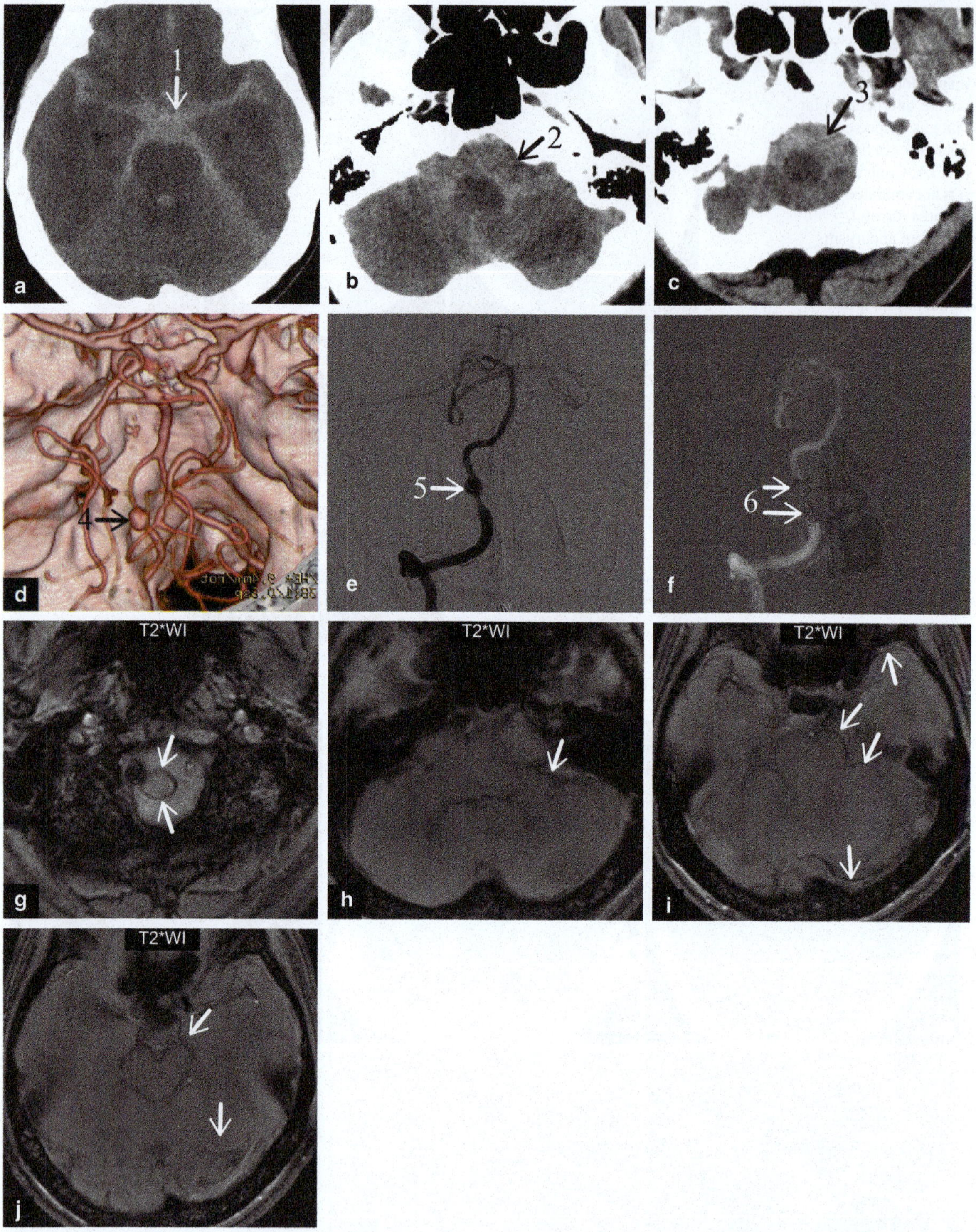

Fig. 4.58 F/43, A vertebral artery aneurysm caused SAH and superficial siderosis. (**a**) CT: Typical SAH in the suprasellar cistern (1). (**b**, **c**) More downward sections of CT: SAH in the cisterns beside the medulla oblongata (2), and even in the subarachnoid space of cervical spine (3), suggesting that the bleeding point should be an aneurysm in the vertebral artery. (**d**) CTA: An aneurysm (4) in the right vertebral artery. (**e**) DSA: Clearly shows the aneurysm (5). (**f**) The neuroradiologist embolized the aneurysm using coils (6), maintaining the flow of the vertebral artery. (**g–j**) Follow-up MRI 1 year later, T2*WI: There is linear hypointensity in the surfaces of the spinal cord, pons, midbrain, and cortex of the cerebellum and cerebrum; these are hemosiderin depositions (arrows), called superficial siderosis

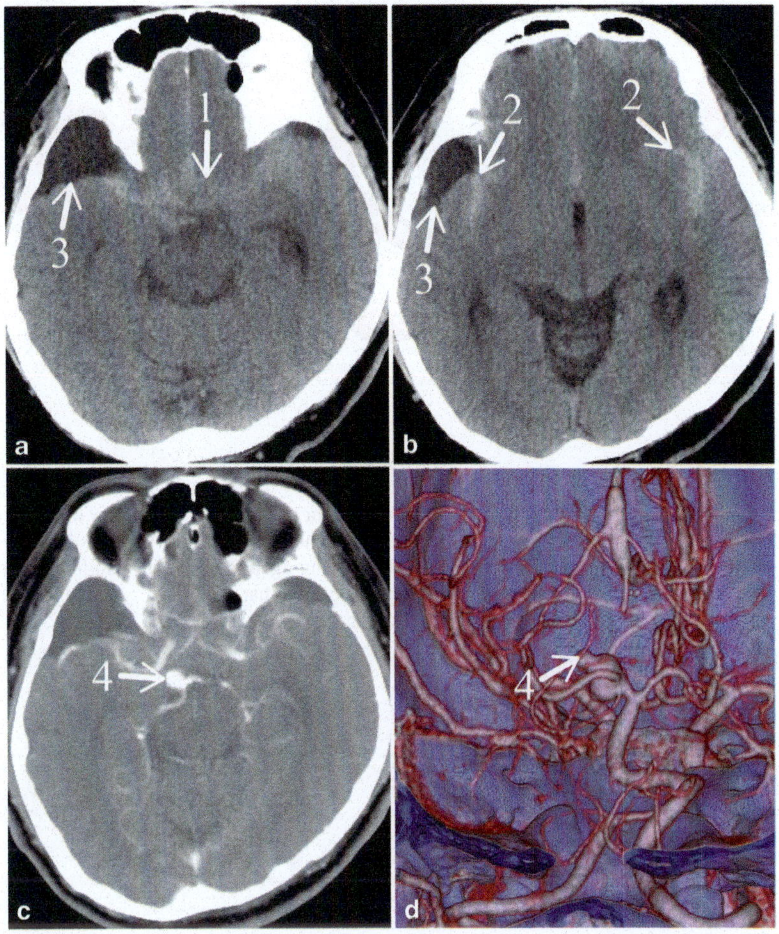

Fig. 4.59 M/56, A PCA aneurysm caused SAH. (**a**, **b**) CT: SAH in the suprasellar cistern (1), Sylvian fissures (2), and, incidentally, an arachnoid cyst (3) in the right middle cranial fossa. (**c**) Source image of CTA: A small contrast medium pooling pocket (4) in the right posterior cerebral artery (PCA), possibly, is an aneurysm. (**d**) CTA: Confirms that this is an aneurysm (4) in the P1 portion of the right PCA, rather than in the tip of the basilar artery

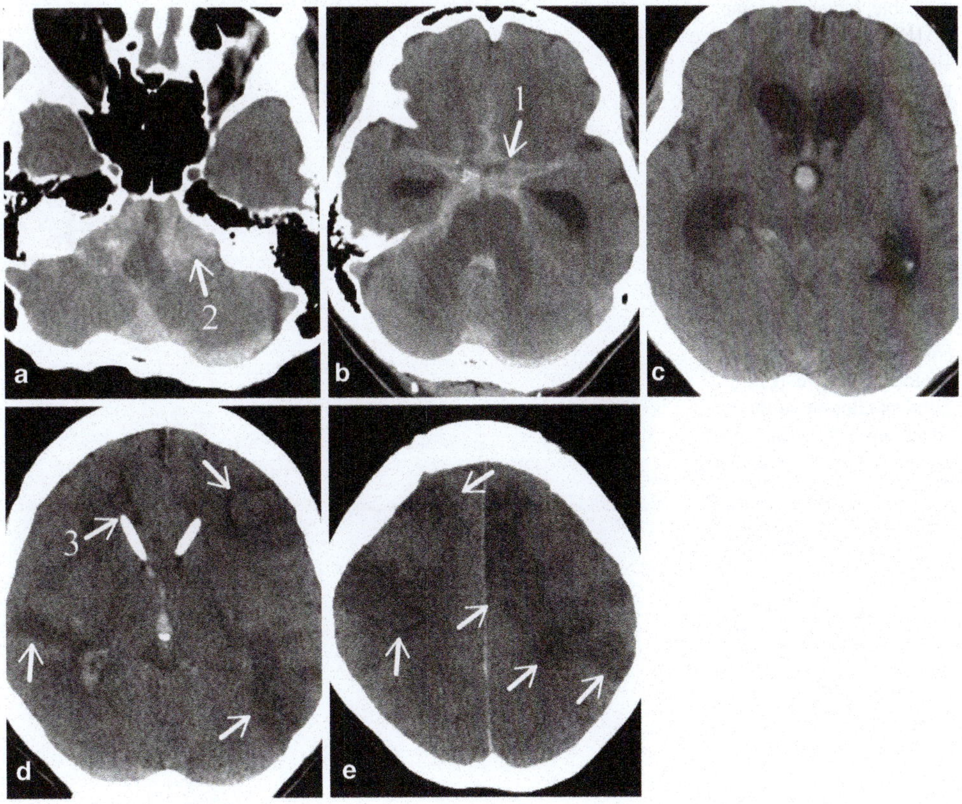

Fig. 4.60 F/69, SAH, no bleeding point found, with vasospasm. (**a–c**) CT: SAH in the suprasellar cistern (1), and also SAH beside the medulla oblongata (2), suggesting that the bleeding source is an aneurysm in the vertebral artery. Hydrocephalus is also noted. However, CTA and later DSA did not find any aneurysm, not even in the bilateral vertebral arteries (not shown). One week later, the patient was in a comatose state. (**d**, **e**) CT: On ventricular drainage tubes (3) in the bilateral lateral ventricles, the hydrocephalus disappears. There are multiple areas of brain tissue edema (arrows) in the bilateral cerebral hemispheres; these are due to arterial infarctions, which are caused by arterial spasms. The vasospasm is a kind of severe complication of SAH

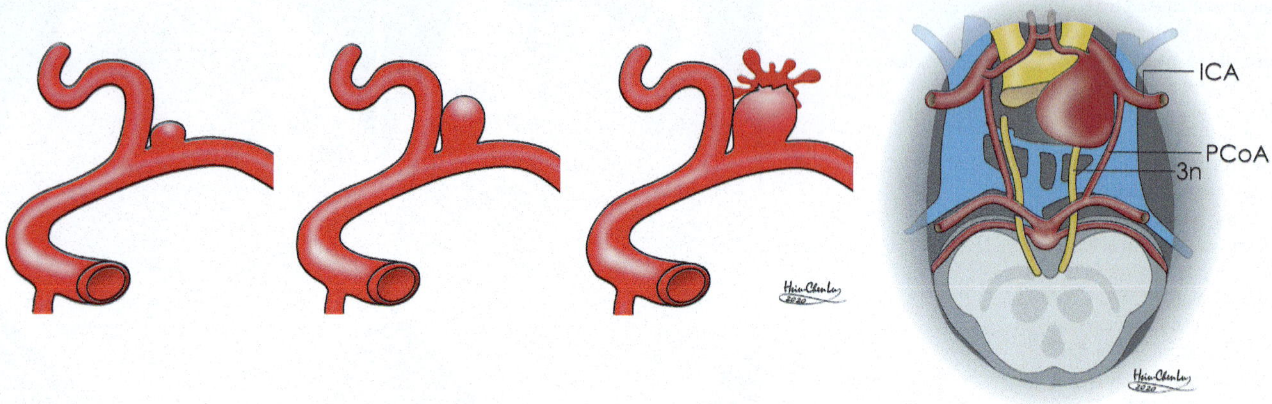

Fig. 4.61 Aneurysm formation. Once an aneurysm has formed, how long does it take to rupture? It is uncertain. An aneurysm is always small; it is unlikely to cause symptoms by pressing against adjacent structures; it is usually only after rupturing and bleeding that symptoms are produced, prompting a medical examination leading to the discovery of an aneurysm. An exception is this aneurysm at ICA/PCoA, compressing the oculomotor nerve (3n) below it, producing ptosis or diplopia. Performing MRA or CTA based on such symptoms allows finding the aneurysm before it ruptures

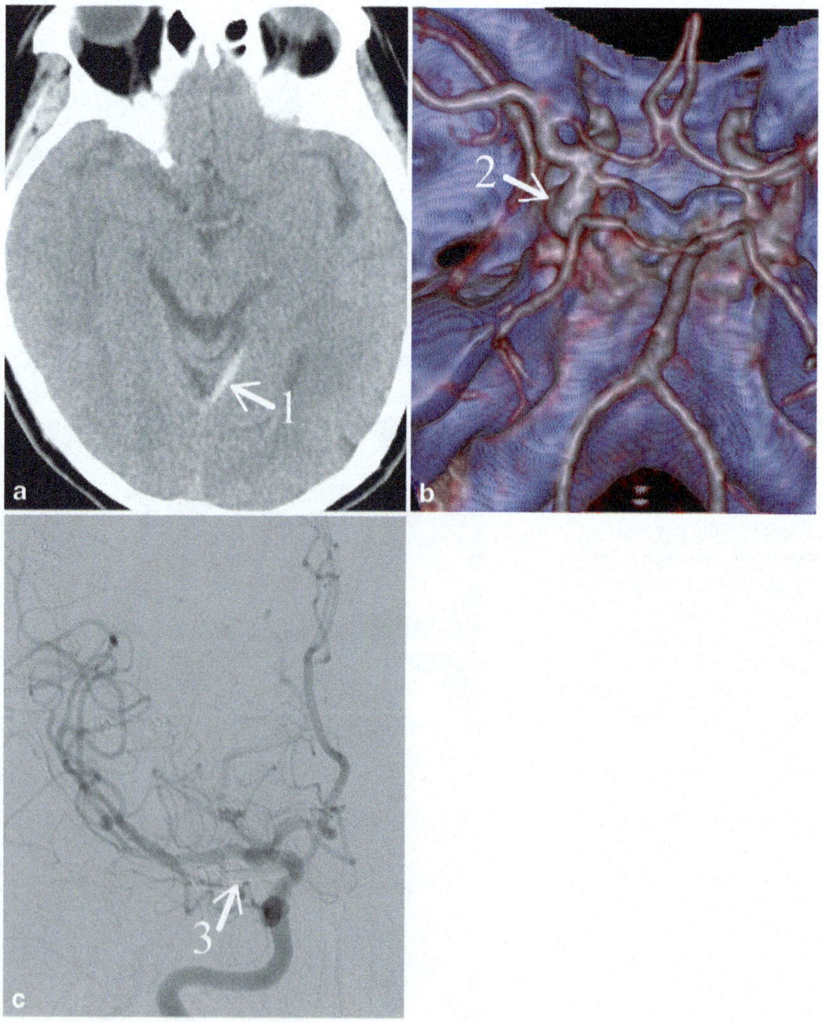

Fig. 4.62 F/63, An aneurysm caused trace SAH and ptosis. The patient suffered a sudden severe headache with diplopia, and right eyelid ptosis occurred in the last week. (**a**) CT: Only a white line (linear hyperdensity) on the left side of the tentorium is visible, indicating some SAH (1) on the tentorial edge. Because there is right eye ptosis, it is highly suspected that an aneurysm in the right ICA/PCoA is compressing the right third cranial nerve (oculomotor nerve), so CTA was done. (**b**) CTA: Confirms a prominent aneurysm (2) at the right ICA/PCoA, which 1 week ago had only a small amount of SAH, but was compressing the right oculomotor nerve. (**c**) Surgical clipping of this aneurysm, DSA: The Aneurysm has been clamped (3)

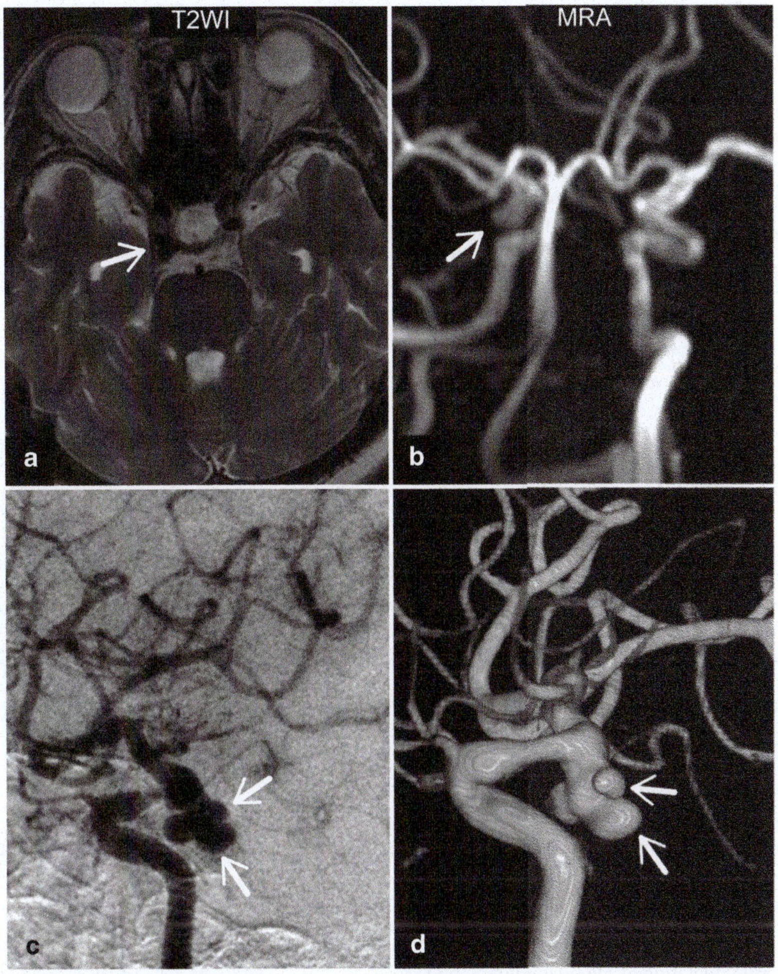

Fig. 4.63 F/66, An unruptured aneurysm compressed the oculomotor nerve. The patient suffered a sudden right eyelid ptosis, so the ophthalmologist arranged for her to have an MRI examination. (**a**) MRI, T2WI: A small protrusion in the cavernous portion of the right ICA, possibly an aneurysm (arrow). (**b**) MRA: Confirms the aneurysm (arrow) in the right ICA/PCoA. (**c**, **d**) DSA and 3D DSA images: Confirm a large aneurysm (arrows) at the right ICA/PCoA, which may be compressing the right oculomotor nerve. Because the shape of this aneurysm is very irregular, it has a high risk of rupture with bleeding, so intra-arterial coil embolization was performed immediately (not shown)

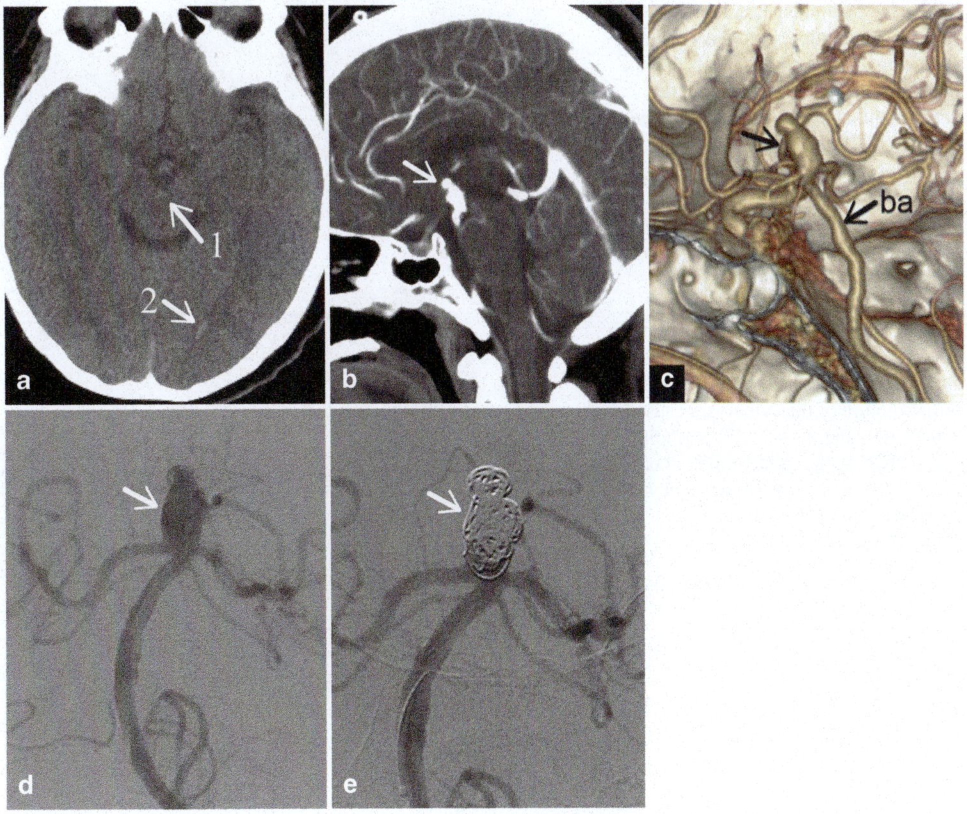

Fig. 4.64 F/66, An aneurysm caused a small amount of SAH. The patient suffered severe headaches for nearly a week. (**a**) CT: Only a small amount of SAH in the interpeduncular fossa (1) of the suprasellar cistern and some IVH in the left lateral ventricle (2). (**b**) Source image of CTA: Shows pooling of contrast medium (arrow) on the top of the basilar artery, suspected to be an aneurysm. (**c**) CTA: Confirms that this is a big aneurysm (arrow) originating at the tip of the basilar artery (ba). (**d**) DSA: Confirms that this is a big aneurysm (arrow) originating at the tip of the basilar artery (ba). (**e**) The neuroradiologist did DSA and embolized this aneurysm with coils (arrow)

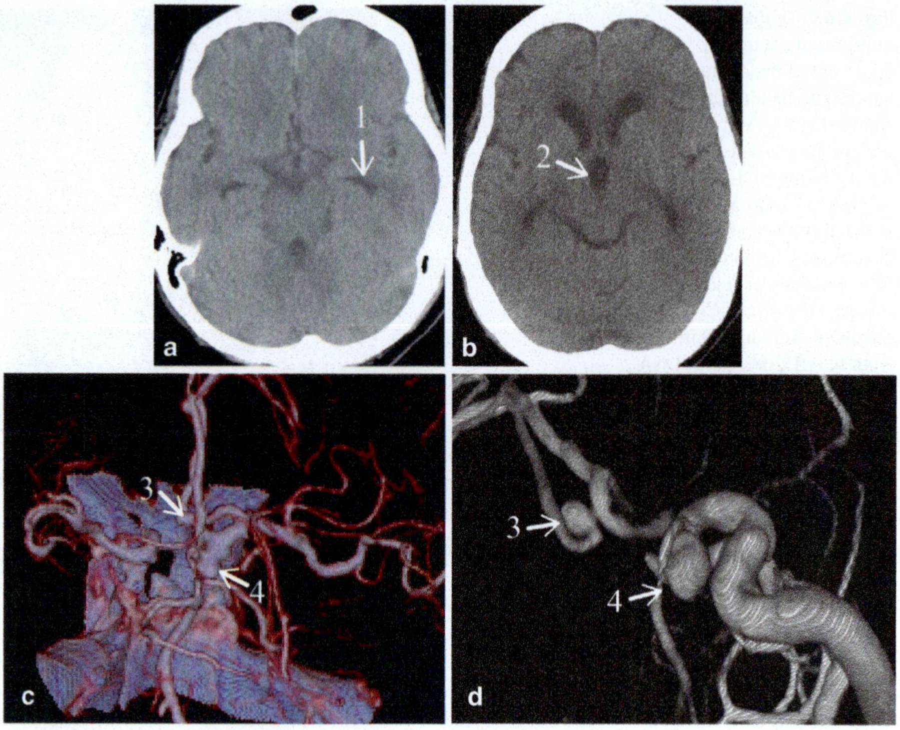

Fig. 4.65 F/67, Two aneurysms, one caused some hemorrhage. The patient had a severe headache with nausea and vomiting for a week; she had a fever for the past 2 days, and the clinician suspected she had meningitis. (**a**, **b**) CT: Only mild dilatation of the temporal horns (1); the third ventricle is also dilated and oval in shape (2), indicating mild hydrocephalus. From the image and clinical symptoms, meningitis was suspected; but it was not possible to rule out the possibility of a small amount of SAH, which may have disappeared in 1 week, so CTA examination was arranged. (**c**) CTA: Shows that the ACoA (3) and left ICA/PCoA (4) each have an aneurysm. (**d**) DSA, 3D image reconstruction: Confirms these two aneurysms (3, 4). In summary, this patient had two aneurysms, one of which leaked and produced a small amount of bleeding, caused headaches. When CT was done a week later, the SAH was invisible; only mild hydrocephalus caused by SAH was visible. Finally, the neurosurgeon surgically clipped the two aneurysms to prevent rebleeding

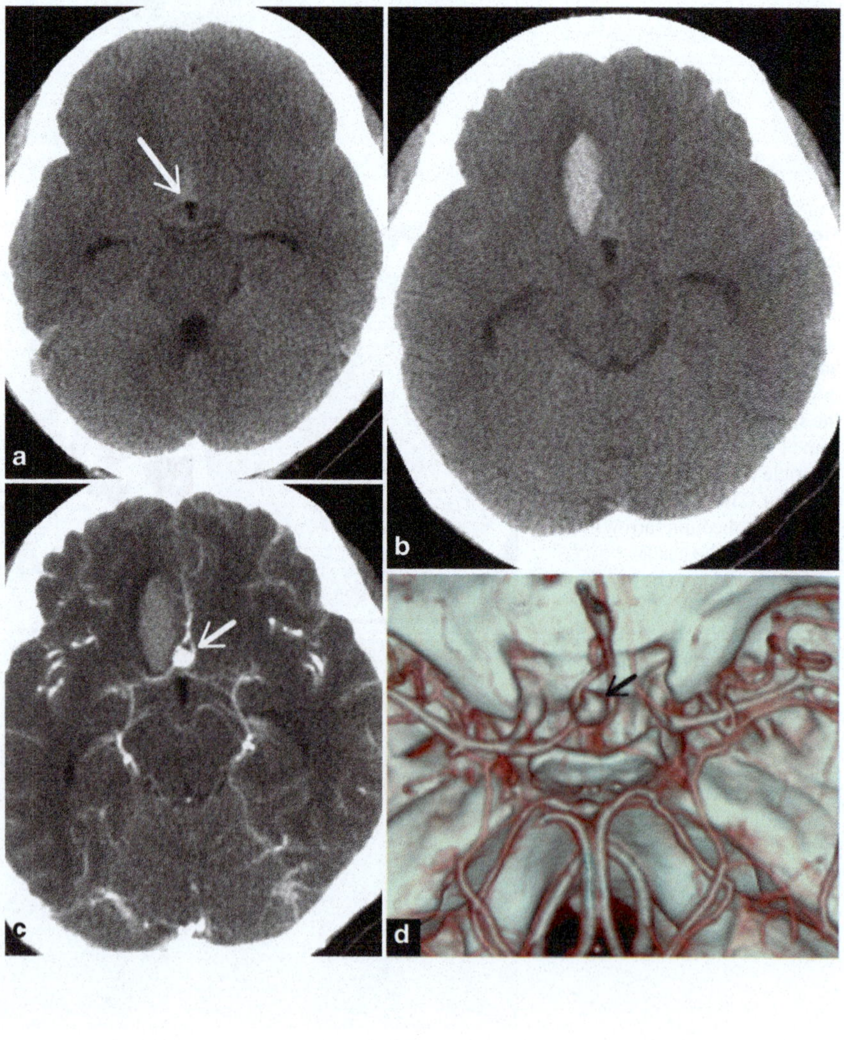

Fig. 4.66 F/33, Rebleeding of an ACoA aneurysm. This patient suffered a sudden severe headache. (**a**) Emergency CT: Small amount of SAH in the suprasellar cistern (arrow), and mild dilatation of the bilateral temporal horns, indicating mild hydrocephalus. After the doctor prescribed medicine to relieve the pain, the patient refused the further examination. Two days later, following another severe headache, the patient came back to the emergency department, and the doctor performed a second CT. (**b**) CT: shows an acute intracerebral hematoma (ICH) in the right frontal lobe; the SAH in the suprasellar cistern is now invisible. (**c**) Source image of CTA: An accumulation of contrast medium in ACoA (arrow), just beside the ICH, so an aneurysm in ACoA is highly suspected. (**d**) CTA: clearly shows that ACoA has an aneurysm (arrow). In summary, the initial rupture of this aneurysm caused some SAH, and the second rebleeding caused ICH in the right frontal lobe. Finally, the neurosurgeon surgically clipped this aneurysm to prevent further bleeding

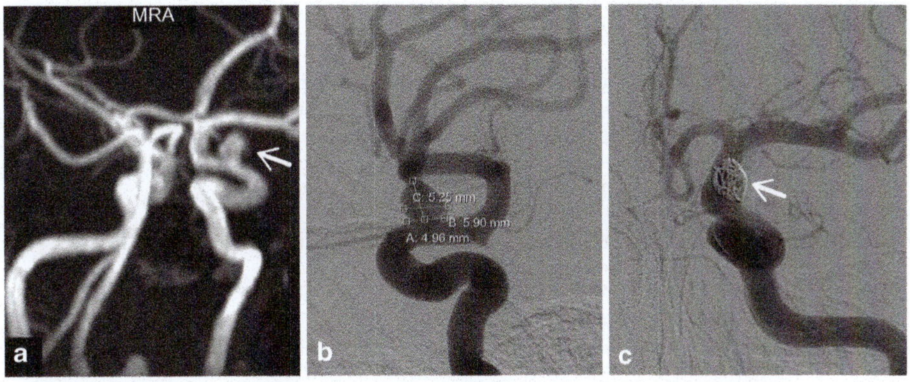

Fig. 4.67 F/38, Unruptured aneurysm. (**a**) When this healthy woman received a health check-up, the MRA happened to find an aneurysm (arrow) in the cavernous portion of the left internal carotid artery (ICA), which is 5 mm broad and had to be proactively treated to prevent rupture and bleeding. (**b**) Neuroradiologists did DSA to measure the size of this aneurysm to prepare for embolization. (**c**) Neuroradiologists used coils (arrow) to embolize this aneurysm

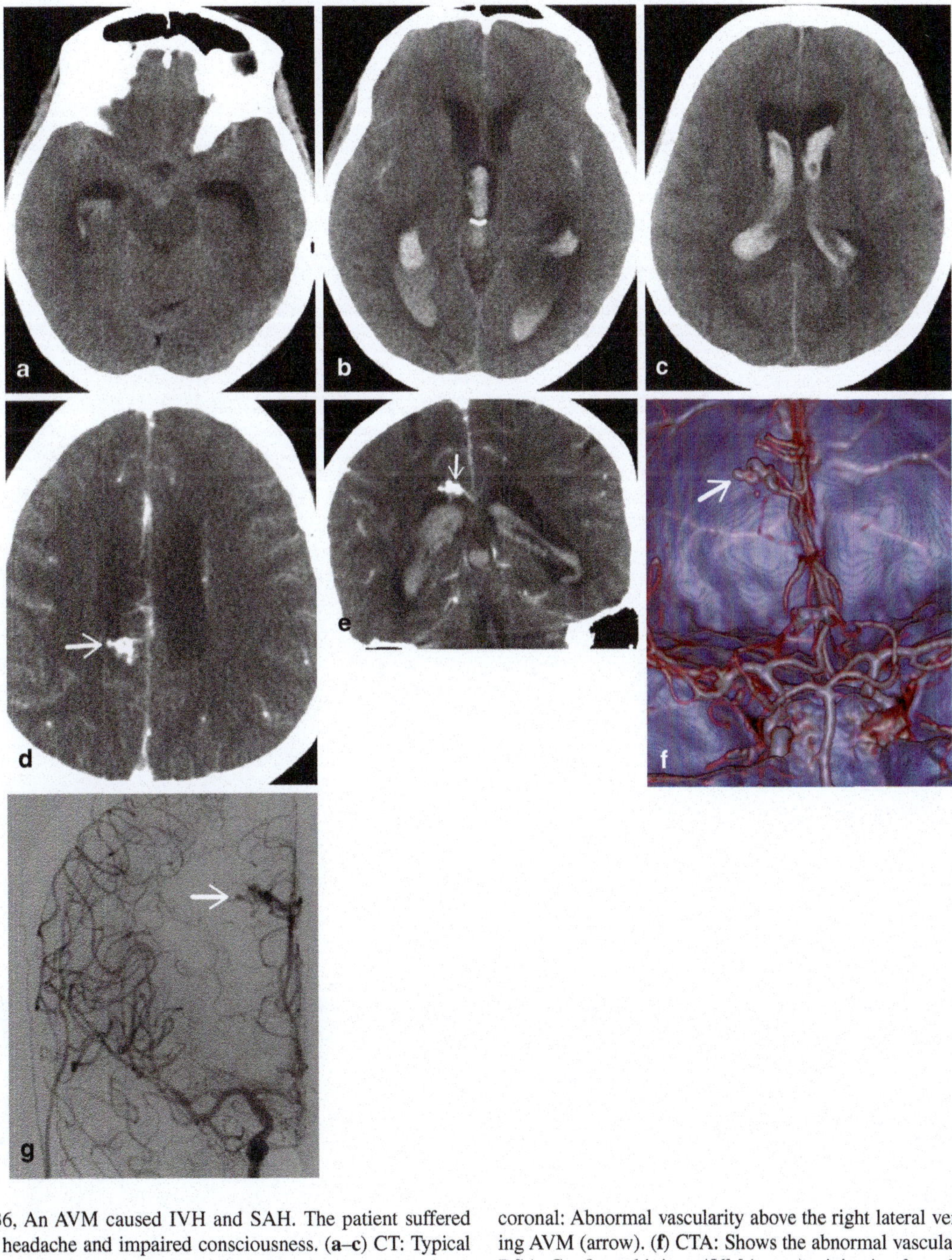

Fig. 4.68 F/36, An AVM caused IVH and SAH. The patient suffered from a severe headache and impaired consciousness. (**a–c**) CT: Typical SAH in the suprasellar cistern and bilateral Sylvian fissures, and a large amount of IVH, hydrocephalus. (**d**, **e**) Contrast-enhanced CT, axial and coronal: Abnormal vascularity above the right lateral ventricle, suggesting AVM (arrow). (**f**) CTA: Shows the abnormal vascularity (arrow). (**g**) DSA: Confirms this is an AVM (arrow) originating from the right ACA. In summary, this AVM bled into the ventricles and caused secondary SAH

References

1. Ripoll MA, et al. Detection and appearance of intraparenchymal haematomas of the brain at 1.5T with spin-echo, FLAIR and GE sequences: poor relationship to the age of the haematomas. Neuroradiology. 2004;46:435–43.
2. Bradley WG. MR appearance of hemorrhage in the brain. Radiology. 1993;189:15–26.
3. Kidwell CS, et al. Comparison of MRI and CT for detection of acute intracerebral hemorrhage. JAMA. 2004;292:1823–30.
4. Macdonald RL, Schweizer TA. Spontaneous subarachnoid hemorrhage. Lancet. 2017;389:655–66.
5. Agid R, et al. Negative CT angiography findings in patients with spontaneous subarachnoid hemorrhage: when is digital subtraction angiography still needed? AJNR Am J Neuroradiol. 2010;31:696–705.
6. Rinkel GJ, et al. Subarachnoid hemorrhage without detectable aneurysm: a review of the causes. Stroke. 1993;24:1403–9.
7. Larsen CC, Astrup J. Rebleeding after aneurysmal subarachnoid hemorrhage: a literature review. World Neurosurg. 2013;79:307–12.
8. Bracchi M, et al. Superficial siderosis of the CNS: MR diagnosis and clinical findings. AJNR Am J Neuroradiol. 1993;14:227–36.
9. Morita A, et al. The natural course of unruptured cerebral aneurysm in a Japanese cohort. N Engl J Med. 2012;366:2474–82.

5 Medical Imaging of Ischemic Stoke

Abstract

CT is the first tool for the diagnosis of acute infarction, but CT is not sensitive to detect early infarction. Several signs of early stages of MCA infarction are noted, including loss of insular ribbon sign, obscuration of lentiform nucleus sign, loss of gray–white matter contrast sign, effacement of cortical sulci sign, and bright MCA sign. The DWI of MRI can accurately diagnose large and small infarctions at a very early stage because the infarct area is cytotoxic edema with diffusion restriction, showing bright (hyperintense) in DWI. CT perfusion is a method to determine whether the infarction is in golden 6 h. Using parameters, such as CBF, CBV, MTT, and DT, can determine the core and penumbra of the hypoperfusion area to determine whether to perform IV thrombolysis and IA thrombectomy. Cerebral vein and venous sinus thrombosis may cause venous infarction edema similar to arterial infarction edema on CT. CT can identify the thrombus as an "empty delta sign." MRI reveals that the venous infarction edema is cytotoxic edema in the middle and combines with peripheral vasogenic edema. The brain damage caused by CO poisoning is primarily in the bilateral globus pallidus, and severe poisoning may involve the centrum semiovale. These brain injuries are also bright in DWI. Moyamoya disease is stenosis and occlusion of the distal ICA with smoke-like collateral circulation vessels in the brain. In adults, it may present ICH and IVH and in children it may present ischemic infarction. Small vessel diseases include leukoaraiosis, microbleeds, and dilated Virchow–Robin spaces. Using variable pulse sequences, MRI is more sensitive than CT in diagnosing small vessel diseases.

5.1 Pathophysiology of Ischemic Stroke

The pathophysiology of ischemic stroke involves the three following mechanisms [1] (Fig. 5.1):

(a) Embolism: obstruction of intracranial arteries caused by a distant embolus. The most common sources of embolus are as follows:
   1. Heart: embolus formed especially by atrial fibrillation, cardiac wall disease, or valve abnormality.
   2. Artery to artery.
      - Carotid bifurcation: atherosclerotic change in the very proximal portion of the internal carotid artery (ICA) near the bifurcation, with embolus formation and flowing into the brain.
      - Embolus in the aortic arch.
      - Dissection of extracranial and intracranial arteries, such as basilar artery and ICA.
      - Such embolism commonly leads to the infarction of major intracranial arteries (such as MCA, ACA, PCA, PICA, and SCA) or their branches, which involves a wide range of brain tissue infarction.

(b) In situ thrombosis of intracranial arteries: Atherosclerosis of large and small arteries, causing stenosis of the arterial lumen and resulting in ischemic infarction in their perfusion area, or small or lacunar infarction of their penetrating arteries.

(c) Hypoperfusion: Atherosclerosis of extracranial arteries (such as ICA) and major intracranial arteries (such as MCA, ACA, and PCA) results in stenosis and steno-occlusion. This condition causes the further formation of watershed ischemic infarction in the arterial perfusion territory. Such infarction occurs in the cortex or subcortical white matter territory across a small and rosary-like area.

Systemic hypotension, such as shock, cardiac arrest, respiratory arrest, and carbon monoxide intoxication, may lead to global hypoxic-ischemic encephalopathy (HIE) in the brain. In such cerebral ischemia, intracranial blood vessels are not genuinely occluded. Brain damage may be found in the watershed territories of the cerebral cortex or deep areas of the brain, including basal ganglia, due to different levels of ischemia.

W.-C. Shen, *Diagnostic Neuroradiology*, https://doi.org/10.1007/978-981-15-4051-6_5

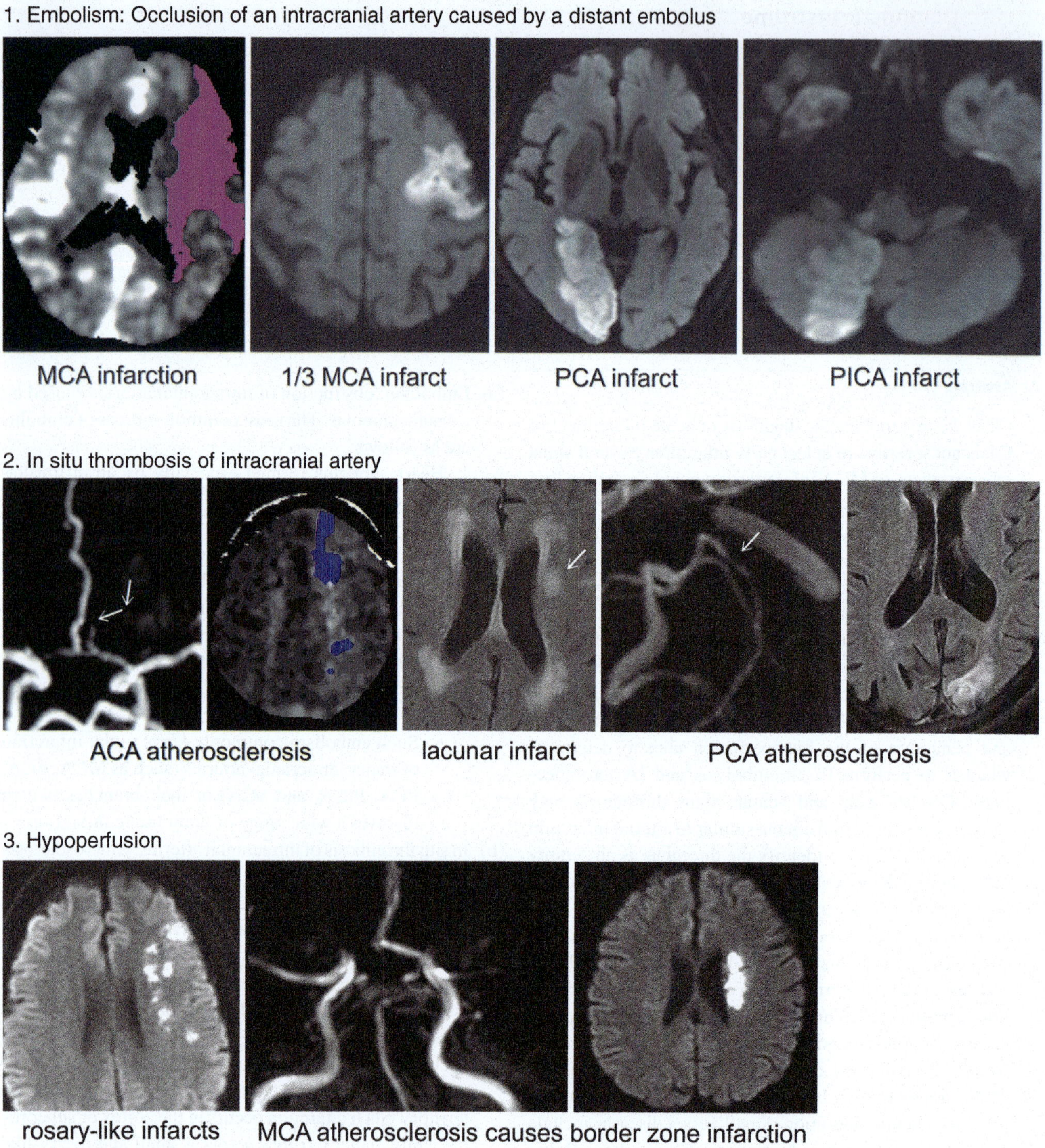

Fig. 5.1 Pathophysiology of ischemic stroke

5.2 Diagnostic Instruments for Brain Infarction

5.2.1 CT

CT is the preferred tool for the diagnosis of cerebral infarction because it is convenient and quick and can be used to detect brain tissue edema, hemorrhagic transformation, and mass effect caused by cerebral infarction. After the advent of multislice CT, CT perfusion and CTA have become important evaluation methods for intravenous (IV) thrombolysis or intra-arterial (IA) thrombectomy in the acute phase of ischemic stroke. However, CT also has disadvantages:

1. CT is insensitive for early brain tissue edema; as such, detection of large infarction takes more than 6–8 h, and detection of small or lacunar infarction takes more than 2 days.
2. Cerebral infarction of medulla oblongata is difficultly detected by CT.
3. CT may fail to reveal small or lacunar infarction.
4. Acute, subacute, and chronic infarction are sometimes difficult to distinguish.

5.2.2 MRI

MRI is more sensitive than CT in detecting cerebral infarction. MRI can detect cerebral infarction that has occurred after several hours. Furthermore, DWI images can even detect changes in cerebral edema in few minutes of infarction. Moreover, MRI is better in detecting brain stem infarction than CT. MRI has a lower chance of failing to detect lacunar infarction at medulla oblongata or any other location of the brain compared with CT. Furthermore, MRI can clearly distinguish among leukoaraiosis, lacunes, microbleeds, and dilated Virchow–Robin spaces caused by small vessel diseases, which are closely related to stroke.

MRA is an MRI examination routine that can assist in the evaluation of major intracranial and extracranial arteries.

MRI pulse sequences for the interpretation of cerebral infarction [2] (Figs. 5.2 and 5.3):

T1WI: Brain tissue edema caused by acute infarction is gray-dark (mild hypointensity) on T1WI and shows mass effect, compressing the adjacent ventricles, cisterns, fissures, and sulci.

T2WI: Cerebral edema in the acute infarct area shows hyperintensity as white color. Chronic cerebral infarction and ischemic demyelination are also hyperintense. Moreover, CSF is whitened, which sometimes brings confusion to the diagnosis of cerebral infarction.

FLAIR: Refers to T2-FLAIR, which is a type of T2WI but inverts the flowing CSF signal into the dark. Thus, on FLAIR, the brain tissue edema is visible but still indistinguishable from chronic infarction and ischemic demyelination.

DWI: Only brain tissue edema with water diffusion restriction shows hyperintensity (bright) in DWI. The acute infarct area is quite prominent. Even very small and low position infarctions, such as in the medulla oblongata, are very clear on DWI.

Moreover, the brightening time for DWI is short. In animal experiments, DWI is brightened 40 s after vascular obstruction. Ordinary MRI is performed at least 1 h after stroke onset. An infarction on T2WI or FLAIR has no signal change but is already apparent on DWI. Thus, DWI is the vital pulse sequence for detecting acute infarction. The high signal of DWI can be maintained in the acute phase for 10–14 days and then gradually weakens. In the chronic phase, if the cavitary change occurs in the infarction area, then it becomes dark.

ADC: ADC reflects the diffusion coefficient value of water molecules. In the acute phase of infarction, the diffusion of water molecules is suppressed. The ADC signal is darkened and can last for 7–10 days. In 10–15 days, the signal is returned to be normal. After 15 days, which refers to the chronic phase, the ADC signal gradually increases and becomes white [3].

T2*WI: It is the most sensitive to the detection of acute and chronic hemorrhage and thus can detect any hemorrhagic transformation in the infarct territory. This method is also very sensitive to microbleeds caused by small vessel diseases.

SWI, SWAN: For the detection of acute and chronic hemorrhage and microbleeds, SWI and SWAN are more sensitive, and it is easier to see changes in intracerebral vessels than T2*WI.

For the above pulse sequence, please also see Chap. 2.

5.2.3 Digital Subtraction Angiography (DSA)

In general, the diagnosis of cerebral infarction only requires CT and MRI. CT and MRI also provide CTA and MRA, which are sufficient to evaluate intracerebral and extracerebral blood vessels. DSA only be performed before or during interventional therapy.

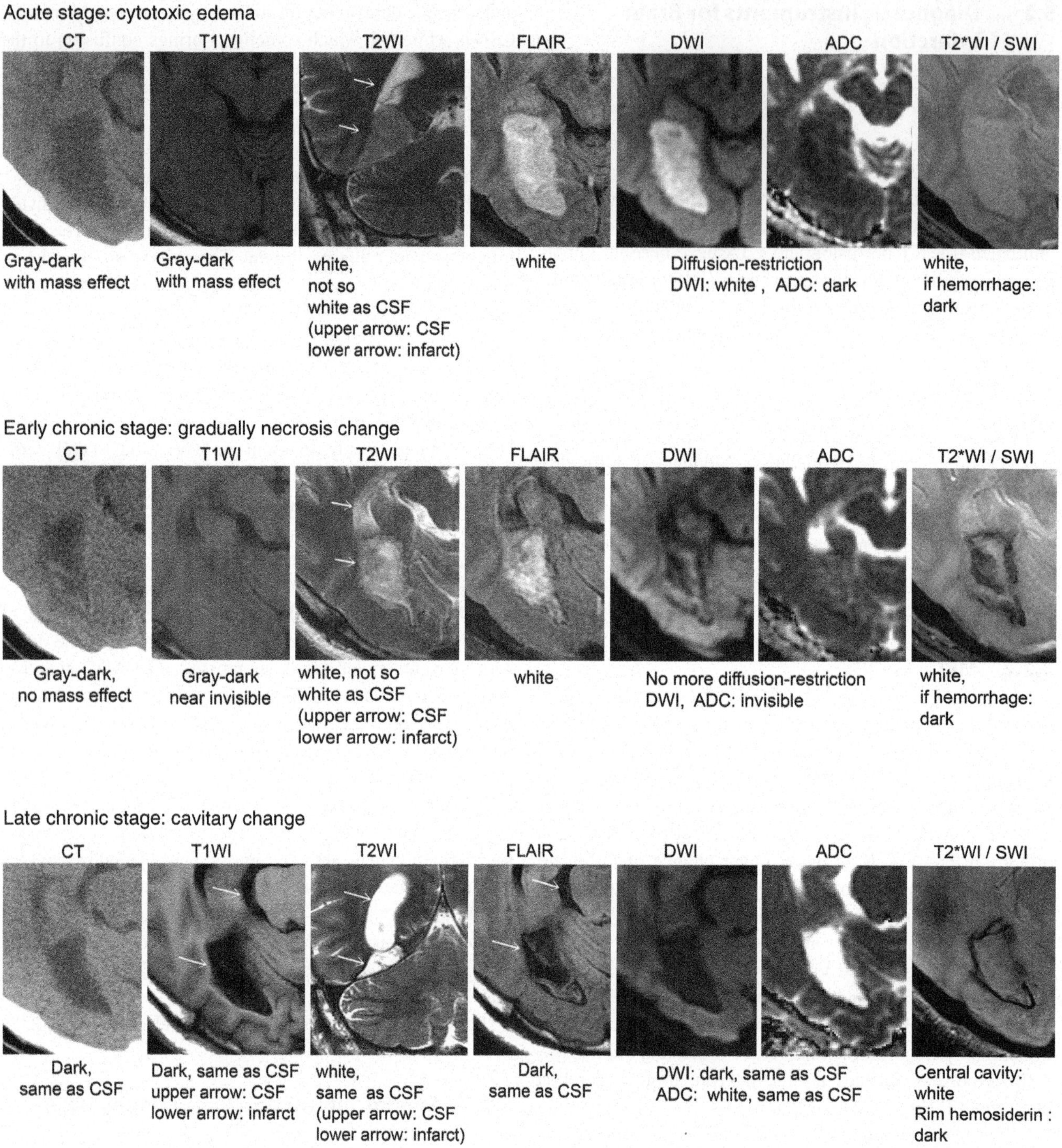

Fig. 5.2 Evolution of Infarction in CT, MRI

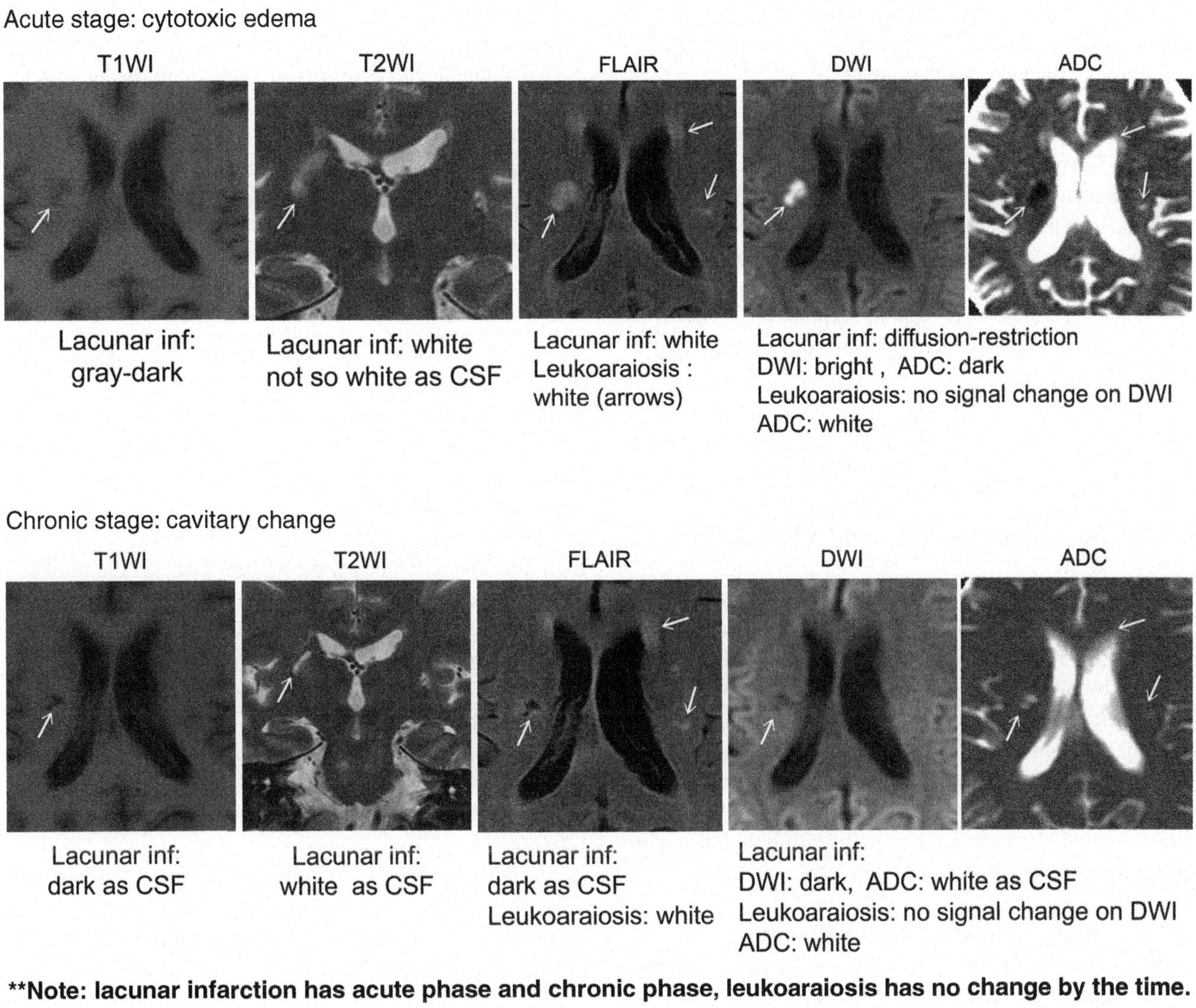

Fig. 5.3 Lacunar infarction and leukoaraiosis, evolution in MRI

5.3 The Evolution of Cerebral Infarction and Image Changes in CT and MRI

5.3.1 Hyperacute Stage

As the incidence of middle cerebral artery (MCA) infarction is the highest and MCA supplies the largest area of brain tissue, it causes the most obvious symptoms. This section mainly describes the MCA infarction.

MCA infarction sometimes involves a large area of brain tissue, which may lead to lifelong disabilities or even cause death. Therefore, the hyperacute infarction of MCA must be identified within a few hours of onset.

A large area of acute cerebral infarction for more than 10 h is easy to diagnose with CT because brain tissue edema in the cerebral infarct territory is gray-dark on CT and shows mass effect, causing sulcal effacement, compressing the adjacent ventricles. However, in the early hours of infarction, brain tissue edema is not apparent, indicating that the density of infarct territory has not been reduced, and with no mass effect, this condition is challenging to diagnose with CT. Even after 6 h, diagnosis with CT remains difficult, though some subtle signs are present. CT is the first-line diagnostic tool for stroke; as such, interpretation of MCA infarction by CT, especially the early signs in the hyperacute stage, is crucial.

The early signs of MCA infarction are as follows:

5.3.1.1 Loss of Insular Ribbon Sign

The normal insular cortex is thin, curved, and ribbon-like. It is gray matter and appears gray on CT (Figs. 5.4, 5.5, 5.6, 5.7, and 5.9). In case of MCA infarction, as the insular cortex is thin, identifying edema is the easiest because insular cortex changes to be gray-dark, which is called "loss of insular ribbon sign." This feature is a meaningful sign to judge MCA infarction in the hyperacute stage [4].

5.3.1.2 Obscuration of the Lentiform Nucleus Sign

Putamen and globus pallidus are collectively called lentiform nucleus, which is gray matter and appears gray on CT. During early edema, the lentiform nucleus is slightly darkened (Figs. 5.5, 5.6, 5.7, 5.9, and 5.12), making it easily recognizable, which is a meaningful diagnostic sign of early infarction MCA [5]. This is called "obscuration of the lentiform nucleus sign."

The putamen changed to be gray-dark from normal gray, is also called "inverted putaminal sign".

The caudate nucleus adjacent to the putamen is also gray matter and will be slightly darkened on the same time.

5.3.1.3 Loss Gray–White Matter Differentiation Sign

This sign is the disappearance of the gray and white matter contrast of brain tissue in the frontal, temporal, and parietal lobes of MCA territory. The gray and white matter in the healthy brain tissue is gray and dark gray on CT, respectively. After 6 h of infarction, brain tissue edema gradually becomes apparent. During this period, the gray matter is sensitive to change in density and appears as dark gray, which is equivalent to the density of white matter. This feature is called "loss gray–white matter differentiation sign" (Figs. 5.5, 5.6, and 5.7).

5.3.1.4 Effacement of Cortical Sulci Sign

This sign involves brain tissue edema in the infarct territory, which begins to produce a mass effect. The sulci become shallow and gradually efface and disappear [6] (Figs. 5.5, 5.6, and 5.7).

5.3.1.5 Hyperdense MCA Sign

Normal MCA has blood flow and is gray on CT. When it contains thrombus, it becomes slightly whiter (Figs. 5.6 and 5.7), which is called "hyperdense MCA sign." However, care must be taken not to mistake vascular wall calcification caused by MCA arteriosclerosis as thrombus [7, 8].

Once CT can reveal the above early sign within 6 h, the prognosis is worse, indicating that these brain tissues will tend to become necrotic due to ischemia in the future *[9, 10].*

For hyperacute infarction of ACA, PCA, or cerebellum, only two signs can be seen, namely **loss gray–white matter differentiation sign** and **effacement of cortical sulci sign**.

Similar to the hyperdense MCA sign, thrombus can also be seen in the basilar artery (Fig. 5.20) and the ICA (Figs. 5.6 and 5.7), making the blood vessels slightly whiter (hyperdense).

The T1WI, FLAIR, and T2WI of MRI may still show no signal changes after several hours of infarction (Fig. 5.6), making the diagnosis difficult. However, ***DWI can detect almost immediately when infarction occurs.***

5.3.2 Acute Stage

The range of cerebral infarction can be seen entirely, which appears as dark gray on CT (approximately 20–25 Hu) and shows a significant mass effect. This stage is easy to diagnose by CT. The long TR image of MRI (T2WI, FLAIR) in the infarct territory shows hyperintensity, which is more apparent than that in CT.

The mass effect rapidly increases on the second day after the infarction and reaches the highest peak on the third and fourth days. The mass effect disappears quickly after 1 week. Thus, the third to seventh day after the infarction is the most critical period. In the case of large infarction, uncal/transtentorial herniations (Fig. 5.8) may occur at any time, making the symptoms worse and even fatal.

5.3.3 Hemorrhagic Infarction

Hemorrhagic infarction is likely to occur in embolic infarction. Hemorrhagic infarction refers to hemorrhage in the infarct territory and is called hemorrhagic transformation (Figs. 5.9, 5.10, and 5.11), namely "red infarction" in pathology. This condition usually leads to bleeding within 2–10 days after infarction, and clinical symptoms aggravate. Clinically, early infarction is often treated by actively performing IV or IA intravascular thrombolytic therapy, and the incidence of hemorrhagic transformation is increased [11].

Hemorrhagic infarction is different from the hypertensive hemorrhagic stroke described in Chap. 4. The two cannot be confused with each other. Their distinctions are as follows:

	Hemorrhagic infarction	Hypertensive ICH
Bleeding location	In the infarct territory	Basal ganglion, thalamus, brain stem, cerebellum
Bleeding time	2–10 days	Immediately
Shape of blood clot	Multiple dot shape or patch shape	One single hematoma
Background	Brain tissue edema in the infarct territory	Slight brain tissue edema around the hematoma

5.3.4 Fogging Effect Stage

In theory, the infarct territory should be less dense, the mass effect should be stronger, and the CT image should be more easily interpreted over time. However, in some cases, the infarction area enters the fogging effect stage at 10–20 days, which is not easy to detect by CT (Fig. 5.12) for the following reasons:

1. The mass effect quickly fades after the eighth day of infarction.
2. The collateral circulation can bring much blood in 10–20 days, showing hyperemia, which increases the density of the infarct territory and making it difficult to interpret.

In the fogging effect stage, the contrast medium should be injected in CT and MRI, and the infarct territory will be enhanced by the contrast medium during this stage.

5.3.5 Enhancement Phenomenon of Contrast Medium in Infarct Territory

Approximately 6–42 days after infarction (peak at 10–20 days), the infarct territory may be enhanced by the contrast medium (Fig. 5.13), and its pathology is as follows:

1. During this stage, the blood–brain barrier (BBB), is temporarily disrupted in the infarct territory, which provides the contrast medium access into the brain tissue.
2. The luxurious perfusion stage occurs, in which collateral circulation brings abundant blood flow and a large amount of contrast medium.

The two following patterns of contrast enhancement occur in the infarction area:

1. Gyral pattern: formation of a gyral pattern through enhancement.
2. Patch pattern: the entire infarct territory is enhanced.

Sometimes, the infarct territory is too strongly enhanced and will be confused with AVM or brain tumor (Fig. 2.14). However, the enhancement of this infarct territory disappears after one and a half months due to the gradual repair of the BBB and the gradual retreat of the collateral circulation.

5.3.6 Chronic (Old) Infarction

After the cerebral infarction territory is re-perfused by the collateral circulation, some areas of brain tissue are indeed rescued, most of which tend to be necrotic. After 2 or 3 months, the infarction becomes chronic and will not be enhanced by the contrast medium. The density of the infarction showing darker on CT is closer to that of CSF. Furthermore, no mass effect occurs. The surrounding brain tissue is atrophied, and the nearby ventricles, cisterns, and sulci are widened (Figs. 5.9, 5.10, and 5.12).

The chronic infarction can be divided into two stages (Fig. 5.2). First, early chronic infarction: the infarct territory becomes darker (hypointensity) on T1WI and whiter (hyperintensity) on T2WI and FLAIR. However, the water-restriction characteristic of DWI disappears, and no signal change is observed on DWI (Fig. 5.21). Second, late chronic infarction: is older infarction, cavitary change occurs in the core of old infarct territory, and showing the same signal of CSF, which is as dark (hypointensity) as CSF on T1WI and FLAIR, as white (hyperintensity) as CSF on T2WI, combined with gliosis of surrounding brain tissue which is white (hyperintensity) on T2WI and FLAIR. The infarct territory and surrounding brain tissue are atrophied, whereas the nearby ventricles, cisterns, and sulcus are widened.

In MRI, even small and lacunar infarctions are evident cavitary change and are sometimes combined with peripheral gliosis of surrounding brain tissues (Fig. 5.3).

5.4 Middle Cerebral Artery Infarction (MCA Infarction)

MCA is the largest and most widely distributed artery in the brain, with the most robust blood flow. Therefore, it is the most likely for the extracranial thrombus to flow to MCA and form the embolic infarction (Figs. 5.4, 5.5, 5.6, 5.7, 5.8, and 5.9). If the occlusion occurs in ICA, then MCA and ACA will be simultaneously infarcted (Figs. 5.5, 5.8, and 5.12). If the occlusion occurs in the M1 segment of MCA, then it may result in extensive cerebral edema involving the basal ganglion and fronto-temporo-parietal lobes (Figs. 5.8 and 5.9), which will form a strong mass effect and cause quite severe clinical symptoms. Uncal/transtentorial herniations may even occur, resulting in brainstem compression and death. Therefore, it is called malignant MCA infarction [10, 12].

If the occlusion is in the branches of MCA, then it will result in the infarction of the anterior, middle, and posterior perfusion territories of the MCA (Figs. 5.11, 5.13, and 5.14).

The MCA itself is also prone to atherosclerosis and becomes stenotic, resulting in insufficient hemodynamic impairment and border zone infarction in the perfusion territory (see next section).

MCA also presents thrombus exfoliation due to its own atherosclerosis, resulting in small infarcts derived from its perforating arteries, which often occur in the corpus striatum, namely striatocapsular infarction (Figs. 5.10 and 5.15) and corona radiata.

5.4.1 Striatocapsular Infarction

Striatocapsular infarction is a unique infarction that is not clinically rare. The infarct area includes the head of the caudate nucleus, anterior limb of internal capsule, and putamen because the blood supply to these structures is the lateral lenticulostriate arteries, which originate from M1 of MCA. If the MCA is stenotic, then these small blood vessels may be occluded, forming a comma-shaped infarction (Figs. 5.10 and 5.15), whose longest diameter can be up to 3 cm. The cerebral cortex supplied by MCA shows no infarction because the cortex tends to have collateral circulation [13]. The main symptoms are hemiparesis of upper limb, dysphasia, neglect, and dyspraxia. This infarction is caused by four factors [14], namely (1) heart emboli occluding the proximal portion of the MCA, (2) severe stenosis of the ICA, (3) stenosis of the proximal portion of the MCA causing occlusion of lateral lenticulostriate arteries, and (4) unknown reason.

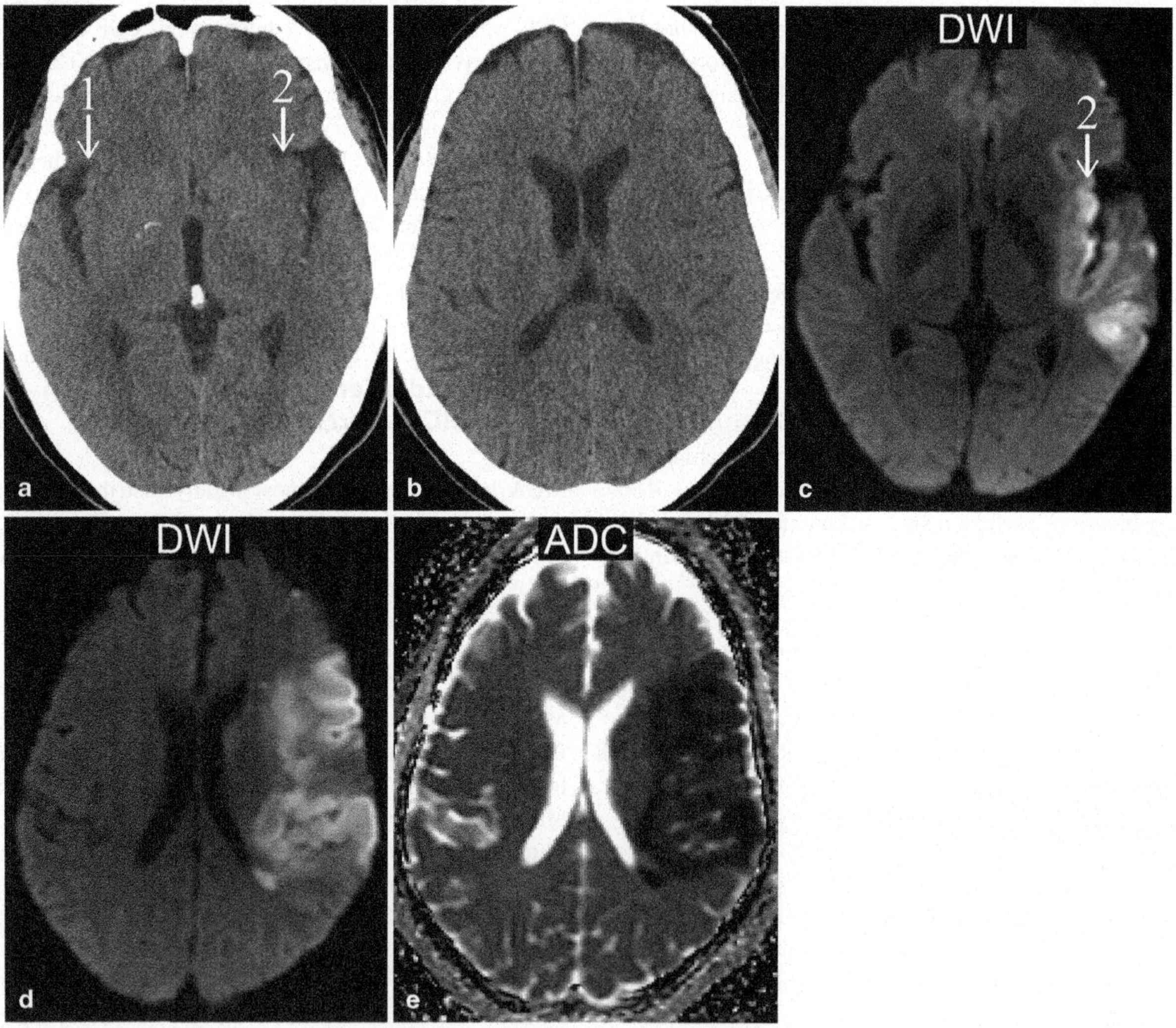

Fig. 5.4 F/70, Early signs of acute infarction. The patient experienced sudden onset of right-sided hemiplegia and alteration of consciousness. (**a**, **b**) CT, 2 h after the onset of symptoms: Compared with the right slightly gray insular cortex (1), the color of the left insular cortex turns slightly dark gray (2), representing early brain tissue edema, which is loss of insular ribbon sign. Although no brain tissue edema can be observed in the left cerebral hemisphere, this finding, combined with clinical symptoms, can be surmised as the very early stage of acute infarction of the left MCA. (**c**, **d**) MRI on the second day, DWI: A large area of brain tissue in the left fronto-parieto-temporal lobe, including insular cortex (2), is bright (hyperintensity), indicating diffusion restriction. This finding suggests cytotoxic edema due to acute infarction of left MCA. (**e**) ADC map: The infarction area is dark (hypointensity) because of the low diffusion coefficient

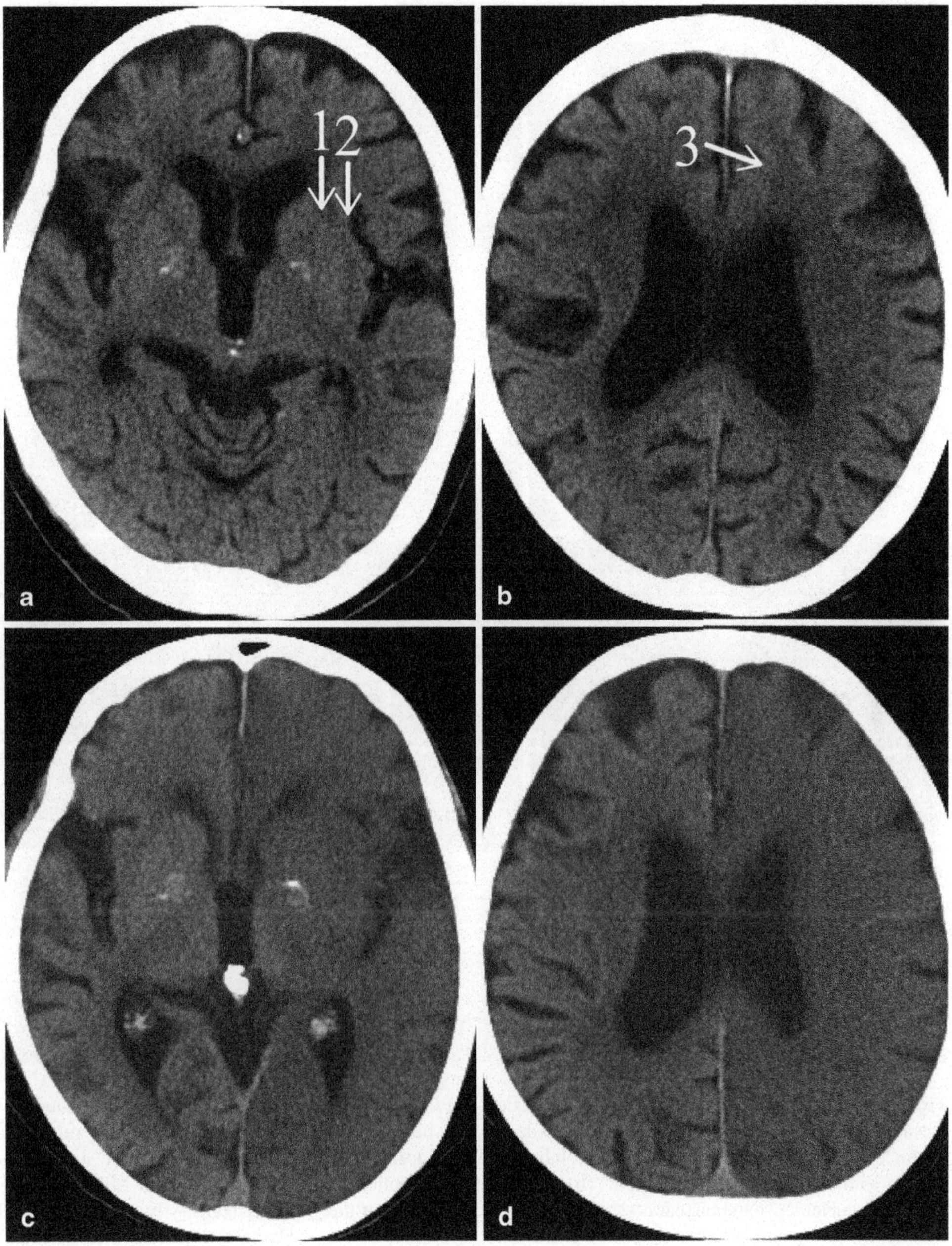

Fig. 5.5 F/91, Early signs of acute infarctions. (**a**, **b**) A CT 1 year ago for comparison: The lentiform nucleus (putamen) is gray (1); the insular cortex is gray (2); the gray matter in the frontal lobe is gray, and the white matter is slightly dark (3). (**c**, **d**) CT, 12 h after an acute stroke: Compared with the above figures, the color of the left lentiform nucleus and the insular cortex changes to dark gray (obscuration of lentiform nucleus sign and loss of insular ribbon sign). The gray matter in the whole left cerebral hemisphere becomes dark gray similar to the white matter (loss of gray–white matter differentiation signs), and effacement of cortical sulci can be observed (sulci effacement sign). Given that the brain edema is in the whole left cerebral hemisphere, the infarction includes the left MCA, ACA, and PCA

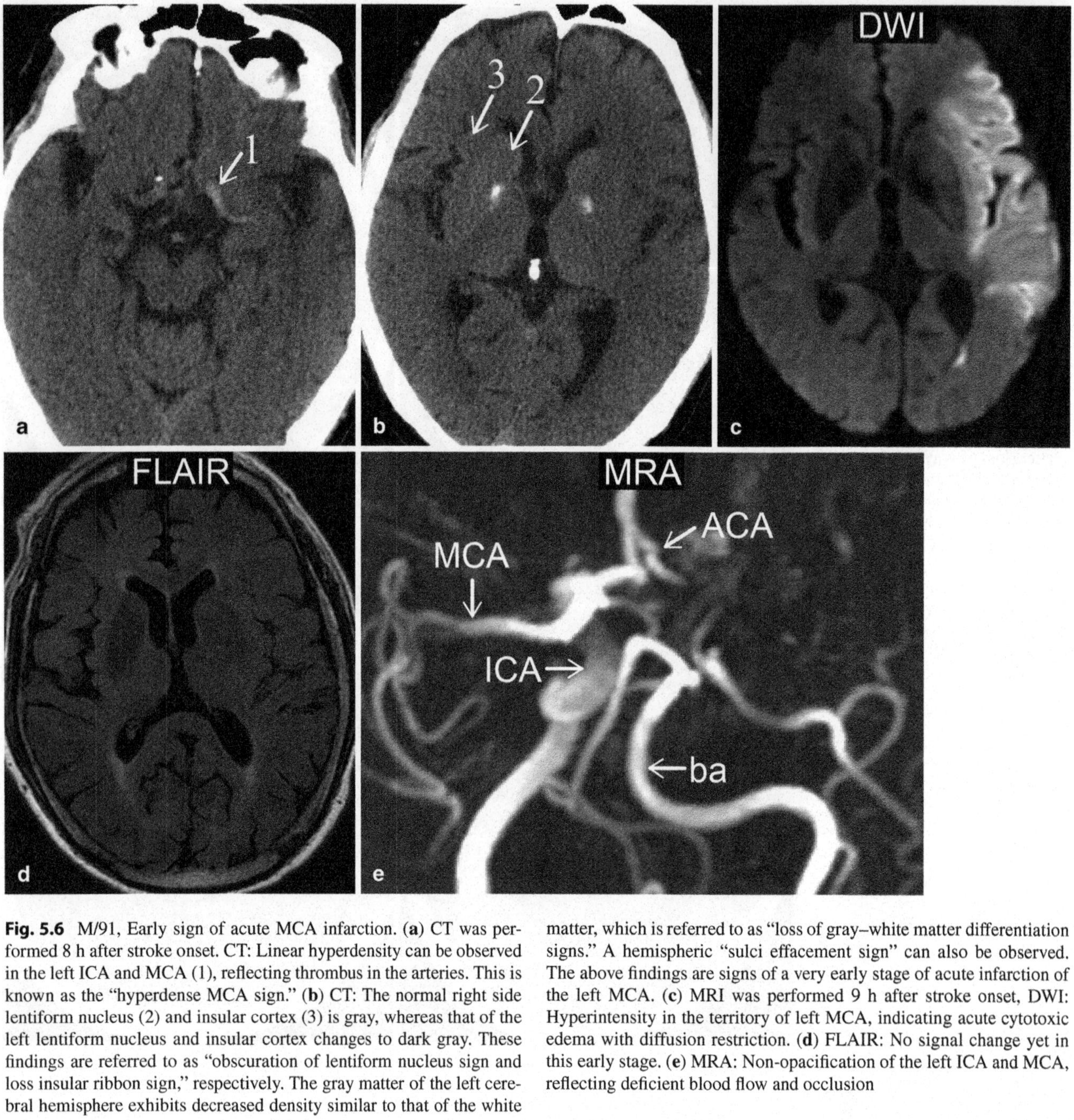

Fig. 5.6 M/91, Early sign of acute MCA infarction. (**a**) CT was performed 8 h after stroke onset. CT: Linear hyperdensity can be observed in the left ICA and MCA (1), reflecting thrombus in the arteries. This is known as the "hyperdense MCA sign." (**b**) CT: The normal right side lentiform nucleus (2) and insular cortex (3) is gray, whereas that of the left lentiform nucleus and insular cortex changes to dark gray. These findings are referred to as "obscuration of lentiform nucleus sign and loss insular ribbon sign," respectively. The gray matter of the left cerebral hemisphere exhibits decreased density similar to that of the white matter, which is referred to as "loss of gray–white matter differentiation signs." A hemispheric "sulci effacement sign" can also be observed. The above findings are signs of a very early stage of acute infarction of the left MCA. (**c**) MRI was performed 9 h after stroke onset, DWI: Hyperintensity in the territory of left MCA, indicating acute cytotoxic edema with diffusion restriction. (**d**) FLAIR: No signal change yet in this early stage. (**e**) MRA: Non-opacification of the left ICA and MCA, reflecting deficient blood flow and occlusion

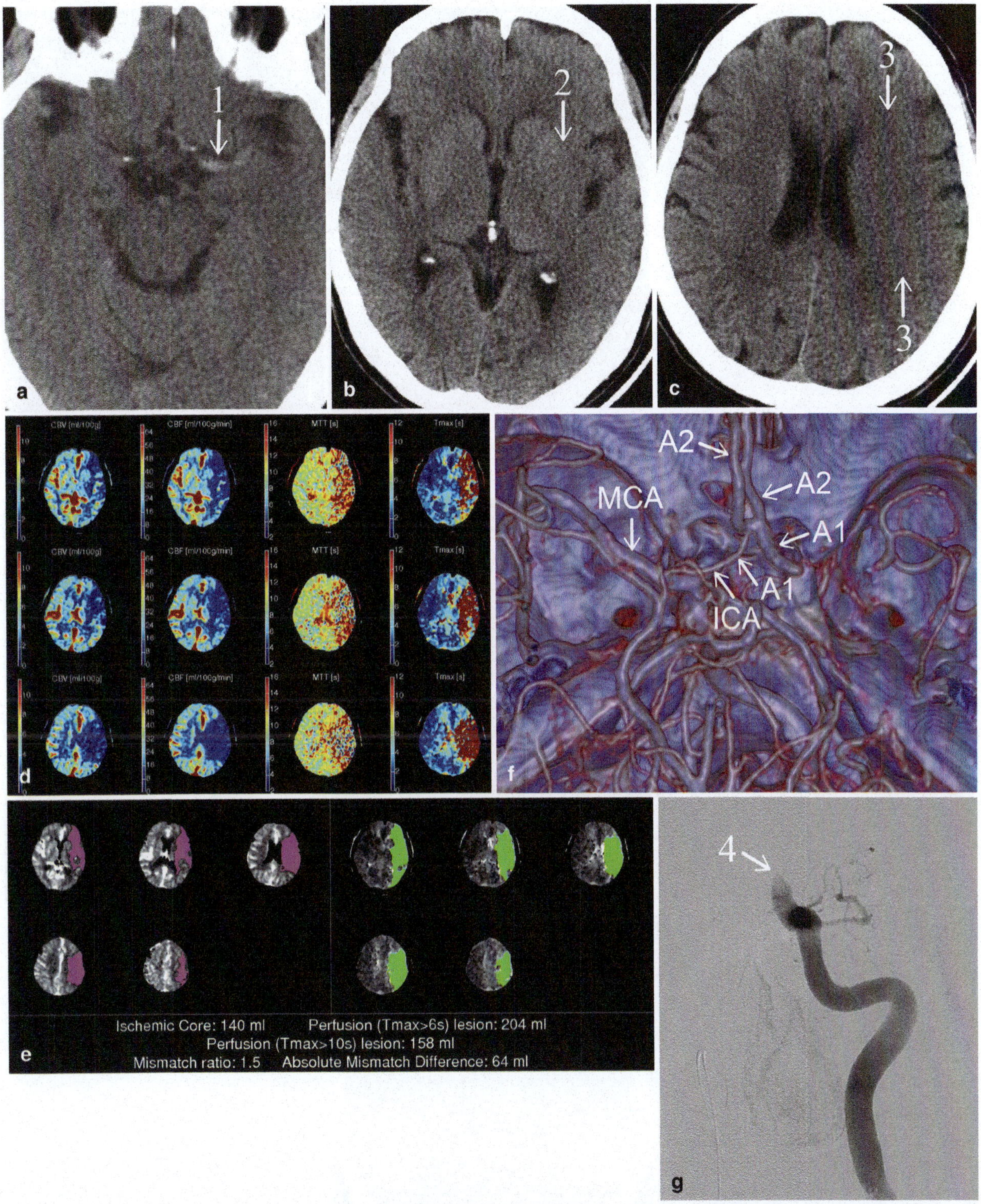

Fig. 5.7 F/68, Total occlusion of the left MCA. The patient suddenly developed right hemiplegia. After being treated in a local hospital, it took more than 6 h to transfer the patient to a medical center. (**a**) CT: Linear hyperdensity can be observed in the left ICA and MCA (1). This is the "hyperdense MCA sign," reflecting thrombus in the arteries. (**b**, **c**) CT: Early signs of acute MCA infarctions, which are associated with the color change in the putamen to dark gray (2), this is inverted putaminal sign. Loss of gray–white matter contrast (3) in the left frontoparietal lobes. Once the early signs appear, the prognosis becomes poor. (**d**, **e**) CT perfusion and summary map: The core area is large, 140 mL. The mismatch (penumbra) is only 64 mL, and the mismatch ratio is 1.5. (**f**) CTA: Well demonstration of the right ICA, MCA, and bilateral ACAs; the left ICA and MCA are non-opacified, reflecting occlusion. (**g**) DSA: Total occlusion of the distal portion of the left ICA due to a thrombus (4). (**h**) DSA soon after IA thrombectomy: Successful retrieval of the thrombus. The blood flow of the left MCA returns to normal. (**i**, **j**) However, clinical symptoms did not improve. MRI was performed on the second day, DWI: The whole left MCA territory is hyperintense, reflecting diffusion restriction with cytotoxic edema. The edema area corresponds to the core area of CT perfusion

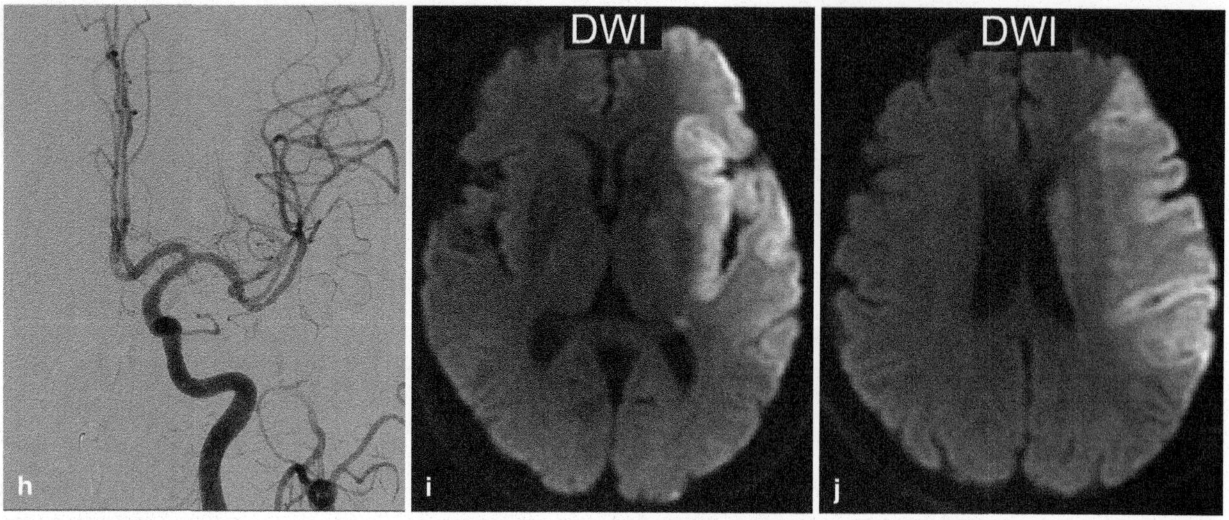

Fig. 5.7 (continued)

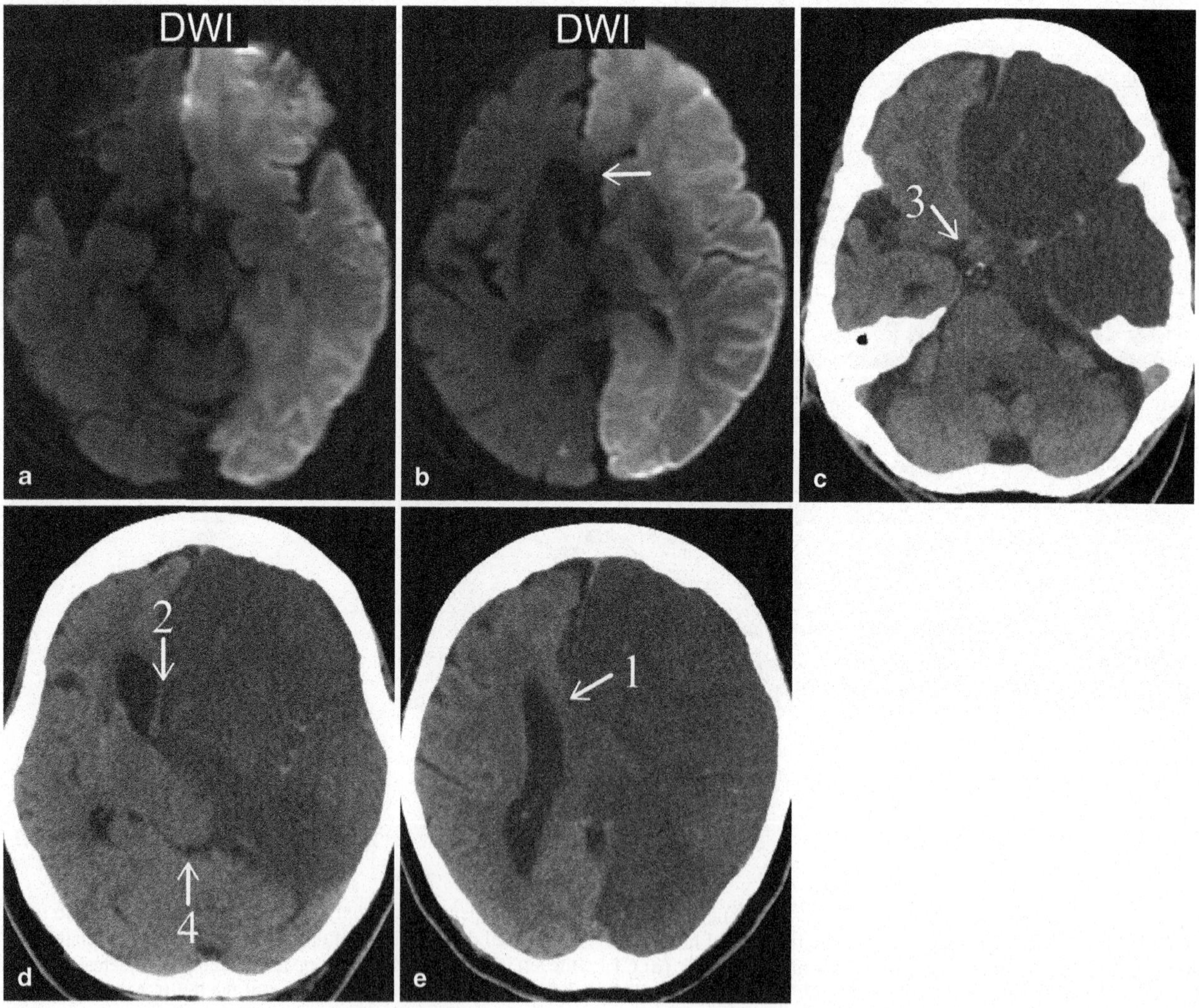

Fig. 5.8 F/94, Large area of acute infarction with strong mass effect. The patient suffered a sudden onset of right hemiplegia, eye deviation to the left side, and loss of consciousness. Urgent CT showed no intracerebral hemorrhage or brain tissue edema (not shown). (**a**, **b**) MRI was performed approximately 3 h after the onset of stroke symptoms, DWI: Hyperintensity in almost the whole left cerebral hemisphere, representing diffused cytotoxic edema. At this early infarction stage, the mass effect is small, and the left ventricle is only slightly compressed (arrow). (**c**–**e**) CT on the third day: Severe brain tissue edema of the whole left cerebral hemisphere with strong mass effect. The left lateral ventricle is compressed and disappeared (1). The midline shifts to the right (2). Deformity of the suprasellar cistern (3) and the quadrigeminal cistern (4), indicating uncal/transtentorial herniations

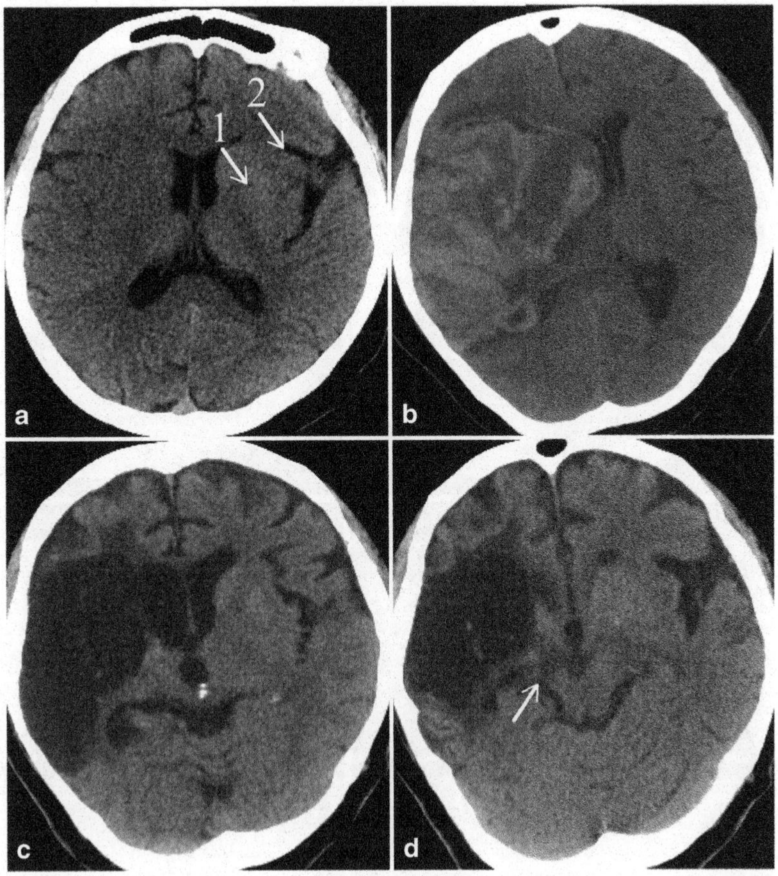

Fig. 5.9 F/76, Hemorrhagic infarction. This patient suffered a sudden onset of left-sided hemiplegia. (**a**) CT was performed 8 h after the onset of symptoms: Compared with the gray left-side normal lentiform nucleus (1) and insular cortex (2), the color of the two anatomic structures on the right side changes to dark gray, which are early signs of acute MCA infarction. (**b**) CT 1 week later: Diffuse hemorrhage can be observed in the infarction area, which is referred to as "hemorrhagic transformation"; hence, this infarction is referred to as "hemorrhagic infarction." The infarction edema, combined with hemorrhage, strengthens the mass effect. The right lateral ventricle is compressed, making it appear small, and the midline shifts to the left side. (**c**, **d**) The patient survived. After 4 years, CT showed that the infarction became an old infarction. The density is dark as CSF, the brain tissue is atrophied, and the right ventricle is large. Given the long-term left hemiplegia, which causes brain stem Wallerian degeneration, the right cerebral peduncle of the midbrain is severely atrophied (arrow)

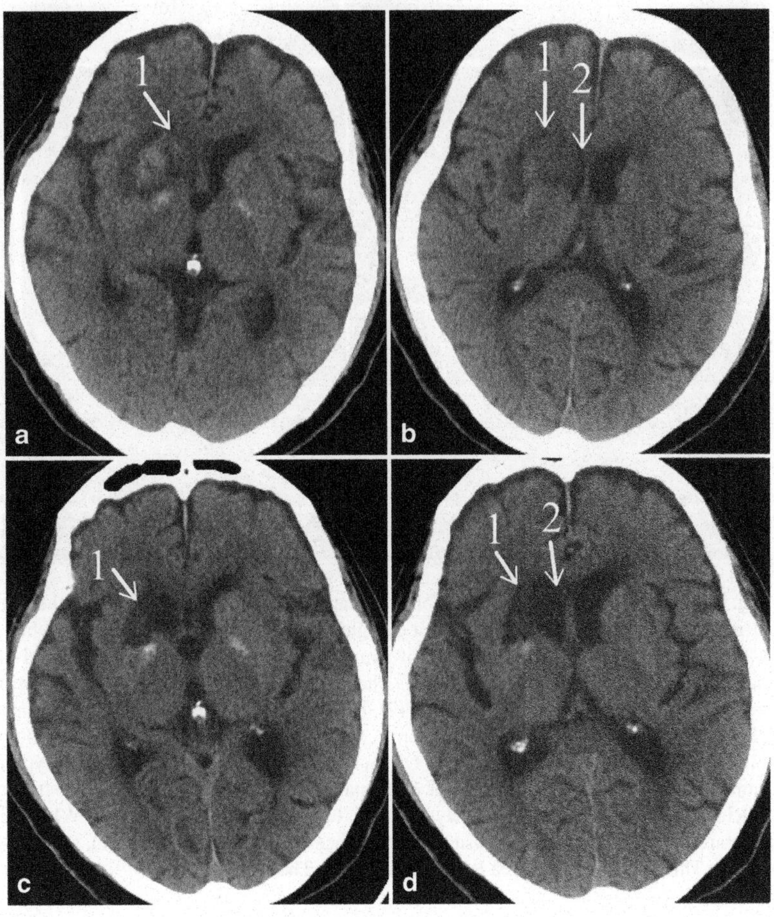

Fig. 5.10 F/84, Hemorrhagic infarction in the corpus striatum. This patient suffered left hemiparesis. (**a**, **b**) CT was performed on the fifth day after symptom onset: Brain tissue edema mixes with some hemorrhage (1) in the right corpus striatum (caudate nucleus and putamen). This finding suggests acute infarction with hemorrhagic transformation. The infarction edema causes a mass effect; the right lateral ventricle is compressed (2). (**c**, **d**) Follow-up CT after 6 months: The infarction area is hypodense (1), and the right lateral ventricle is dilated (2) because the infarction is in the chronic stage with brain tissue necrosis and atrophy

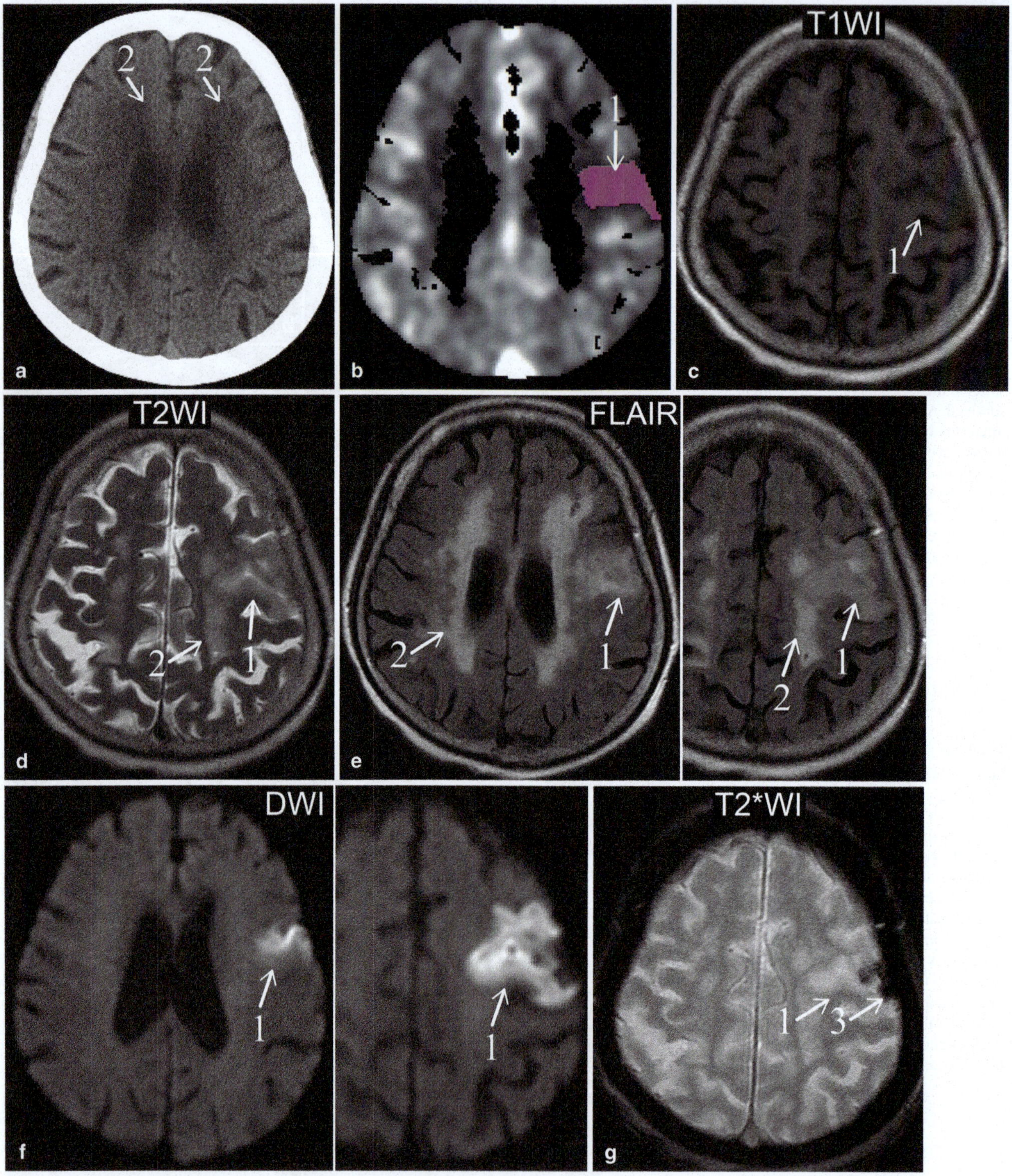

Fig. 5.11 F/87, Hemorrhagic infarction. The patient with a history of atrial fibrillation suffered a sudden onset of right-sided hemiplegia. (**a**) CT was performed 6 h after the onset of symptoms; no intracerebral hematoma or brain tissue edema is seen. The density in the bilateral periventricular white matter is decreased (2), indicating chronic demyelination (leukoaraiosis). (**b**) CT perfusion: A small area of brain tissue in the left frontal lobe shows decreased CBV (1), reflecting hypoperfusion, which is a possible indication of early stage of acute infarction. MRI was performed on the second day. (**c**) MRI, T1WI: The hypoperfusion area exhibits mild hypointensity (1) and effacement of sulcus. (**d**) T2WI: This hypoperfusion area is hyperintense (1). The demyelination (2) in the centrum semiovale and CSF in the sulci are also hyperintense; all are white and difficult to distinguish from one another. (**e**) FLAIR: The signal intensity of CSF is attenuated, which appears dark, and the hypoperfusion area is hyperintense (1). The demyelination (leukoaraiosis) (2) is also hyperintense. The hypoperfusion area and the leukoaraiosis are both difficult to distinguish. (**f**) DWI: Only the hypoperfusion area is hyperintense (1) because only the acute infarction area has diffusion restriction. The demyelination shows no signal change on DWI. (**g**) T2*WI: Some hypointensity (3) can be observed in the infarction area (1), which is a hemorrhagic transformation

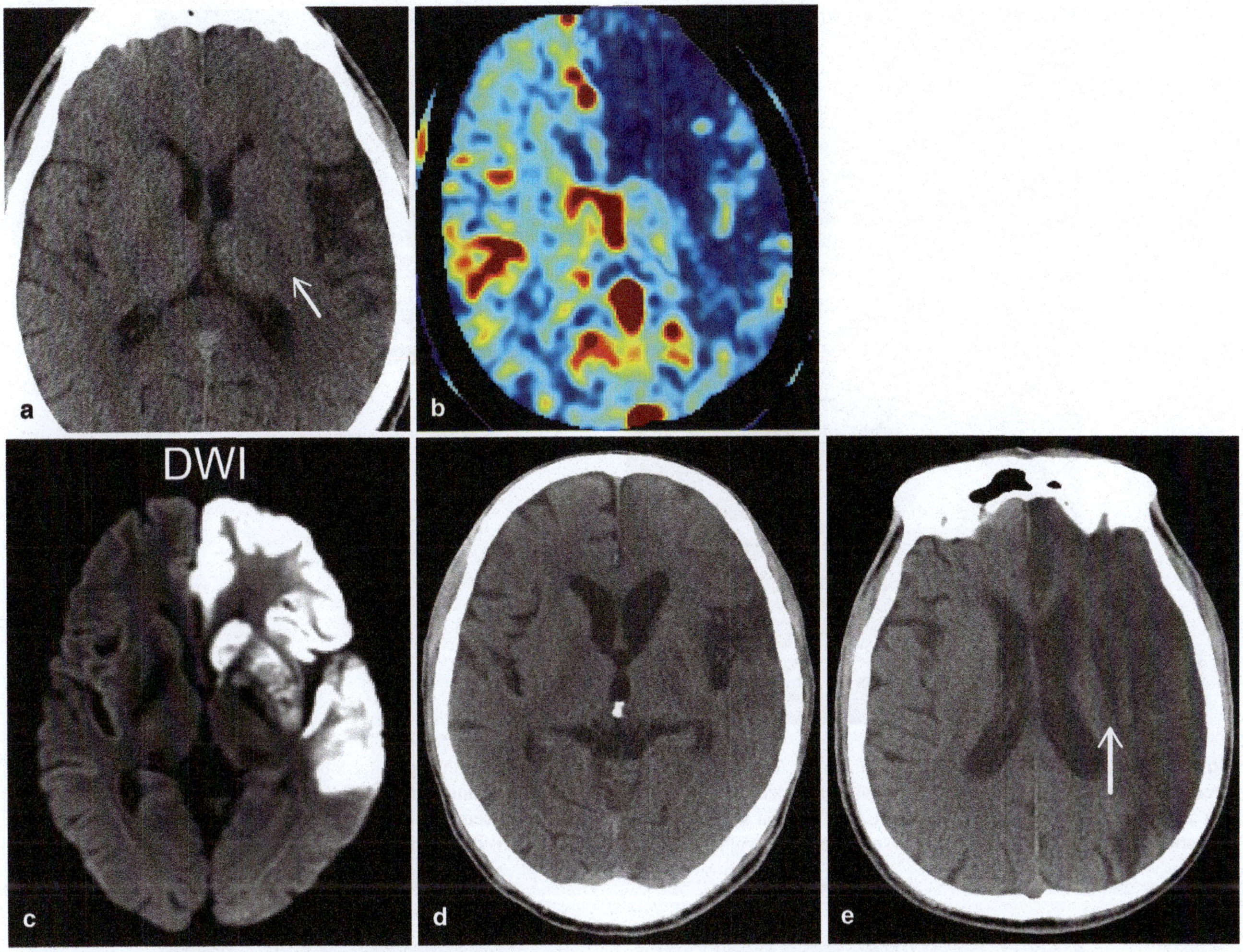

Fig. 5.12 M/61, Left MCA, ACA infarctions, with fogging effect. The patient suffered a sudden onset of right hemiplegia and then a coma. (**a**) Emergency CT: The left putamen (arrow) showing dark gray is an early sign of acute MCA infarction, this is inverted putaminal sign. (**b**) CT perfusion, cerebral blood flow (CBF) map: The blue color in the left ACA and MCA territories reflects deficient CBF. (**c**) MRI on the second day, DWI: The left ACA and MCA territories and left corpus striatum are bright (very hyperdense), indicative of cytotoxic edema with diffusion restriction. (**d**) Follow-up CT on the 14th day: Theoretically, the density of the infarct should decrease day by day, which can be easily observed by CT. However, on the 14th day, CT revealed no apparent brain tissue edema, only effacement of the sulci of the left frontal lobe. This occurrence is the so-called fogging effect stage of infarction, which is due to the hyperperfusion after recanalization of the occluded blood vessel or due to collateral circulation. (**e**) Right hemiplegia is persistent. Follow-up CT was performed after 6 months. A large area of the brain tissue in the left frontoparietal lobes and corpus striatum (arrow) is hypodense, which indicates old infarction

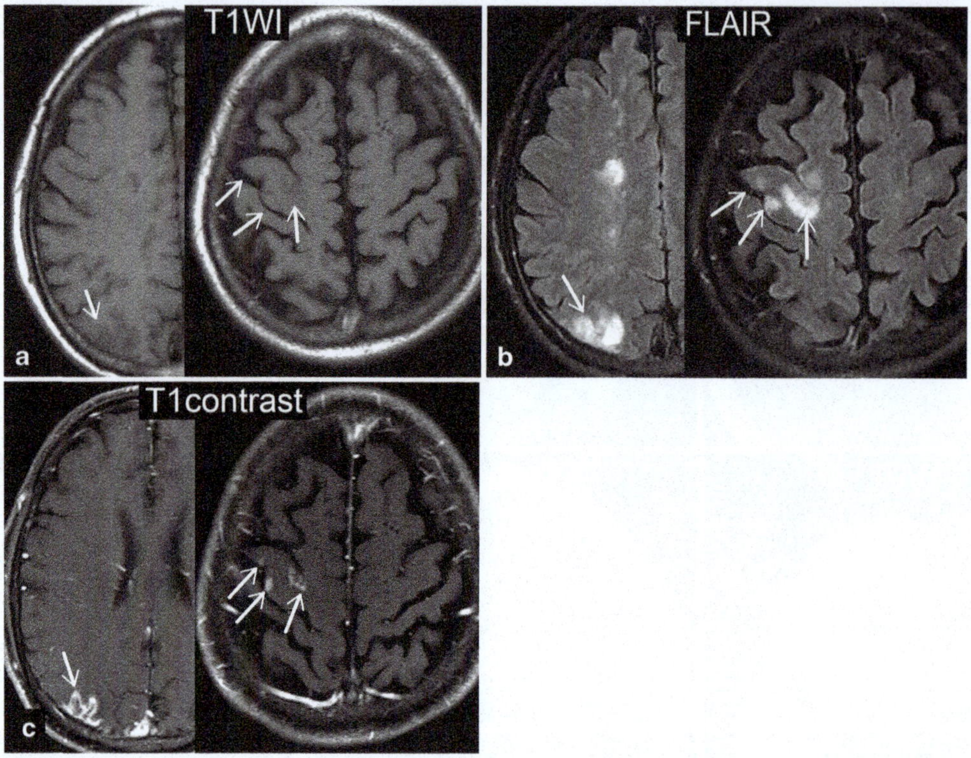

Fig. 5.13 M/63, Enhancement of the infarction area. The patient suffered from left-sided hemiparesis. MRI was performed on the fifth day after symptom onset. (**a, b**) T1WI, FLAIR: Several small acute infarctions can be observed in the cortex/subcortex of the right frontal lobe and cortex of the occipital lobe, showing mild hypointensity on T1WI and hyperintensity on FLAIR (arrows). (**c**) Contrast T1WI: Contrast enhancement of the above infarction areas is seen (arrows), indicating BBB destruction

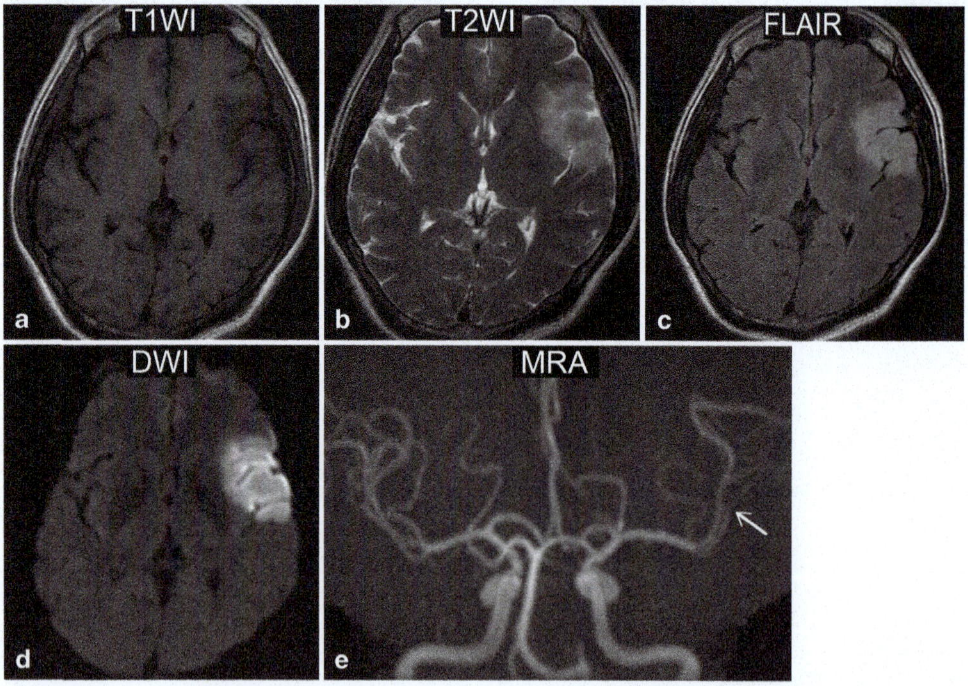

Fig. 5.14 M/41, Acute infarction in the anterior one-third of the MCA territory. This patient suffered a sudden onset of right hemiparesis and dysphonia. MRI was performed on the fifth day after symptom onset. (**a**) T1WI: A hypointense area can be seen in the left frontotemporal lobes. (**b, c**) T2WI, FLAIR: The above area shows hyperintense. (**d**) DWI: this area showing hyperintensity on DWI confirms diffusion restriction, which suggests cytotoxic edema caused by acute infarction. The infarction area is located in the anterior one-third territory of the left MCA. (**e**) MRA: Stenosis (arrow) is detected in a branch of the left MCA

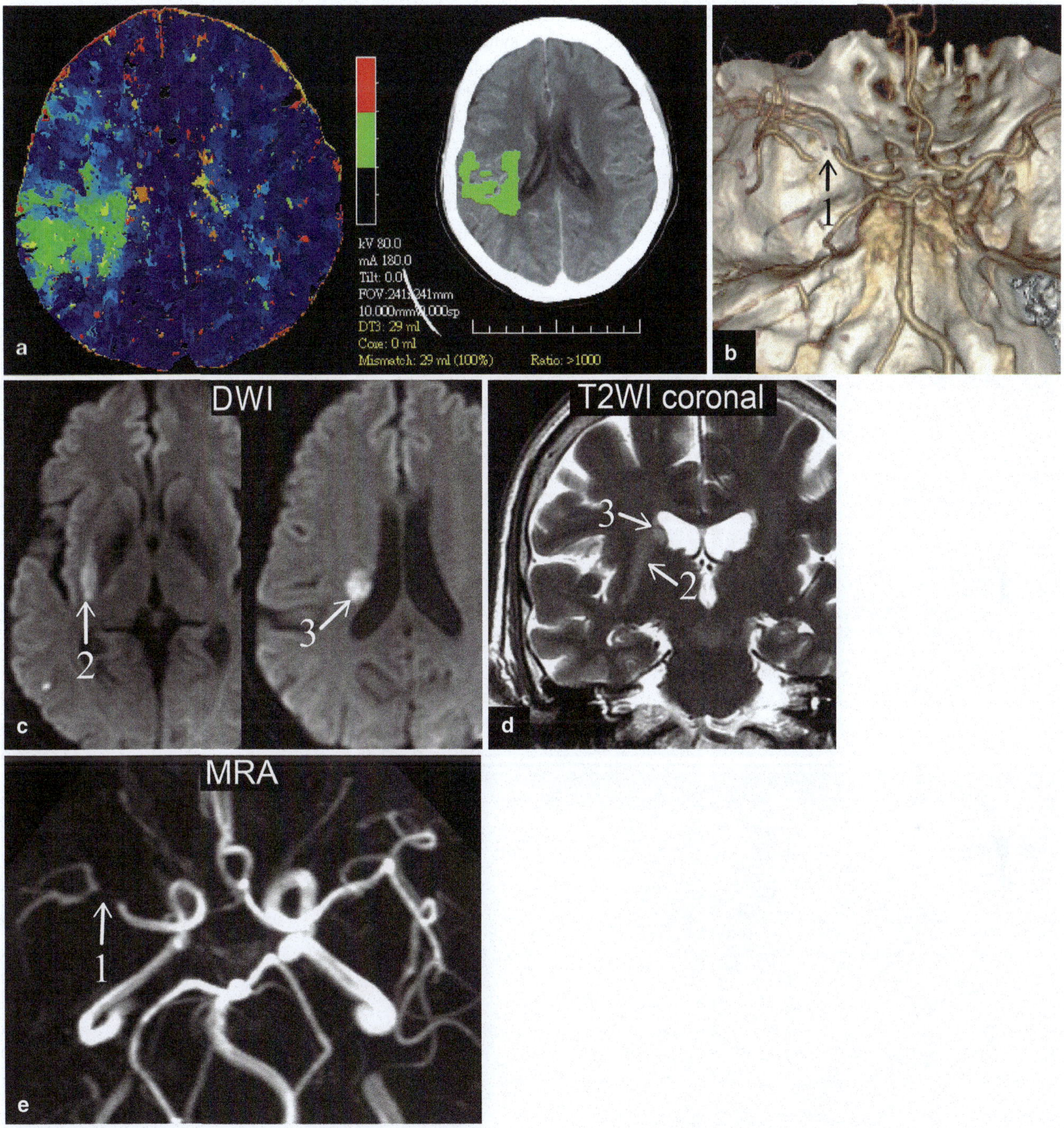

Fig. 5.15 F/72, Corpus striatum acute infarction. The patient with hyperlipidemia and no history of a stroke suffered a sudden onset of left hemiparesis. CT was performed 4 h after symptom onset. No visible brain tissue hemorrhage or edema was observed. Thus, CT perfusion and CTA were performed immediately. (**a**) CT perfusion, time to peak map: An area in the right MCA territory shows hypoperfusion; all are penumbra, without a core. (**b**) CTA: Segmental steno-occlusion (1) can be seen in the transverse portion of the right MCA. The patient received intravenous tPA treatment, but the symptoms persisted. MRI was then performed. (**c**) DWI: Hyperintensity is seen in the right putamen (2) and caudate nucleus (3), reflecting diffusion restriction, which is indicative of acute cytotoxic edema due to infarction. (**d**) T2WI, coronal section: The infarction showing hyperintensity in the corpus striatum, that is putamen (2) and caudate nucleus (3), appears as "comma shape." (**e**) MRA: Steno-occlusion in the transverse portion of the right MCA

5.5 Anterior Cerebral Artery Infarction (ACA Infarction)

ACA infarction is far less frequent than MCA and PCA infarction.

The infarction area is in the inner side of the frontal lobe, the front part of the corpus callosum, the anterior limb of the internal capsule, and the lower part of the caudate nucleus.

The most common cause is ICA remote obstruction in synergy with MCA infarction (Figs. 5.5, 5.8, and 5.12). Single ACA infarction is less frequent (Fig. 5.16) as the collateral circulation will support ACA perfusion territory.

ACA itself will also be stenotic due to atherosclerosis [15], causing hemodynamic impairment and resulting in subcortical rosary-like infarction and cortical infarction (Fig. 5.17).

Subfalcine herniation will compress ACA, resulting in ACA infarction (Fig. 3.31).

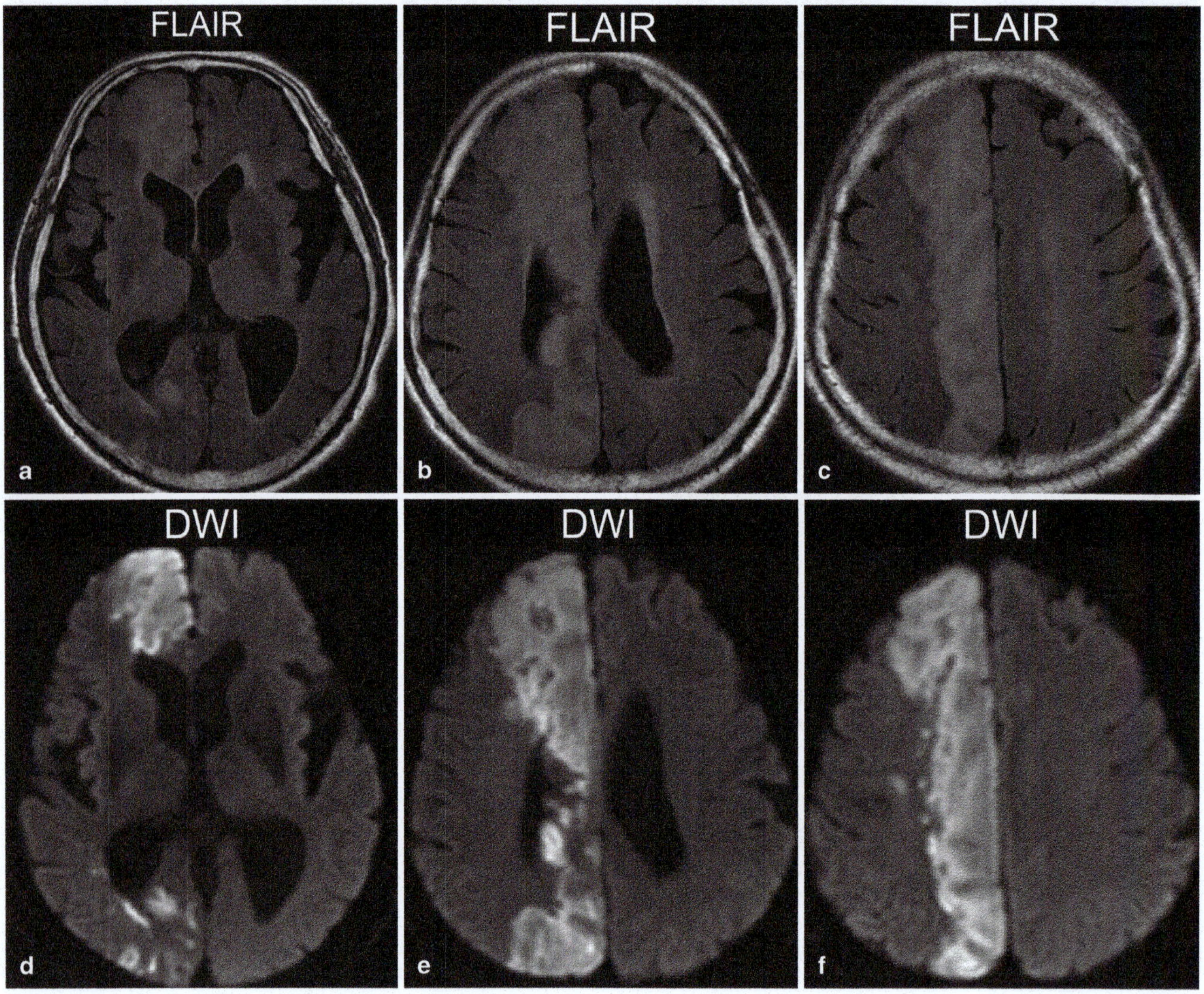

Fig. 5.16 M/67, ACA and PCA acute infarctions. A hypertensive and diabetic patient with a history of myocardial infarction had a sudden onset of left lower limb weakness, inability to speak, and dull response. MRI was performed on the tenth day after the onset of symptoms. (**a–c**) FLAIR: Hyperintensity is seen in the right frontoparietal lobes and the whole corpus callosum, which is the entire right ACA irrigation territory. Hyperintensity is also detected in the right occipital lobe, which is the PCA territory. (**d–f**) DWI: The above areas show hyperintensity, reflecting diffusion restriction, which is typical for acute infarct cytotoxic edema

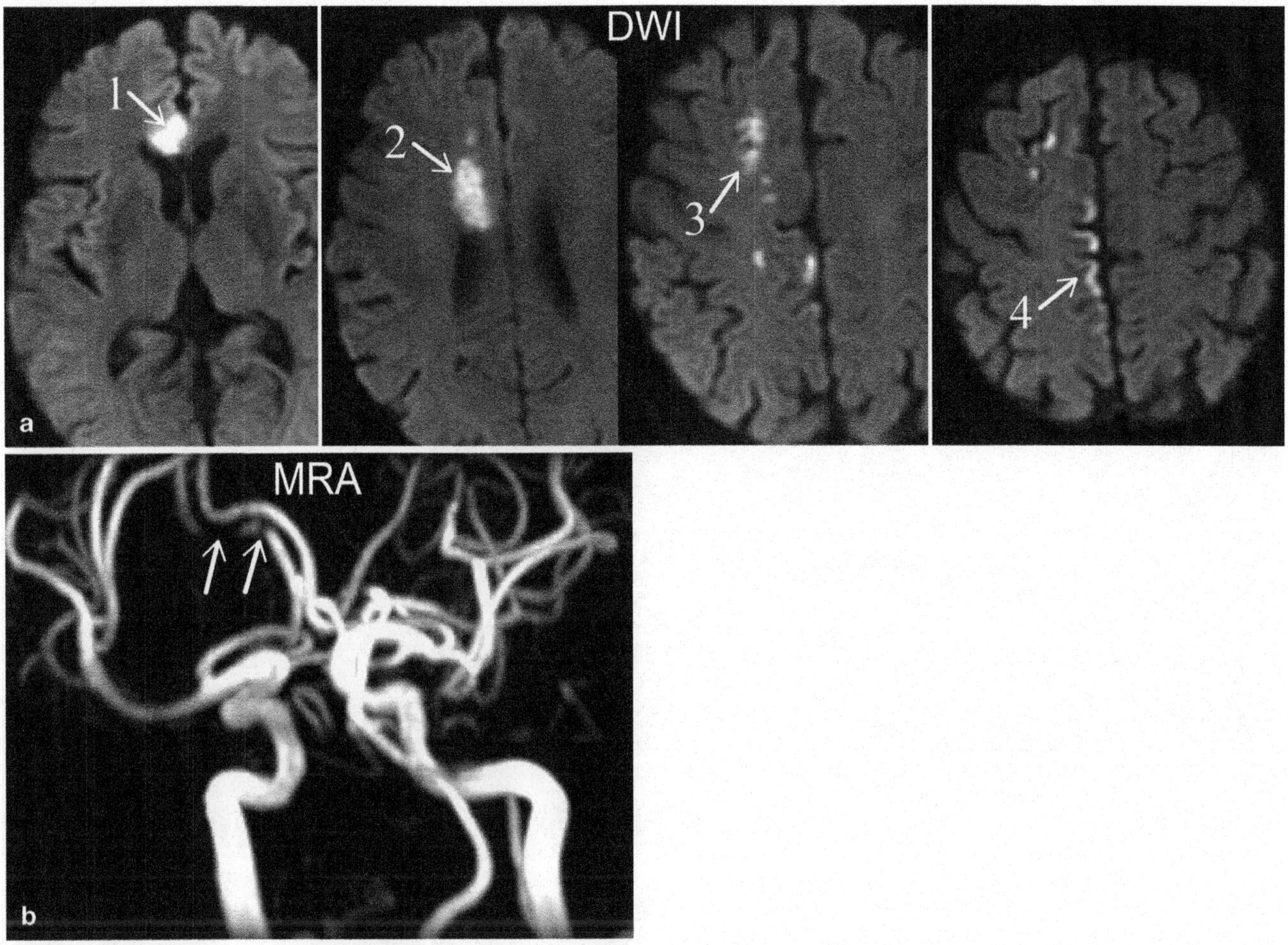

Fig. 5.17 F/60, ACA stenosis causes border zone infarction. The patient with hypertension and hyperglycemia suffered a sudden onset of left hemiparesis and truncal ataxia. MRI was performed on the third day after symptom onset. (**a**) DWI: Hyperintense lesions on the right side of the genu of corpus callosum (1). At the medial part of the right frontal lobe, confluent (2) and rosary-like (3) hyperintense lesions are present. The linear hyperintense lesion is also present in the deep cortex (4). All the above hyperintense lesions are acute cytotoxic edemas with diffusion restriction. This finding indicates acute infarction of the right ACA territory. (**b**) MRA: Severe stenosis (arrows) is seen in the right ACA. This finding is indicating severe atherosclerosis. Thus, the above infarctions are a kind of border zone infarction caused by hemodynamic impairment due to severe atherosclerosis of the right ACA

5.6 Posterior Cerebral Artery Infarction (PCA Infarction)

PCA infarction can cause edema in occipital and temporal lobes (Figs. 5.16, 5.18, 5.19, 5.20, and 5.21), which can lead to visual field defects because of the visual pathway and visual cortex locate in the occipital lobe. The blood supply to the thalamus is from the thalamoperforating artery, which is also derived from PCA. Therefore, thalamic infarction (Figs. 5.19 and 5.20) occurs at the same time, causing thalamic syndrome (opposite limb numbness and tingling) [16].

Most of the PCA infarctions are derived from extracranial thromboembolism. Given that PCA is usually derived from the basilar artery, the obstruction of the basilar artery can also affect PCA (Fig. 5.20).

PCA itself also will be stenotic due to atherosclerosis, causing infarction in its perfusion territory (Fig. 5.21).

Uncal/transtentorial herniation will compress PCA, resulting in PCA infarction (Fig. 3.31).

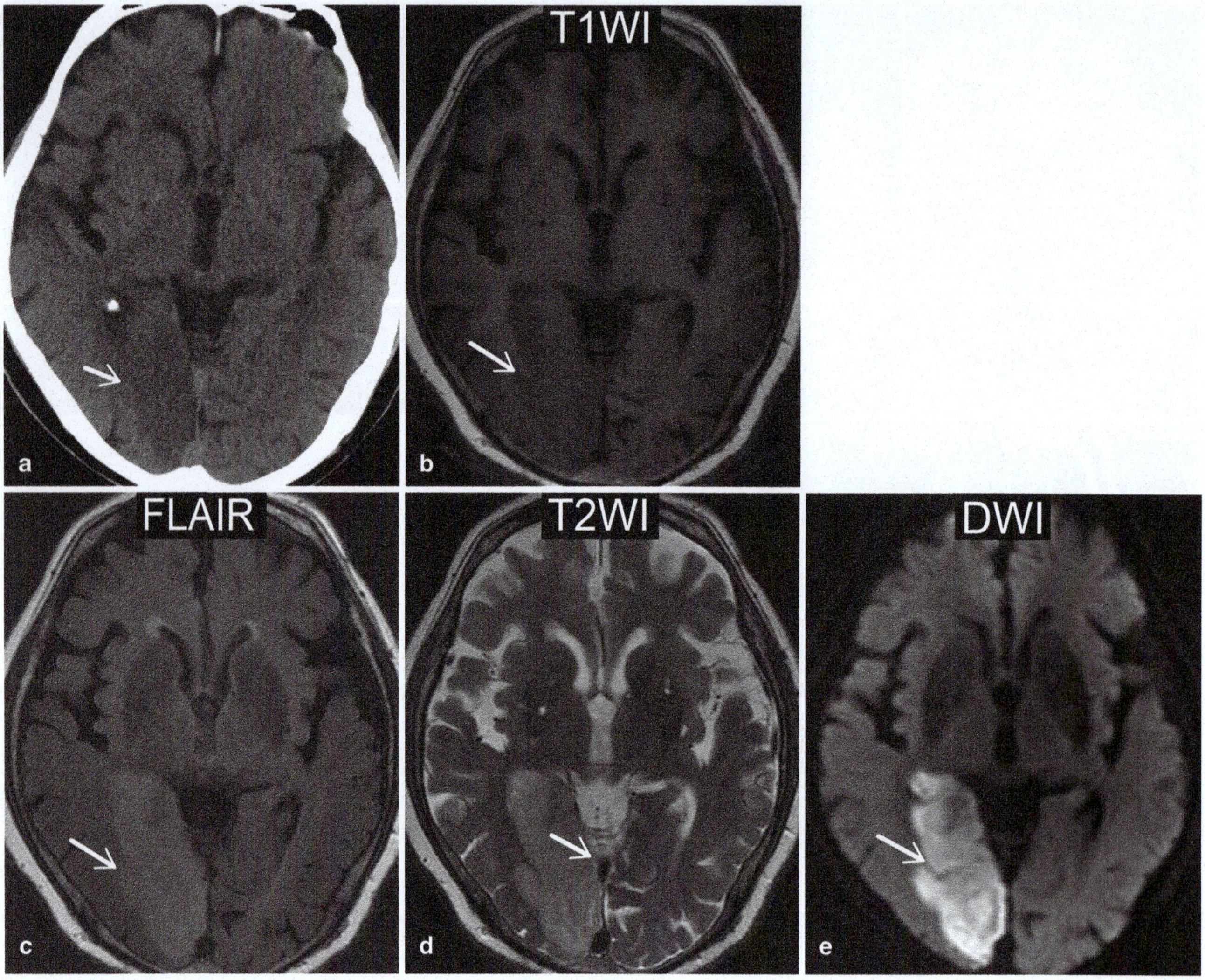

Fig. 5.18 M/82, PCA infarction. The patient suffered a sudden onset of left-side blurred vision; the ophthalmologist found he had left-side hemianopia. (**a**) CT: Acute brain tissue edema (arrow) in the right occipital lobe, reflecting right PCA acute infarction. (**b–e**) MRI T1, FLAIR, T2, and DWI: Acute cytotoxic edema in the right occipital lobe, a typical feature of acute PCA infarction

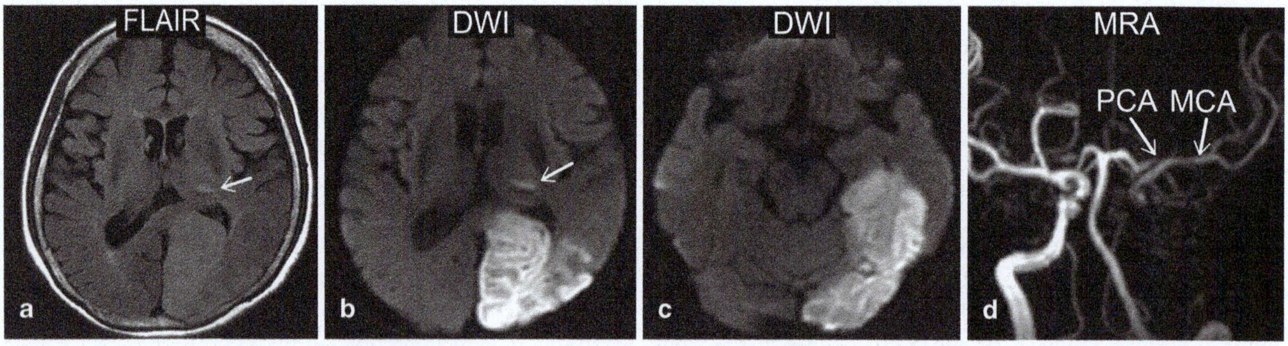

Fig. 5.19 F/79, Acute PCA infarction. The patient with hypertension and a history of atrial fibrillation suffered a sudden onset of severe vertigo, hemianopia, and right limb dysmetria. (**a–c**) MRI, FLAIR, DWI: An area with cytotoxic edema with diffusion restriction is seen in the left temporo-occipital lobes, which indicates acute infarction of the left PCA. Small acute infarction edema is also detected in the left thalamus (arrow). (**d**) MRA: Occlusion of the left PCA (arrow)

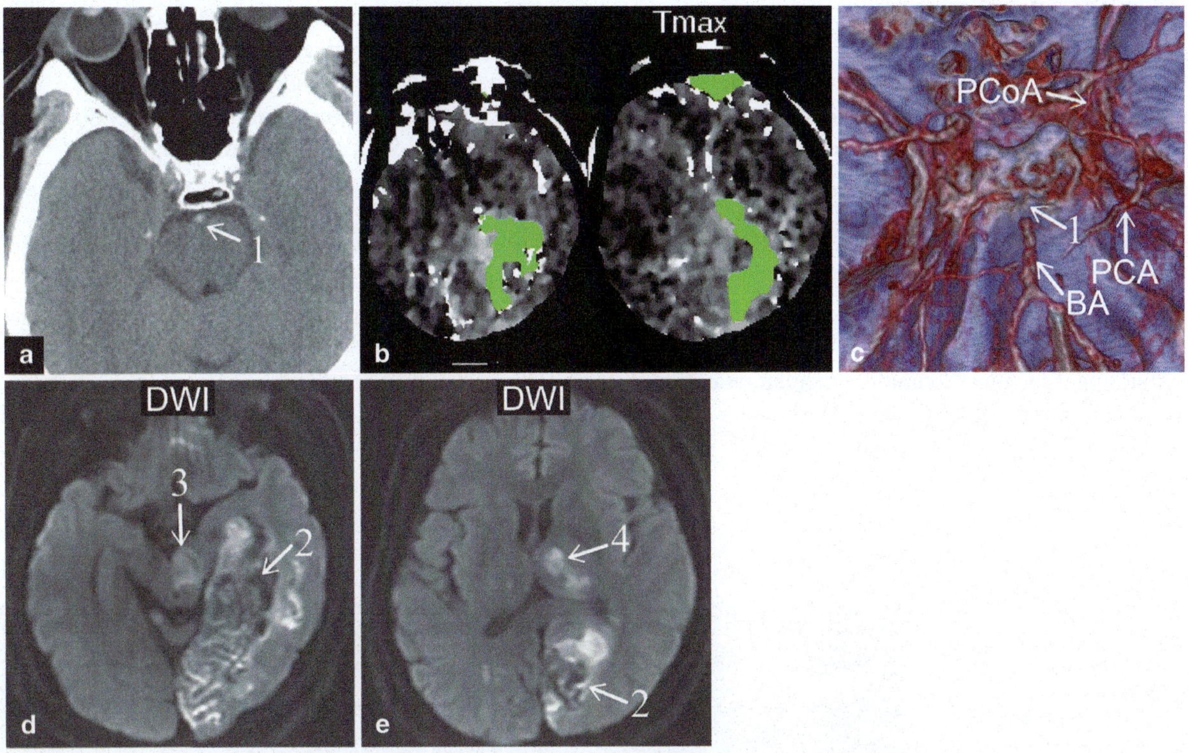

Fig. 5.20 M/55, Basilar artery occlusion causes acute infarction. A diabetic patient with a history of myocardial infarction due to cardiovascular stenosis complained of sudden onset of dizziness and vomiting. CT was performed 10 h after symptom onset. (**a**) CT: A small white spot (1) is seen in the basilar artery, which is suspected to be a thrombus. (**b**) CT perfusion, T_{max}: In the territory of the left PCA, the green-colored area is T_{max} >6″, reflecting hypoperfusion. (**c**) CTA: Occlusion of the basilar artery (1). Opacification of the left PCA is seen, and the blood flow is from the PCoA. The neuroradiologist performed IA thrombectomy to retrieve the thrombus in the basilar artery, but the clinical symptoms did not improve. MRI was performed on the second day. (**d**, **e**) DWI: Acute cytotoxic edema in the left temporo-occipital lobes with the hemorrhagic transformation (2) and infarction cytotoxic edema in the left side of the midbrain (3) and thalamus (4)

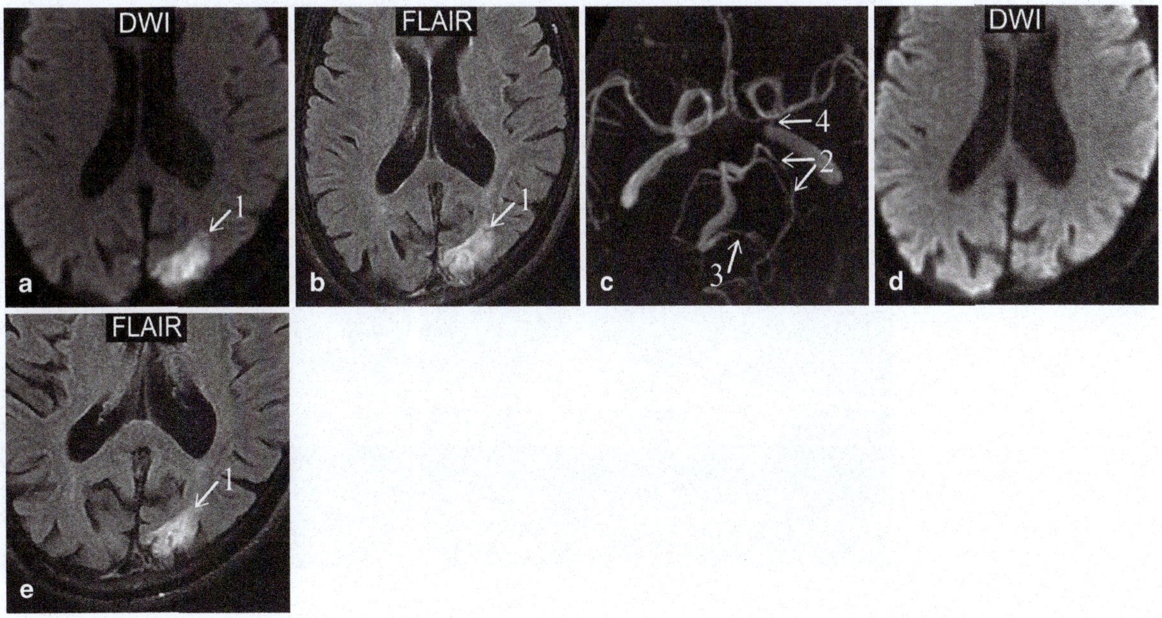

Fig. 5.21 M/73, Atherosclerosis of PCA causes occipital lobe infarction. The patient with diabetes, hypertension, and hyperlipidemia suddenly suffered dizziness. MRI was performed on the fourth day after symptom onset. (**a**) DWI: Diffusion restriction area in the left occipital lobe, which indicates acute cytotoxic edema due to infarction in the PCA territory. (**b**) FLAIR: Hyperintensity is also noted in the infarction area. (**c**) MRA: Two segmental stenoses (2) in the left PCA and stenosis in the left vertebral artery (3) and left ICA (4). (**d**, **e**) Follow-up MRI after 7 weeks: No signal change is seen in DWI. Thus, no diffusion restriction of the infarction area in this time, but FLAIR still exhibits hyperintensity. Therefore, this infarction is in the early chronic stage

5.7 Cerebellar Infarction

The cerebellum has three major blood vessels. The incidence of infarction is the highest in the superior cerebellar artery (SCA), followed by the posterior inferior cerebellar artery (PICA) and the anterior inferior cerebellar artery (AICA) (Fig. 5.22) [16, 17].

5.7.1 SCA Infarction

SCA infarction is the most common cerebellar infarction that affects the cerebellar vermis and a part of the midbrain (Fig. 5.23).

SCA infarction can cause ipsilateral cerebellar symptoms (ataxia, dysarthria, nystagmus) as well as brainstem symptoms, such as Horner's syndrome.

The causes include vertebral/basilar artery dissection, distant emboli, and SCA atherosclerosis.

5.7.2 PICA Infarction

PICA infarction affects the posterior inferior cerebellum, inferior cerebellar vermis, and lateral medulla oblongata (Fig. 5.24).

Clinically, this condition presents dizziness, vomiting, and truncal ataxia. If the infarction area includes the inferior cerebellar peduncle of the medulla oblongata, then lateral medullary syndrome (Wallenberg syndrome) occurs.

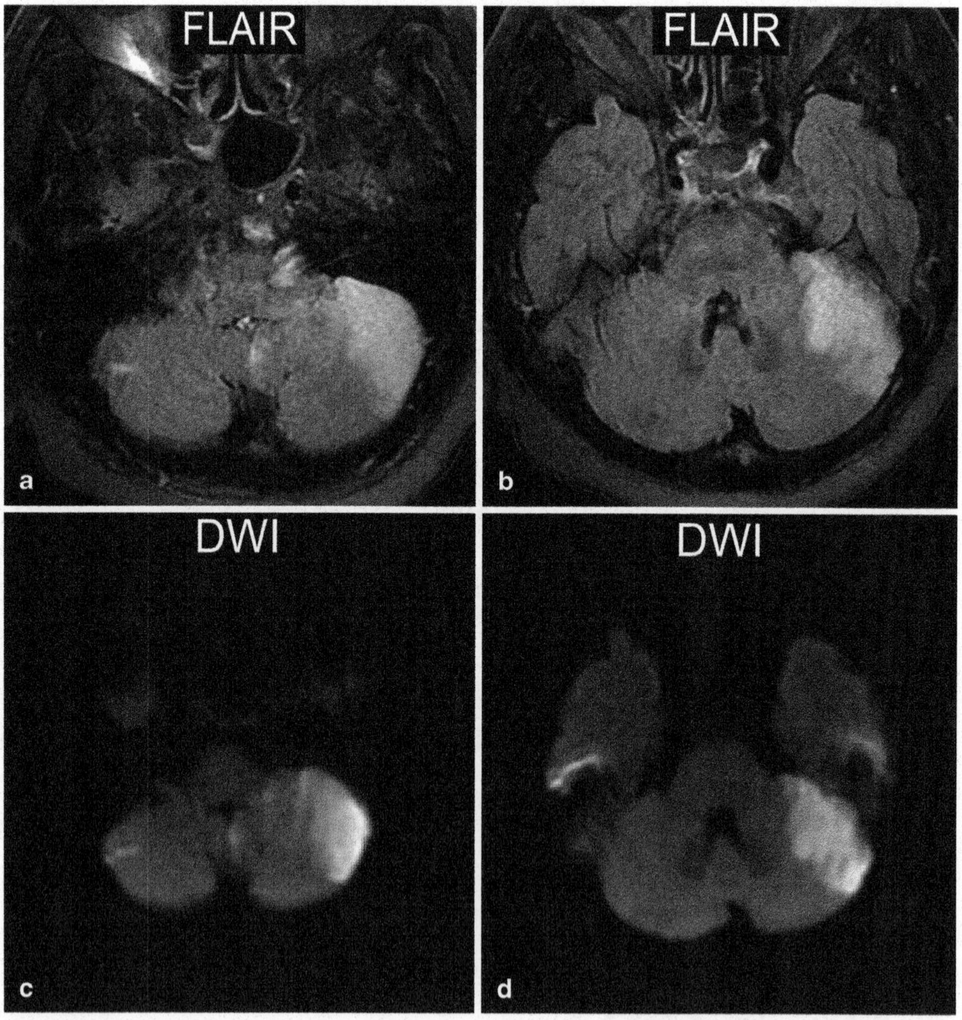

Fig. 5.22 F/81, Anterior inferior cerebellar artery (AICA) acute infarction. The patient suffered a sudden onset of vertigo and bilateral tinnitus; neurological examination revealed nystagmus of both eyeballs. Emergency CT revealed no findings (not shown). MRI was performed on the second day. (**a**, **b**) MRI, FLAIR: An area of hyperintensity in the left cerebellum. (**c**, **d**) DWI: DWI reveals hyperintensity, confirming that this area has diffusion restriction, which indicates acute cytotoxic edema due to acute infarction of the left AICA. The other two small acute infarctions are detected in the vermis and right cerebellum

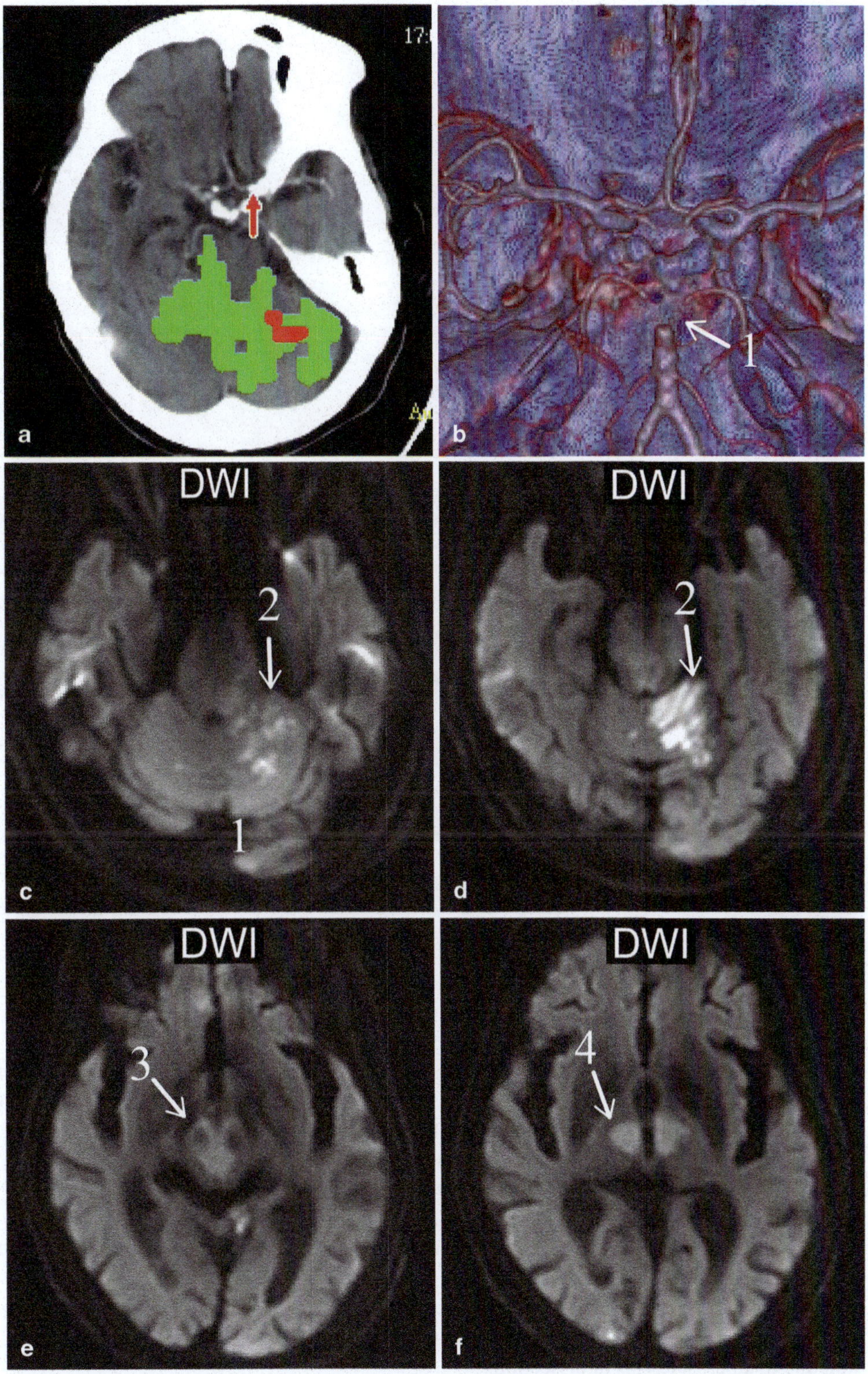

Fig. 5.23 F/85, Acute occlusion of the basilar artery. The patient with hypertension and a history of atrial fibrillation suffered a sudden onset of consciousness disturbance. CT was performed 2 h after symptom onset, and no brain tissue hemorrhage or edema was observed (not shown). CTA and CT perfusion were performed immediately. (**a**) CT perfusion: A large area of hypoperfusion in the cerebellum; most of the area is the penumbra, and the core area is small. (**b**) CTA: Total occlusion of the basilar artery (1). Given the patient's old age, the family was reluctant to conduct active treatment; hence, no IA thrombectomy was performed. (**c**–**f**) MRI was performed 2 days later: DWI demonstrated hyperintensities in the superior cerebellar artery (SCA) territory in the left cerebellum (2), midbrain (3), and bilateral thalami (4), representing acute cytotoxic edemas with diffusion restriction. These are acute infarctions due to occlusion of the basilar artery

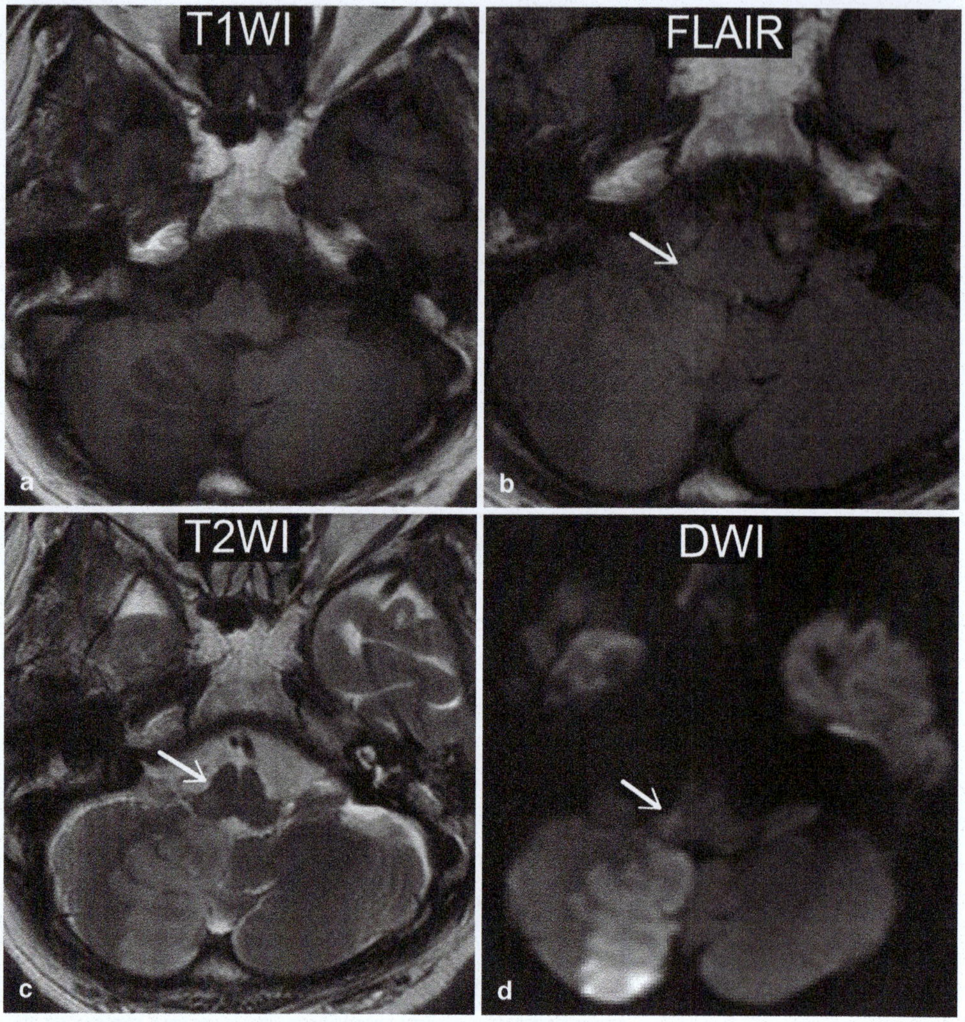

Fig. 5.24 M/62, Posterior inferior cerebellar artery (PICA) acute infarction. The patient suffered a sudden onset of vertigo, dizziness, vomiting, and numbness on the right side of the body. Emergency CT showed no abnormality (not shown); MRI was performed on the second day. (**a**) MRI, T1WI: An area of hypointensity is seen in the right cerebellum, reflecting acute brain tissue edema. (**b**, **c**) FLAIR, T2WI: Hyperintensity in the above area and slight hyperintensity in the right inferior cerebellar peduncle (arrows) of medulla oblongata are detected. The above areas are located in the territory of the right PICA. (**d**) DWI: The above areas are hyperintense on DWI, which confirms that such areas exhibit diffusion restriction, indicating acute cytotoxic edemas due to acute infarction of the right PICA

5.8 Brainstem Ischemic Stroke

Brainstem ischemic stroke accounts for approximately 10% of all ischemic strokes, occurring mostly at the pons (Figs. 5.25, 5.26, and 5.27), followed by medulla oblongata (Figs. 5.24, 5.29, and 5.30) and midbrain (Figs. 5.20 and 5.23) [18].

The basilar artery is stenotic due to artherosclerosis or produces a thrombus that causes infarction of the pons, midbrain, and cerebellum.

The vertebral artery causes medulla and cerebellar infarction due to atherosclerosis or dissection.

The penetrating artery from the basilar artery to the brainstem will also be obstructed due to atherosclerosis itself, causing the lacunar infarction of the brainstem, mostly at pons.

5.8.1 Pontine Infarction

Pontine infarction is mostly paramedian (Figs. 5.25, 5.26, and 5.27), with sharp edges [18] and less lateral infarction (Fig. 5.27).

Pontine infarction can be combined with cerebellar infarction. However, pure pontine lacunar infarction (Figs. 5.25, 5.26, and 5.27) caused by the atherosclerosis of its penetrating artery is also common [19].

Bilateral pontine infarction also occurs. If edema occurs in the middle of the pons, then it may be pontine myelinolysis (Fig. 5.28) [20] which is not real infarction.

5.8.2 Medullary Infarction

Lateral medullary infarction is more frequent than medial medullary infarction and also with a sharp margin [18]. The causes include vertebral artery atherosclerosis and dissection. Medulla infarction can be associated with cerebellar infarction (Fig. 5.24). However, pure medulla lacunar infarction (Figs. 5.29 and 5.30) caused by atherosclerosis of its penetrating artery is also common.

Lateral medullary infarction causes Wallenberg syndrome, whereas medial medullary infarction causes Dejerine syndrome [18].

5.8.3 Midbrain Infarction

Blood supply to the midbrain comes from PCA, basilar artery, and SCA. Midbrain infarction is often associated with the cerebellum, thalamus, and pons infarction (Figs. 5.20 and 5.23). Pure midbrain infarction is rare [21].

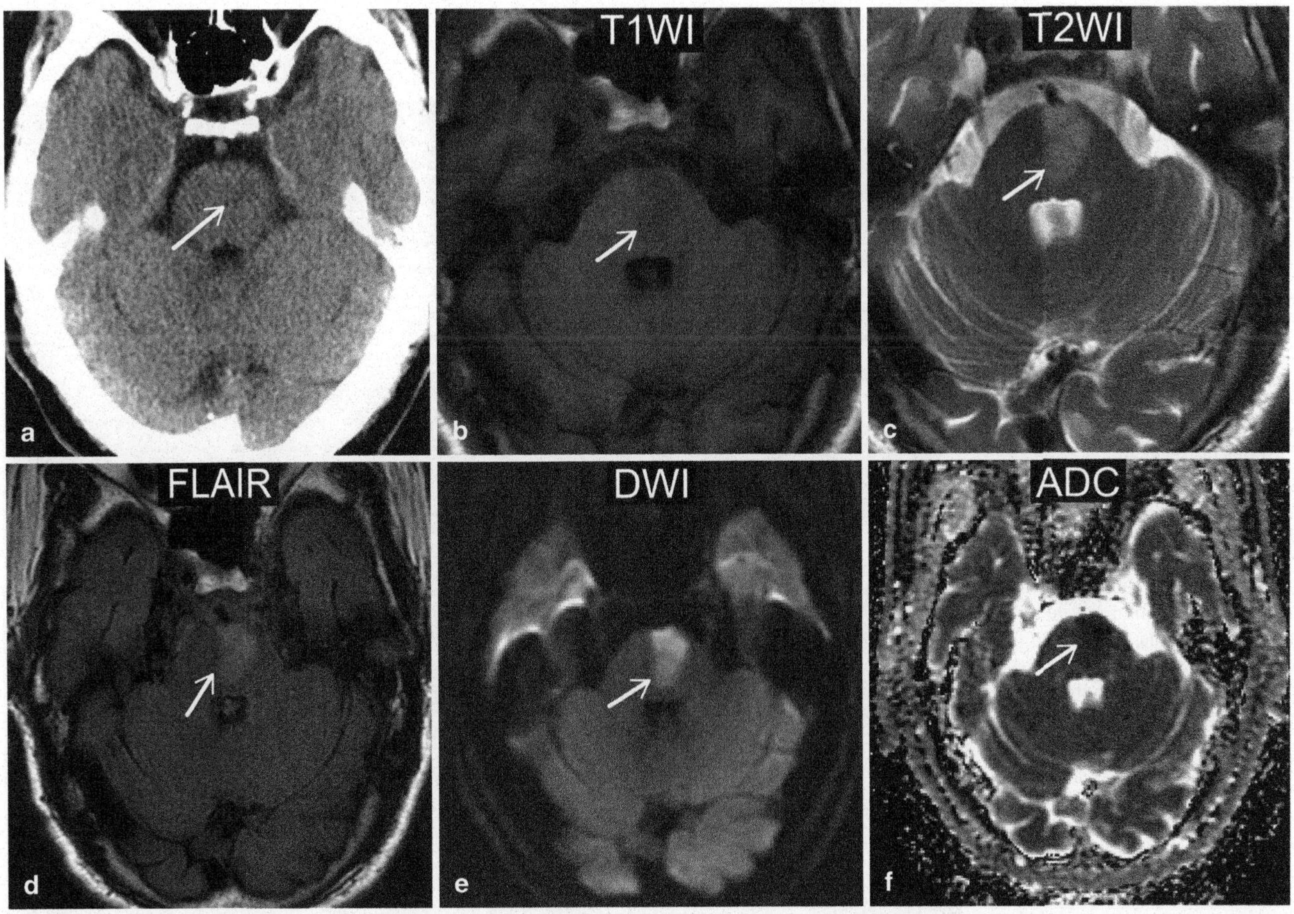

Fig. 5.25 M/67, Acute pontine infarction. The patient with hypertension and diabetes suffered a sudden onset of right hemiparesis, dysarthria, and mild dysphagia. No brain tissue hemorrhage or edema was observed during emergency CT (not shown). (**a**) Follow-up CT on the second day: A suspicious hypodense lesion (arrow) on the left side of pons. (**b–f**) MRI was performed on the same day: T1WI shows a hypointense lesion on the left side of the pons, and T2WI and FLAIR exhibit hyperintensity. DWI and ADC show hyperintensity and hypointensity, respectively. DWI and ADC confirm that the edema exhibits diffusion restriction; hence, this case is acute cytotoxic edema due to acute pontine infarction. This pontine infarction is in paramedian, and the margin is sharp

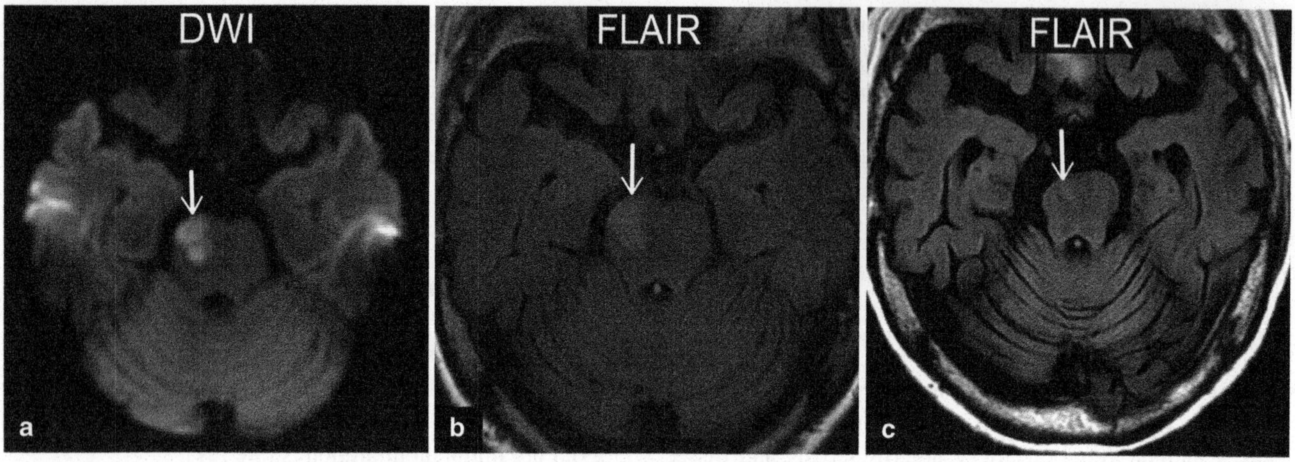

Fig. 5.26 F/75, Pontine infarction, acute and chronic stage. The patient suffered a sudden onset of left hemiplegia. MRI was performed 2 days later. (**a**) MRI, DWI: A hyperintense lesion on the right side of the pons (arrow). This finding suggests acute cytotoxic edema with diffusion restriction due to acute infarction. (**b**) FLAIR: FLAIR also shows a hyperintense lesion on the right side of pons (arrow). (**c**) Follow-up MRI after 8 years, FLAIR: The infarction became an old infarction (arrow) with two small necroses and brain tissue atrophy

Fig. 5.27 F/78, Acute pontine infarctions. The patient with hypertension suffered a sudden onset of left hemiparesis and dizziness. CT was performed on the second day after symptom onset. (**a**) CT: Three small hypodense lesions (arrows) on the right side of the pons, which are suspected to be small acute infarction edemas. (**b–d**) MRI on the same day: These three lesions (arrows) are hyperintense on FLAIR, bright (very hyperintense) on DWI, and hypointense on ADC, reflecting acute brain tissue cytotoxic edema with diffusion restriction caused by acute infarctions. Among the three acute lacunar infarctions, two are in the paramedian location, and one is located in a lateral site

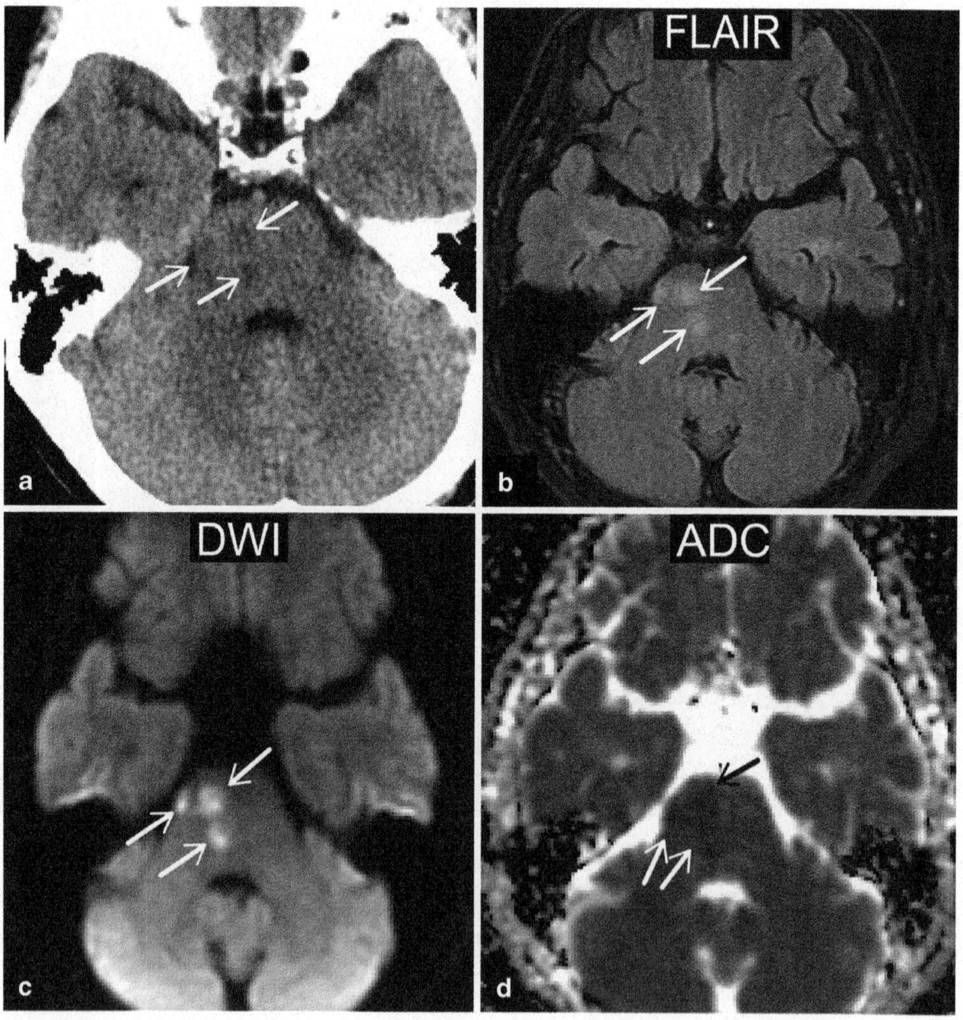

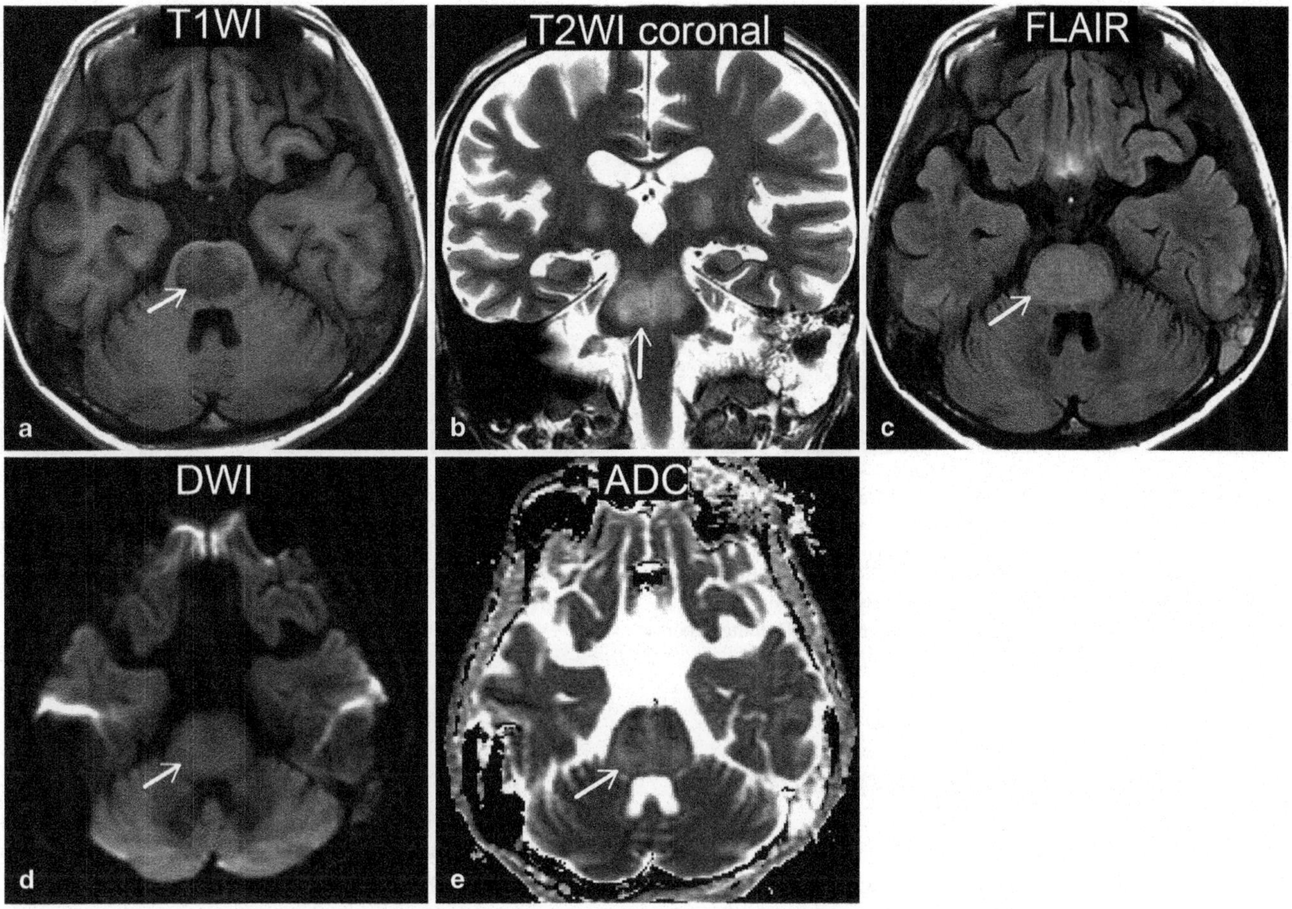

Fig. 5.28 F/33, Central pontine myelinolysis (CPM). The patient with alcoholism suffered a sudden onset of consciousness disturbance. MRI was conducted on the 12th day. (**a–c**) MRI: Most of the pons (arrows) show hypointensity on T1WI and hyperintensity on T2WI and FLAIR, which are indicative of acute pontine edema. However, edema is present in the middle area, crossing over the right and left sides, so this case is not pontine infarction, which always occurs on one side. (**d**, **e**) DWI, ADC: No bright signal change on DWI, and hyperintensity on ADC, these findings representing no diffusion restriction; hence, this case is CPM, not cytotoxic edema. CPM is caused by a sudden elevation of serum osmolality, which induces brain tissue destruction of myelin sheath in the pons, this is a kind of demyelination, not cytotoxic edema

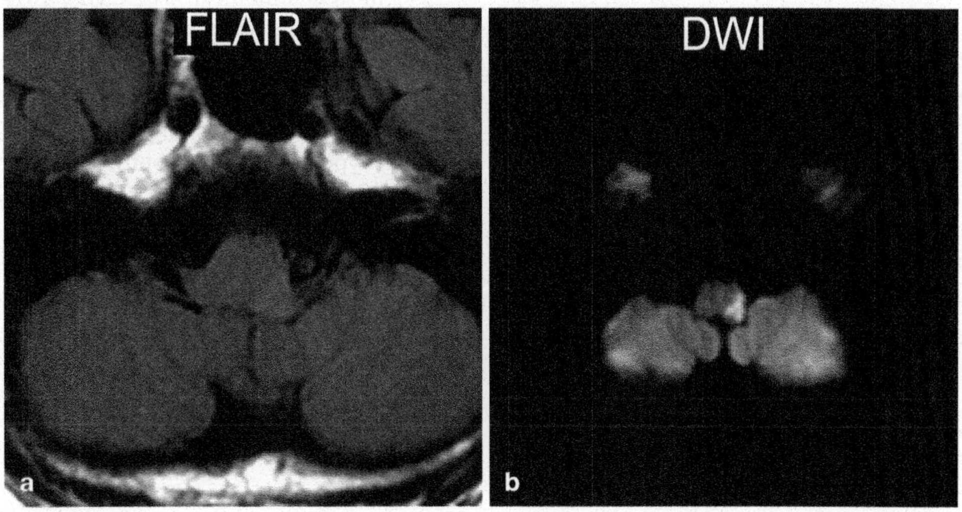

Fig. 5.29 M/70, Acute infarction of the medulla oblongata. The patient with hypertension and diabetes suffered a sudden onset of vertigo, unsteady gait, and dysphagia. MRI was performed 10 h after symptom onset. (**a**) MRI, FLAIR: The abnormality is difficult to recognize. (**b**) DWI: Definite hyperintensity is seen in the left inferior cerebellar peduncle of the medulla oblongata, reflecting diffusion restriction; hence, this case is acute cytotoxic edema caused by infarction. Infarction or hemorrhage in the inferior cerebellar peduncle may cause Wallenberg syndrome or lateral medullary syndrome

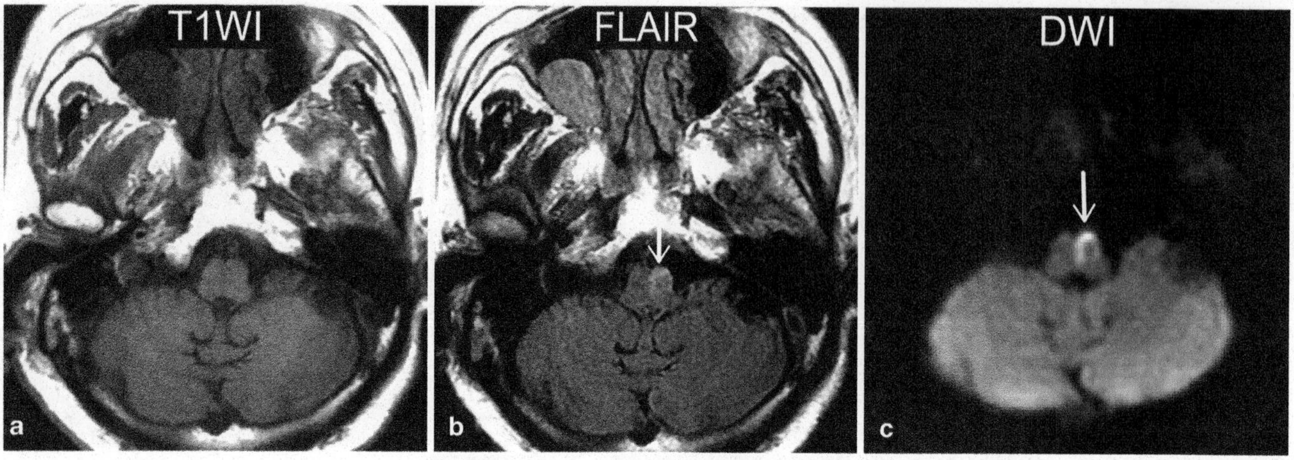

Fig. 5.30 M/75, Acute infarction of the medulla oblongata. The patient suffered a sudden onset of right hemiplegia. Emergency CT was performed, but no hemorrhage or edema was noted (not shown). MRI was conducted on the second day. (**a**) MRI, T1WI: No visible abnormality is seen in the medulla oblongata. (**b**) FLAIR: Hyperintensity (arrow) is seen on the left side of the medulla oblongata. (**c**) DWI: Definite hyperintensity (arrow) is noted on the left side of the medulla oblongata, reflecting diffusion restriction; hence, this case is acute cytotoxic edema caused by infarction. The infarction includes the pyramid, which is the course of the corticospinal tract; thus, it causes contralateral-side hemiplegia

5.9 Border Zone (Watershed) Infarction

Border zone or watershed refers to the territory between two major blood vessels or at the end of the blood flow of the major blood vessels. Supplying blood to this territory is relatively low. In case of stenosis or occlusion of proximal blood vessels, such as ICA (Figs. 5.31, 5.33, and 5.36) and MCA (Figs. 5.32, 5.34, and 5.35), the watershed territory is the most susceptible to ischemia and ischemic infarction [22–26], which accounts for approximately 10% of all infarct strokes [22].

Such infarction can be divided into three categories:

1. Cortical or external infarction (Figs. 5.31 and 5.32). Cortical infarction is often located between the boundaries of ACA/MCA or MCA/PCA and is triangular in shape.
2. Subcortical or internal infarct. Internal border zone infarct mainly occurs in the centrum semiovale and corona radiata, and the symptoms are apparent (Figs. 5.17, 5.31, 5.32, 5.33, 5.34, and 5.35). Subcortical infarction has two shapes, namely rosary-like with a series of small infarctions (Figs. 5.17, 5.32, and 5.33) and confluent-like (Figs. 5.17, 5.34, and 5.35).
3. Mixed type, combining cortical and subcortical infarctions (Figs. 5.31 and 5.32).

This infarction is hypoperfusion in distant brain tissue in case of typical hemodynamic impairment, especially the subcortical border zone infarction. The cortical border zone infarct is related to embolization, indicating that in case of hypoperfusion, microemboli are impossible to wash out, resulting in embolization.

The most common cause of such border zone infarcts is severe stenosis or occlusion of ICA (Figs. 5.31, 5.33, and 5.36). Moreover, the severe stenosis or occlusion of MCA (Fig. 5.32, 5.34, and 5.35) and ACA (Fig. 5.17) can cause hemodynamic impairment in their blood supply territories, causing hypoperfusion and border zone infarction.

Heart diseases reduce blood flow, which leads to decreased systemic perfusion and hypoperfusion in the brain. Microemboli from the heart cannot be washed out, which also may result in border zone infarct in the brain.

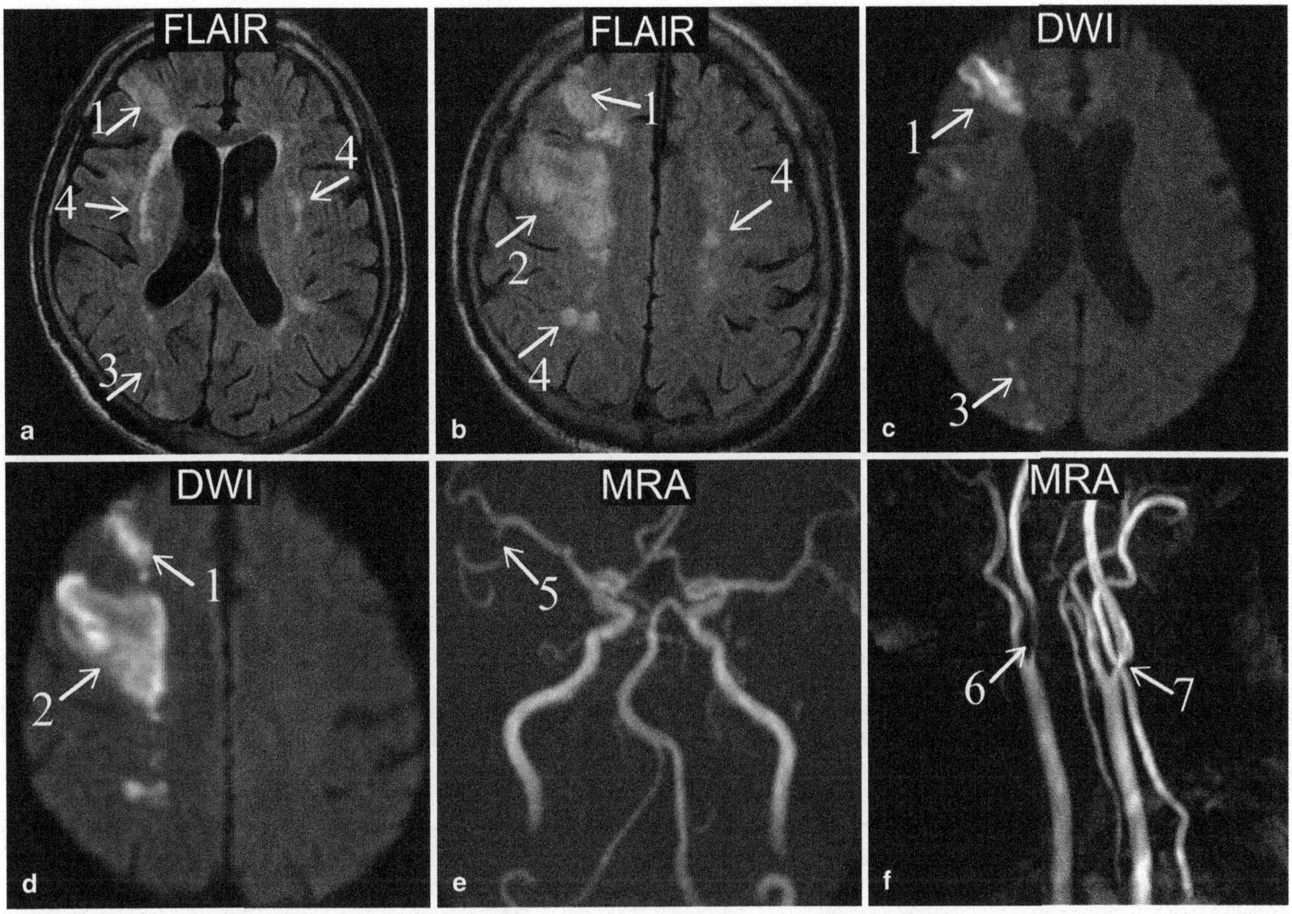

Fig. 5.31 M/72, Watershed infarctions, and MCA infarction. The patient with diabetes and chronic renal failure had several instances of right-side minor strokes in the past decade. During this time, he suffered a sudden onset of left hemiparesis and dysphonia. (**a**, **b**) FLAIR: Multiple hyperintense lesions with variable sizes are observed in the right fronto-parieto-occipital lobes and right corona radiata (1–4). Distinguishing between old and new infarctions and leukoaraiosis is difficult. (**c**, **d**) DWI: Two areas (1, 2) of hyperintensity are seen in the frontal lobe with diffusion restriction, indicating cytotoxic edema of acute infarctions. One is located in the watershed of MCA and ACA (1), and the other is in the anterior one-third territory of MCA (2). Such infarction (2) is due to embolism. Also, rosary-like small acute infarctions are found in the right occipital lobe (3), which is the watershed infarction of the right MCA–PCA. In FLAIR, the hyperintense lesions in left corona radiata (4) shows invisible on DWI, because of no diffusion restriction, and these are leukoaraiosis. (**e**) MRA revealed stenosis in one branch (5) of the right MCA. (**f**) Neck MRA: Approximately 90% stenosis (6) in the proximal portion of the right ICA, and 80% stenosis (7) in the proximal portion of the left ICA. In summary, this patient had anterior and posterior border zone infarctions, all caused by severe stenosis of right ICA near the bifurcation. *Rt.* ICA stenosis is symptomatic, *Lt.* ICA stenosis is asymptomatic

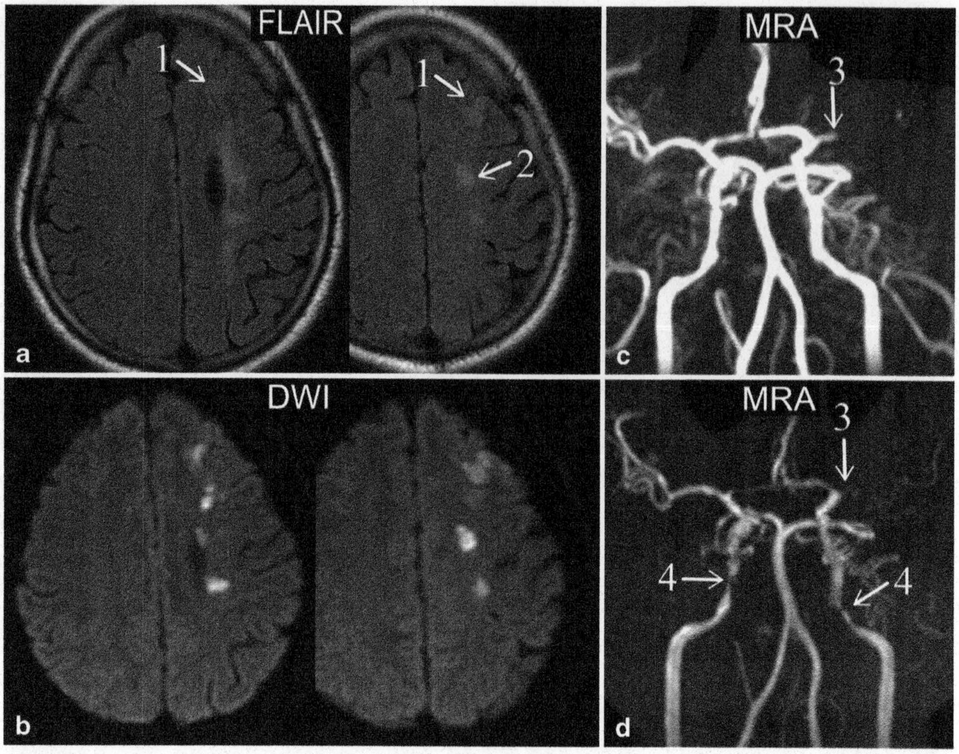

Fig. 5.32 F/39, MCA border zone infarction. The patient had diabetes for 12 years, which was not adequately controlled. She also has hyperlipidemia and hypertension. She suffered a sudden onset of right hemiparesis. MRI was conducted on the third day after symptom onset. (**a**) MRI, FLAIR: Several small hyperintense lesions (1, 2) in the watershed area between left MCA and ACA. (**b**) DWI: Hyperintense lesions are present, reflecting diffusion restriction; hence, all of them are acute cytotoxic edemas due to acute infarction. These are cortical-border-zone (1) associated subcortical (2) rosary-like infarctions, which are always due to severe stenosis of MCA or ICA. (**c**) MRA: Confirms severe steno-occlusion (3) of the left MCA. (**d**) Follow-up MRA after 3 years: In addition to the steno-occlusion (3) of the left MCA, stenoses are found in the bilateral ICAs (4)

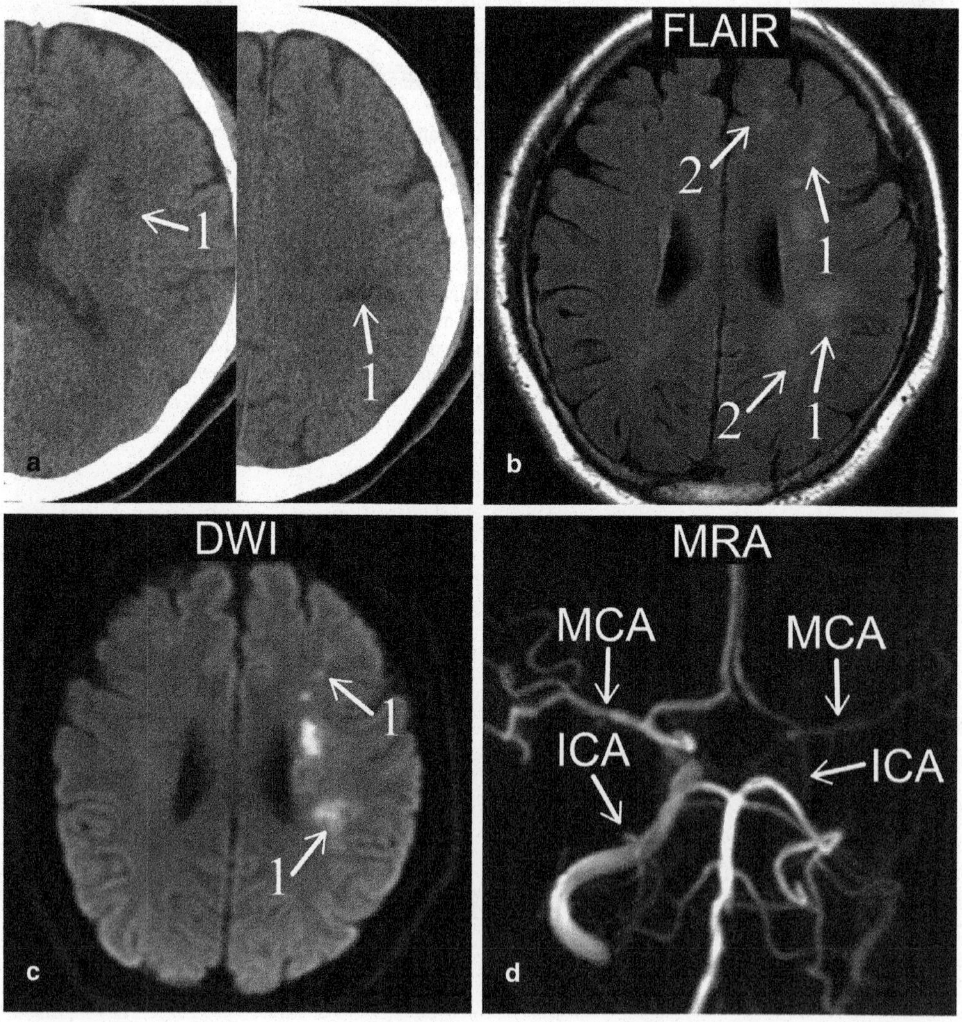

Fig. 5.33 M/45, ICA occlusion causes internal border zone infarcts. The patient has hypertension and hyperlipidemia. He suffered repeated right limb weakness in the last 4 days, and the latest attack was associated with speechlessness; thus, he was rushed to the emergency room of a medical center. (**a**) CT: Several small hypodense lesions (1) in the left centrum semiovale, which are suspected for acute infarctions. (**b**) MRI was performed immediately. FLAIR: The hypodense lesions in CT show hyperintensity (1); other small hyperintense lesions (2) are also present. (**c**) DWI: Multiple small rosary-like lesions with diffusion restriction are seen (1), which are acute cytotoxic edema, possibly are internal border zone infarctions. Other hyperintense lesions are observed on FLAIR (2), but no signal change is noted on DWI, these are leukoaraiosis. (**d**) MRA: Total occlusion of the left ICA; only the distal portion is opacified. The left MCA is patent, but the blood flow is relatively low compared with the right MCA

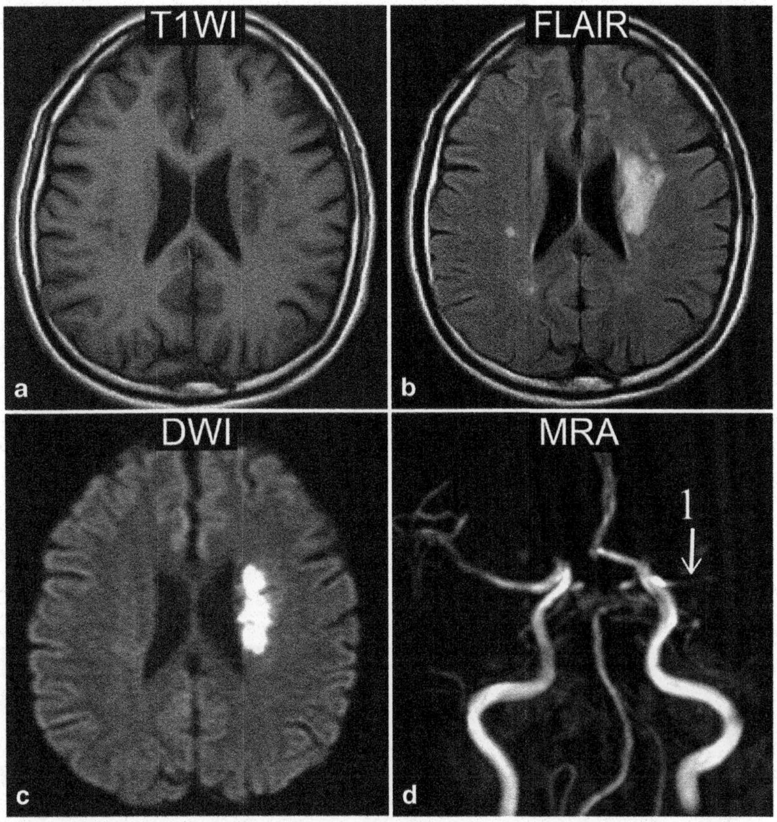

Fig. 5.34 M/57, Internal border zone infarction, confluent pattern. The patient with hypertension and alcoholism suffered a sudden onset of right hemiparesis and dysarthria for 4 days. (**a–c**) MRI: Brain tissue edema is noted in the left corona radiata, showing mild hypointensity on T1WI, hyperintensity on FLAIR, and brightness on DWI, reflecting diffusion restriction; thus, this is a case of acute cytotoxic edema due to acute infarction. (**d**) MRA: Severe stenosis and occlusion (steno-occlusion) of the left MCA (arrow). This is a typical internal border zone infarction, confluent type, due to hemodynamic impairment caused by the steno-occlusion of the left MCA

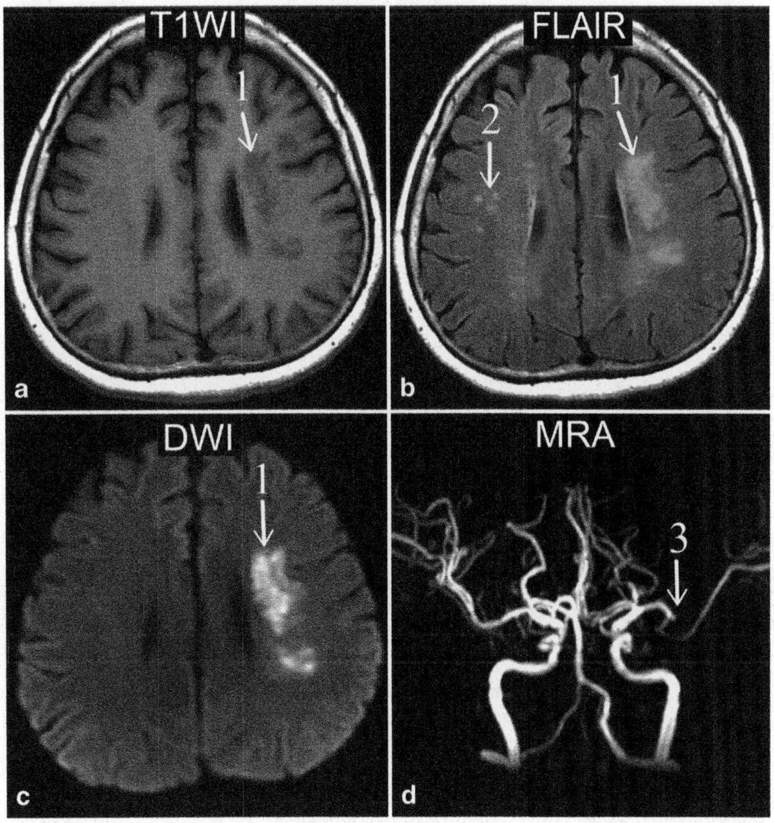

Fig. 5.35 F/62, Internal border zone infarct, confluent type. The patient with hypertension and hyperlipidemia suffered a sudden onset of right hemiparesis, dull response, and dysarthria. MRI was performed on the fifth day. (**a**) MRI, T1WI: A hypointense lesion (1) is seen in the left corona radiata. (**b**) FLAIR: Several hyperintense lesions (1, 2) are seen in the bilateral corona radiata. (**c**) DWI: The lesion in the left corona radiata (1) is bright, showing diffusion restriction, this is cytotoxic edema caused by acute infarction. The lesions in the right corona radiata show no signal change, which is indicative of leukoaraiosis. (**d**) MRA: Occlusion of the left MCA (3); thus, this is a case of confluent-type internal border zone infarction caused by MCA steno-occlusion with hemodynamic impairment

5.10 Lacunar Infarction

Lacunar infarction is caused by the occlusion of penetrating branches of major blood vessels, such as MCA, PCA, basilar artery, ACA, and vertebral artery. The lacunar infarctions are located in the deep brain and brainstem, with a diameter ranging from 3–4 to 15–20 mm [27]. Large lacunar infarction is more susceptible to symptoms than small ones. Small lacunar infarction shows no symptoms, unless locates in the sensory or motor pathways [28, 29]. The vulnerable locations are the putamen (Fig. 5.36), caudate nucleus (Fig. 5.37), thalamus (Fig. 5.38), pons (Fig. 5.27), internal capsule (Figs. 5.39 and 5.40), and cerebral subcortical white matter, such as corona radiata (Figs. 5.36, 5.41, and 5.42). Various lacunar syndromes will occur due to different locations [29].

The pathophysiology of lacunar infarction involves the two following mechanisms [28, 30]:

1. Lipohyalinosis of the single penetrating artery, which is a cerebrovascular disease caused by hypertension.
2. It is occluded by the small thrombus from the heart or its parent artery.

Detecting acute lacunar infarction in several days by CT is not easy. Infarction for few days of a stroke may show hypodensity on CT and can be detected. However, distinguishing new lacunar infarction from old lacunar infarction is sometimes difficult in CT.

Through DWI, MRI is very definite in diagnosing acute lacunar infarct [30], even if a lacunar infarction occurs in a very low location, such as in the medulla oblongata (Figs. 5.29 and 5.30). Chronic lacunar infarction shows visible cavitary change, which can be clearly diagnosed by MRI T1WI plus FLAIR. T1WI shows small lacune, and peripheral gliosis shows hyperintensity on FLAIR (Figs. 5.3, 5.59, and 5.61).

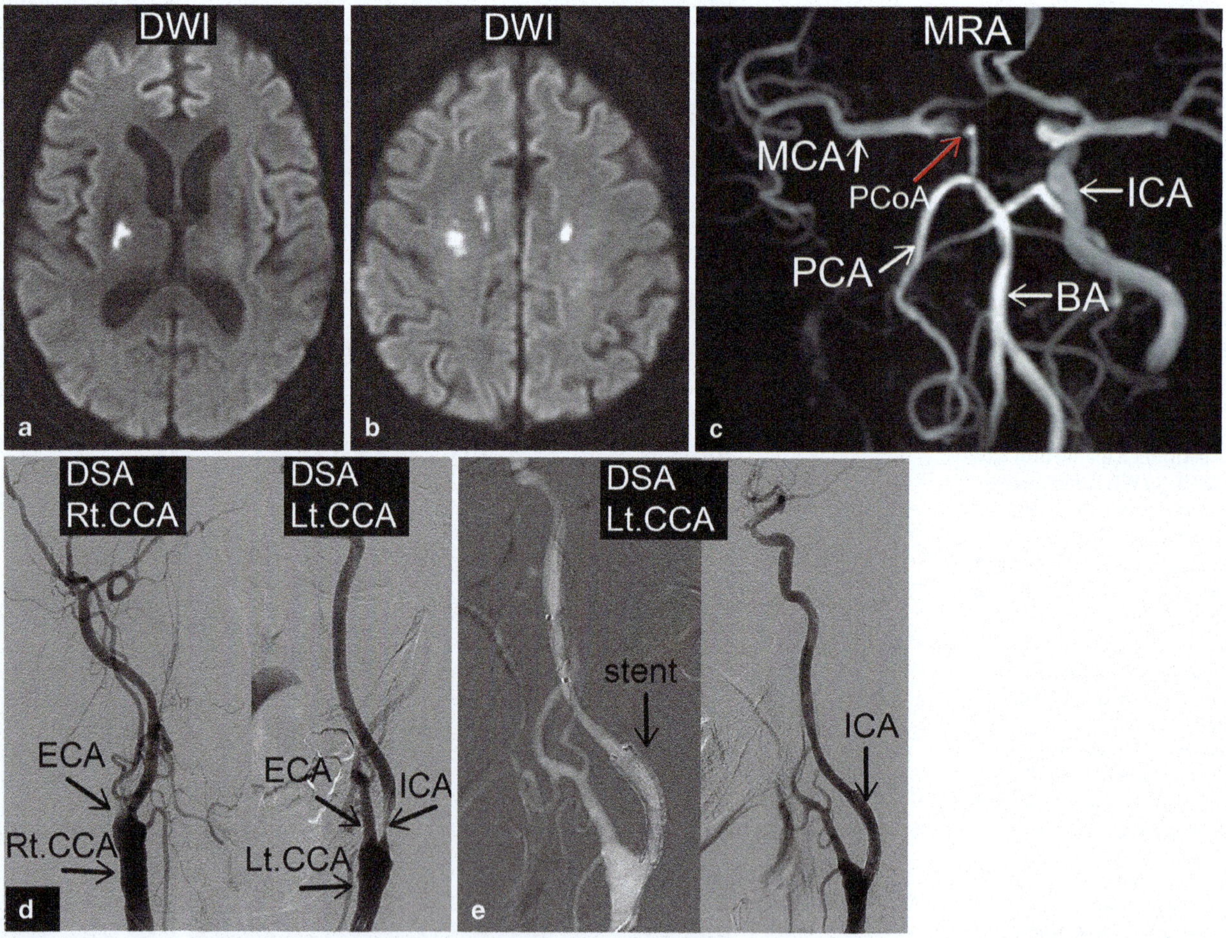

Fig. 5.36 M/73, Acute lacunar infarction caused by ICA stenosis and occlusion. The patient with hypertension and diabetes and a history of arrhythmia suffered a sudden onset of left hemiparesis. MRI was performed on the second day. (**a**) MRI, DWI: A small hyperintense lesion is seen in the right putamen, reflecting diffusion restriction; this is acute lacunar infarction. (**b**) DWI: Several small lesions with diffusion restriction are observed in the bilateral corona radiata; these are terminal zone infarctions representing hemodynamic insufficiency. This is always caused by severe stenosis of the internal carotid artery (ICA) or MCA. (**c**) MRA: Non-opacification of the right ICA, reflecting total occlusion. However, the right MCA is normal because the blood supply comes from the right PCA via the PCoA (red arrow). BA: basilar artery. (**d**) DSA: Right carotid angiogram shows total occlusion of the right ICA. At the same time, the left carotid angiogram shows severe stenosis in the bifurcation of the left ICA. *ECA* external carotid artery, *CCA* common carotid artery. (**e**) The patient received angioplasty with stent (arrow) for the left ICA, and the follow-up DSA shows no more stenosis of left ICA

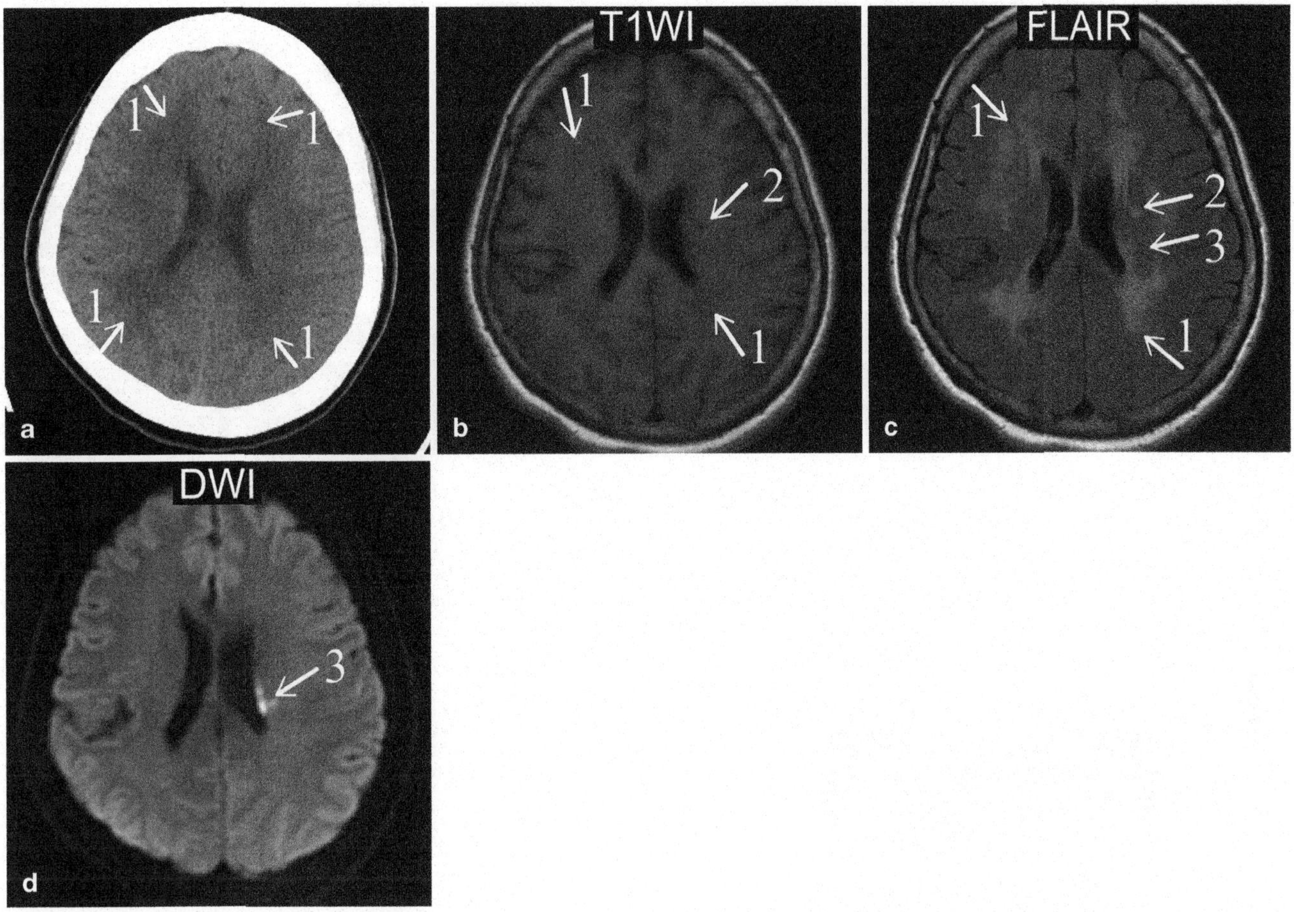

Fig. 5.37 F/48, Caudate nucleus acute lacunar infarction. The patient with hypertension and hyperlipidemia suffered a sudden onset of right hemiparesis. (**a**) CT: Periventricular low-attenuation areas are seen (1), which are indicative of white matter disease (leukoaraiosis). MRI was performed on the fourth day. (**b**) MRI, T1WI: Periventricular hypointensity (1), and an old lacunar infarction (2) in the left corona radiata are observed. (**c**) FLAIR: Periventricular leukoaraiosis (1); the old lacunar infarction (2) and a small acute infarction (3) are all hyperintense but cannot be distinguished. (**d**) DWI: Only a small lesion in the left caudate nucleus is bright (3), reflecting diffusion restriction; this is cytotoxic edema caused by acute infarction. The other lesions (1, 2) exhibit no signal change on DWI

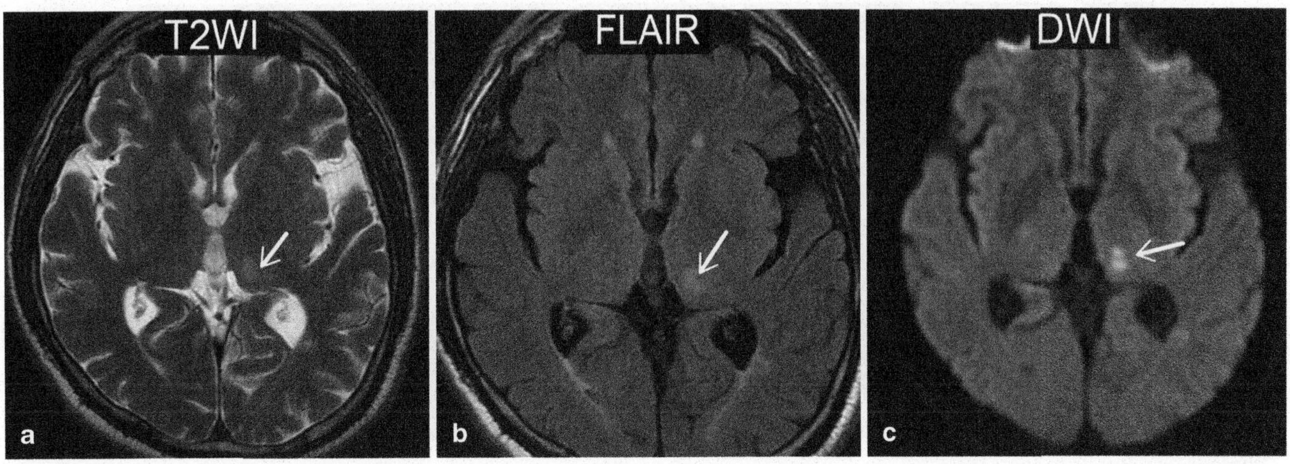

Fig. 5.38 M/67, Acute lacunar infarction of the left thalamus. The patient suffered a sudden onset of right hemiparesis and numbness of the right face and right hand. Emergency CT showed no brain tissue hemorrhage or edema (not shown). MRI was performed on the fifth day. (**a**, **b**) MRI, T2WI, FLAIR: A small hyperintense lesion (arrow) is seen in the left thalamus; however, whether it is an acute or chronic infarction cannot be determined. (**c**) DWI: The lesion shows hyperintensity (arrow), indicating diffusion restriction; thus, this is acute cytotoxic edema caused by acute infarction

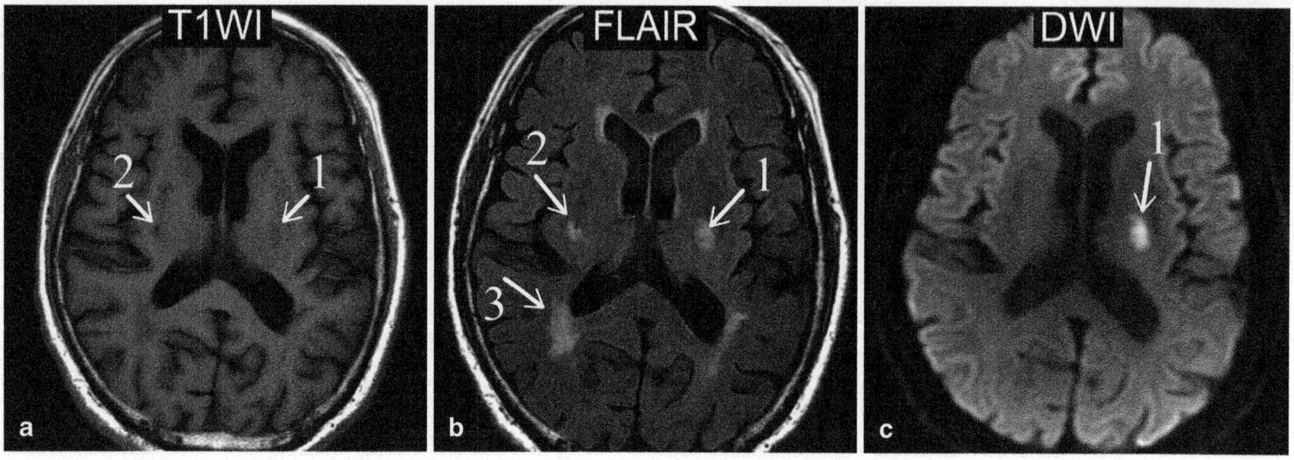

Fig. 5.39 M/77, Acute lacunar infarction in the internal capsule. The patient suffered a sudden onset of right hemiparesis. No infarction or hemorrhage was observed in CT (not shown). MRI was performed on the fourth day. (**a**) MRI, T1WI: A suspicious hypointense lesion is seen in the posterior limb of the left internal capsule (1). An old lacunar infarction is noted in the right putamen (2). (**b**) FLAIR: The two lesions, as mentioned above (1, 2), are hyperintense on FLAIR; periventricular hyperintensity (PVH) is also observed (3). (**c**) DWI: Only the lesion in the left internal capsule is bright, demonstrating diffusion restriction. Thus, this is an acute lacunar infarction. The old infarction and PVH show no signal change on DWI because they have no diffusion restriction

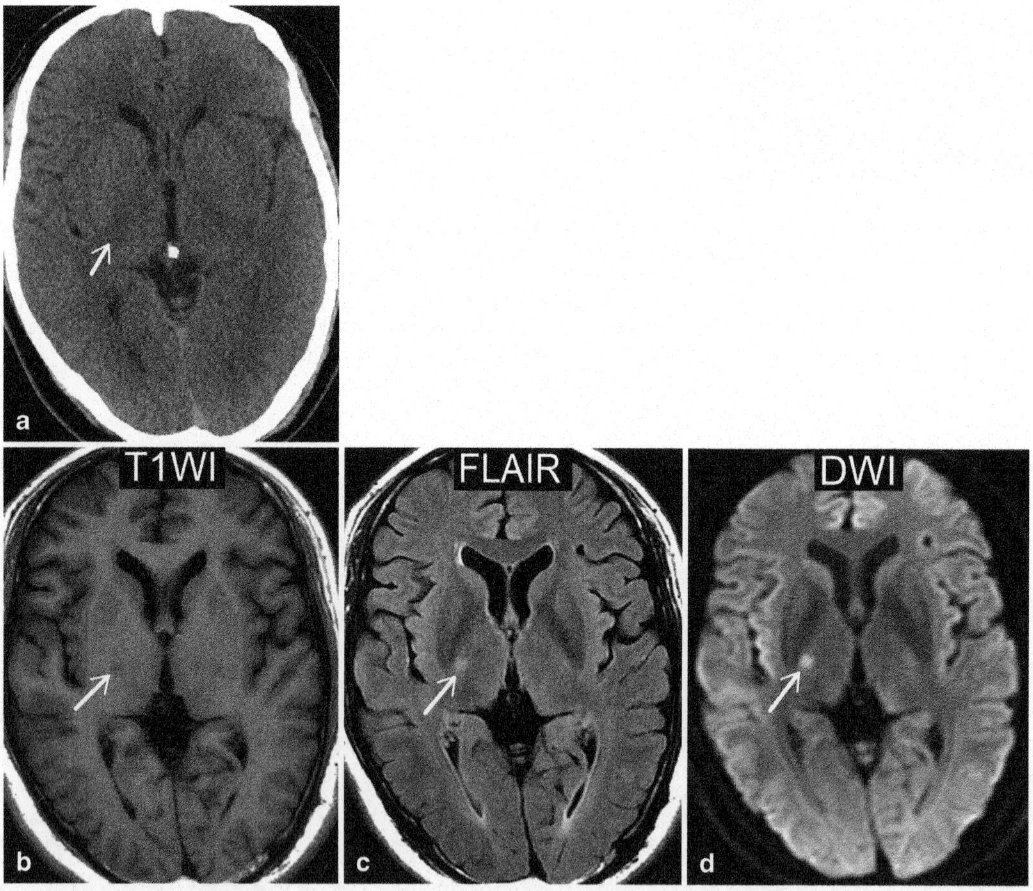

Fig. 5.40 M/46, Internal capsule acute lacunar infarction. A hypertensive patient suffered a sudden onset of left hemiparesis for 2 days. (**a**) CT: No abnormality is seen. The bilateral internal capsules are white matter, showing mild hypodensity (arrow) in CT. MRI was performed 2 h after CT. (**b**) MRI, T1WI: No signal change is noted; the bilateral corticospinal tracts (arrow) show mild hypointensity on T1WI. (**c**) FLAIR: The posterior limb of the right internal capsule show hyperintensity (arrow), which is suspected to be an acute lacunar infarction. (**d**) DWI: The lesion is bright (arrow), confirming that this small lesion has diffusion restriction. This finding suggests acute cytotoxic edema caused by acute infarction. Although this infarction is small, it is present in the course of the corticospinal tract, thereby clinically presenting significant left-sided hemiparesis

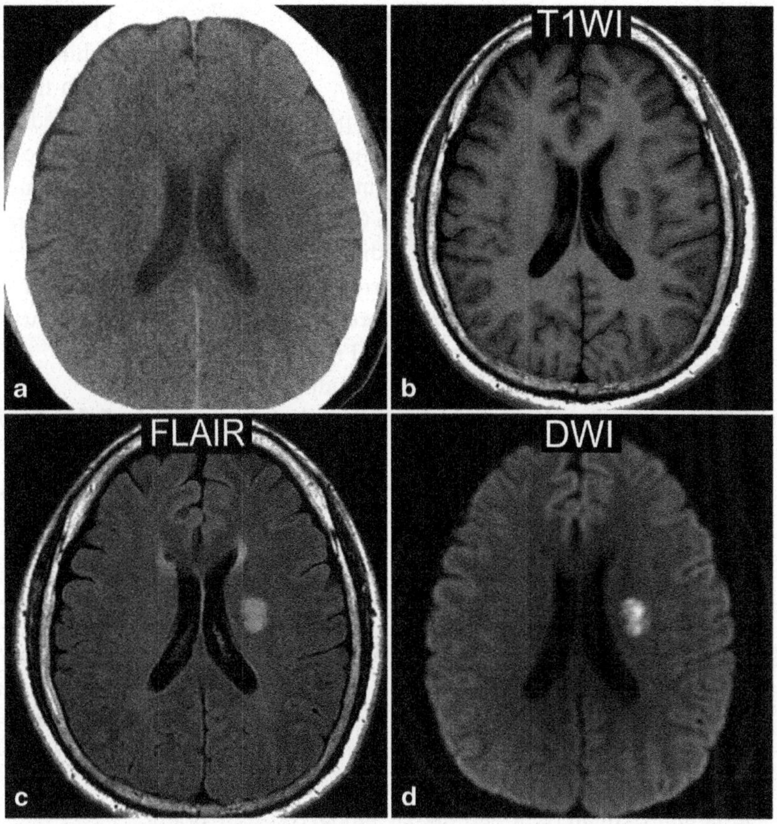

Fig. 5.41 M/53, Corona radiata acute lacunar infarction. The patient with diabetes suffered a sudden onset of right-sided hemiparesis. CT was conducted on the third day. (**a**) CT: A small hypodense lesion is seen in the left corona radiata, suggesting acute infarction edema. MRI was performed on the seventh day after symptom onset. (**b, c**) MRI: This lesion exhibits hypointensity on T1WI and hyperintensity on FLAIR. (**d**) DWI confirms that this lesion has diffusion restriction because it is bright; hence, this is acute cytotoxic edema due to acute infarction. The length of this lesion is 1.5 cm; thus, it is a lacunar infarction

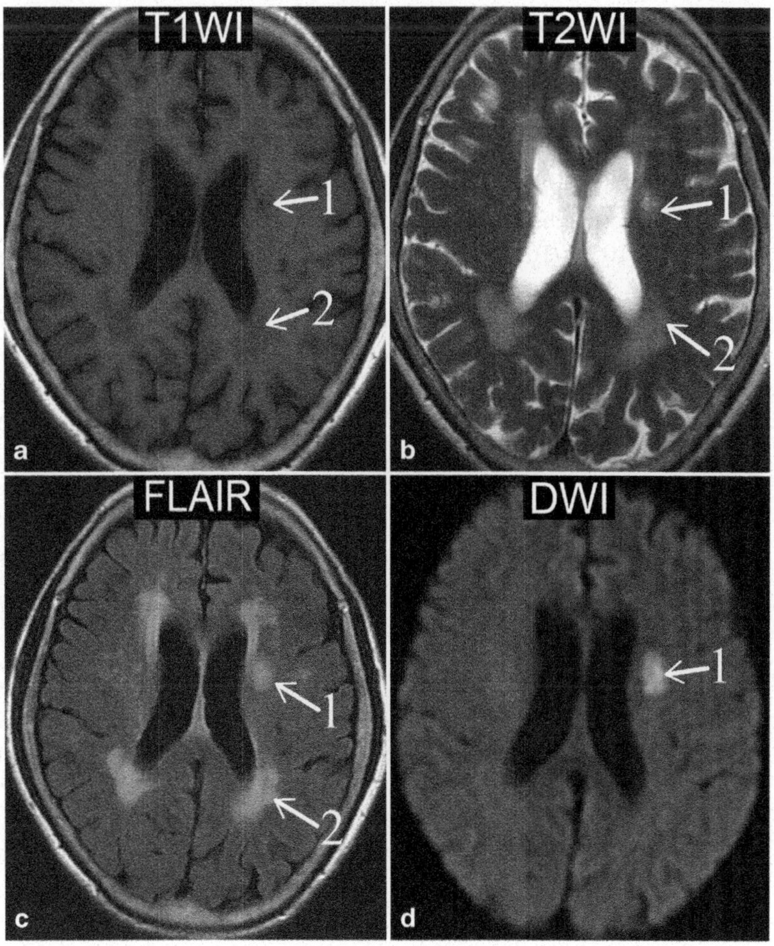

Fig. 5.42 F/76, Left corona radiata acute lacunar infarction. The patient with a history of atrial fibrillation suffered a sudden onset of right-sided hemiparesis. No infarction or hemorrhage was observed upon emergency CT (not shown). MRI was performed on the third day after symptom onset. (**a**) MRI, T1WI: A suspicious hypodense lesion (1) is seen in the left corona radiata, and periventricular hypointensity (2) is noted. (**b, c**) T2WI, FLAIR: A small hyperintense lesion (1) is seen in the left corona radiata, and periventricular hyperintensity (PVH) (2) is present. (**d**) DWI: Only the lesion (1) in the left corona radiata is bright, representing diffusion restriction and indicating acute cytotoxic edema caused by acute infarction. The PVH has no diffusion restriction; thus, no signal change is seen on DWI

5.11 CT Perfusion, Imaging, and Interpretation

CT perfusion and CT angiography are performed simultaneously and involve an intravenous injection of 40–50 mL of iodine-containing contrast medium at a rate of 5 mL/s to rapidly obtain source images. The CT machine will first produce CT perfusion images, including CBF, CBV, MTT, T_{max}, or DT (detailed below). The current CT machine will automatically calculate the area of core and penumbra and then present it as a summary map (Figs. 5.7, 5.44 and 5.46) so that all the physicians, including the general practitioner and medical students, can easily interpret it.

Immediately following CT perfusion, another injection of contrast medium is administered, and the source images are reused to form a CTA images (Figs. 5.7, 5.15, 5.20, 5.23, 5.43, 5.44, 5.45, and 5.46).

5.11.1 Cerebral Blood Flow (CBF)

CBF is the most crucial parameter of CT perfusion. CBF can indicate the blood flow of brain tissue in a specific time period. The CBF of gray matter of healthy brain tissue is approximately 50–80 mL of blood/100 g of brain/min. The CBF of white matter is approximately 20 mL of blood/100 g of brain/min. The CBF of the cerebral cortex or basal ganglia gray matter is 2–3 times that of white matter.

The diameter of cerebral blood vessels can be adjusted to keep the blood flow of the brain constant due to the autoregulation function of the brain. When the blood pressure is too high, blood vessels dilate. When the blood pressure drops too much, blood vessels constrict. When CBF drops below 20 mL/100 g/min, the autoregulation of blood vessels is not sufficient to regulate blood flow. Thus, brain tissue is hypoxic but still reversible. When CBF is lower than 10–15 mL/100 g/min, the threshold of hypoxia in brain tissue is reached. Approximately 2–10 min of brain tissue hypoxia causes irreversible damage. The area with blood flow lower than 10–15 mL/100 g/min is called infarct ***core***, and the area with CBF higher than 20 mL/100 g/min is called infarct penumbra and which involves reversible damage. As long as the blood flow is opened, the ***penumbra*** territory can still return to normal, which is the territory where doctors want to perform thrombolysis to salvage [31, 32].

5.11.2 Cerebral Blood Volume (CBV)

Normal gray matter in the cerebral cortex and basal ganglia contains high CBV due to abundant blood vessels. The white matter has low CBV due to few blood vessels. CBV also exhibits autoregulation.

In the infarct territory, CBF in the core and penumbra is reduced. However, CBV is increased in the penumbra territory due to autoregulation. The infarct core territory loses vessel autoregulation, and CBV is reduced, so the acute infarction territory is subjected to irreversible damages (e.g., infarct core) and reversible damages (e.g., infarct penumbra, which is also known as salvageable tissue). Physicians must decide whether or not to perform thrombolysis therapy.

5.11.3 Mean Transit Time (MTT)

MTT reflects the time of blood flow through the capillary of the brain tissue.

MTT = CBV/CBF.

Normal MTT is 4.0 s in gray matter and 4.8 s in white matter.

When vascular stenosis or occlusion causes ischemia in the perfusion territory, the cerebral perfusion pressure is reduced to the threshold of brain tissue autoregulation. As a result, the CBF is diminished and the MTT is prolonged.

5.11.4 Time to Peak (TTP) or Time to Maximum (T_{max}) or Delayed Time (DT)

TTP is the time in which the brain tissue in a particular territory is enhanced to the peak after the contrast medium is injected in seconds.

Some software programs use T_{max} or delayed time *(DT)*.

5.11.5 Core and Penumbra

When the blood flow in the cerebral ischemia territory is reduced to lower than 30%, the brain tissue may become necrotic, forming a true infarction, which is called **core**. The core is when the CBF is lower than 25–30%, the T_{max} is greater than 6 s, and the DT (delay time) is greater than 3 s.

Although CBF is declining in the periphery of the core and the brain tissue is in ischemia, the brain tissue can still return to normal as long as the blood vessels are opened and the blood flow is restored. This territory is **penumbra**.

5.11.5.1 Interpretation of Core and Penumbra

The CT machine can automatically generate colored pictures of CBV, CBF, MTT, T_{max}, and DT.

In general, CBV is used as the core territory, and MTT with CBV deducted as mismatch territory, which refers to penumbra [33]. In another theory, CBV with CBF deducted is a mismatch (penumbra) [34].

The interpretation of CT perfusion was previously based on visually observing the colored map produced by CT, which is not accurate or objective. Current CT software can generate a summary map and present it with data. Even doctors with insufficient training can easily interpret it.

MIStar software uses the territory with CBF < 25% as the ischemic core and the territory with DT > 3 s deducting the mismatch territory with CBF < 25% as the penumbra. A summary map is then automatically generated (Figs. 5.15, 5.45, and 5.46), which is convenient for interpretation.

RAPID software uses the territory with CBF < 30% as the ischemic core and the mismatch territory with T_{max} >6″ deducting the area with CBF < 30% as penumbra [35] (Figs. 5.7 and 5.44).

If the core is more extensive than 60 mL or if the core is close to the penumbra, then it is not suitable for IV tPA thrombolysis or IA thrombectomy; however, the principles of each hospital vary greatly [36].

The Stanford Stroke Center uses RAPID software for large-scale transnational clinical trials [35]. The recommended CT-perfusion principle for thrombectomy is as follows:

Core range <70 mL.

Ratio of ischemic tissue to infarction core >1.8.

Penumbra >15 mL.

CT perfusion is valuable in the diagnosis of the anterior circulation, namely the judgment of ischemia in ACA and MCA perfusion territories. Especially sensitive for MCA, only one branch (Fig. 5.11) or its perforating artery (Fig. 5.15) can also present hypoperfusion territory of infarction. The diagnostic sensitivity to posterior circulation, such as perfusion territory of PCA and vertebro-basilar artery, is low [34] (Figs. 5.20 and 5.23). Some research reported that the sensitivity to lacunar infarction is good [37]. For patients with TIA, CT perfusion can be used to assess cerebral ischemia territory, whereas CTA can be used to evaluate the presence of stenosis or occlusion of major intracranial and extracranial arteries (Fig. 5.43).

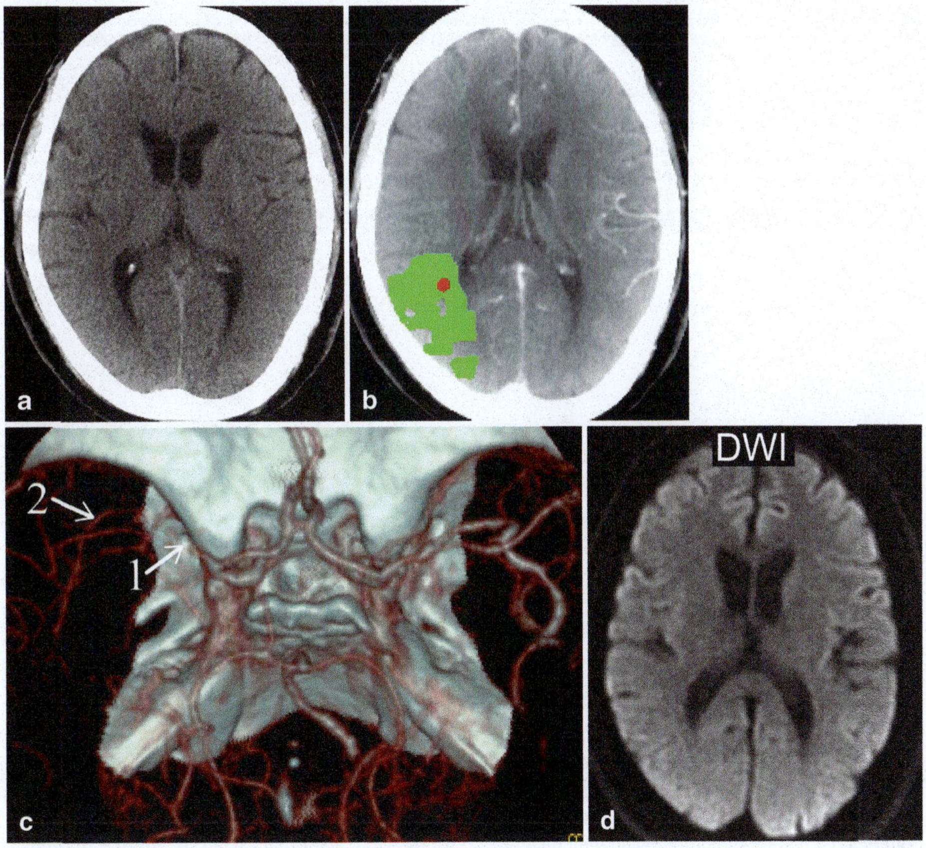

Fig. 5.43 M/64, Severe arteriosclerosis of MCA, causing transient ischemic attack (TIA). The patient suffered a sudden onset of left limb weakness, which persisted for 2 h. (**a**) CT: No brain tissue edema or hemorrhage is seen. (**b**) CT perfusion: A small area of hypoperfusion is seen in the posterior of the right parietal lobe; this area is the posterior one-third territory of the right MCA. (**c**) CTA: Severe stenosis of the transverse portion of the right MCA due to severe atherosclerosis (1); however, well opacification of its branches (2) indicates that the collateral circulation has been established. (**d**) MRI was performed on the second day: DWI shows no water-restriction area, meaning that no real infarction occurred

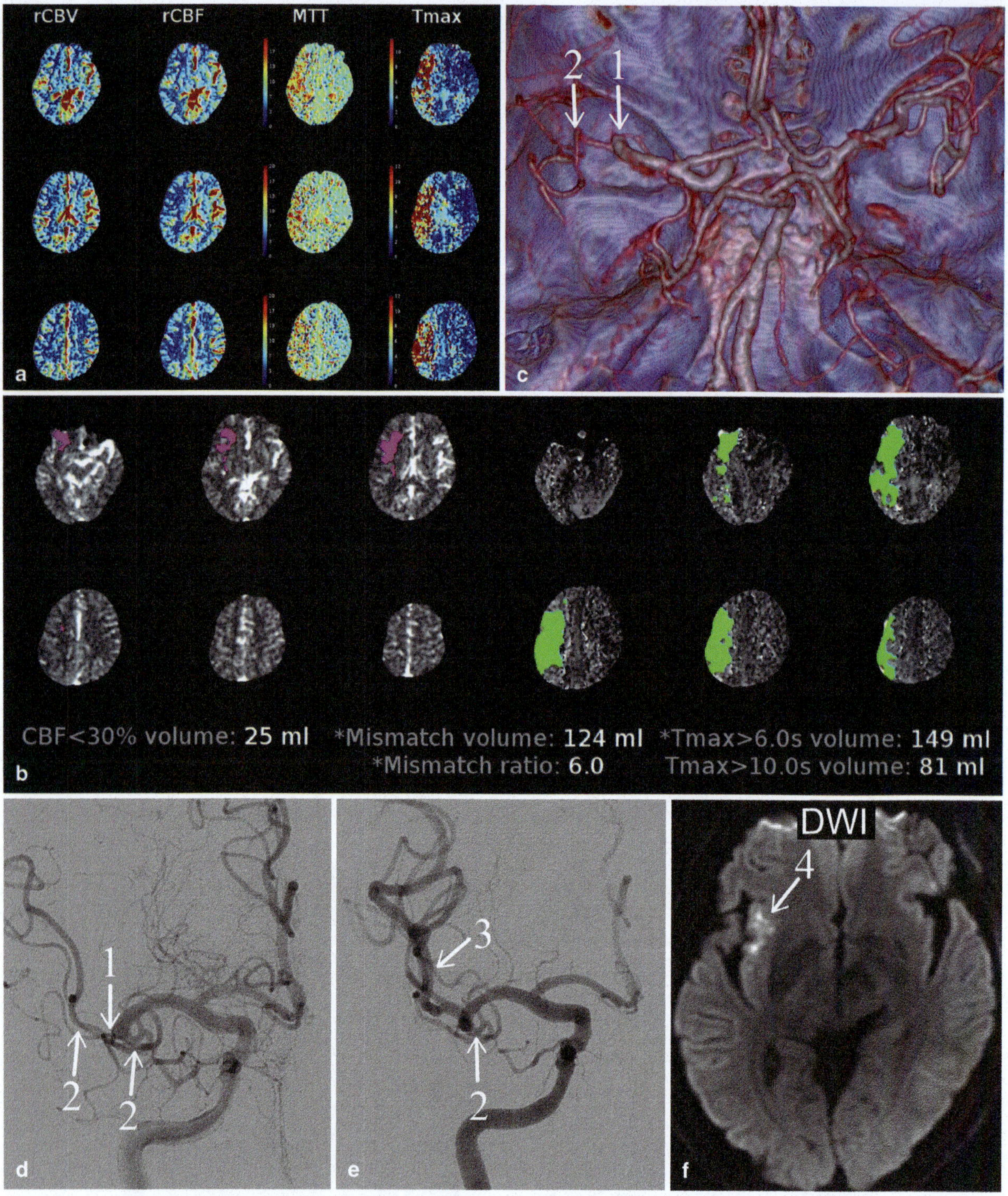

Fig. 5.44 M/61, Rt. MCA acute infarction, successful IA thrombectomy. The patient with hypertension and diabetes and a history of atrial fibrillation suffered a sudden onset of left hemiplegia and aphasia. Emergency CT was conducted 2 h after symptom onset, which showed no intracerebral hemorrhage or infarction (not shown); CT perfusion and CTA were performed immediately. (**a**) CT perfusion: An area of hypoperfusion in the right F-P lobes is observed in rCBV, rCBF, MTT, and T_{max}, but judging the core and penumbra with the naked eyes is difficult. (**b**) A summary map was created using RAPID software. The area CBF < 30% is marked in pink, which is approximately 25 mL, representing the core. The T_{max} >6″ area is 149 mL. T_{max} − rCBF = 124 mL is a mismatch, that is the penumbra area. The mismatch ratio is 6.0. From the above data, this patient is suitable for IV tPA and IA thrombectomy. (**c**) CTA: Total occlusion of a branch (1) of the right MCA, another branch (2), is normal. (**d**) DSA: Similar findings to CTA. (**e**) DSA after IA thrombectomy: The entire right MCA was opened (3). (**f**) Follow-up MRI on the second day: DWI shows that only a small area in the right insular cortex is hyperintense, representing diffusion restriction (4) due to infarction. This is the core area displayed on the CT perfusion. The penumbra area was salvaged, and no cytotoxic edema is observed in this area. Clinically, the symptoms disappeared after thrombectomy

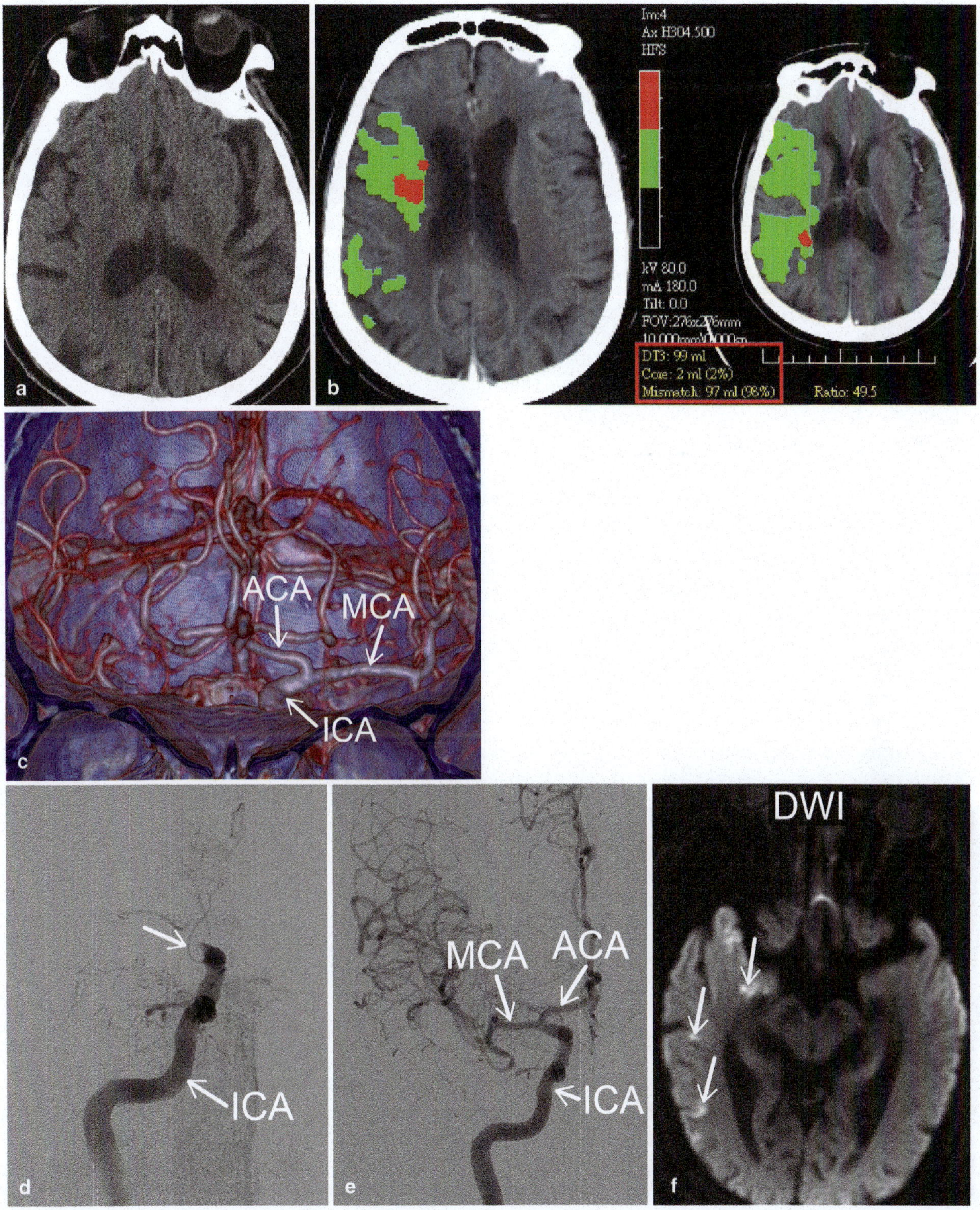

Fig. 5.45 M/77, MCA infarction, successful IA thrombectomy. The patient suffered a sudden onset of left hemiparesis. CT was performed 2 h after symptom onset. (**a**) CT: The right insular cortex and putamen are slightly grayed out, which is a possible early sign of acute infarction. (**b**) CT perfusion: The left lower corner shows that the MIStar software immediately calculates DT3 (delayed time > 3 s) as 99 mL, CBF <25% as 2 mL (core), and mismatch (penumbra) as 97 mL. Thus, the patient is suitable for IV tPA and IA thrombectomy. (**c**) CTA: Well opacification of the left ICA, MCA, and ACA, while non-opacification of the right ICA and MCA, reflecting occlusion. (**d**) DSA was performed immediately after CT, CTA, and CT perfusion: Total occlusion of the distal portion of the right ICA, a thrombus in the occlusion site (arrow). (**e**) IA thrombectomy was performed, and the thrombus was successfully removed. Follow-up DSA: well opacification of the right ICA, MCA, and ACA. (**f**) Follow-up MRI on the second day, DWI: Only several small acute infarction cytotoxic edemas (arrows) be observed in the right temporal lobe, rather than in the entire right MCA territory because most of the penumbra area was successfully salvaged. Clinically, the patient recovered to only slight weakness on the left limb alone

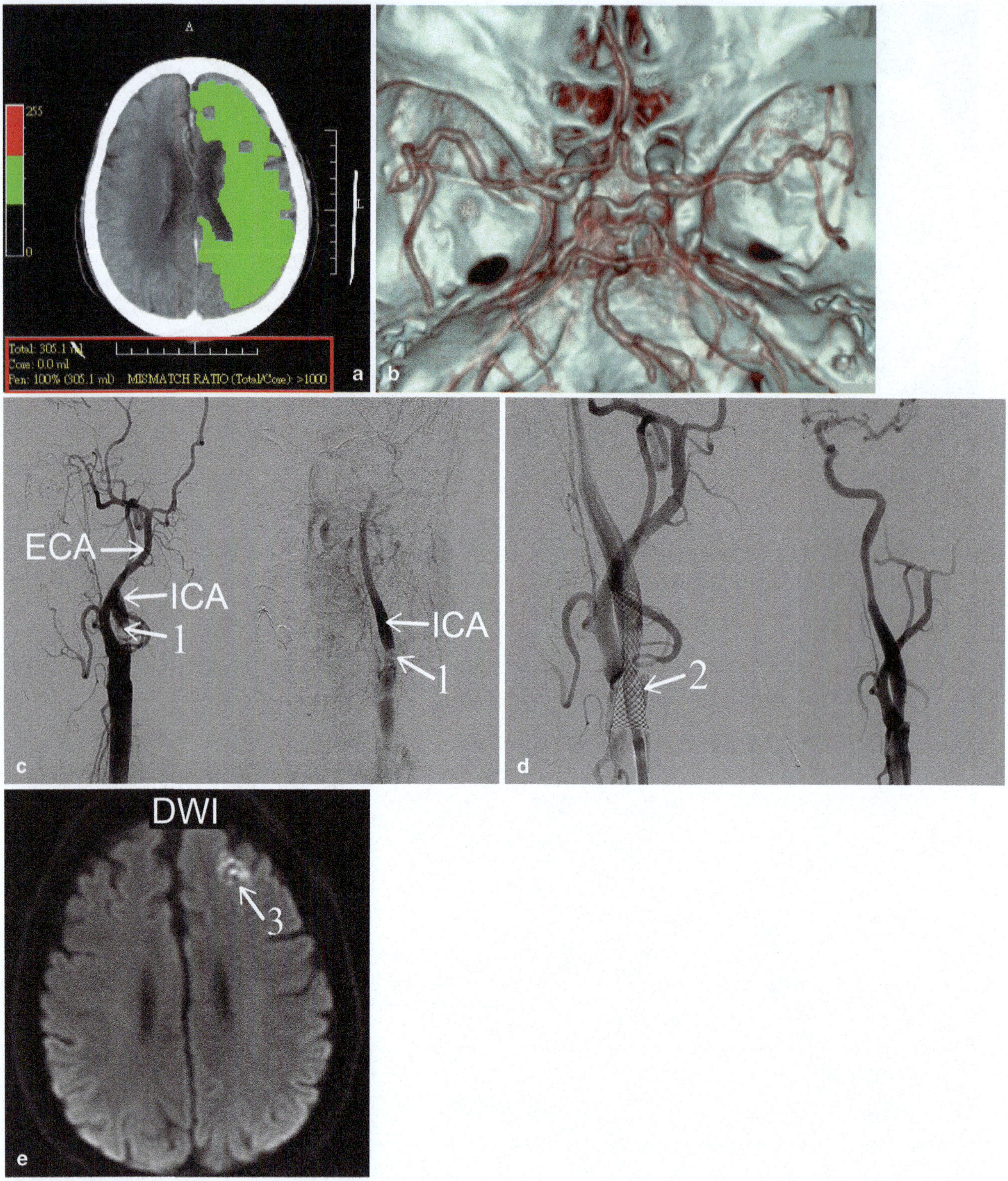

Fig. 5.46 M/80, ICA occlusion, IA thrombectomy, and stenting. A colon cancer patient. After surgery for colon cancer, the patient was found to have right hemiplegia and aphasia in the recovery room. Given that it occurred in the hospital, emergency CT was performed within 30 min, which revealed no intracranial hemorrhage or brain tissue edema (not shown). (**a**) CT perfusion showed a large area of hypoperfusion in the left cerebral hemisphere. The map generated by MIStar showed that the green area, which is DT > 3 s, is 305 mL and that no area where CBF is lower than 25% was detected, indicating that no core area; all the hypoperfusion area is the penumbra. (**b**) CTA showed that the left MCA and ACA are well opacified, and angiography was performed immediately. (**c**) DSA showed a thrombus (1) in the very proximal portion of the left ICA. Compared with ECA, ICA blood flow is very slow. (**d**) A neuroradiologist conducted IA thrombectomy immediately and successfully retrieved the thrombus; stenosis was observed in the proximal portion of the left ICA, and a stent (2) was placed for dilatation of the stenosis. (**e**) Follow-up MRI on the next day: Only a small area of brain tissue in the left frontal cortex showed diffusion restriction (3), which was a watershed infarction between MCA and ACA. Most of the MCA and ACA supply areas were rescued

5.12 Hypoxic-Ischemic Encephalopathy (HIE)

Arrhythmia and a decline in blood pressure may cause temporary hypoxia in the brain, resulting in syncope symptoms.

Cardiac arrest, respiratory arrest, and shock may cause a lack of oxygen in the brain for a long time, causing watershed infarction between major blood vessels.

If the brain is deprived of oxygen for too long, then the brain is severely hypoxic, which causes global hypoxia-ischemia and extensive brain damage, which is called HIE [1, 38].

The prognosis of HIE is poor, and patients usually enter a long-term coma.

5.12.1 HIE Imaging

CT shows a decreasing density of gray matter in the cerebral cortex, effacement of the sulci, and slightly decreased density of the basal ganglia (putamen and caudate nuclei) (Fig. 5.47). However, the density change in CT is not apparent and is easily ignored [38].

If the patient has been in a coma, then an MRI will be performed (Fig. 5.48). DWI and FLAIR can clearly reveal the brain damage areas. The most commonly affected areas by HIE are the cerebral cortex and deep gray matter of the caudate nucleus, putamen, and thalamus, also the white matter of centrum semiovale [39].

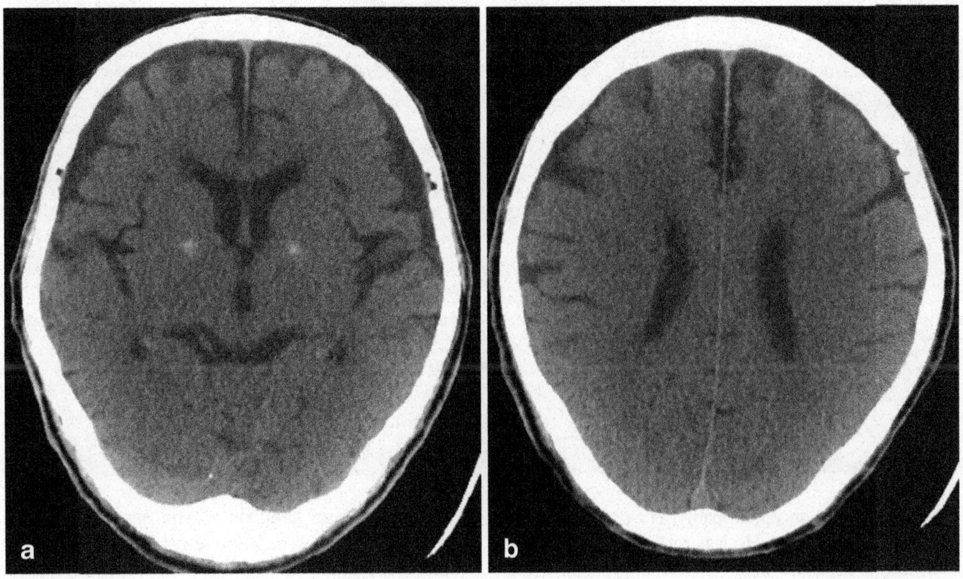

Fig. 5.47 M/83, Hypoxic-ischemic encephalopathy. The patient has diabetes and parkinsonism. The family found the patient in a coma and respiratory arrest. The patient was rushed to the hospital for an emergency. (**a**) CT: The putamen and caudate nuclei of the bilateral basal ganglia lose normal grayish density. (**b**) The higher section of CT showed that the gray matter of the cerebral hemisphere becomes gray-dark as the white matter, losing normal gray–white matter contrast. Effacement of the cortical sulci of bilateral cerebral hemispheres. The above findings indicate early brain tissue edema of the whole brain. The findings are indicating diffuse brain tissue edema was due to respiratory arrest

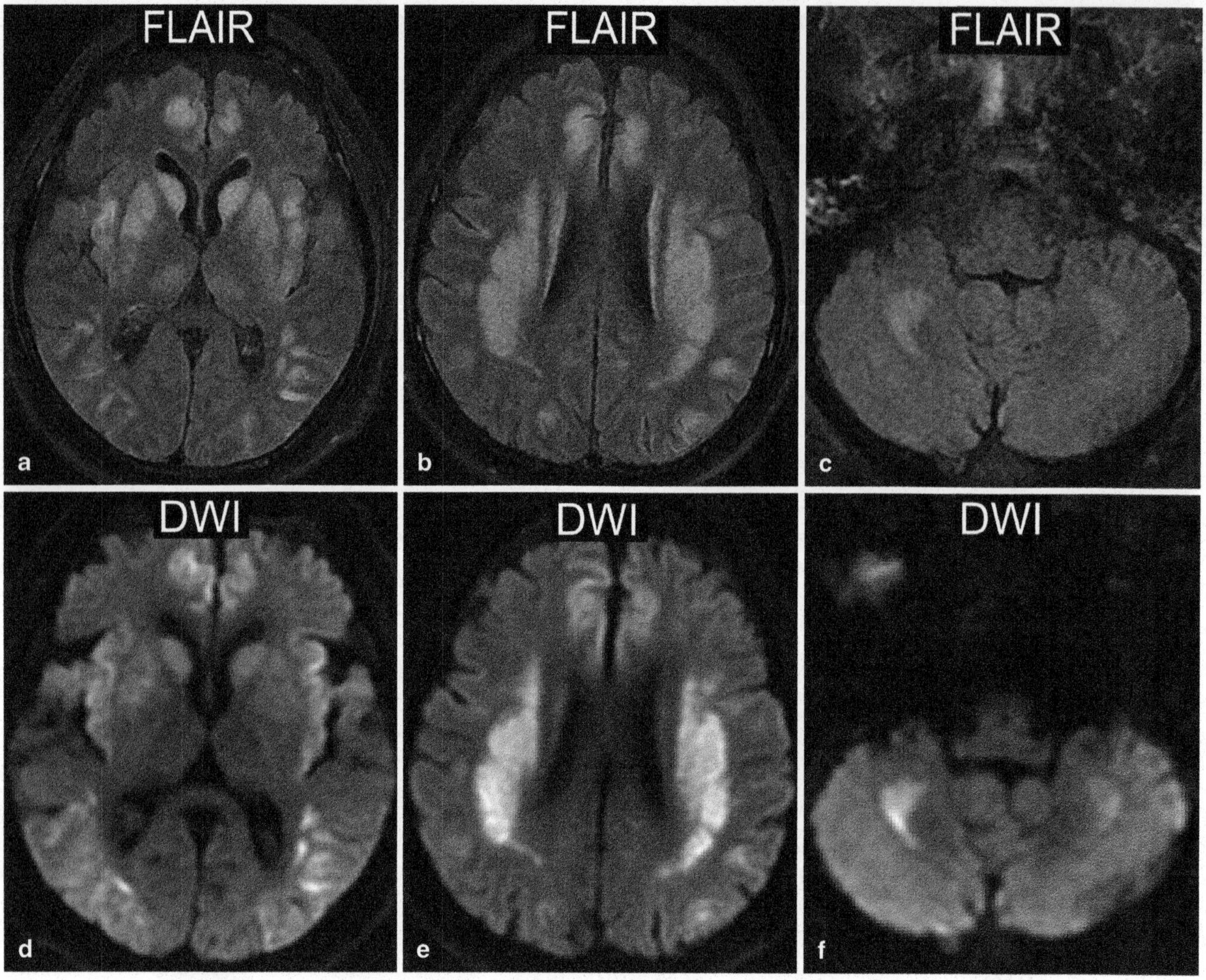

Fig. 5.48 M/67, Hypoxic-ischemic encephalopathy. The patient with fulminant hepatitis suffered a cardiac arrest. He was rescued, and his heartbeat was restored; however, he became comatose. MRI was performed on the third day. (**a–c**) MRI, FLAIR: Symmetrical hyperintensities are seen in the bilateral basal ganglia, thalami, insular cortexes, frontal lobes, temporo-occipital lobes, centrum semiovale, and dentate nuclei of the cerebellum. (**d–f**) DWI: The above areas show diffusion restriction except for the bilateral thalami. This finding is indicative of cytotoxic edema

5.13 White Matter Edema

White matter edema is vasogenic edema. In particular, white matter edema caused by brain tumors (Fig. 5.49) or brain abscess sometimes have sudden symptoms, such as hemiparesis and dysphonia, which are very similar to stroke symptoms. Given that CT is the preferred tool for diagnosing stroke and usually does not require contrast medium, vasogenic edema is easily mistaken for cytotoxic edema caused by infarction. Notably, if edema occurs only in white matter and is palm-shaped, this condition may not be infarction. Furthermore, the contrast medium must be injected to enhance the visualization of the lesion within the white matter edema.

In MRI, white matter edema is more explicit as vasogenic edema caused by tumor or abscess. White matter edema shows hypointense on T1WI and hyperintense on T2WI and FLAIR, this feature is the same as that of cytotoxic edema caused by infarction. However, white matter edema has no signal change on DWI because vasogenic edema has no water diffusion restriction. Therefore, DWI can clearly distinguish between the two types of brain tissue edema (see Chap. 2 and Fig. 2.8).

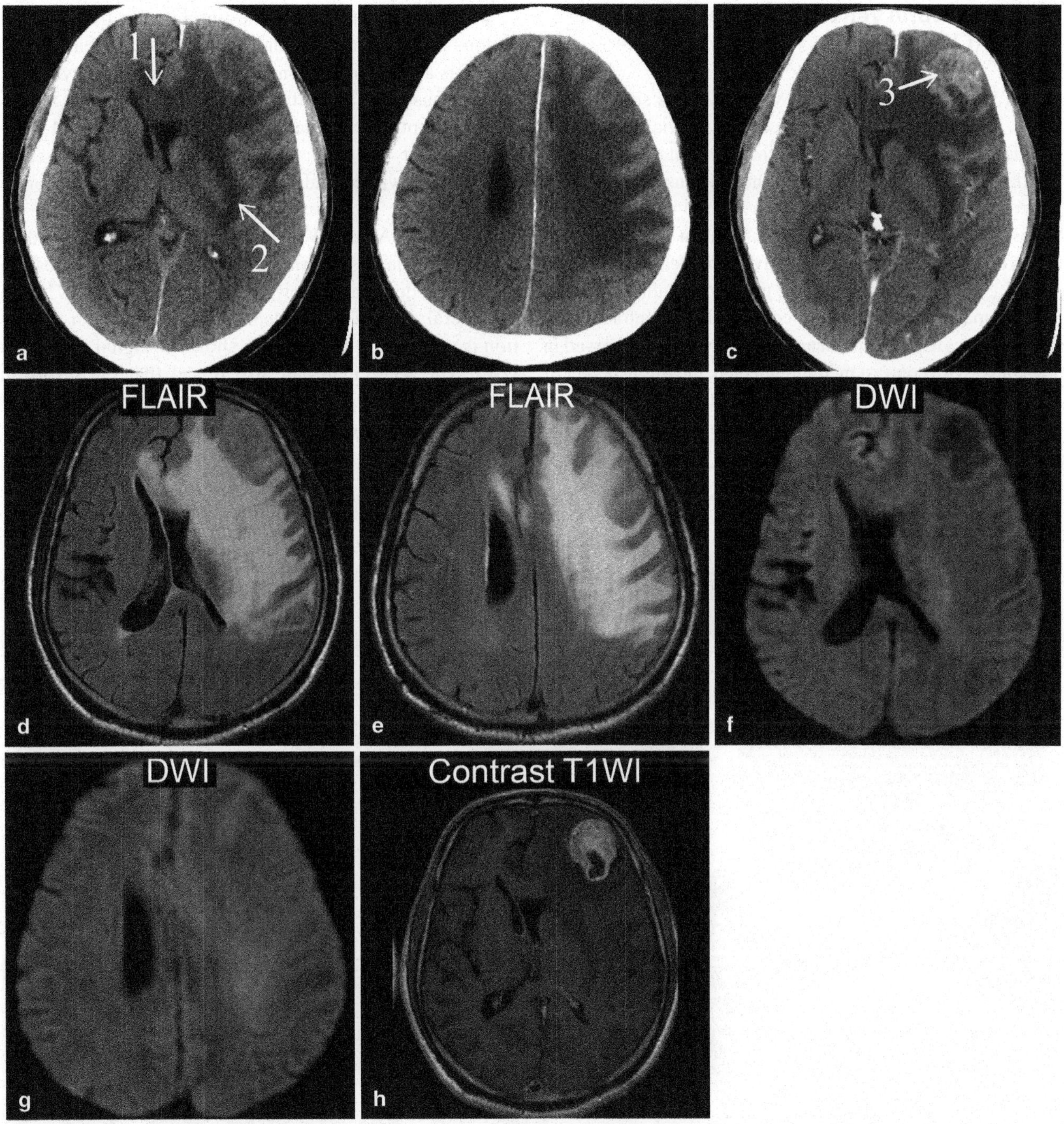

Fig. 5.49 M/76, Brain tumor causes white matter edema. The patient suffered right limb weakness, dysphonia, and was suspected stroke. (**a**, **b**) CT: A large area of brain tissue edema is observed in the left frontal lobe, which extends to the genu of the corpus callosum (1) and left external capsule (2). The brain edema is mainly in the white matter, forming a palm-like shape. The appearance of palm-like white matter edema necessitates contrast medium injection because tumors may be present inside; without contrast enhancement, the tumor may not be easy to analyze. (**c**) Contrast CT: A tumor is enhanced (3) in the left frontal lobe. MRI was performed on the same day. (**d**, **e**) MRI, FLAIR: The brain edema shows hyperintensity. (**f**, **g**) DWI: No signal change is seen on DWI because no diffusion restriction is present; hence, this is vasogenic edema, not cytotoxic edema. (**h**) Contrast-enhanced T1WI: The tumor is enhanced by Gd-DTPA. After surgical removal of this tumor, pathology proved that this is a metastatic tumor from pulmonary adenocarcinoma

5.14 Cerebral Venous Sinus Thrombosis (CVST)

CVST refers to the intracranial vein or venous sinus thrombosis. CVST has lower incidence than arterial thrombosis but is still common. The clinical manifestations include headache, limb weakness, disturbance of consciousness, and other neurological symptoms, even seizure or coma. Many types of etiology are involved in CVST. In young women, the primary etiology is contraceptive complications.

CT is the preferred diagnostic tool for revealing brain tissue edema. Few cases occur combined with intracerebral hemorrhage (ICH). Hyperdense thrombus can be observed in the sinus. With contrast medium injected, the filling defect of the thrombus in the sinus can be detected, which is called "empty delta signs" (Fig. 5.50). This sign makes the definite diagnosis of CVST on CT [40].

MRI can directly reveal the thrombus in the vein and venous sinus. Although brain tissue edema caused by CVST is also an infarction, it is not the same as cytotoxic edema caused by arterial infarction. The edema is a mixture of cytotoxic edema and vasogenic edema [41, 42]. The flow of drainage vein is obstructed due to sinus thrombosis, which leads to venous congestion and brain tissue edema. The entire edema area is hyperintense on T2WI and FLAIR. DWI can demonstrate that the middle area of edema has restricted diffusion, which represents cytotoxic edema and shows hyperintensity on DWI. The peripheral area of brain edema with no diffusion restriction is vasogenic edema, which shows no signal change on DWI. The ADC map can also reveal that the diffusion restriction territory is dark, and the vasogenic edema territory is white (Fig. 5.50).

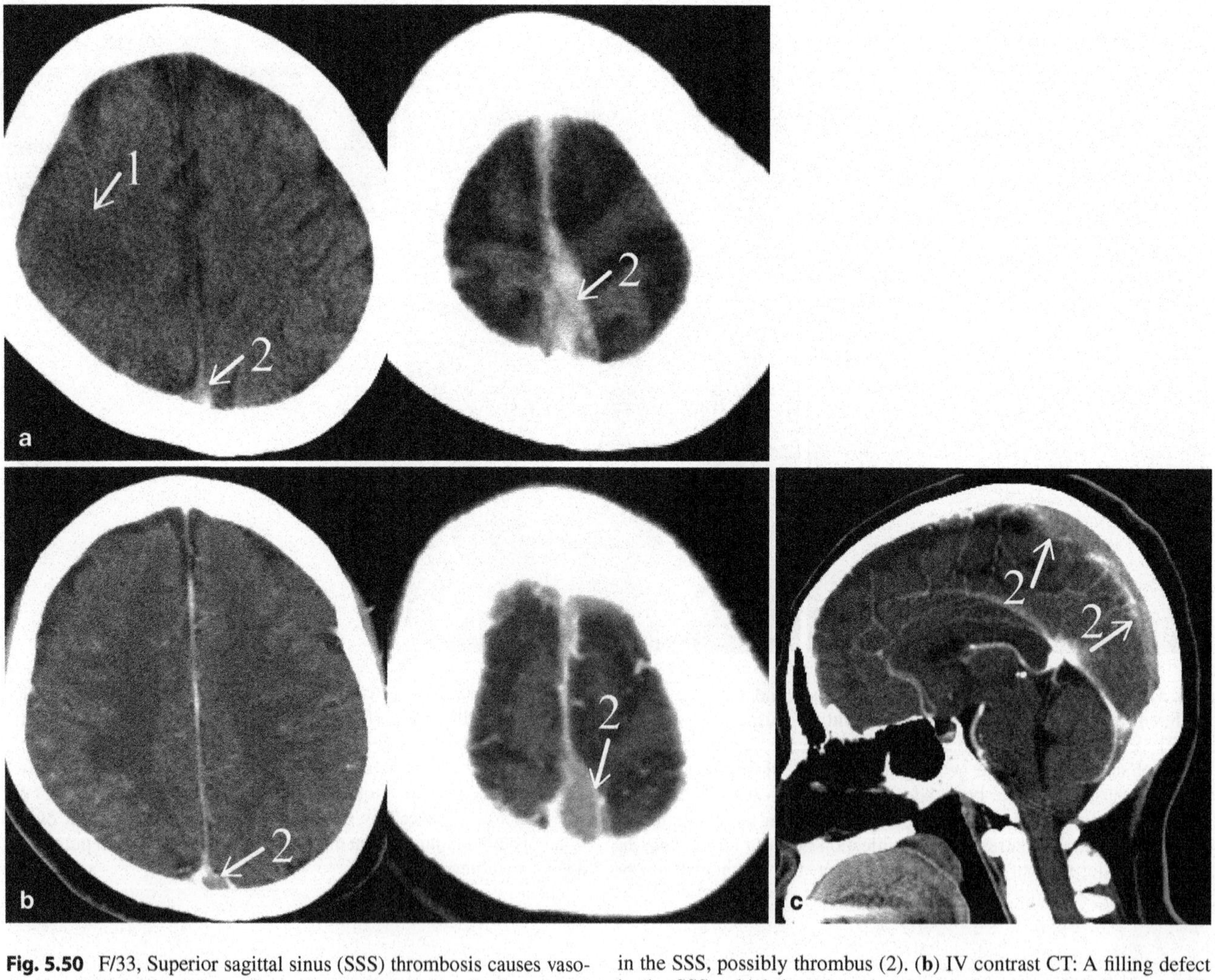

Fig. 5.50 F/33, Superior sagittal sinus (SSS) thrombosis causes vasogenic and cytotoxic edemas. The patient had a migraine for 2 years and suffered a sudden onset of left hemiparesis for 2 days. (**a**) CT: An area of brain tissue edema (1) in the right frontoparietal lobes. Hyperdensity in the SSS, possibly thrombus (2). (**b**) IV contrast CT: A filling defect in the SSS, which is a thrombus in the sinus, a typical "empty delta signs" (2). (**c**) Contrast CT, sagittal reconstruction: All the posterior segment of SSS has thrombus (2). MRI was performed on the third day.

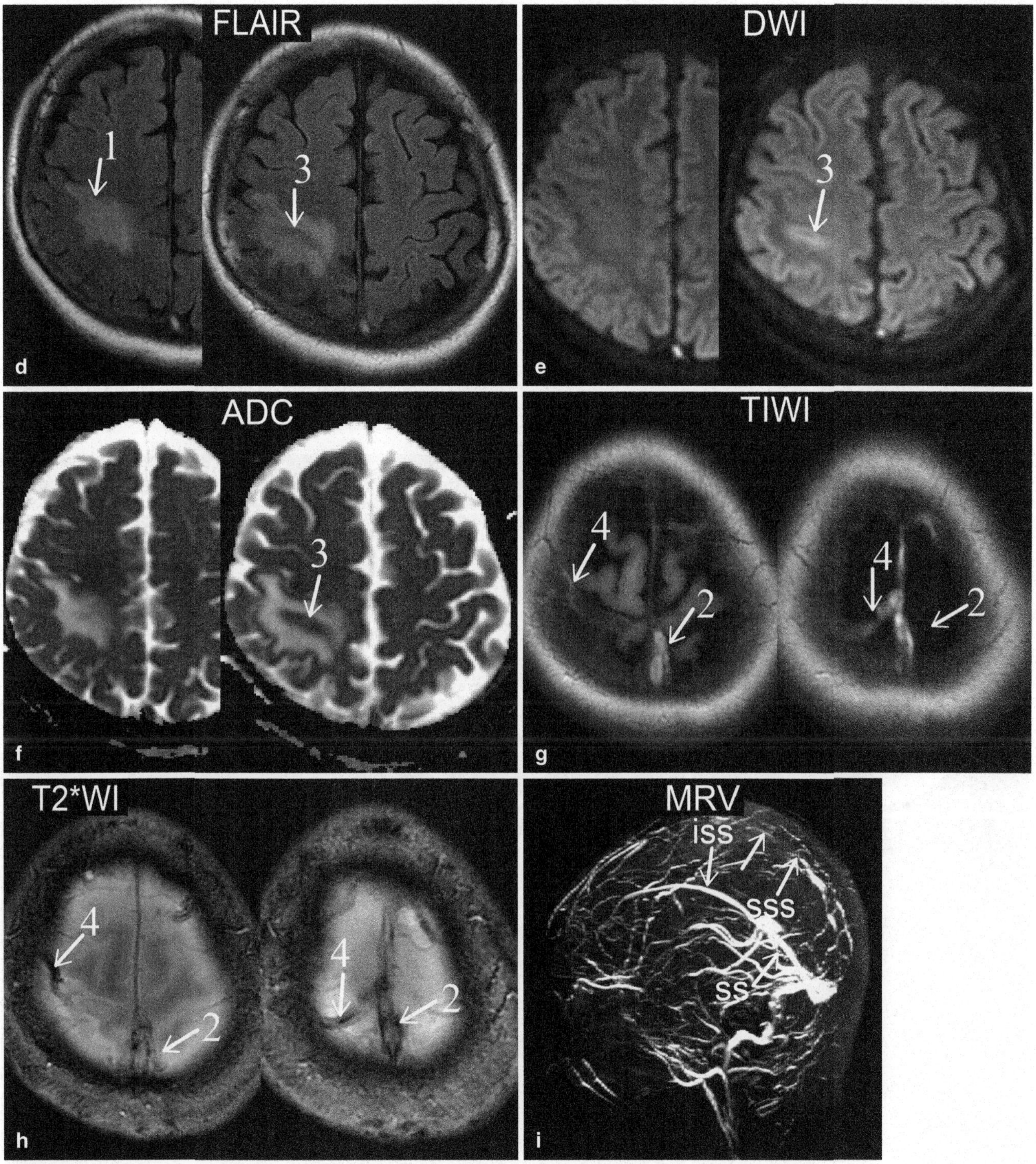

Fig. 5.50 (continued)
(**d**) MRI, FLAIR: The brain tissue edema on CT shows hyperintensity (1) on FLAIR but has hypointensity (3) in the middle of edema. (**e**) DWI: Only the middle area of edema shows hyperintensity on DWI (3), reflecting diffusion restriction; this is cytotoxic edema. The other part of edema shows no signal change on DWI, which is vasogenic edema. (**f**) ADC: Similar to DWI, only the middle area shows a decreased ADC value, indicating hypointensity (3); hence, diffusion restriction occurs, and this is cytotoxic edema. Other parts of the edema show hyperintensity, exhibiting increasing ADC value; this is vasogenic edema. (**g**) T1WI: Hyperintensity in the SSS (2) and a cortical vein (4), which are indicative of thrombus. (**h**) T2*WI: Thrombus in the SSS (2) and a cortical vein (4), showing hypointensity in T2*WI. (**i**) MRV: Poor opacification of the SSS because of thrombosis. The inferior sagittal sinus (ISS) and straight sinus (ss) are well opacified, indicating normal venous flow

5.15 Carbon Monoxide (CO) Poisoning

CO poisoning is common due to accident or suicide. This phenomenon causes hypoxia because CO binds to hemoglobin 230–270 times stronger than O_2. The brain and heart are the organs with the highest oxygen demand in the body. Therefore, CO poisoning often causes brain damage and decreased heart function. The main location of brain damage is globus pallidus (Figs. 5.51 and 5.52), which lacks anastomotic vascular supply. The heme iron of the globus pallidus is the most abundant, which is the most easily taken away by CO, causing hypoxia and cytotoxic edema [43]. In addition to the globus pallidus, the white matter in centrum semiovale (Fig. 5.52), cerebellum, and splenium of the corpus callosum can also be involved.

CT is the preferred diagnostic tool for emergent examination. CT reveals that the bilateral globus pallidus are hypodense (Fig. 5.51). However, in the acute stage, the sensitivity of CT is low. Hypodensity in the globus pallidus is revealed after few days.

MRI is the most important diagnostic tool for CO poisoning (Figs. 5.51 and 5.52). The bilateral globus pallidus become hypointense on T1WI and hyperintense on T2WI and FLAIR. And they show diffusion restriction on DWI and ADC (hyperintensity on DWI and hypointensity on ADC). On the ADC map, a thin rim of hyperintensity can be identified on the margin of the lesion in the globus pallidus, indicating vasogenic edema around the cytotoxic edema. Approximately 80% of the patients have a dark spot in the globus pallidus, which represents petechial hemorrhage [44].

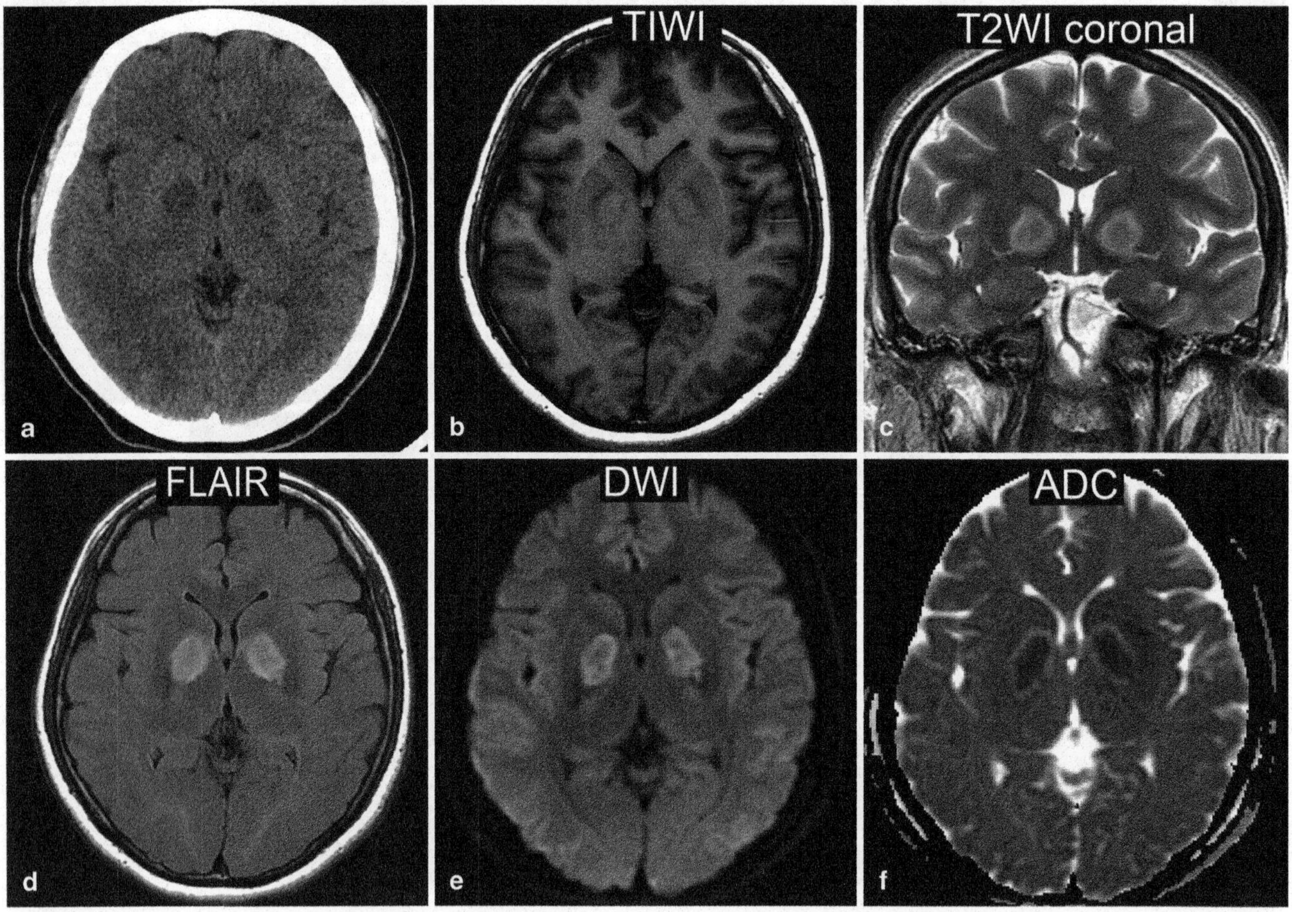

Fig. 5.51 F/31, CO poisoning. A patient with depression who committed suicide by burning charcoal was found in a state of coma. (**a**) CT: Symmetrical hypodensity in the bilateral globus pallidus, which is a typical CT pattern of CO poisoning. MRI was performed on the second day after CT. (**b–d**) MRI: The bilateral globus pallidus shows mild hyperintensity on T1WI and hyperintensity on T2WI and FLAIR, reflecting brain tissue edema. (**e, f**) DWI, ADC: The bilateral globus pallidus shows hyperintensity on DWI and hypointensity on ADC, indicating diffusion restriction; this is cytotoxic edema. A thin-rim hyperintensity is seen on ADC; this is vasogenic edema

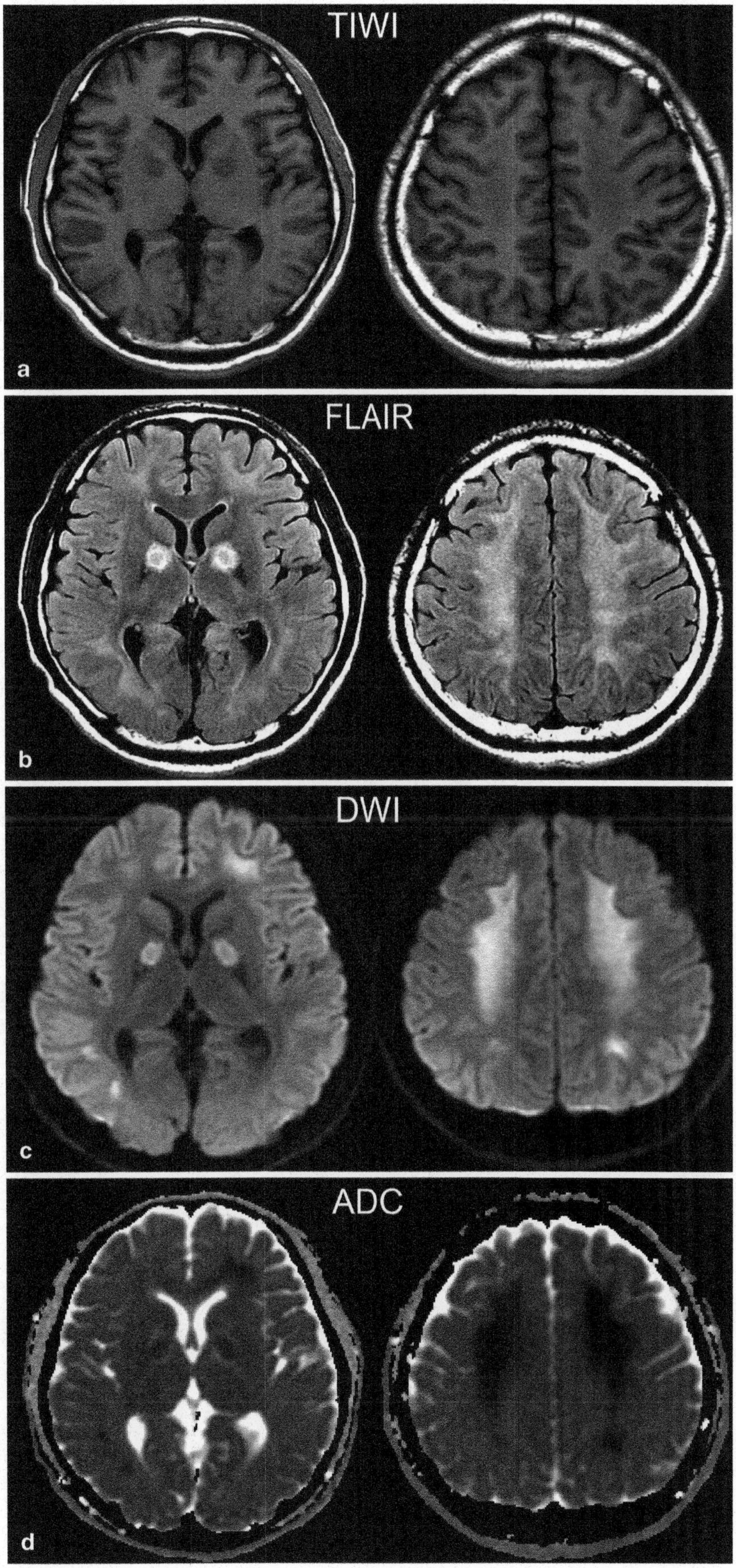

Fig. 5.52 M/22, CO poisoning. The patient committed suicide by burning charcoal in a closed room and was found in a state of coma. In the emergency department, CT revealed no findings (not shown). Laboratory data showed CoHb of 36.6%. MRI was performed on the third day. (**a–d**) MRI: The bilateral globus pallidus and centrum semiovale show mild hypointensity on T1WI, hyperintensity on FLAIR, hyperintensity on DWI, and hypointensity on ADC, indicating diffusion restriction, all are cytotoxic edemas. In ADC, a thin-rim hyperintensity is seen in the bilateral globus pallidus; this is vasogenic edema. The above features are typical of CO poisoning damage to the brain

5.16 Moyamoya Disease

Moyamoya disease was first proposed by the Japanese in 1957. As the distal portion of the internal carotid artery is stenotic and occluded, which creates many smoke-like small collateral circulation vessels in the brain, the Japanese word "moyamoya" for smoke is used as the name of the disease.

This disease is common in Asians. Children are more susceptible than adults. The distal portions of bilateral ICAs are stenotic and occluded. The blood flow cannot reach MCA and ACA, resulting in the collateral circulation of many moyamoya vessels. The collateral circulation also comes from the external carotid artery. In addition to the stenosis of distal ICA, the proximal portions of MCA, ACA, and PCA and the distal portion of basilar artery may have stenosis [45].

Clinical symptoms include headache, TIA, weakness of hands and feet, paralysis, visual field defects, syncope, personality changes, and epilepsy.

Moyamoya disease in adults often presents intracerebral hemorrhage (ICH) and intraventricular hemorrhage (IVH) (Fig. 5.53). In children, this disease is mostly characterized by ischemic stroke (Fig. 5.54).

CT: In case of stroke, CT can reveal typical cerebral edema of infarction, ICH, or IVH. CT with an injection of contrast medium can show blurred MCA, ACA, and ICA, with smoky enhancement on the periphery of MCA.

MRI: New and old infarcts can be revealed. Many fine collateral circulations are visible on FLAIR and contrast T1WI. Numerous small blood vessels occur in the cisterns and sulci, similar to the ivy climbing on the stone, which is called "ivy sign."

DSA: DSA can clearly show the stenosis and occlusion at the distal portion of ICA, the smoky collateral circulations (Figs. 5.53 and 5.54), and the collateral circulation from ECA.

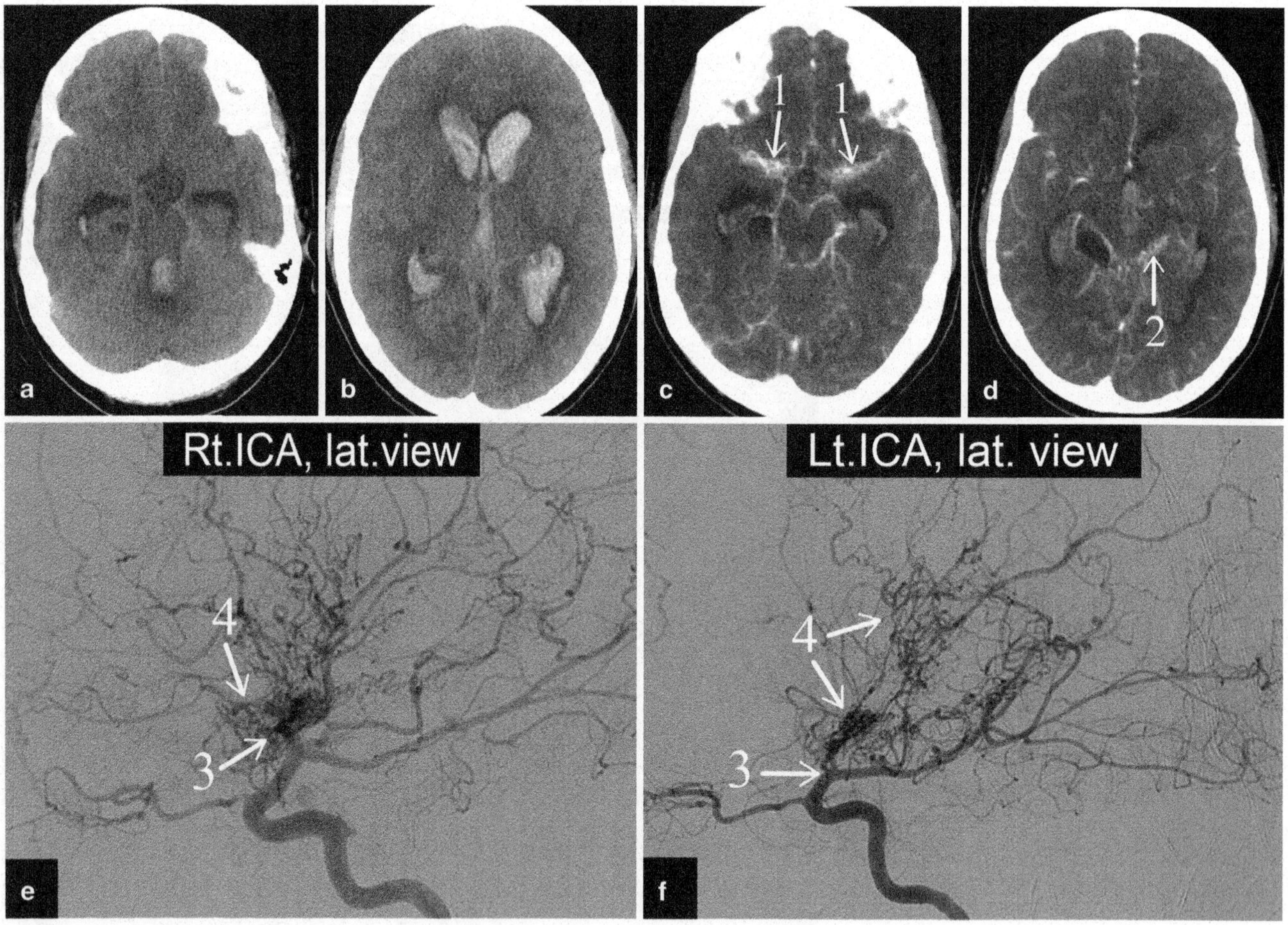

Fig. 5.53 F/32, Intraventricular hemorrhage (IVH) due to moyamoya disease. The patient suffered a sudden onset of severe headache and then lost consciousness. (**a**, **b**) CT: Massive amount of IVH and mild hydrocephalus with dilatation of bilateral temporal horns. (**c**, **d**) Contrast CT: Smokey enhancement around the bilateral MCAs (1) and abnormal enhancement in the left ambient cistern (2). The above findings possibly indicate moyamoya disease. (**e**, **f**) DSA, lateral view: Total occlusion of the distal portions of bilateral ICAs (3) and with "puff of smoke" appearance of collateral circulation (4)

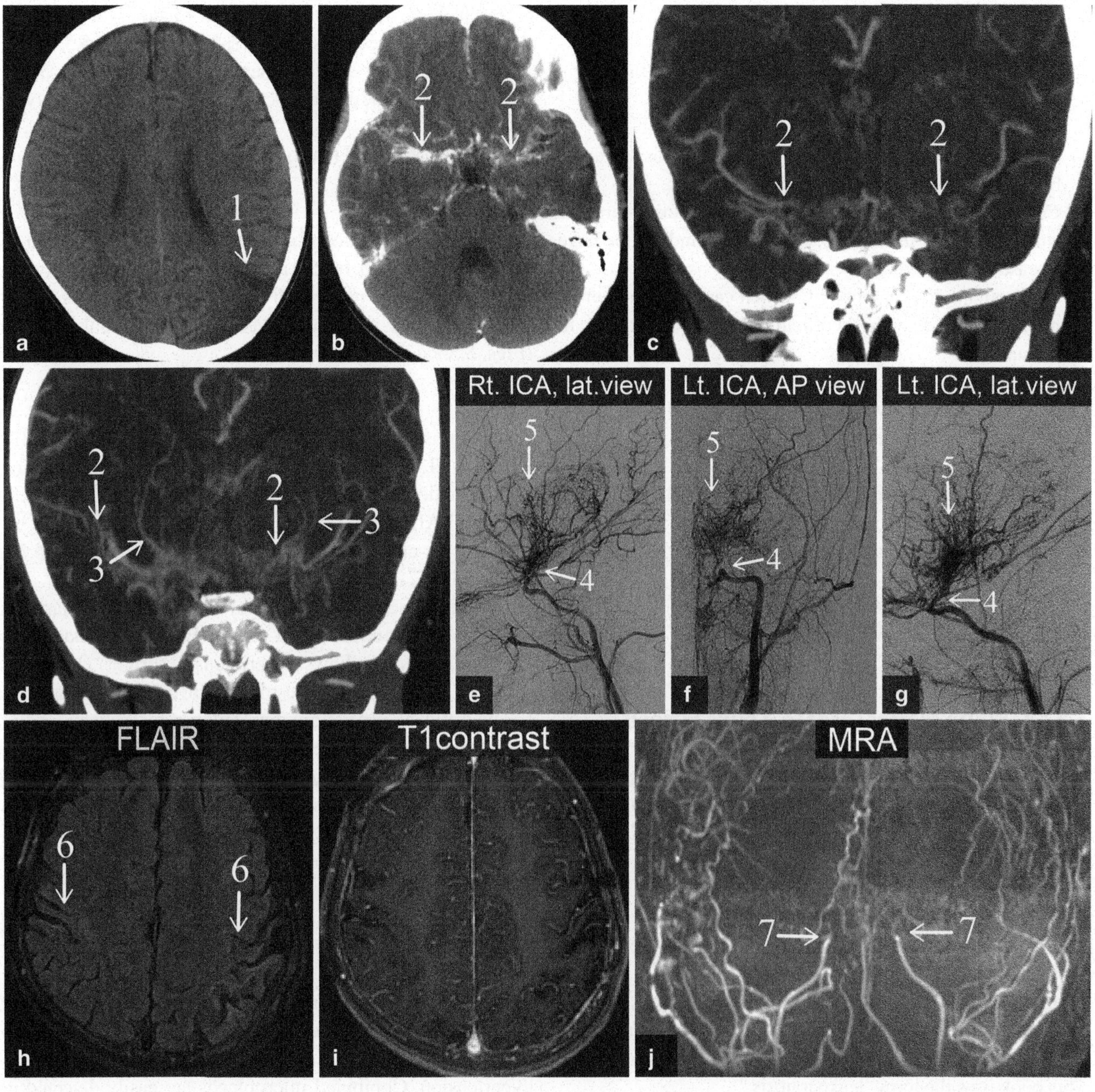

Fig. 5.54 F/9, Moyamoya disease. The patient suffered from left limb weakness three times; the symptom disappeared after several hours. A transient ischemic attack (TIA) was considered, and CT was performed. (**a**): CT: A small old infarction (1) is seen in the left parietal lobe. (**b–d**) Contrast CT: Bilateral MCAs are opacified but not clear, with smoky enhancement around the bilateral MCAs (2). The lenticulostriate arteries in the bilateral basal ganglia are dilated and visible (3). (**e**) Right carotid angiogram and (**f, g**) left carotid angiogram: Stenosis and occlusion are seen in the distal portions of bilateral ICAs (4), with "puff of smoke" appearance of collateral circulations (5). A follow-up MRI was performed after 1 year and 2 months. (**h**) FLAIR: Two small areas of old infarctions (6) are seen in the bilateral parietal lobes. (**i**) Contrast T1WI: Linear leptomeningeal enhancement is seen in the sulci of bilateral frontoparietal lobes; this is the "ivy sign." (**j**) MRA: Occlusion in the distal portions (7) of the bilateral internal carotid arteries. No opacification of the bilateral MCAs is observed. Many collateral circulations are built from the bilateral ECAs

5.17 Small Vessel Diseases

Three significant changes occur in degenerative intracerebral vessel disorders with increasing age [46, 47]:

1. Small vessel diseases, which cause leukoaraiosis, microbleeds, and dilated perivascular spaces.
2. Cerebral vascular atherosclerosis, which causes large or small or lacunar infarctions, even rupture and hemorrhage in case of hypertension (Chap. 4).
3. Cerebral amyloid angiopathy, which causes intracerebral microbleed and cerebral cortical hemorrhage in the brain (Chap. 4).

In MRI, compared with the pathology, small vessel diseases present three patterns [48]:

1. White matter hyperintensities, which are leukoaraiosis.
2. Lacunes, ranging from 3 to 15 mm and containing water in MRI, including old lacunar infarcts (Figs. 5.59 and 5.61), old small hemorrhage (microbleed) (Fig. 5.58), and dilated perivascular space.
3. Microbleeds (Figs. 5.58 and 5.60).

5.17.1 White Matter Disease (Leukoaraiosis)

In interpreting the routine CT and MRI of the adult brain, the white matter often shows abnormal density, which is mild hypodense on CT and hyperintensity on MRI T2WI and FLAIR. The incidence increases with age. White matter disease was reported in the nineteenth century by Binswanger and Alzheimer and was considered to be a small vessel disease in the brain [49]. On CT and MRI, this disease can often be identified in living people. On CT, it is called periventricular lucency (PVL). On MRI, it has many terms, such as leukoaraiosis, unknown bright object (UBO), periventricular hyperintensity (PVH), and white matter hyperintensity (WMH). This book uses the term "leukoaraiosis."

5.17.1.1 Pathology

The pathogenesis of leukoaraiosis caused by small vessel disease is vascular endothelial changes and stenosis due to hypertension and atherosclerosis of the small blood vessels, which reduces the blood flow and leads to brain tissue ischemia and cerebral vascular barrier (BBB) breakdown. Therefore, the toxic substances of the plasma component flow into the brain tissue, resulting in leukoaraiosis. The lacunar infarct is also caused by the occlusion of small perforating vessels, which often coexist [46, 50–52].

Leukoaraiosis occur in two types:

1. Periventricular leukoaraiosis (Figs. 5.11, 5.37, 5.42, 5.56, 5.57, 5.59, 5.60, and 5.61).
2. Deep white matter leukoaraiosis, which is divided into individual leukoaraiosis (Figs. 5.31, 5.33, 5.35, 5.55, 5.56, 5.59, and 5.61) and confluent leukoaraiosis (Fig. 5.57), wherein even the entire subcortical white matter is involved.

5.17.1.2 Medical Imaging

CT

CT shows leukoaraiosis around the ventricles, which is called PVL (Figs. 5.10, 5.37, 5.56, and 5.57). For leukoaraiosis of deep white matter, CT can only detect confluent leukoaraiosis (Fig. 5.57) or severe individual leukoaraiosis (Figs. 5.55 and 5.56) [49].

MRI

Leukoaraiosis shows hyperintensity on T2WI and FLAIR. Notably, FLAIR has attenuated the CSF signal, allowing easy detection of leukoaraiosis. Even a small lesion is definite on FLAIR.

The PVL on CT is called PVH on MRI (Figs. 5.11, 5.37, 5.56, and 5.57).

The difference between leukoaraiosis and acute infarction must be assessed based on DWI (Figs. 5.42 and 5.56). Because DWI only shows hyperintensity (bright) in the area of acute infarction with restricted diffusion, leukoaraiosis has no diffusion restriction; thus, leukoaraiosis shows no signal change on DWI, which can be used to rule out acute infarction. However, small chronic infarction is difficult to distinguish. MRI can also distinguish very old infarction in which cavitary change occurs (Figs. 5.3 and 5.60), but leukoaraiosis never has cavitary change.

5.17.2 Microbleeds

The incidence of cerebral microbleeds in the elderly can reach 11.1–23.5%. It is a type of small blood vessel disease in the brain and often occurs in patients with uncontrollable hypertension. Combined microbleeds are easily detected in patients with hypertensive hemorrhagic stroke [53].

Microbleeds include two types of vascular diseases [54]:

1. Hypertensive vasculopathy, which is caused by hypertensive lipohyalinotic changes. Such microbleeds are mostly located in the basal ganglia, thalamus, brain stem, and cerebellum (Figs. 5.57, 5.58, and 5.60).
2. Amyloid angiopathy, which occurs mostly in the cerebral cortex, is also prone to hemorrhage, thus resulting in real hemorrhagic stroke (Figs. 4.24 and 4.25).

Microbleeds are not easy to detect on CT. MRI T2*WI (T2*gradient echo GRE) and susceptibility-weighted image (SWI, SWAN) are the best pulse sequences in diagnosing the microbleeds because they are sensitive to hemosiderin deposition (Figs. 4.24, 4.25, 5.57, 5.58, and 5.60).

5.17.3 Dilated Virchow–Robin Space

Dilated (or enlarged, widened) perivascular space (Virchow–Robin space) is also a type of small vessel disease. In CT, it is difficult to distinguish from old lacunar infarction but is easy to be distinguished in MRI. As this dilated perivascular space contains CSF, the signal changes are consistent with CSF (Figs. 5.59 and 5.60) [55].

5.17.4 CADASIL

Cerebral autosomal dominant arteriopathy with subcortical infarcts and leukoencephalopathy (CADASIL) is a small intracranial vascular disorder caused by abnormal mutations in a single chromosome (NOTCH3) [56, 57]. It occurs mostly in the age of 40–50 years and poses no risks of hypertension, diabetes, high blood lipids, and other factors. However, it is often accompanied by minor stroke and gradual intelligence and memory decline and has a family disease history.

CADASIL presents three common cerebral small vessel diseases in MRI: (1) white matter hyperintensities (leukoaraiosis), especially in the white matter of anterior temporal lobe, which is a unique sign; (2) lacunar infarcts; and (3) microbleeds (Fig. 5.61) [58].

White matter hyperintensities can also be found in the periventricular brain tissue, deep white matter, and brain stem.

On the basis of clinical symptoms and imaging, many CADASIL patients have been previously misdiagnosed with multiple sclerosis or other neurodegenerative diseases. A skin biopsy can be made to confirm genetic mutations. A combination with MRI findings can confirm the diagnosis.

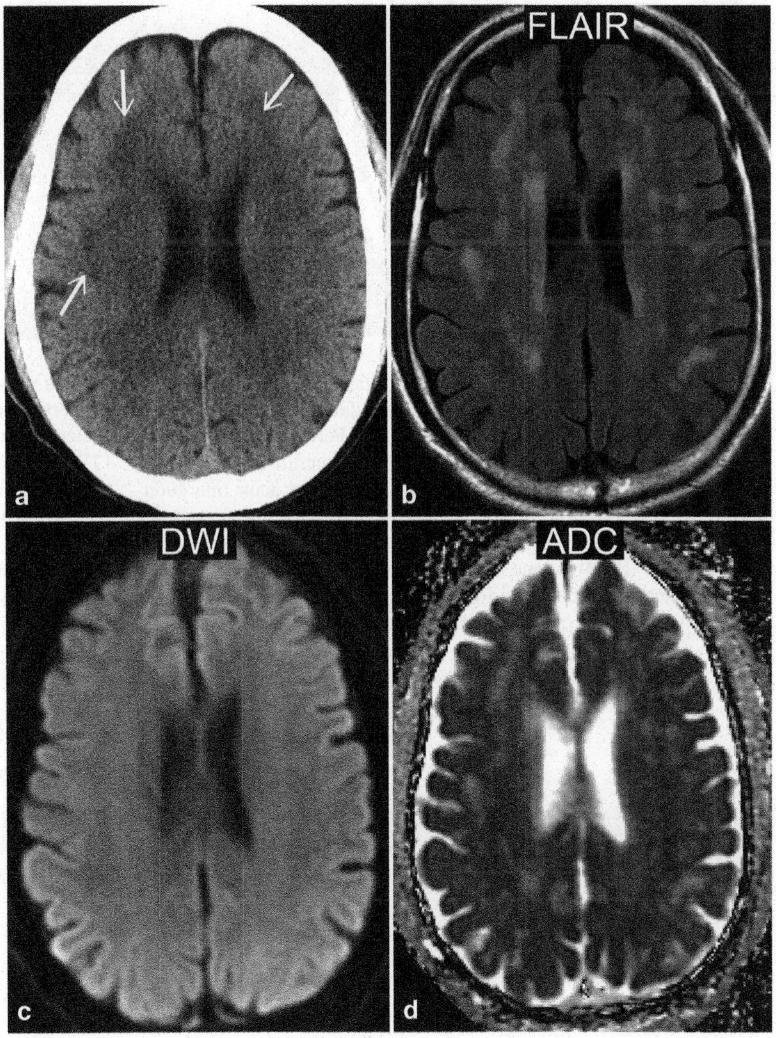

Fig. 5.55 M/67, Leukoaraiosis. (**a**) CT: Several areas of mild hypodensity are seen in the bilateral centrum semiovale; these findings are indicative of white matter disease, that is, leukoaraiosis. But CT cannot clearly and accurately detect leukoaraiosis. (**b**) MRI, FLAIR: Many hyperintense lesions are observed in the bilateral centrum semiovale; all are leukoaraiosis, and every lesion is apparent and distinct. FLAIR is the best pulse sequence to show leukoaraiosis. (**c**) DWI: The leukoaraiosis shows no diffusion restriction; thus, no signal change is seen on DWI. (**d**) ADC: The ADC value of leukoaraiosis is high, indicating hyperintensity on the ADC map

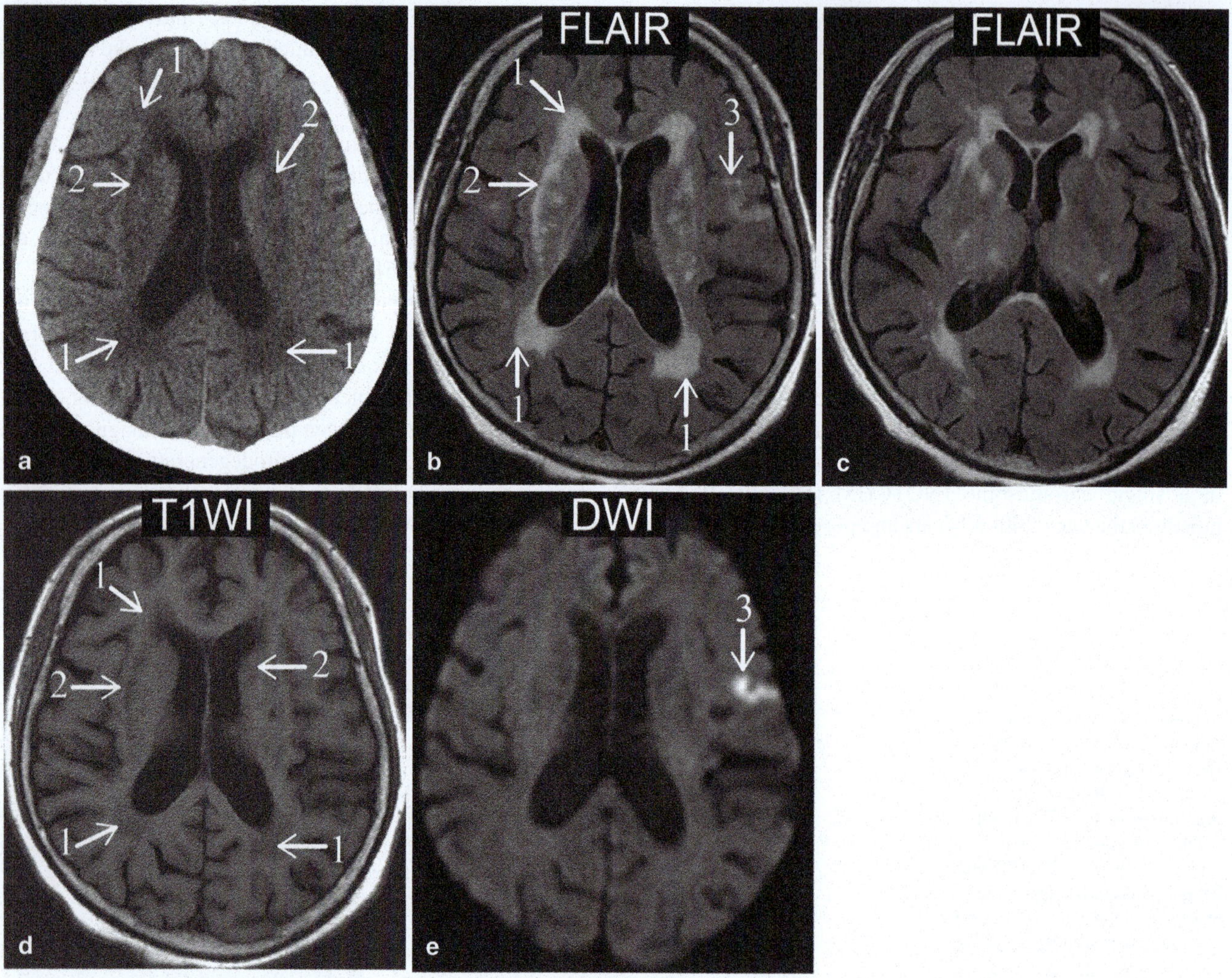

Fig. 5.56 F/87, Leukoaraiosis, and acute infarction. The patient with hypertension and atrial fibrillation suffered a sudden onset of right hemiparesis. Emergency CT was conducted. (**a**) CT: Periventricular lucency (PVL) (1) and decreased density in the bilateral centrum semiovale (2) are seen; these are suspected leukoaraiosis, but whether acute infarction edema is present within the left centrum semiovale remains unclear. MRI was conducted on the second day. (**b**) MRI, FLAIR: Periventricular hyperintensity (PVH) (1) and multiple hyperintense lesions (2) are seen in the bilateral centrum semiovale; these are leukoaraiosis. A small hyperintense lesion is observed in the cortex (3) of the left frontal lobe; this is a possible acute infarction because leukoaraiosis is not found in the cortex. (**c**) FLAIR: Multiple hyperintense spots are present in the bilateral basal ganglia, which are also indicative of leukoaraiosis. (**d**) T1WI: all the PVH and punctate leukoaraiosis show mild hypointensity on T1WI. (**e**) DWI: Only the lesion in the cortex of the left frontal lobe is hyperintense (3), representing diffusion restriction; this is acute cytotoxic edema due to acute infarction. The other lesions, including PVH and hyperintense lesions in the centrum semiovale and basal ganglia, exhibit no signal change on DWI; these are leukoaraiosis

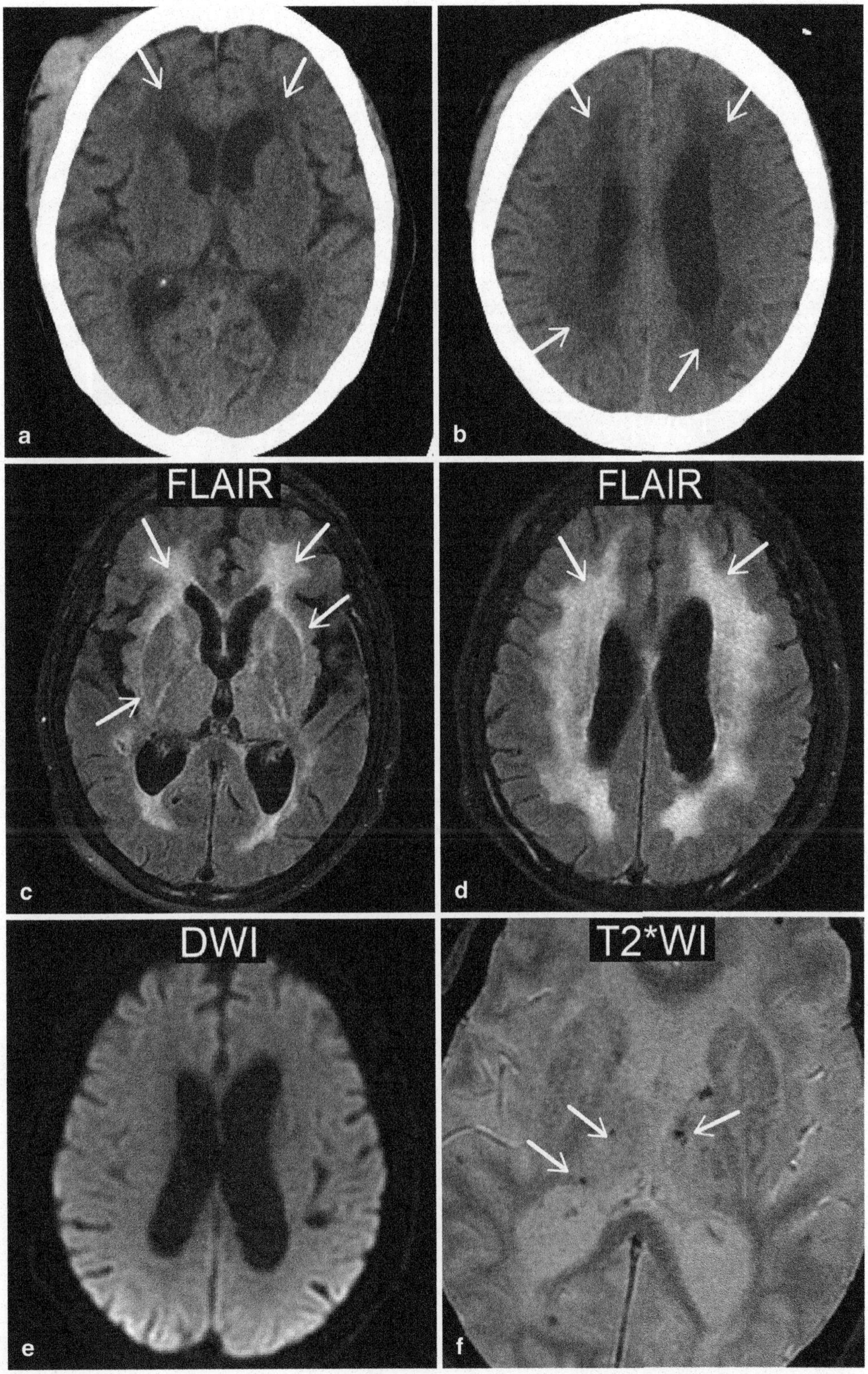

Fig. 5.57 M/77, Diffused leukoaraiosis, and microbleeds. A dementia patient who hit his head after a fall. (**a**, **b**) CT: In addition to scalp swelling, periventricular lucency (PVL) and hypodensity of the white matter are unexpectedly seen in the bilateral centrum semiovale, which are indicative of severe leukoaraiosis (arrows). MRI was conducted on the second day. (**c**, **d**) MRI, FLAIR: The periventricular white matter, centrum semiovale, and even internal and external capsules are hyperintense (arrows), showing diffuse periventricular hyperintensity (PVH), actually this is a confluent type of leukoaraiosis. (**e**) DWI: All the above hyperintensity on FLAIR shows no signal change on DWI because of the absence of diffusion restriction. (**f**) T2*WI: Several microbleeds are seen in the bilateral thalami (arrows)

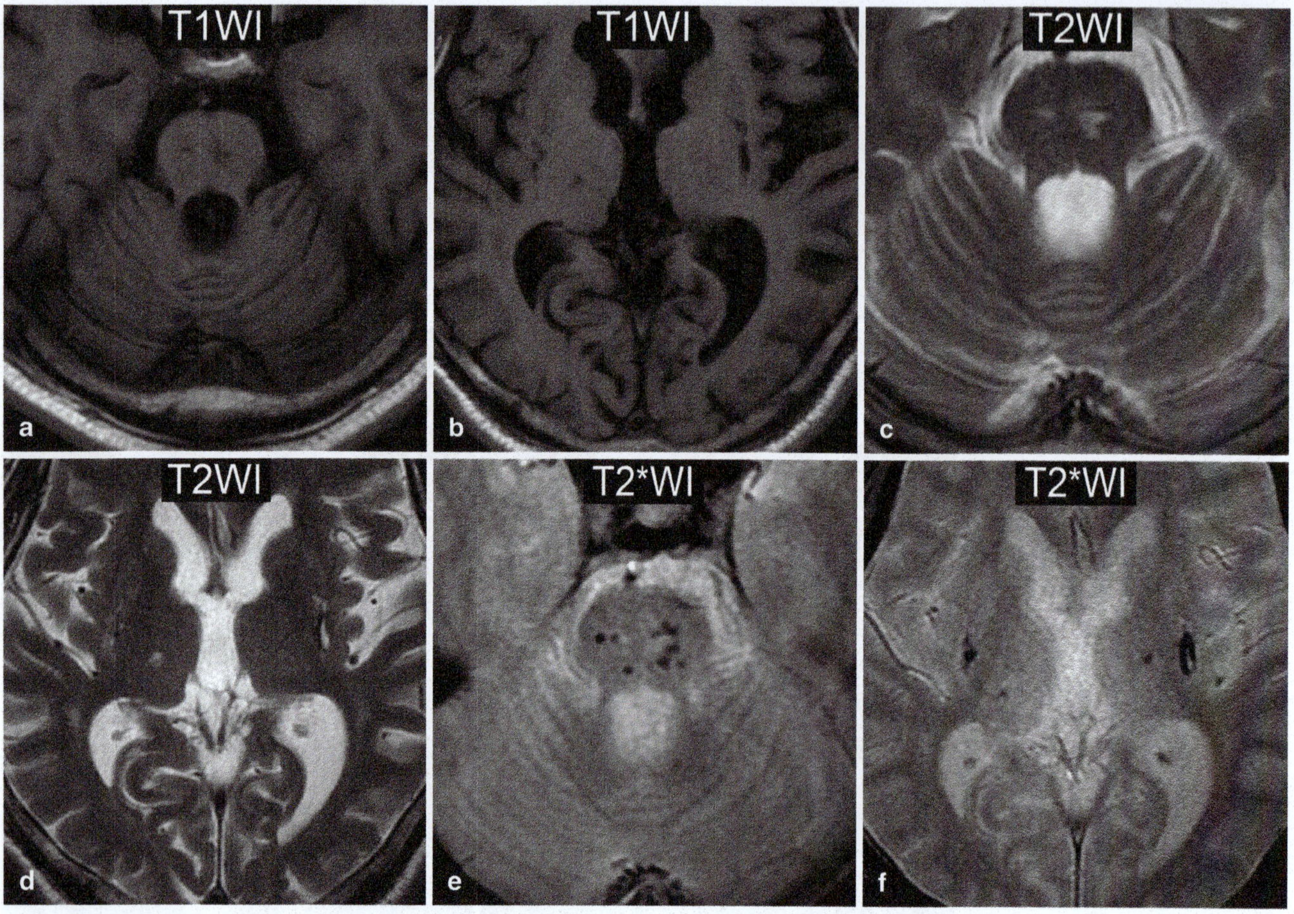

Fig. 5.58 M/66, Microbleeds, and lacunes. The patient with diabetes and hypertension experienced several transient ischemic attacks (TIAs). (**a–d**) MRI, T1WI, and T2WI: T1WI shows that multiple small hypointense spots are present in the pons and bilateral basal ganglia. These lesions are hyperintense on T2WI, appearing white as CSF; these are small cavities, which are called "lacunes." (**e, f**) T2*WI: Some of the above lacunes have hemosiderin depositions, which are known as microbleeds. More microbleeds are detected in the pons, which are showed only on T2*WI

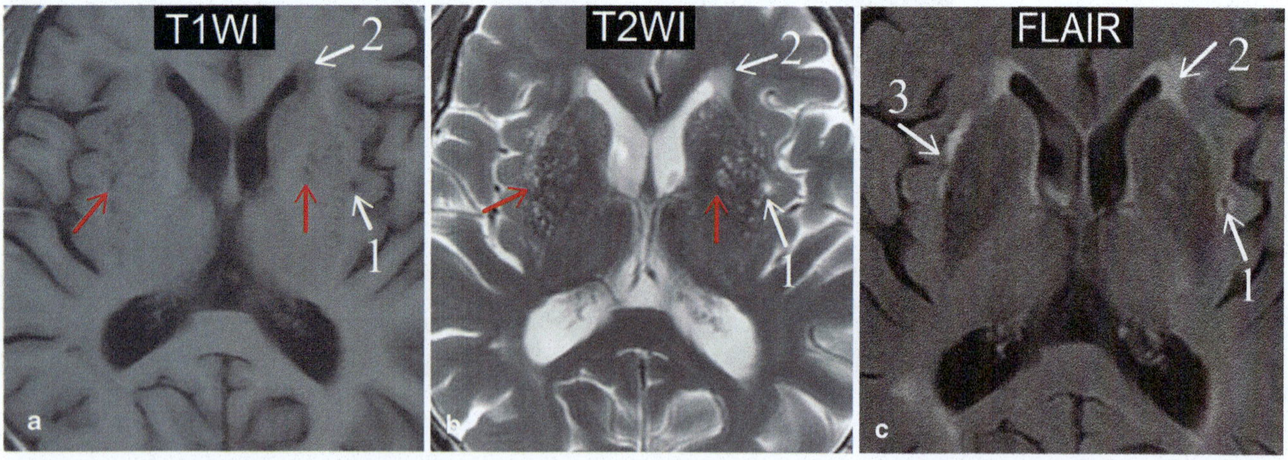

Fig. 5.59 M/70, Dilated Virchow–Robin Space. No specific clinical symptoms. MRI was performed for a healthy examination. (**a**) T1WI: Many tiny cavities (red arrows) are seen in the bilateral lentiform nuclei. The one beside the left putamen is possibly an old lacunar infarction (1). Mild hypointensity of the periventricular white matter (2) indicates leukoaraiosis. (**b**) T2WI: Numerous tiny hyperintense spots (red arrows) are observed in the bilateral lentiform nuclei. They are white as CSF in the ventricles, appearing as "état criblé." These are typical dilated perivascular spaces or Virchow–Robin spaces. (**c**) FLAIR: The content of the dilated perivascular space is CSF and thus attenuated as CSF, which is difficult to be recognized on FLAIR. A small lacune (1) is detected beside the left putamen; the periphery has a circle of gliosis, indicative of old lacunar infarction. Periventricular hyperintensity (PVH) (2) is observed, which is indicative of leukoaraiosis. A linear hyperintensity (3) beside the right putamen is also observed, which is also indicative of leukoaraiosis

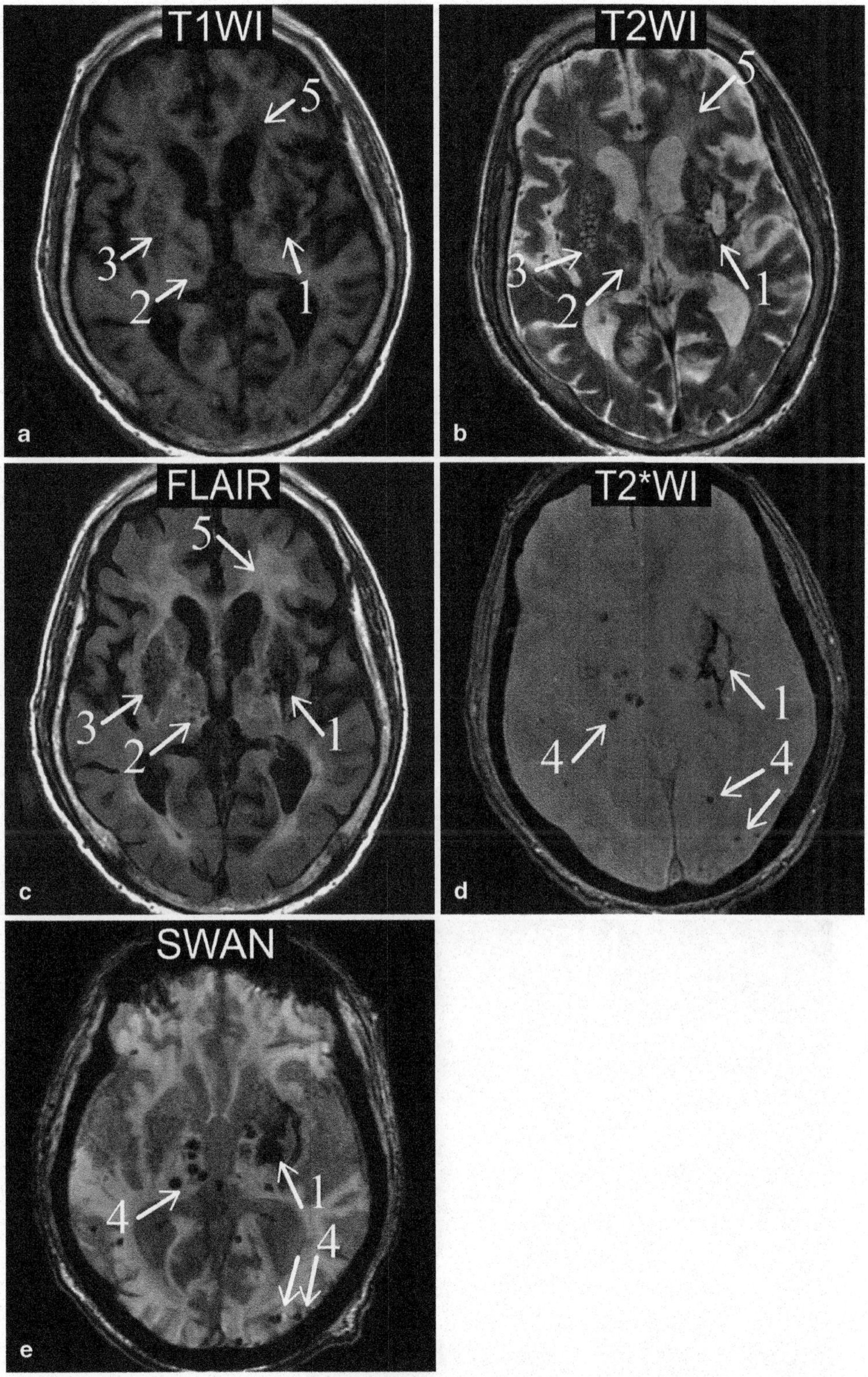

Fig. 5.60 M/78, Old ICH, microbleeds, dilated Virchow–Robin spaces, and leukoaraiosis. The patient has hypertension, diabetes, and history of hypertensive stroke with hemorrhage on the left side of the brain that occurred 25 years ago. (**a**–**e**) MRI: A cavitary lesion (1) is seen in the left putamen, showing hypointensity on T1WI and FLAIR and hyperintensity on T2WI, T2*WI, and SWAN. Hemosiderin deposition is observed in the periphery of this cavity shown on T2*WI and SWAN. This is a sequela of previous intracerebral hematoma (ICH), which is the hypertensive stroke that occurred 25 years ago. Several old lacunar infarctions (2) in the bilateral thalami exhibit hypointensity on T1WI and hyperintensity on T2WI and FLAIR. Many tiny cavities (3) are found in the bilateral putamina; these are état criblé, which are dilated Virchow–Robin spaces. On T2*W and SWAN, many microbleeds (4) are observed in the bilateral thalami and left occipital lobe. On T2WI and FLAIR, periventricular hyperintensity (PVH) (5) is seen, which is hypointense on T1WI. This finding indicates leukoaraiosis

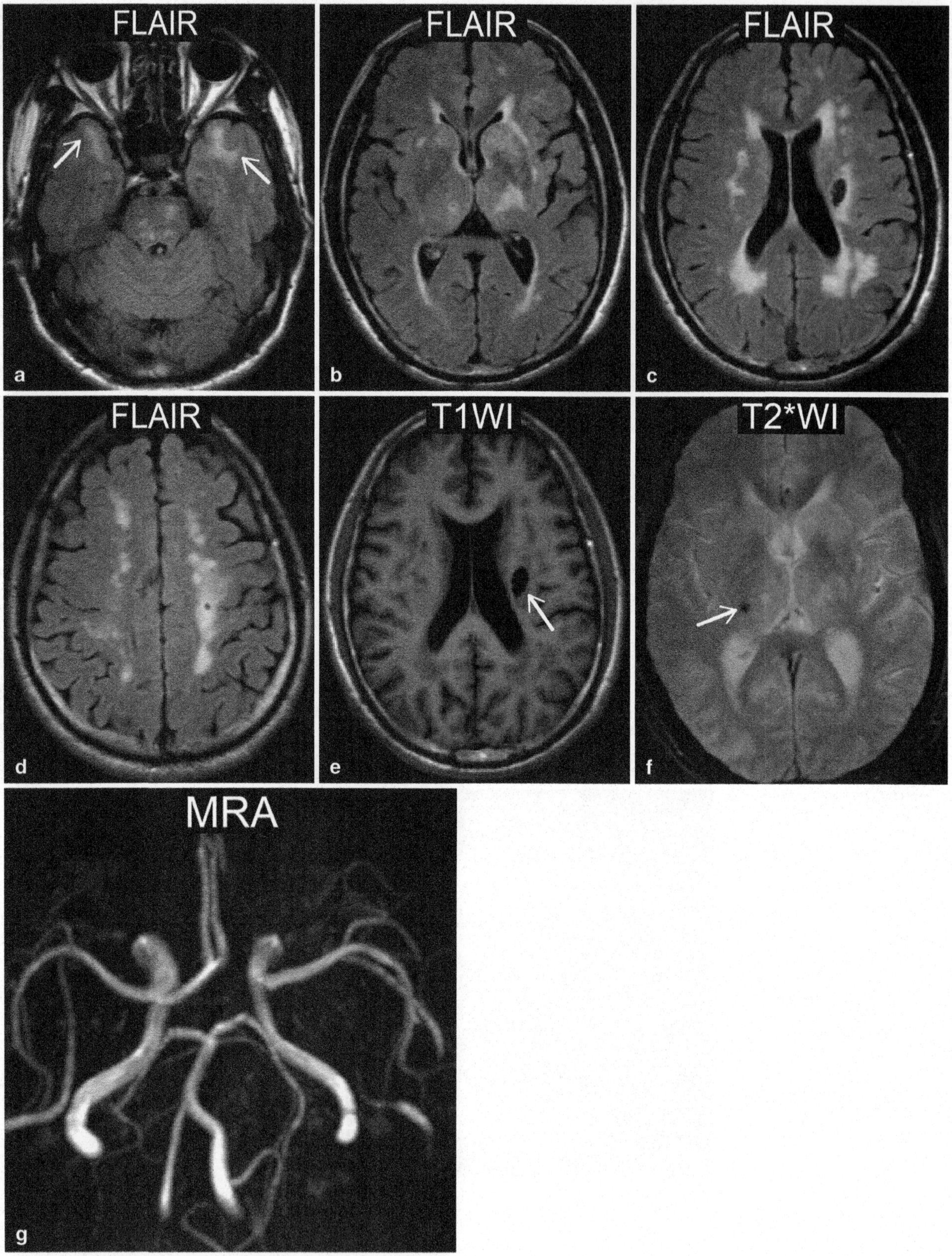

Fig. 5.61 M/50, CADASIL. The patient's mother, brother, and sister have histories of stroke. In recent years, the patient reported unsteady gait, memory decline, urinary incontinence, and right limb weakness. The patient has no hypertension and no diabetes. (**a–d**) MRI, FLAIR: Many hyperintense lesions are seen in the subcortical white matter, including pons and thalamus. These lesions exhibit no signal change on DWI (not shown); all are leukoaraiosis. Leukoaraiosis in the temporal lobe (arrows in **a**) is especially specific for CADASIL. (**e**) T1WI: A 1.5 cm lacune (arrow) in the left corona radiata. (**f**) T2*WI: A microbleed (arrow) in the right thalamus. (**g**) MRA: No abnormality of the great vessels. From the above imaging findings and clinical presentation, CADASIL should be considered for middle-aged people with small vessel diseases, especially leukoaraiosis in the temporal lobe

References

1. Smith WS, et al. Cerebrovascular diseases. In: Harrison's principle of internal medicine. 18th ed. New York: McGraw-Hill; 2012. p. 3275.
2. Allen LM, et al. Sequence-specific MR imaging findings that are useful in dating ischemic stroke. Radiographics. 2012;32:1285–97.
3. Shen JM, et al. The use of MRI apparent diffusion coefficient (ADC) in monitoring the development of brain infarction. BMC Med Imaging. 2011;11:1–4.
4. Truwit CL, et al. Loss of the insular ribbon: another early CT sign of acute middle cerebral artery infarction. Radiology. 1990;176:801–6.
5. Tomura N, et al. Early CT finding in cerebral infarction: obscuration of the lentiform nucleus. Radiology. 1988;168:463–7.
6. Moulin T, et al. Early CT signs in acute middle cerebral artery infarction: predictive value for subsequent infarct locations and outcome. Neurology. 1996;47:366–75.
7. Pressman BD, et al. An early sign of ischemic infarction: increased density in a cerebral artery. AJNR. 1987;8:645–8.
8. Schuierer G, Huk W. The unilateral hyperdense middle cerebral artery: an early CT-sign of embolism or thrombosis. Neuroradiology. 1988;30:120–2.
9. Von Kummer R, et al. Early prediction of irreversible brain damage after ischemic stroke at CT. Radiology. 2001;219:95–100.
10. Treadwell SD, Thanvi B. Malignant middle cerebral artery (MCA) infarction: pathophysiology, diagnosis and management. Postgrad Med J. 2010;86:235–42.
11. Jaillard A, et al. Hemorrhagic transformation in acute ischemic stroke. The MAST-E Study. MAST-E Group. Stroke. 1999;30:1326–32.
12. Arboix A, et al. Malignant middle cerebral artery infarction: a clinical study of 32 patients. Rev Investig Clin. 2015;67:64–70.
13. Bladin PF, Berkovic SF. Striatocapsular infarction: large infarcts in the lenticulostriate arterial territory. Neurology. 1984;34:1423–30.
14. Donnan GA, et al. The stroke syndrome of striatocapsular infarction. Brain. 1991;114:51–70.
15. Kumral E, et al. Spectrum of anterior cerebral artery territory infarction: clinical and MRI findings. Eur J Neurol. 2002;9:615–24.
16. Merwick Á, Werring D. Posterior circulation ischaemic stroke. BMJ. 2014;348:28–34.
17. Tohgi H, et al. Cerebellar infarction, clinical and neuroimaging analysis in 293 patients. Stroke. 1993;24:1697–701.
18. Ortiz de Mendivil A, et al. Brainstem stroke: anatomy, clinical and radiological findings. Semin Ultrasound CT MRI. 2013;34:131–41.
19. Kumral E, et al. Clinical spectrum of pontine infarction, clinical-MRI correlation. J Neurol. 2002;249:1659–70.
20. Benders P, et al. Central pontine myelinolysis: case report and short overview. Neth J Crit Care. 2017;25:129–32.
21. Kim JS, Kim J. Pure midbrain infarction, clinical, radiologic and pathophysiologic findings. Neurology. 2005;64:1227–32.
22. Mangla R, et al. Border zone infarcts: pathophysiologic and imaging characteristics. Radiographics. 2011;31:1201–14.
23. Wong KS, et al. Mechanisms of acute cerebral infarctions in patients with middle cerebral artery stenosis: a diffusion-weighted imaging and microemboli monitoring study. Ann Neurol. 2002;52:74–81.
24. Derdeyn CP, et al. Severe hemodynamic impairment and border zone-region infarction. Radiology. 2001;220:195–201.
25. Kim DE, et al. Association of internal border zone infarction with middle cerebral artery steno-occlusion. Eur Neurol. 2010;64:178–85.
26. Moustafa RR, et al. Microembolism versus hemodynamic impairment in rosary-like deep watershed infarcts: a combined positron emission tomography and transcranial Doppler study. Stroke. 2011;42:3138–43.
27. Fisher GM. Lacunes. Small, deep cerebral infarcts. Neurology. 1965;15:774–84.
28. Fisher GM. Lacunar strokes and infarcts: a review. Neurology. 1982;32:871–6.
29. Gerraty RP, et al. Examining the lacunar hypothesis with diffusion and perfusion magnetic resonance imaging. Stroke. 2002;33:2019–24.
30. Schonewille WJ, et al. Diffusion-weighted MRI in acute lacunar syndromes: a clinical-radiological correlation study. Stroke. 1999;30:2066–9.
31. Gonzalez RG. Imaging-guided acute ischemic stroke therapy: from "time is brain" to "physiology is brain". AJNR Am J Neuroradiol. 2006;27:728–35.
32. Campbell BC, et al. Cerebral blood flow is the optimal CT perfusion parameter for assessing infarct core. Stroke. 2011;42:3435–40.
33. de Lucas EM, et al. CT protocol for acute stroke: tips and tricks for general radiologist. Radiographics. 2008;28:1673–87.
34. Wing SC, Markus HS. Interpreting CT perfusion in stroke. Pract Neurol. 2019;190:136–42.
35. Albers GW, et al. Thrombectomy for stroke at 6 to 16 hours with selection by perfusion imaging. N Engl J Med. 2018;378:708–18.
36. Bivard A, et al. Perfusion computer tomography: imaging and clinical validation in acute ischemic stroke. Brain. 2011;134:3408–16.
37. Rudilosso S, et al. Perfusion deficits and mismatch in patients with acute lacunar infarcts studied with whole-brain CT perfusion. AJNR Am J Neuroradiol. 2015;36:1407–12.
38. Muttikkal TJ, Wintermark M. MRI pattern of global hypoxic-ischemic injury in adults. J Neuroradiol. 2013;40:164–71.
39. Arbelaez A, et al. Diffusion-weighted MR imaging of global cerebral anoxia. AJNR Am J Neuroradiol. 1999;20:999–1007.
40. Lee EJ. The empty delta sign. Radiology. 2002;224:788–9.
41. Lovblad K-O, et al. Diffusion-weighted MR in cerebral venous thrombosis. Cerebrovasc Dis. 2001;11:169–76.
42. Wasay M, et al. Diffusion-weighted magnetic resonance imaging in superior sagittal sinus thrombosis. J Neuroimaging. 2002;12(3):267–9.
43. Varrassi M, et al. Advanced neuroimaging of carbon monoxide poisoning. Neuroradiol J. 2017;30:461–9.
44. Kim DM, et al. Acute carbon monoxide poisoning: MR imaging findings with clinical correlation. Diagn Interv Imaging. 2017;98:299–306.
45. Scott RM, Smith ER. Moyamoya disease and moyamoya syndrome. N Engl J Med. 2009;360:1226–37.
46. Grinberg LT, Thal DR. Vascular pathology in the aged human brain. Acta Neuropathol. 2010;119:277–90.
47. Lammie GA. Hypertensive cerebral small vessel disease and stroke. Brain Pathol. 2002;12:358–70.
48. Gouw AA, et al. Heterogeneity of small vessels disease: a systematic review of MRI and histopathology correlations. J Neurol Neurosurg Psychiatry. 2011;82:126–35.
49. Grueter BE, Schulz UG. Age-related cerebral white matter disease (leukoaraiosis), a review. Postgrad Med J. 2012;88:79–87.
50. Pantoni L, Garcia JH. Pathogenesis of leukoaraiosis: a review. Stroke. 1997;28:652–9.
51. Fazekas F, et al. Pathologic correlates of incidental MRI white matter signal hyperintensities. Neurology. 1993;43:1683–9.
52. Wardlaw JM, et al. Mechanisms of sporadic cerebral small vessel disease: insights from neuroimaging. Lancet Neurol. 2013;12:483–97.
53. Roob G, et al. Frequency and location of microbleeds in patients with primary intracerebral hemorrhage. Stroke. 2000;31:2665–9.

54. Greenberg SM, et al. Cerebral microbleeds: a guide to detection and interpretation. Lancet Neurol. 2009;8:165–74.
55. Barkohof F. Enlarged Virchow-Robing spaces: do they matter? J Neurol Neursurg Psychy. 2004;75:1516–7.
56. Joutel A, et al. Notch3 mutation in CADASIL, a hereditary adult-onset condition causing stroke and dementia. Nature. 1996;383:707–10.
57. Chen YC. Cerebral autosomal dominant arteriopathy with subcortical infarcts and leukoencephalopathy. Acta Neurol Taiwanica. 2014;23:64–74.
58. Stojanov D, et al. Imaging characteristics of cerebral autosomal dominant arteriopathy with subcortical infarcts and leukoencephalopathy (CADASIL). Bosn J Basic Med Sci. 2015;15:1–8.

6 Medical Imaging of Intracranial Tumors

Abstract

The intracranial tumors can be divided into three categories according to the location of tumor growth: (1) Intra-axial tumors, including astrocytic tumors, medulloblastoma, lymphomas, hemangioma, and metastasis. (2) Intraventricular tumors, tumors arising from the ventricular wall, such as ependymoma, tumor arising from choroid plexus, such as papilloma and meningioma. (3) Extra-axial tumors, such as meningioma, pituitary adenoma, and schwannoma. The names of the intracranial tumors using 2016 WHO CNS tumor classification. The diagnosis of intracranial tumors is mainly based on CT and MRI imaging features. Some tumors have specific anatomical locations, and some tumors have specific clinical symptoms. New MRI technologies such as DWI and ADC, and the use of MRS, provide valuable assistance in the diagnosis of CNS tumors. Based on the above, 70–80% of the tumor diagnosis of intracranial tumors using CT and MRI can be consistent with surgery and pathology, and the other 20–30% need to wait for the pathological examination. Low-grade astrocytomas showed changes in the density and signal intensity of the brain tissue on CT and MRI; the BBB is not damaged, so the contrast agent does not enhance it. Glioblastoma is irregular in shape, severely central necrosis, cauliflower-like shape, and usually large of tumor size. Medulloblastoma is common in children; most of them grow in the cerebellar vermis, which will compress the fourth ventricle and aqueduct and cause hydrocephalus. Lymphoma is often multiple and less necrosis, with higher DWI signals and more elevated MRS lipids. Metastases may be intra-axial, extra-axial, or even in the skull, and some are leptomeningeal metastases. Hemangioblastomas may have a mural nodular sign; solid hemangioblastoma shows hypointensity on DWI due to high vascularity; this is a characteristic sign. Meningiomas are always solid; less cystic change and may have calcifications, hyperostosis of the adjacent skull, and "dural tail sign" seen in MRI. If the tumor has central necrosis and adjacent bone erosion, it is atypical or anaplastic meningioma. Pituitary adenomas are in the sella turcica, and may extend upward to compress the optic chiasm, and are very easy to diagnose using CT or MRI. But functional microadenoma needs coronal section and contrast enhancement to see the delayed enhancement at the microadenoma. The acoustic neuroma is the highest incidence of cranial nerve schwannomas. The tumor grows in the CP angle cistern and will extend into the internal auditory canal, to form a "fruit stalk sign." Germ cell tumors display a characteristic of growing in the midline, such as the pineal region and suprasellar region.

Intracranial tumors include central nervous system (CNS) tumors, which have numerous types of tumors. This chapter discusses only common clinical cases of intracranial tumors.

6.1 Classification of CNS Tumors

CNS tumors were first classified histologically by Bailey and Cushing in 1926. Their classification has been applied for almost a century. In 2016, the WHO classification of CNS tumors initiated the era of molecular medicine. Because of challenges in genetic and epigenetic development over the past 20 years, the most recent WHO classification of CNS tumors comprises the following three layers: the name of the disease, genetic alteration, and grading [1, 2].

From the perspective of imaging, the classification of tumor location facilitates diagnosis. Therefore, this chapter provides a self-defined classification of tumor location (Table 6.1).

1. Intra-axial tumors, which are tumors grown from or within the brain parenchyma.
2. Intraventricular tumors.
3. Extra-axial tumors, which are tumors grown outside the brain parenchyma.

W.-C. Shen, *Diagnostic Neuroradiology*, https://doi.org/10.1007/978-981-15-4051-6_6

Table 6.1 Classification of intracranial tumors based on the anatomical locations and 2016 WHO CNS tumor classification

Intra-axial tumors	Intraventricular tumors	Extra-axial tumors
Diffuse astrocytic and oligodendroglial tumors: Diffuse astrocytoma (Figs. 6.1–6.3) Anaplastic astrocytoma (Figs. 6.3 and 6.4) Glioblastoma (Figs. 6.5–6.8) Oligodendroglioma (Fig. 6.9) **Other astrocytic tumors:** Pilocytic astrocytoma (Fig. 6.10) Subependymal giant cell astrocytoma (Fig. 6.11) **Embryonal tumors:** Medulloblastoma (Figs. 6.12–6.14) **Primary CNS lymphomas** (Figs. 6.15 and 6.16) **Mesenchymal, non-meningothelial tumors:** Hemangioma (Figs. 6.17 and 6.18) Hemangioblastoma (Figs. 6.19–6.21) **Metastasis**[a] (Figs. 6.22– 6.29)	**Tumors of ventricular wall (ependymal tumors):** Subependymoma Ependymoma (Figs. 6.30 and 6.31) Subependymal giant cell astrocytoma (Fig. 6.11) **Tumor of the choroid plexus:** Choroid plexus papilloma (Figs. 6.33 and 6.34) and carcinoma. Choroid meningioma (Fig. 6.35) **Neuronal and mixed neuronal-glial tumors:** Central neurocytoma (Fig. 6.32)	**Tumor of meninges:** Meningioma (Figs. 6.36–6.47) **Mesenchymal, non-meningothelial tumors:** Hemangiopericytoma (Figs. 6.48 and 6.49) Intracranial lipoma (Figs. 6.76 and 6.77) **Tumors of sellar region:** Pituitary adenoma[b] (Figs. 6.50–6.57) Pituicytoma Craniopharyngioma (Figs. 6.58 and 6.59) Rathke's cleft cyst[b] (Fig. 6.60) **Tumors of cranial and paraspinal nerves** Schwannoma (Figs. 6.61–6.67) Neurofibroma (Fig. 6.66) **Tumors of the pineal region:** Pineocytoma/pineoblastoma (Fig. 6.71) **Germ cell tumors**[c] Germinoma (Figs. 6.68 and 6.69) Teratoma (Fig. 6.70) **Others:** Arachnoid cyst[b] (Figs. 6.72 and 6.73) Dermoid/epidermoid cyst[b] (Figs. 6.74 and 6.75) **Metastasis**[a] (Figs. 6.23 and 6.28) **Skull base tumors:** Chordoma[b] (Fig. 6.78)

[a]Metastases occur in intra-axial and extra-axial locations and even in the skull
[b]Pituitary adenoma, Rathke's cleft cyst, arachnoid cyst, dermoid/epidermoid cyst, and chordoma are not listed in 2016 WHO classification of CNS tumors
[c]Germ cell tumors develop in extra- and intra-axial locations

6.2 Diagnosis of CNS Tumors

The main examination tools for diagnosing intracranial tumors are CT with contrast and MRI, which includes T1WI, T2WI, FLAIR, DWI, MRS, and contrast enhancement. These tools are used to observe the anatomical location and appearance of tumors as the basis for diagnosis.

MRI provides images of the axial, sagittal, and coronal planes with excellent resolution. At the skull base, no artifacts exist, and most tumors are sensitive to gadolinium contrast medium in the MRI, thereby have better contrast enhancement. Therefore, in the diagnosis of intracranial tumors, MRI outperforms CT. However, CT is superior to MRI in certain situations. (1) CT is sensitive to calcification, which is an essential reference for the diagnosis of certain tumors. (2) CT shows bone erosion and hyperostosis more clearly than MRI does. (3) Performing CT is more convenient than performing an MRI when the patient is unconscious or requires sedation.

Most intracranial tumors present no specificity in CT and MRI images. Therefore, the primary tasks of CT and MRI are the detection of tumor location, the scope of invasion, and tumor invasion of surrounding structures. The final diagnosis requires surgical and histopathological determination. However, there are some concerns regarding this determination.

1. Some tumors have a unique appearance and unique CT and MRI images.
2. Some tumors have specific locations, such as acoustic schwannoma in the CP angle cistern, pituitary adenoma in the sella turcica, craniopharyngioma in the suprasellar region.
3. Some tumors have particular clinical symptoms such as pituitary adenoma and acoustic schwannoma.
4. Some tumors tend to occur at specific ages.

Therefore, according to tumor appearance, anatomical location presented in CT and MRI images, and to clinical symptoms, patient's age, experienced physicians can confirm diagnoses of tumor type with the results identical to surgical findings and final pathology reports in approximately 70% of cases. For the remaining 20–30% of diagnoses, a final pathology report is required to confirm the diagnosis.

Some characteristics of intracranial tumors require special attention:

1. Most tumors induce edema in peripheral brain tissues, especially white matter, and this is called peritumoral (perifocal) white matter edema. Intra-axial, extra-axial, and intraventricular tumors all can induce peritumoral white matter edema.
2. Some tumors often contain calcifications such as meningioma, oligodendroglioma, craniopharyngioma, and ependymoma.
3. Some tumors may hemorrhage and exhibit symptoms of a stroke.
4. Some malignant tumors demonstrate leptomeningeal infiltration of the CSF spaces and even spread to the spinal canal and spinal cord.
5. Some tumors have central necrosis, especially malignant tumors. Some tumors exhibit cystic changes such as pituitary adenoma and acoustic schwannoma.

Diagnosis of CNS tumors is also challenged by the confusion of nonneoplasms, including abscesses, tumefactive demyelinating lesions, encephalitis, and some subacute intracerebral hematoma. Sometimes infarction in the subacute stage exhibits mass effects and contrast-enhanced BBB disruption and thus resembles CNS tumors.

6.3 Application of New MRI Technology in Diagnosing CNS Tumors

In the last 20 years, new MRI technology has been widely applied in the diagnosis of CNS tumors. This technology provides satisfactory assistance, particularly in excluding nonneoplasms. New MRI technology includes MR spectroscopy (MRS), DWI, ADC mapping, and blood flow volume (rTBV) of perfusion imaging [3–5].

6.3.1 MRS

In CNS primary tumors, metastasis, and lymphoma, Cho is increased, and NAA is decreased (Figs. 6.1, 6.2, 6.3, 6.6, 6.8, 6.31, 6.32, and 6.38).

Lac/Lip in high-grade tumors and lymphoma are increased (Figs. 2.9, 6.5, 6.6, 6.15, 6.24, and 6.25), *especially, the Lip in lymphoma is increased* (Fig. 6.15).

mI in low-grade tumors is increased (Figs. 6.1, 6.2, and 6.31).

6.3.2 DWI for Solid Tumors

Primary CNS tumors: Great difference; most DWI images appear mild hyperintensity (whitish) which reflect diffusion-restriction (Figs. 6.2, 6.3, 6.4, 6.6, 6.14, 6.15, 6.37, 6.39, 6.47, 6.71, and 6.74); *the ADC value is decreased slightly and appears slightly dark* (Figs. 6.3, 6.5, 6.74).

Metastases: Most DWI images appear whitish; the ADC value is decreased slightly and appears slightly dark (Fig. 6.25).

Lymphoma: DWI images appear white; the ADC value is decreased slightly and appears dark (Figs. 6.15 and 6.16).

*Hemangioblastoma: DWI images appear dark (*Fig. 6.19*); this is a unique sign for hemangioblastoma. Hemangiopericytoma also shows hypointensity on DWI* (Fig. 6.48) *due to hypervascularity.*

6.3.3 DWI for Tumor Necrosis or Cystic Change

Necrosis of primary CNS tumors and metastasis: Most DWI images appear dark (Figs. 6.5, 6.7, 6.24, 6.25, 6.26, and 6.27); *the ADC value is increased and appears white* (Figs. 6.5, 6.25, and 6.26).

Abscess: Contains pus and appears white because pus has strong diffusion restriction, and the ADC value is decreased (Chap. 7).

Table 6.2 compares intra-axial tumors, metastasis, lymphoma, and intra-axial lesions that are not neoplasms (e.g., demyelination, abscess, and encephalitis).

Table 6.2 Intra-axial lesion expressions in new MRI technology

	Primary tumors	Metastasis	Lymphoma	Demyelination	Abscess	Encephalitis
MRS/lipid	Increased, particularly for high-grade tumors	Increased	Considerably increased	—	Increased	—
Lactate	Increased, particularly for high-grade tumors	Increased	Increased	—	Increased	Increased
NAA	Decreased, particularly for high-grade tumors	Decreased	Decreased	Decreased	Absent	Decreased
Choline	Increased	Increased	Increased	Increased	Absent	Decreased
Myoinositol	Increased, particularly for low-grade tumors	—	—	—	—	Increased
DWI	Variable	Necrosis: DWI dark ADC white	DWI gray-white ADC gray-dark	No signal change	DWI bright ADC dark	Variable

6.4 Intra-axial Tumors

Diffuse Astrocytic and Oligodendroglial Tumors:

- Diffuse astrocytoma. Gr II** (Figs. 6.1, 6.2, and 6.3).
- Anaplastic astrocytoma. Gr III (Figs. 6.3 and 6.4).
- Glioblastoma. Gr IV (Figs. 6.5, 6.6, 6.7, and 6.8).
- Oligodendroglioma. Gr II (Fig. 6.9).
- Anaplastic oligodendroglioma. Gr III.

Other Astrocytic Tumors

- Pilocytic astrocytoma. Gr I (Fig. 6.10).
- Subependymal giant cell astrocytoma. Gr I (Fig. 6.11).

** According to 2016 WHO CNS tumor grading.

Gliomas

- Glial cells include astrocytes, oligodendrocytes, microglial cells, and ependymal cells. They are the most abundant cells in brain tissues and prone to tumor growth. Therefore, gliomas are the most crucial brain tumors.

6.4.1 Diffuse Astrocytoma Gr II

Also called low-grade astrocytoma.

Morphology: Possibly an integral solid tumor or infiltrating tumor (Figs. 6.1, 6.2, and 6.3).

Position: All brain tissues and the spinal cord.

Age: Children and young adults.

CT: Either isodense or hypodense. Because the BBB is not disrupted, the appearance of most tumors is not enhanced by an iodine-containing contrast medium. If an area of brain tissue shows irregularity and low density, and it lacks contrast enhancement, this is commonly a low-grade astrocytoma.

MRI: Astrocytoma present hyperintensity on FLAIR and T2WI, and MRI is more sensitive than CT to detect the abnormal high-signal area in brain tissues. Contrast enhancement is often absent after the injection of Gd-DTPA.

In MRS, myoinositol (mI) increase can be observed.

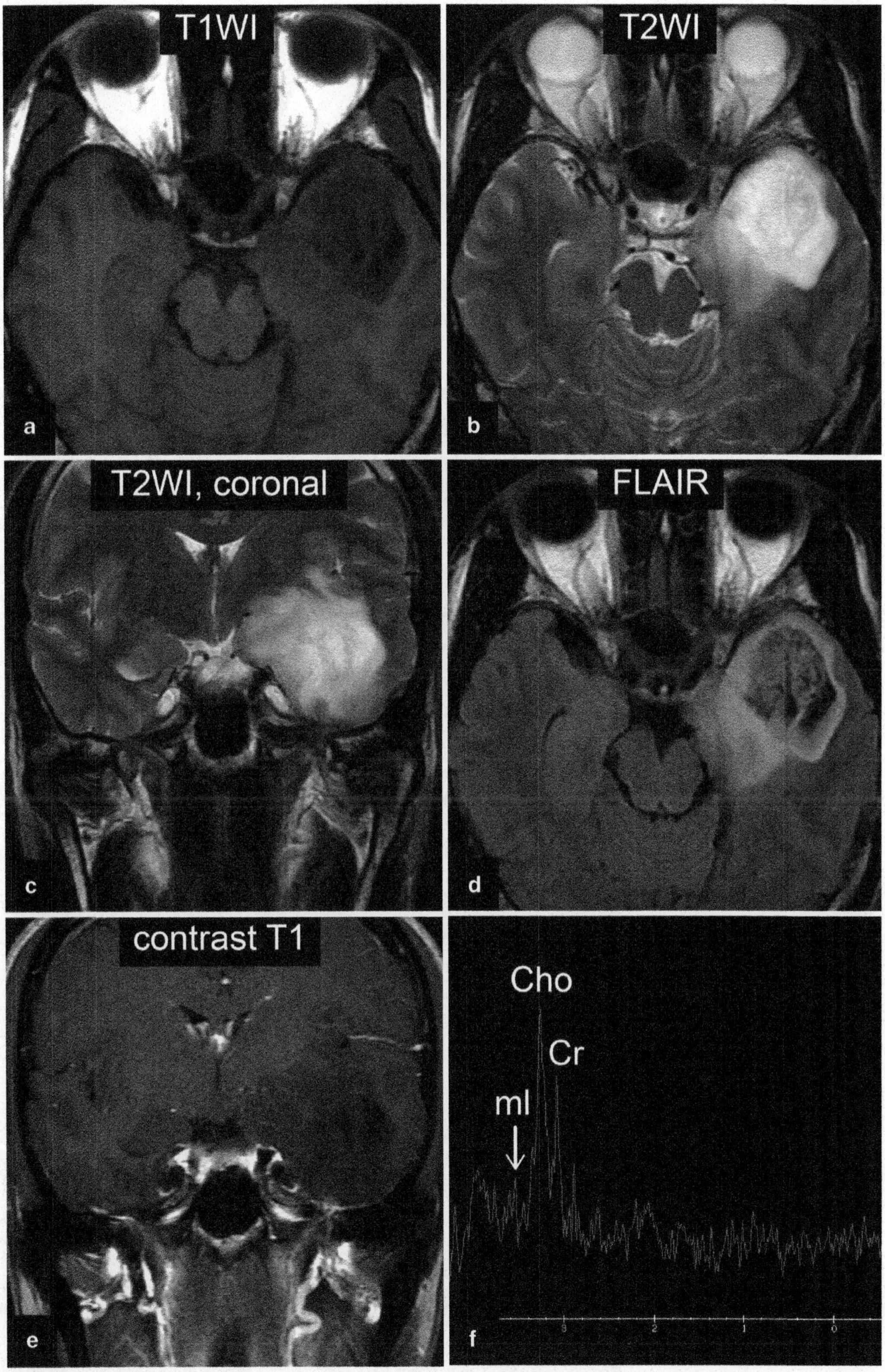

Fig. 6.1 M/46, Diffuse astrocytoma, grade II. The patient suffered from dizziness for 1 year. (**a**–**e**) MRI: An area of brain tissue in the left temporal lobe shows hypointensity on T1W, hyperintensity on T2WI, heterogeneous intensity on FLAIR, and no enhancement by the contrast medium. For the above findings, low-grade astrocytoma should be considered. (**f**) MRS (TE 144 ms): The levels of choline (Cho; 3.2 ppm) is elevated, and creatine (Cr; 3.0 ppm) is slightly reduced, NAA (2.0 ppm) has disappeared, myoInositol (mI; 3.5 mm) is slightly elevated (arrow), and lactate is absent. This MRS is a sign of low-grade astrocytoma. Surgical removal of this mass and astrocytoma (grade II) is confirmed by pathological examination

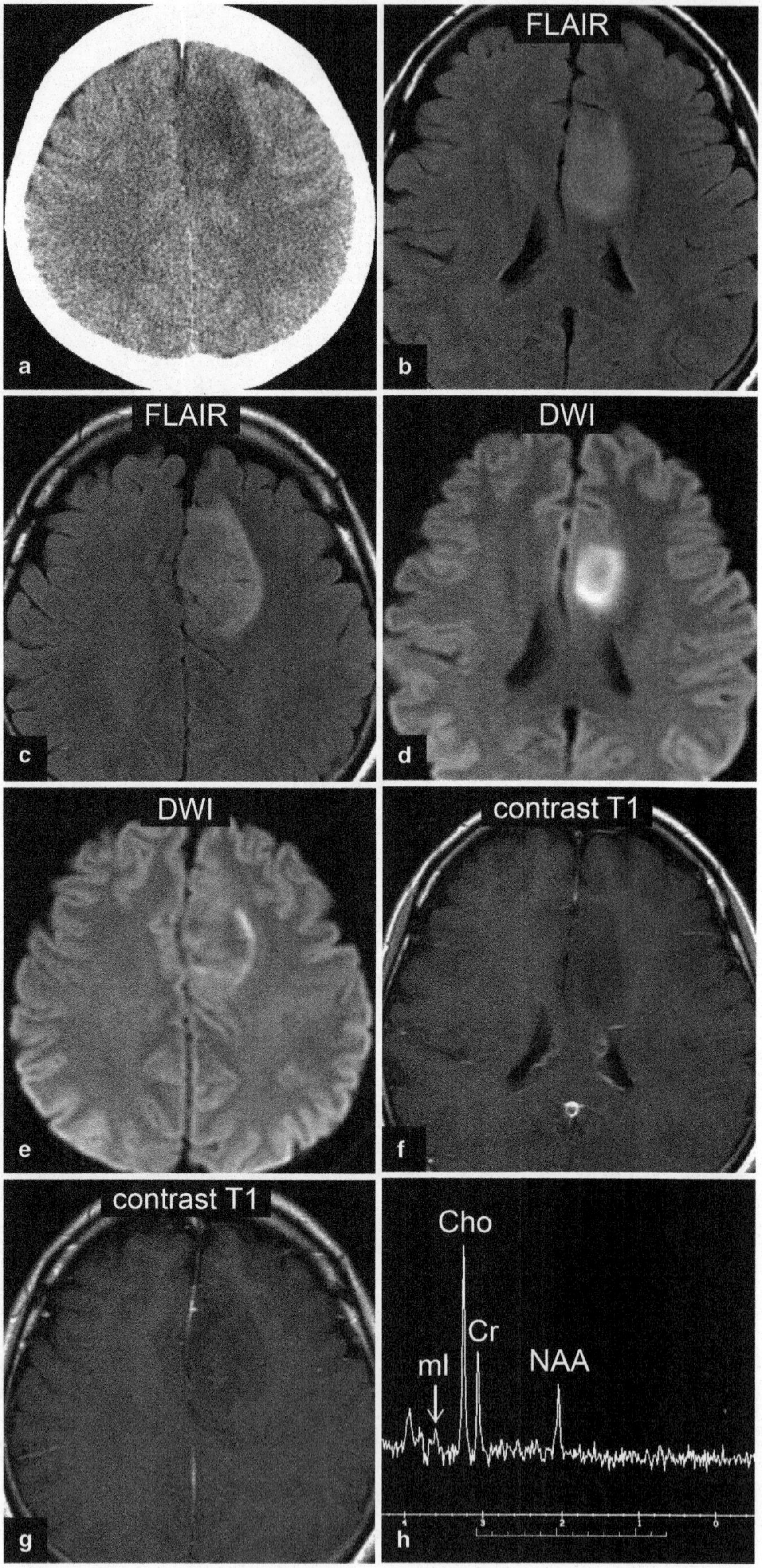

Fig. 6.2 F/20, Diffuse astrocytoma, grade II. CT and MRI were performed for seizure. (**a**) CT: One area of the brain tissue in the left frontal lobe shows hypodensity. No contrast enhancement (not shown) is present. (**b–g**) MRI: This lesion shows hyperintensity on FLAIR. A portion of the lesion shows hyperintensity on DWI and is not enhanced by the contrast medium. (**h**) MRS (TE 144 ms): Cho is elevated, NAA is reduced, mI is slightly elevated (arrow), and lactate is absent. The MRS reflects the possibility of low-grade astrocytoma. Surgical removal of this mass and diffuse astrocytoma (WHO grade II) was confirmed by pathological examination

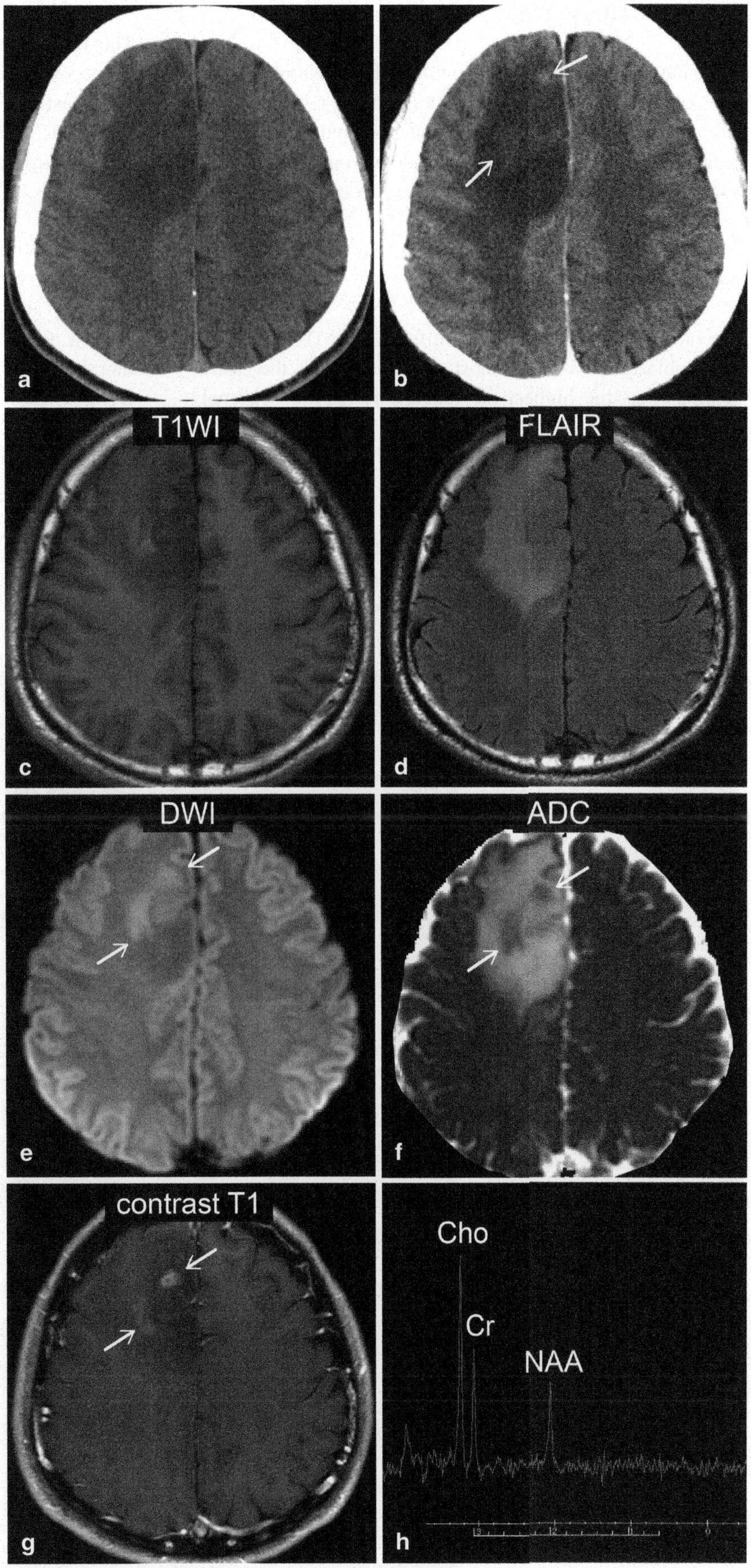

Fig. 6.3 M/45, Astrocytoma, grades II and III. (**a**) CT (**b**) contrast CT: An area of brain tissue in the right frontal lobe shows hypodensity and also shows mild enhancement (arrows) by contrast medium. (**c–g**) MRI: The lesion showing hypointensity on T1WI and hyperintensity on FLAIR. A small portion of the lesion (arrows) shows mild hyperintensity on DWI, mild hypointensity on DAC, reflecting mild diffusion restriction. Only this portion has contrast enhancement (arrows). (**h**) MRS (TE 144 ms): Cho is elevated, NAA is reduced, and no lactate appears. Surgical removal of this tumor, grades II and III astrocytomas were confirmed by pathological examination. The enhanced parts in CT and MRI possible are the Gr III areas

6.4.2 Anaplastic astrocytoma Gr III

CT and MRI: Tumors that exhibit irregular density and intensity and can be enhanced by contrast media (Fig. 6.3). The tumor may be solid or has irregular necrosis and cystic change. This type of tumor is indistinguishable from glioblastoma. Some are not enhanced, such as diffuse astrocytoma (Fig. 6.4).

6.4.3 Glioblastoma Gr IV

The old term is glioblastoma multiform (GBM).

Glioblastoma is the most aggressive of the astrocytomas, has the highest incidence, and has an extremely undesirable prognosis.

2016 WHO CNS tumor classification further divides glioblastoma into the following types:

- **Glioblastoma isocitrate dehydrogenase (IDH) wild type** accounts for 90% of glioblastomas. It is clinically defined as primary or de novo glioblastoma, which means that the tumor is destined to be Grade IV once it develops. This type of tumor is likely to occur in patients aged older than 55 years old (Figs. 6.5, 6.6, and 6.7).
- **Glioblastoma IDH mutant** accounts for 10% of glioblastomas. It transforms from diffuse astrocytoma or anaplastic astrocytoma and often occurs in young adults (Fig. 6.8).

Position: White matter in the cerebral hemisphere, particularly at the frontal and temporal lobes. Glioblastoma may also develop at the basal ganglia. Glioblastoma in the frontal lobe often penetrates the corpus callosum to reach the contralateral hemisphere.

CT and MRI: The tumor volume is usually large, with an irregular outline. The contrast enhancement is apparent. There is severe irregular central necrosis. The above features are giving the tumor the shape of a cauliflower. In most cases, peritumoral white matter edema is apparent.

In MRS, Lac/Lip is increased.

Glioblastoma can spread along the CSF and even metastasize into the spinal canal through the CSF.

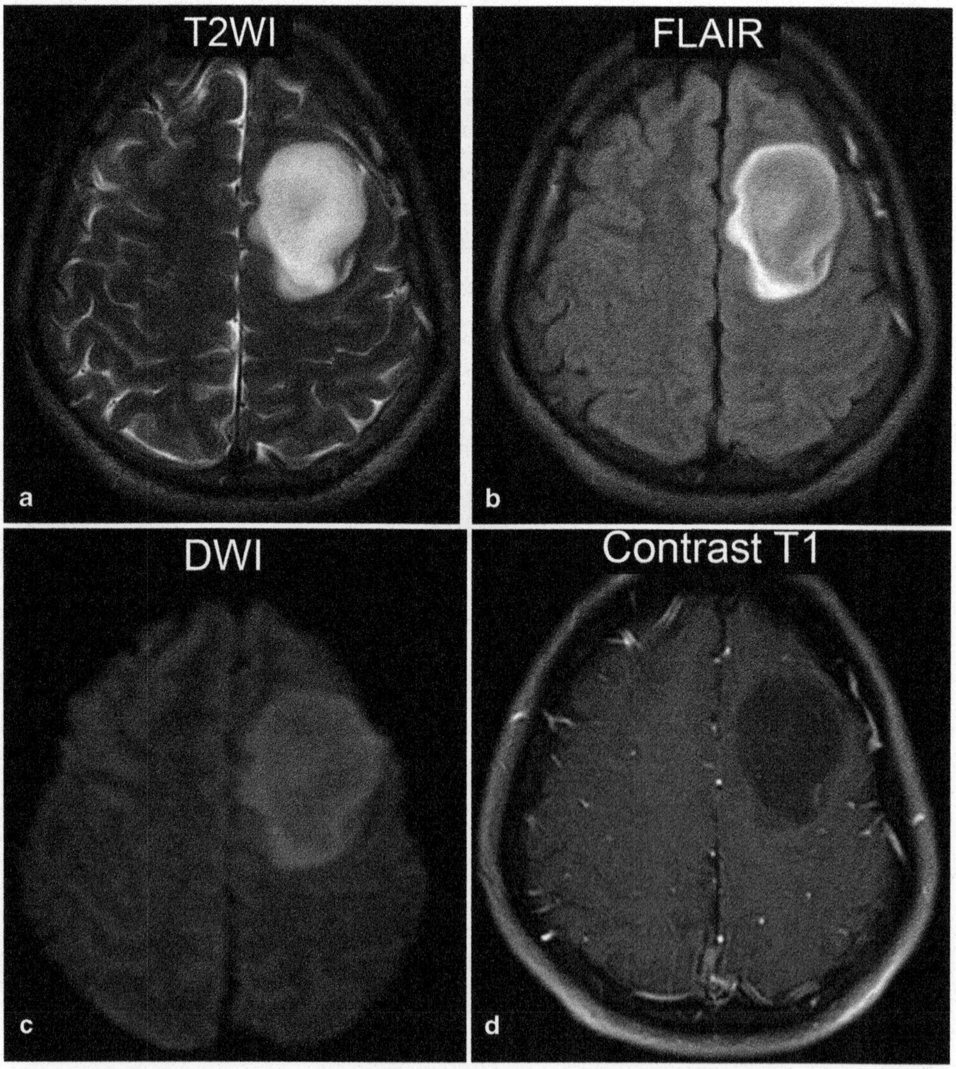

Fig. 6.4 M/24, Anaplastic astrocytoma, grade III. The patient suffered from several seizure attacks in the last 2 months. (**a–c**) MRI: A lesion in the left frontal lobe shows hyperintensity on T2WI, FLAIR, and also hyperintensity on DWI. (**d**) Contrast T1WI: No enhancement by contrast medium is observed. Surgical removal of this tumor and pathology proved this is anaplastic astrocytoma (WHO grade III)

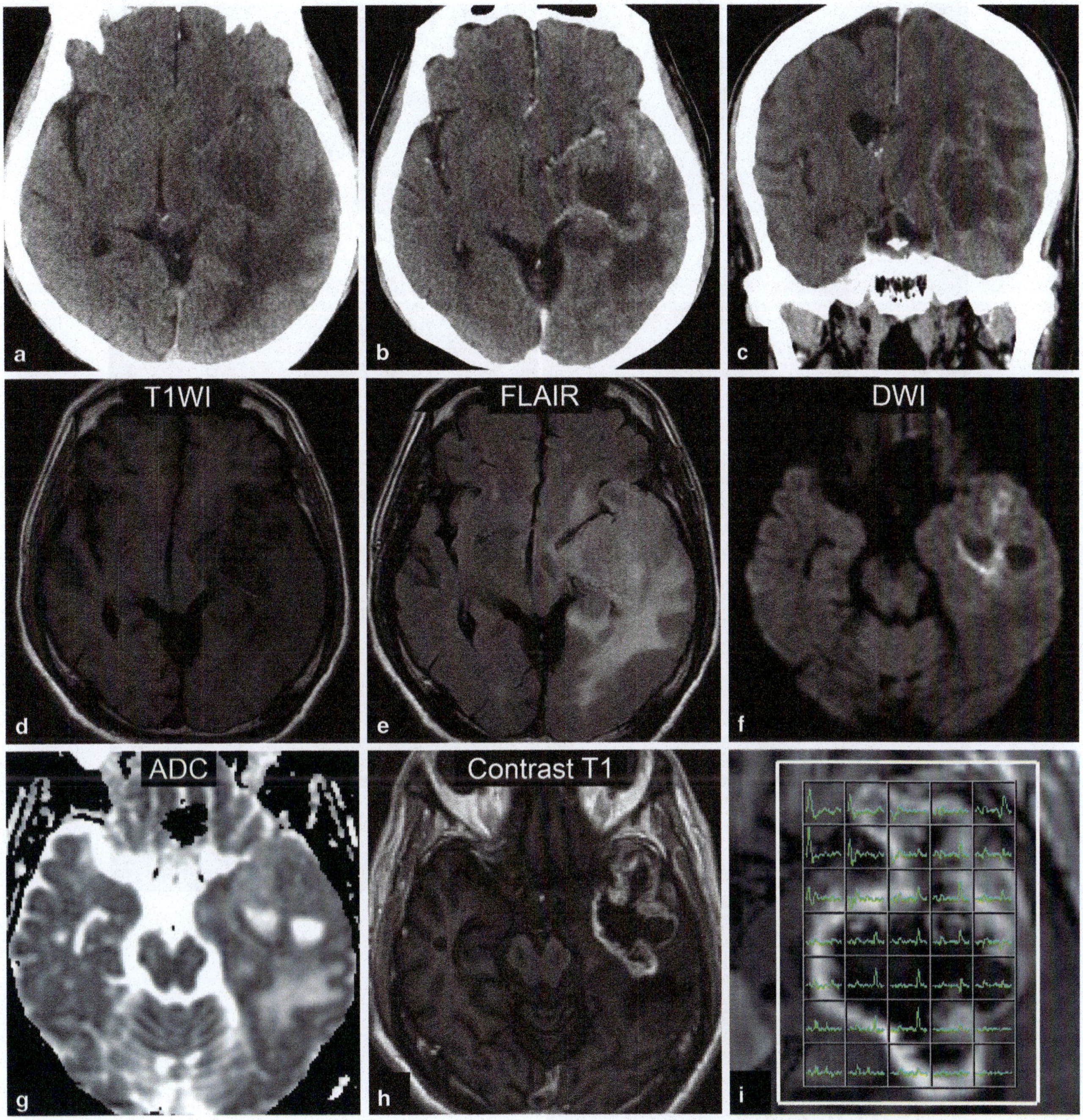

Fig. 6.5 M/66, Glioblastoma. (**a**) CT: A hypodense lesion with peripheral white matter edema is observed in the left temporal lobe. (**b**, **c**) Contrast CT: This lesion shows irregular marginal enhancement. CT features are similar to those of glioblastoma with severe central necrosis. (**d–h**) MRI: This mass shows hypointensity on T1WI and hyperintensity on FLAIR with peripheral white matter edema. Contrast T1WI presents irregular marginal enhancement with severe central necrosis, giving the tumor the shape of a cauliflower. A portion of the necrosis demonstrates hypointensity on DWI and hyperintensity on ADC, and only a small portion shows hyperintensity on DWI and mild hypointensity on ADC. (**i**) Multivoxel MRS (TE:22.8 ms): Certain areas exhibit high Cho level, and some areas show elevated lactate/lipid levels. The features indicate malignancy in the tumor; the first consideration is glioblastoma. This tumor was surgically removed and confirmed to be a glioblastoma by pathological examination

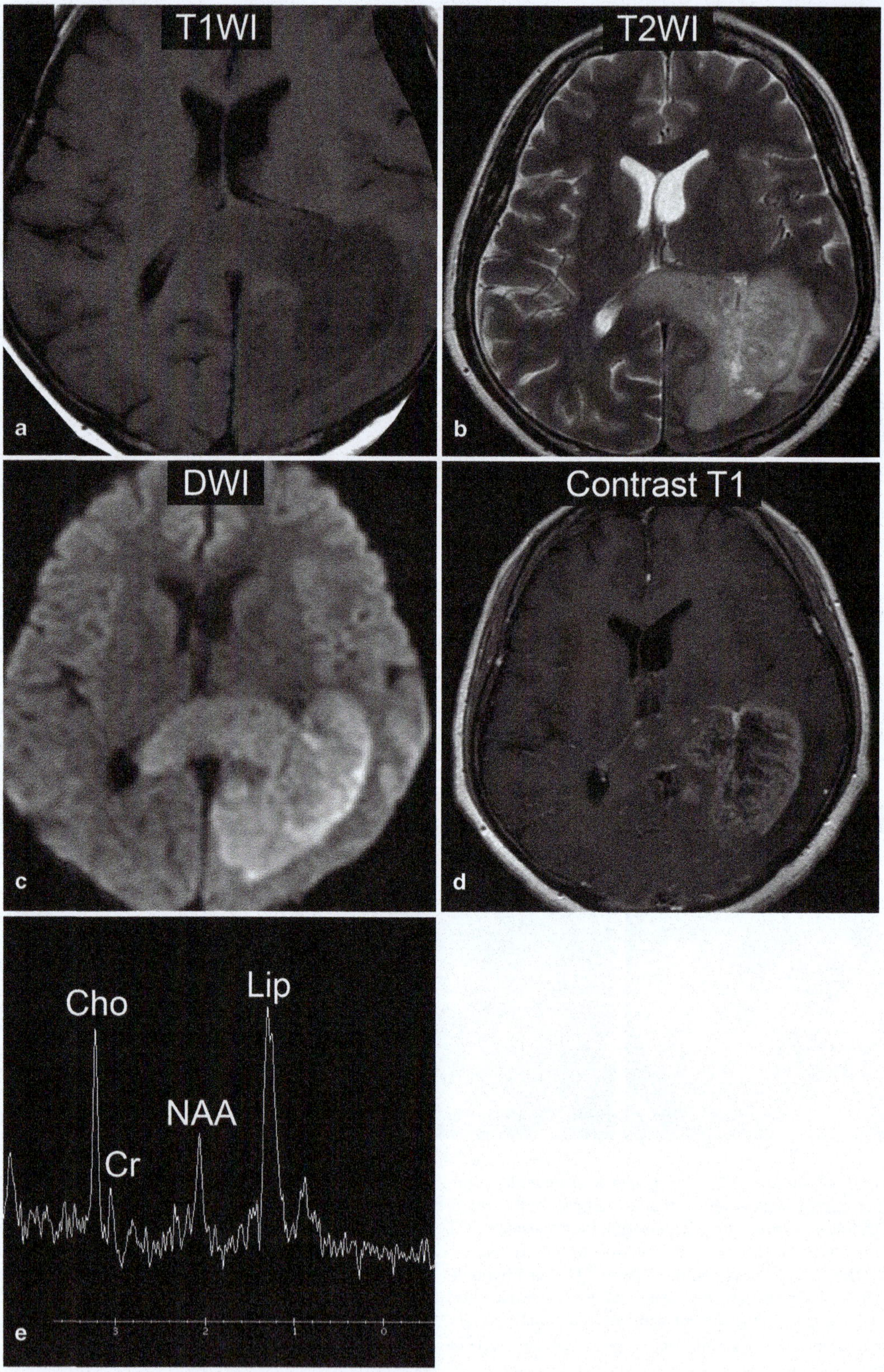

Fig. 6.6 F/49, Glioblastoma. The patient suffered from severe headaches and memory loss. (**a–d**) MRI: A large lesion in the left occipital lobe and splenium of the corpus callosum shows hypointensity on T1WI, hyperintensity on T2WI, and mild hyperintensity on DWI. Contrast T1WI presents irregular central necrosis. The features indicate typical glioblastoma. (**e**) MRS (144 ms): NAA is reduced, and Cho and lipid levels are elevated. The MRS features indicate typical glioblastoma. A portion of this tumor was surgically removed and was confirmed to be a glioblastoma by pathological examination

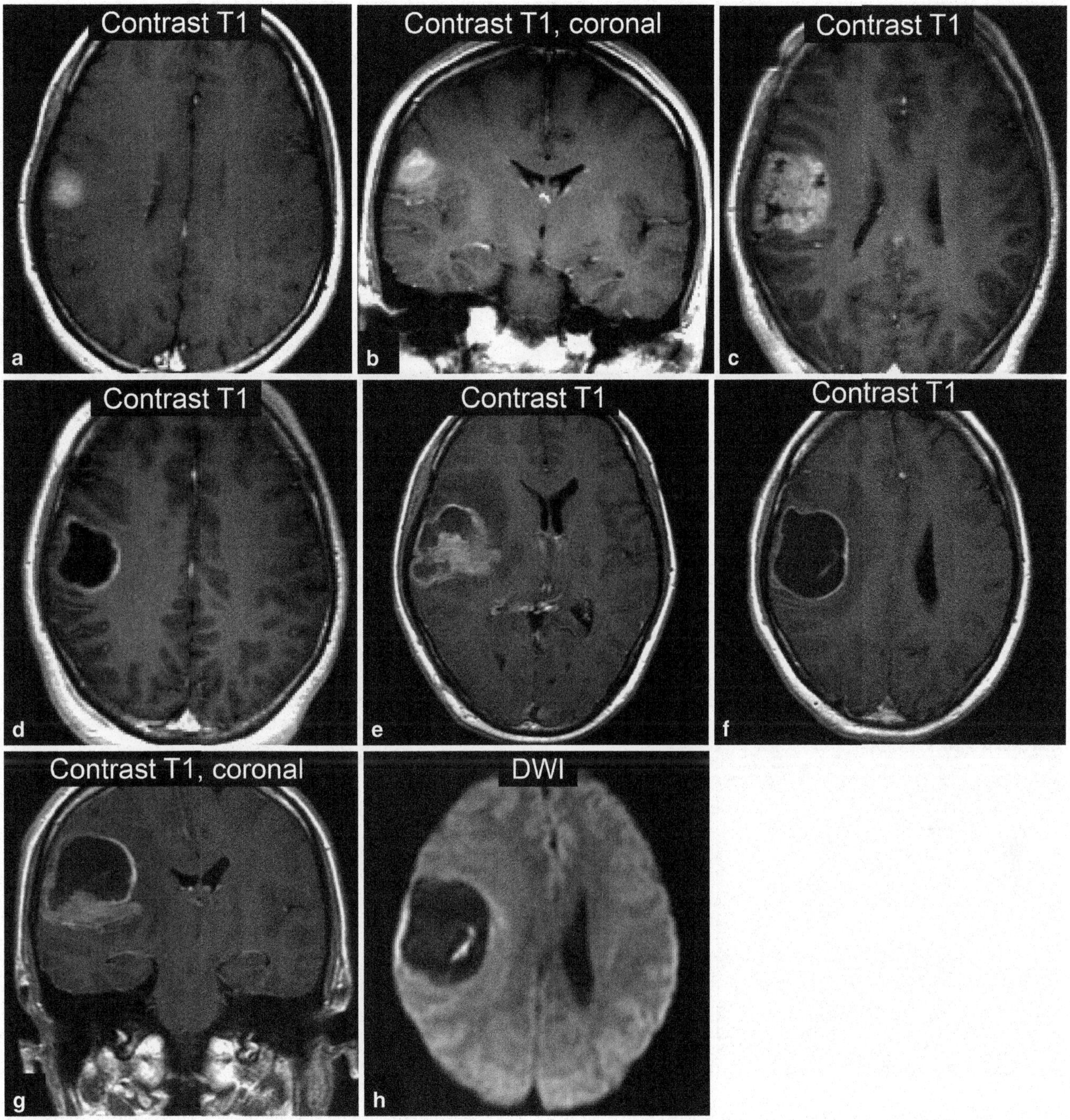

Fig. 6.7 F/34, de novo glioblastoma. (**a**, **b**) First MRI, contrast T1WI: A small solid mass with homogenous enhancement without central necrosis is observed in the right parietal lobe. (**c**, **d**) Repeat MRI after 50 days, contrast T1WI: The upper part of the tumor shows severe central necrosis. (**e**–**h**) Follow-up MRI after another 55 days: Tumor size increases with heterogeneous enhancement, and severe central necrosis is observed. The necrotic portion shows hypointensity on DWI. The tumor is surgically removed and confirmed to be a glioblastoma by pathological examination. In summary, the features indicate typical primary glioblastoma (de novo glioblastoma) . As soon as the tumor grew small, it was destined to be high-grade glioma (develop de novo)

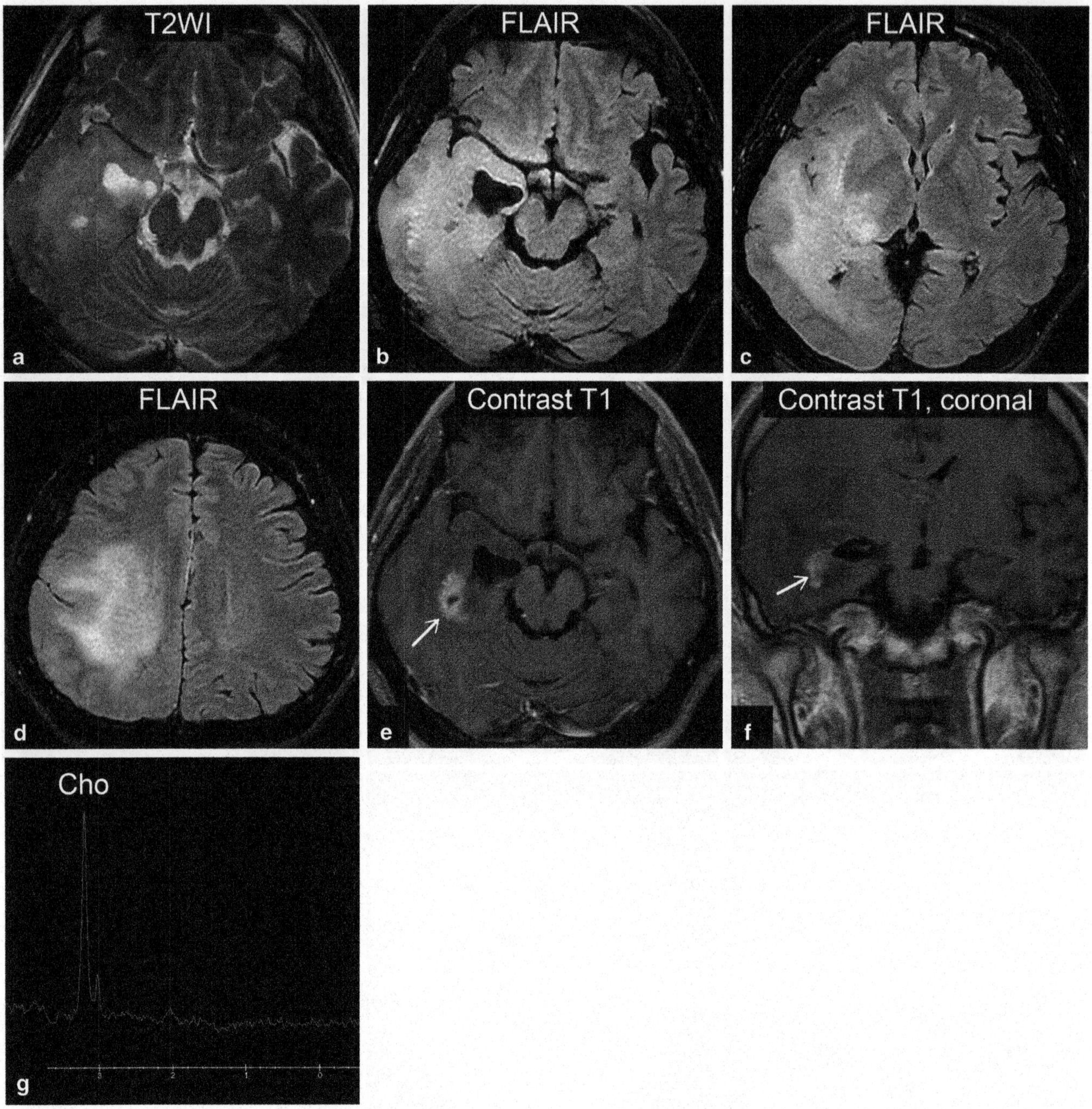

Fig. 6.8 M/44, Glioblastoma. (**a–d**) MRI, T2WI, and FLAIR: An area of the brain tissue in the right temporal lobe shows hyperintensity with a certain degree of peripheral white matter edema. (**e, f**) Contrast T1WI: Only a small portion of the lesion is enhanced (arrow). (**g**) MRS (TE 144 ms): Cho level is significantly elevated, NAA disappears, and lactate is absent. The abnormal brain tissue was surgically removed and confirmed to be a glioblastoma by pathological examination. This tumor may be a low-grade astrocytoma gradually transforming into glioblastoma, which is the so-called secondary glioblastoma

6.4.4 Oligodendroglioma

Oligodendroglioma Gr II.

Anaplastic oligodendroglioma Gr III.

Oligodendroglioma develops from oligodendrocytes. It mostly occurs in the frontal lobe and white matter of the other cerebral hemisphere. Some originate from lateral ventricles.

Age: Adults, with few cases in children.

CT: In 70–90% of cases, speckled and nodular calcification is observed (Fig. 6.9). Soft tissue parts are enhanced by contrast medium. Cystic degeneration is often observed.

MRI: Heterogeneous signal intensity; injection of Gd-DTPA may enhance the tumor; however, calcification is not as evident as in CT.

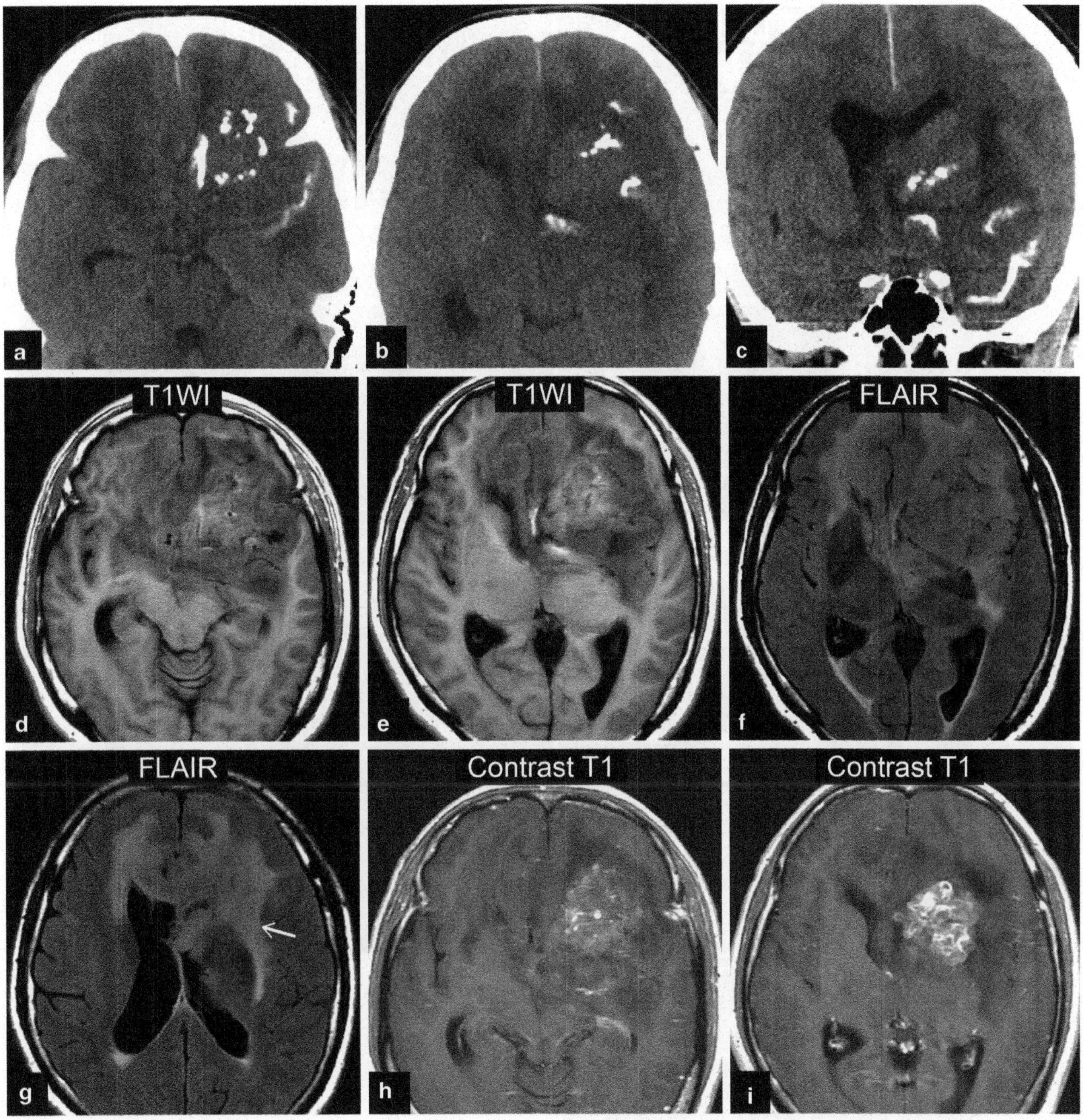

Fig. 6.9 M/55, Oligodendroglioma. (**a**, **b**) CT axial (**c**) CT coronal: A large tumor with considerable calcifications in the left frontotemporal lobes. The margin of the tumor is unclear. (**d**–**i**) MRI: This tumor shows hypointensity on T1WI and hyperintensity on FLAIR and has contrast enhancement. Peripheral white matter edema (arrow) is observed. The margin of the tumor and calcifications are hardly observed in the MRI. The tumor was surgically removed and confirmed to be an anaplastic oligodendroglioma by pathological examination

6.4.5 Pilocytic Astrocytoma

Age: Children and young adults.

Location: Near the fourth and third ventricles, hypothalamus, and cerebellar vermis (Fig. 6.10).

Morphology: Cystic pattern with a clear outline.

CT and MRI: Because pilocytic astrocytoma contains many tiny cysts, CT and MRI T1WI show that the cysts have a higher liquid component. Therefore, CT demonstrates hypodensity, whereas MRI T1WI shows hypointensity. MRI T2WI shows the hyperintensity of liquid signals. Because pilocytic astrocytoma contains soft tissues, enhancement of the soft tissues becomes observable after injection of contrast media.

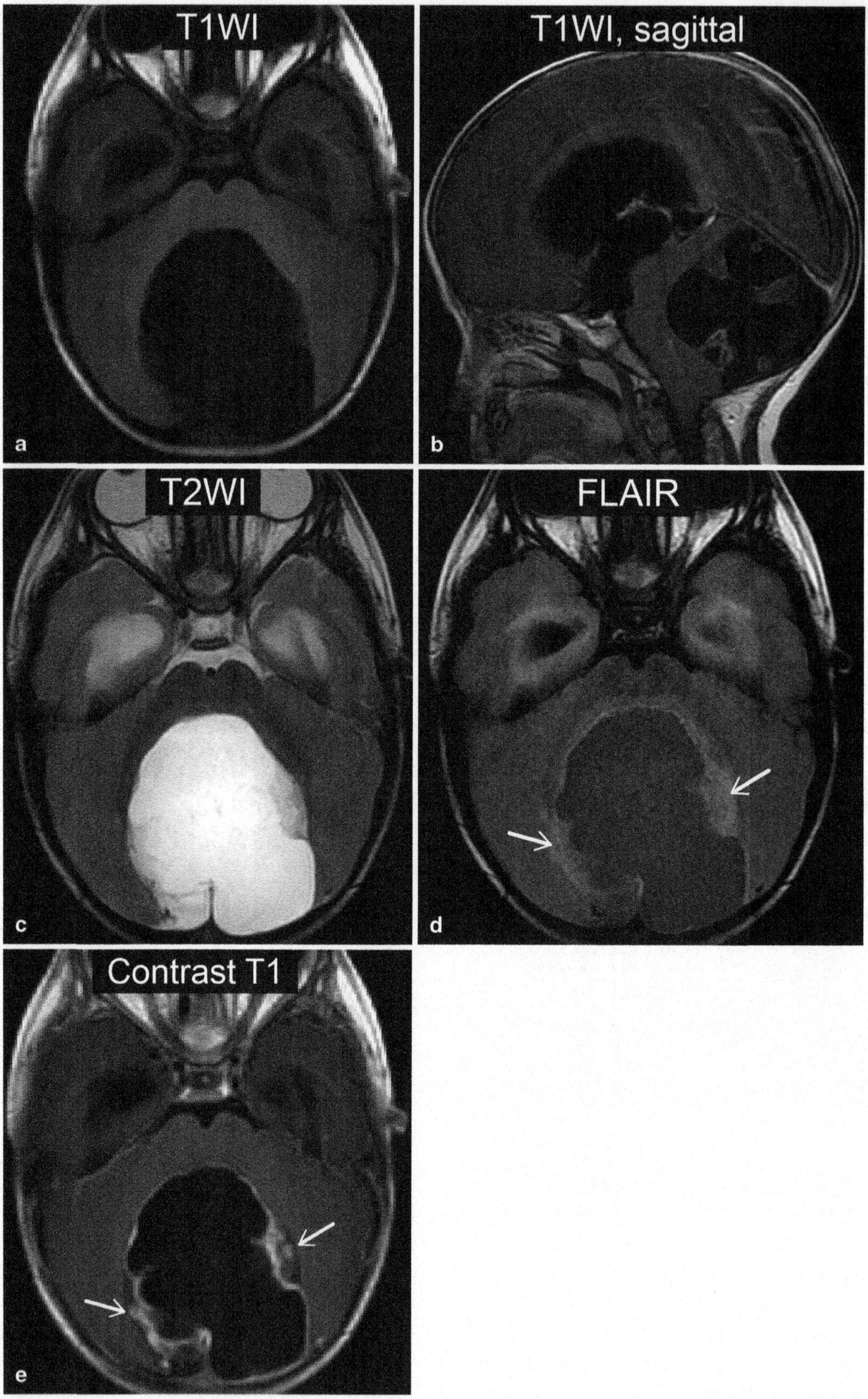

Fig. 6.10 F/25, Pilocytic astrocytoma. The patient suffered from unsteady gait and lethargy in the last 10 days. (**a**–**d**) MRI: A large tumor is found in the middle of the cerebellum. Signal intensities on T1WI and T2WI are similar to those of CSF, indicating a cystic mass. FLAIR shows some soft tissue components (arrows) in the cystic wall. (**e**) Contrast T1WI: The soft tissue components are enhanced by the contrast medium (arrows). After the successful removal of the tumor by surgery, the tumor was confirmed to be a pilocytic astrocytoma (WHO Gr I) by pathological examination

6.4.6 Subependymal Giant Cell Astrocytoma

This type of tumor occurs in patients with tuberous sclerosis. Multiple small and calcified hamartomas exist around the ventricles. A hamartoma near the foramen of Monro may develop into a more massive tumor, which is subependymal giant cell astrocytoma and compresses the foramen of Monro, causing obstructive hydrocephalus (Fig. 6.11).

CT: Tumors near the foramen of Monro with calcification and multiple calcified nodules identified on the ventricular wall can be diagnosed as tuberous sclerosis combined with giant cell astrocytoma.

MRI: The image is similar to that of CT; however, calcification is difficult to determine.

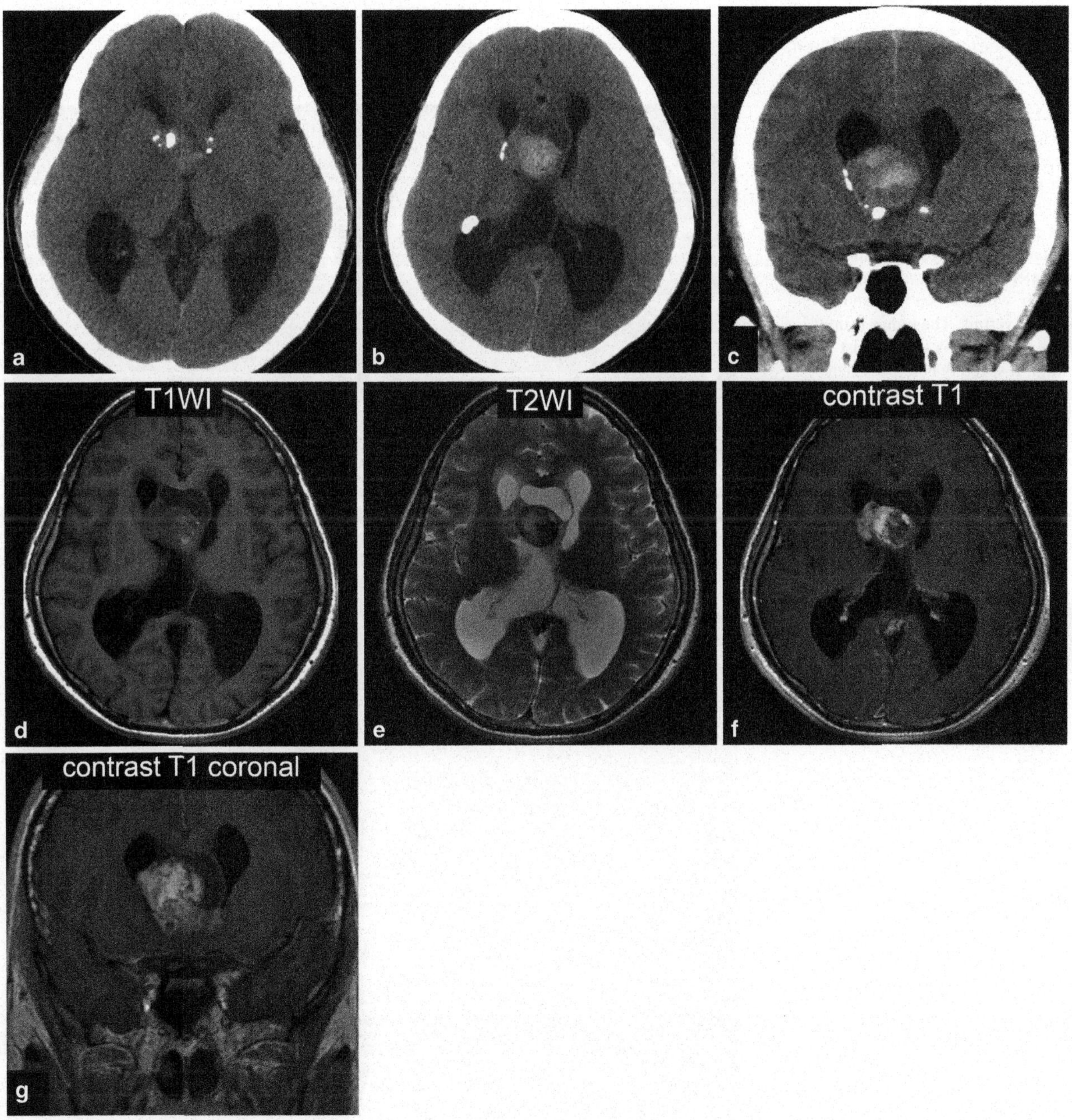

Fig. 6.11 M/30, Giant cell astrocytoma. The patient complained about severe headaches in the last 10 days. (**a–c**) CT: Multiple calcifications are observed in the ventricular wall. The feature is a pathognomonic sign of tuberous sclerosis (TS). A hyperdense tumor is present between the bilateral lateral ventricles and causes obstructive hydrocephalus. Several calcifications are in the margin of this tumor. For a TS patient with a tumor in this location, the giant cell astrocytoma is considered. The high density of this tumor is possibly due to tumor bleeding. (**d–g**) MRI: The tumor shows intermediate signal intensity on T1WI, and a small portion of hypointensity on T2WI represents hemorrhage. The tumor is well enhanced by the contrast medium. The tumor was surgically removed and found it originated from septum pellucidum and confirmed to be a subependymal giant cell astrocytoma by pathological examination

6.4.7 Medulloblastoma Gr IV

Medulloblastoma only develops at the posterior cranial fossa. The incidence of medulloblastoma accounts for 15–25% of the intracranial tumors among children and 1% of those among adults.

Age: 75% of cases are in children, and the rest are in young adults.

Position: Mostly at the cerebellar vermis (Figs. 6.12, 6.13, and 6.14), especially in children. In adults, the tumor develops in the cerebellar hemisphere. Few cases develop in the cerebellar hemisphere in children.

CT and MRI: Rare calcification (Fig. 6.12) and cystic change. Because medulloblastoma mostly develops at the vermis, if a solid tumor with minimum cystic change is identified at the vermis of a child, the doctor should consider the tumor to be medulloblastoma. Development at the vermis easily compresses the fourth ventricle and causes obstructive hydrocephalus. If the tumor develops in the cerebellar hemisphere, cystic changes are likely to occur and it can be confused with astrocytoma.

Medulloblastoma is a malignant tumor that can easily spread into the subarachnoid space or even seeds in the spinal canal through the CSF.

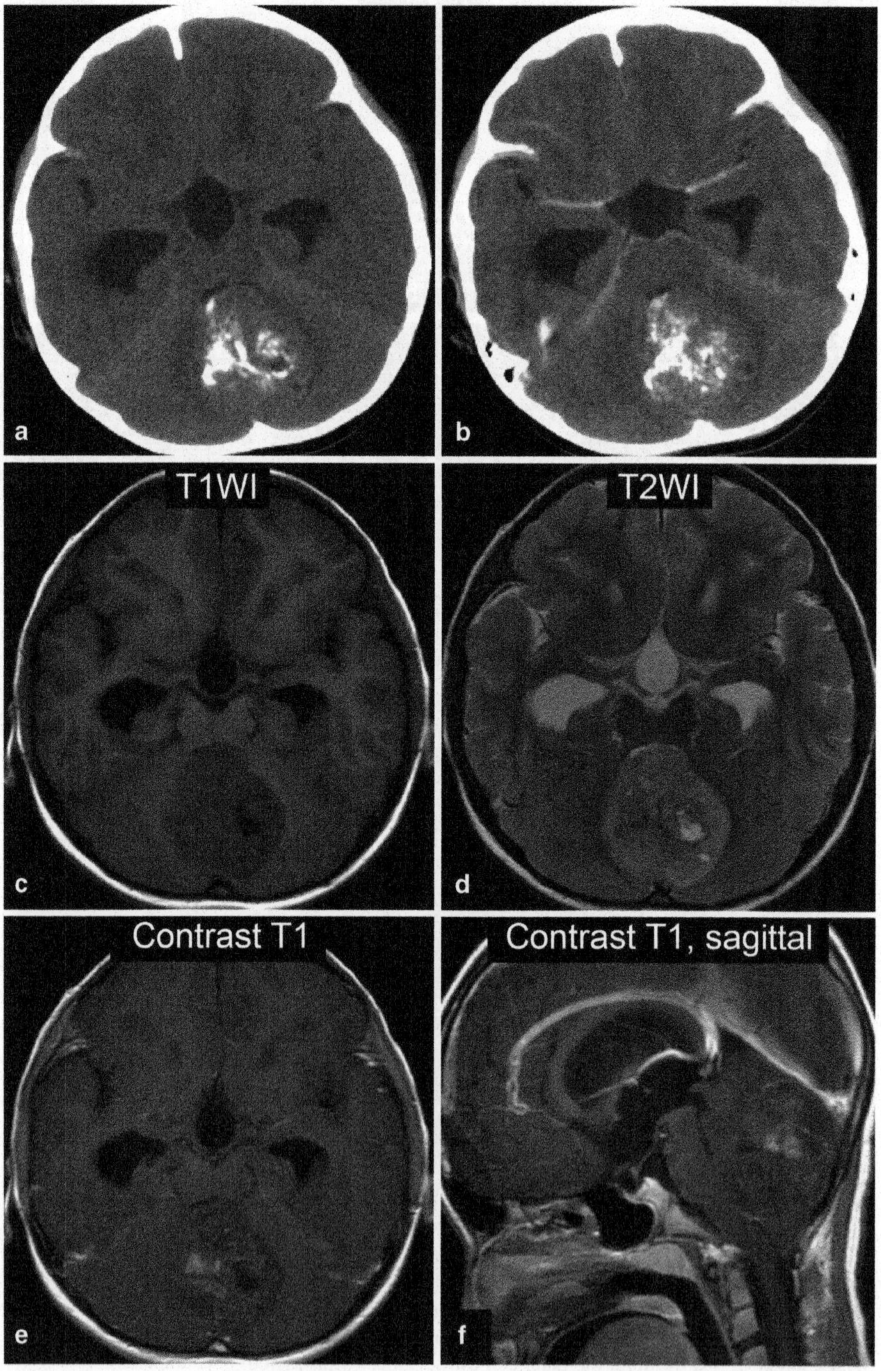

Fig. 6.12 F/7, Medulloblastoma. The patient suffered from headaches and unsteady gait for a month. (**a**, **b**) CT: A tumor mass in the middle of posterior fossa contains dense calcification, compresses the fourth ventricle, and causes obstructive hydrocephalus. (**c**–**f**) MRI: MRI clearly shows the margin of the tumor, which arises from the cerebellar vermis. The tumor is only slightly enhanced by the contrast medium. It severely compresses the fourth ventricle and causes obstructive hydrocephalus. The tumor was surgically removed and confirmed to be a large-cell medulloblastoma by pathological examination

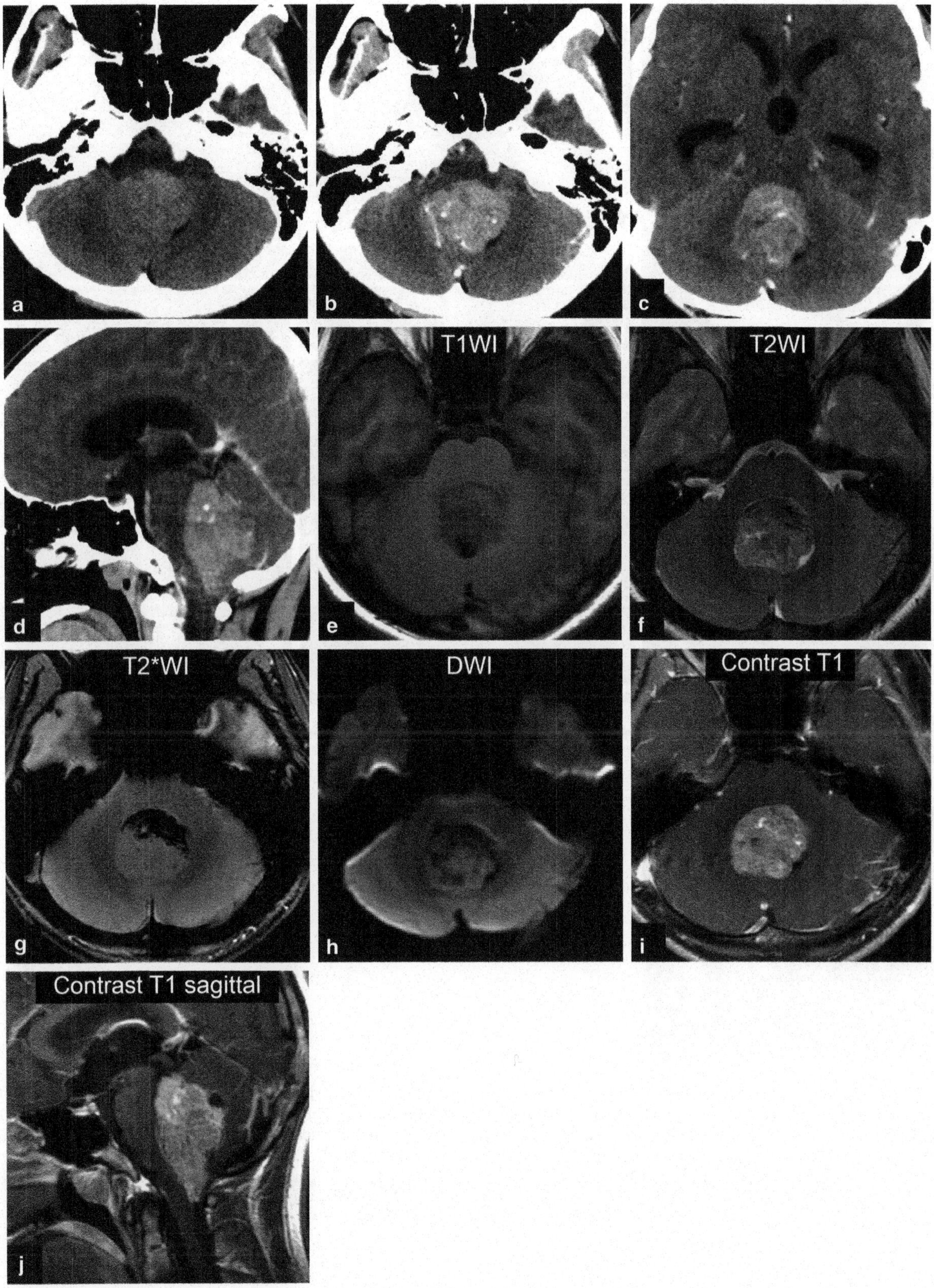

Fig. 6.13 M/13, Medulloblastoma. The patient suffered from dizziness and vomiting for 2 weeks. (**a**) CT: A tumor mass in the middle of the posterior fossa shows mild hyperdensity, possibly due to tumor bleeding. (**b–d**) Contrast CT: This tumor is well enhanced by the contrast medium. Dilatation of the third ventricle and temporal horns of bilateral lateral ventricles reflects hydrocephalus because this tumor compresses the fourth ventricle. (**e–h**) MRI: This tumor shows intermediate signal intensity on T1WI and mild hyperintensity on T2WI. The hypointensity of T2*WI in the anterior part of the tumor indicates tumor bleeding. (**i, j**) Contrast T1WI: This tumor has well enhancement by contrast medium. This tumor was surgically removed and confirmed to be a medulloblastoma by pathological examination

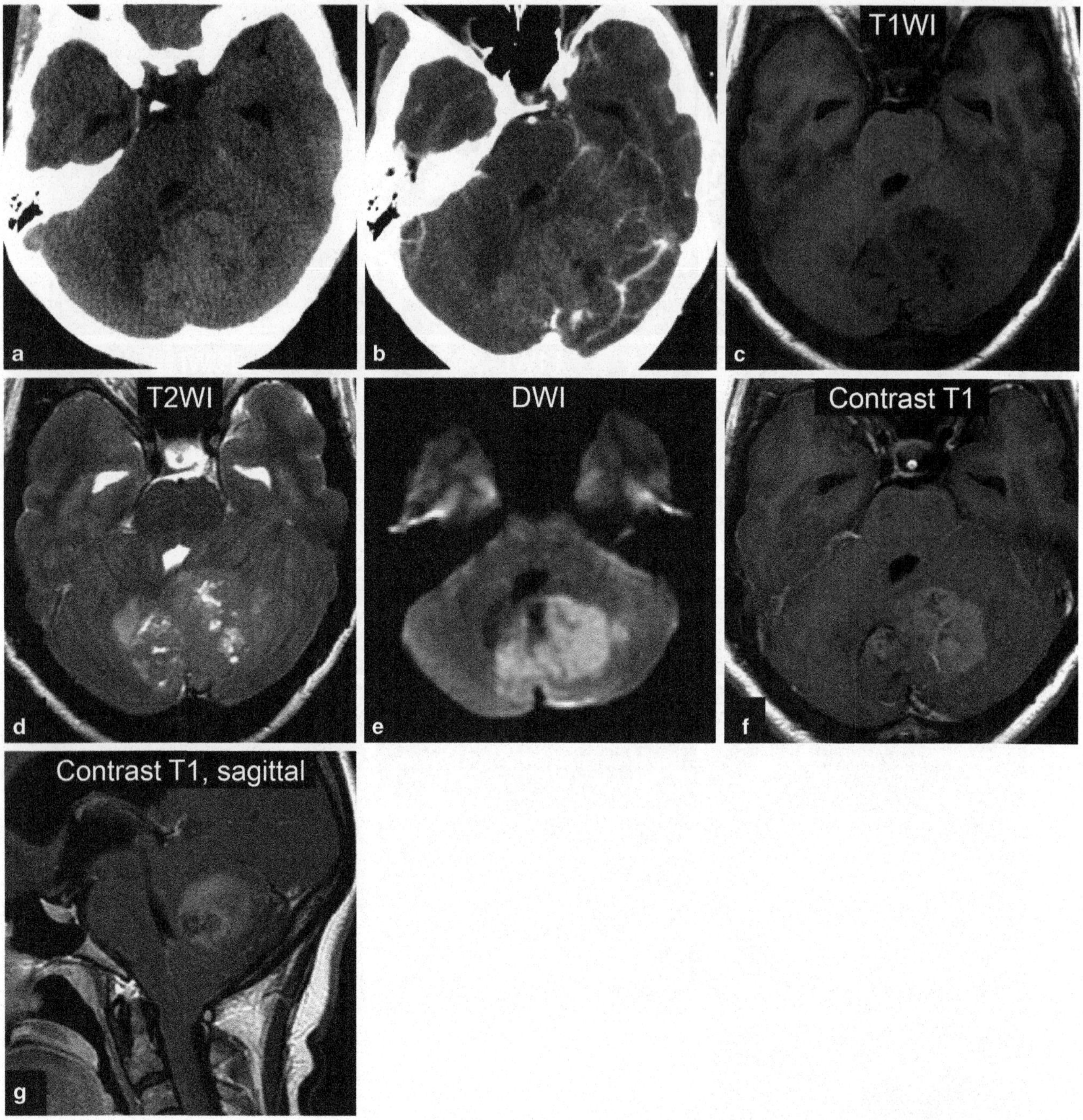

Fig. 6.14 F/32, Adult medulloblastoma. This patient suffered from headaches for 2 months. (**a**) CT (**b**) contrast CT: A big tumor mass is observed in the cerebellar vermis and extends to the left cerebellum with only mild enhancement. (**c–g**) MRI: This tumor shows mild hypointensity on T1WI, heterogeneous hyperintensity on T2WI, possibly contains many small cysts, hyperintensity on DWI, and moderate enhancement by contrast medium. This tumor was surgically removed, and medulloblastoma from vermis extending into the cerebellum was confirmed by pathological examination. The adult-type medulloblastoma may have cystic change and often migrates into the cerebellar hemisphere from vermis

6.4.8 Primary CNS Lymphomas

In 2016 WHO classification of CNS tumors, lymphomas consist of eight types, one of which is related to immune deficiency. These lymphomas appear similar in imaging and are thus consistently called primary CNS lymphomas.

The incidence rates of lymphomas are high. In Taiwan, many lymphomas occur not in patients with immunodeficiency but ordinary patients (Figs. 6.15 and 6.16).

Lymphomas exhibit several characteristics in CT and MRI:

1. Single or several tumor masses.
2. Solid tumors with minimum central necrosis and excellent contrast enhancement.
3. Peritumoral white matter edema in most incidences.
4. In MRI, DWI shows diffusion restriction (DWI white).
5. MRS: Cho is increased; the Cho/Cr ratio is reversed; NAA is low; the lactate/lipid peak appears.
6. PET: fluorodeoxyglucose uptake is high with a strong signal.

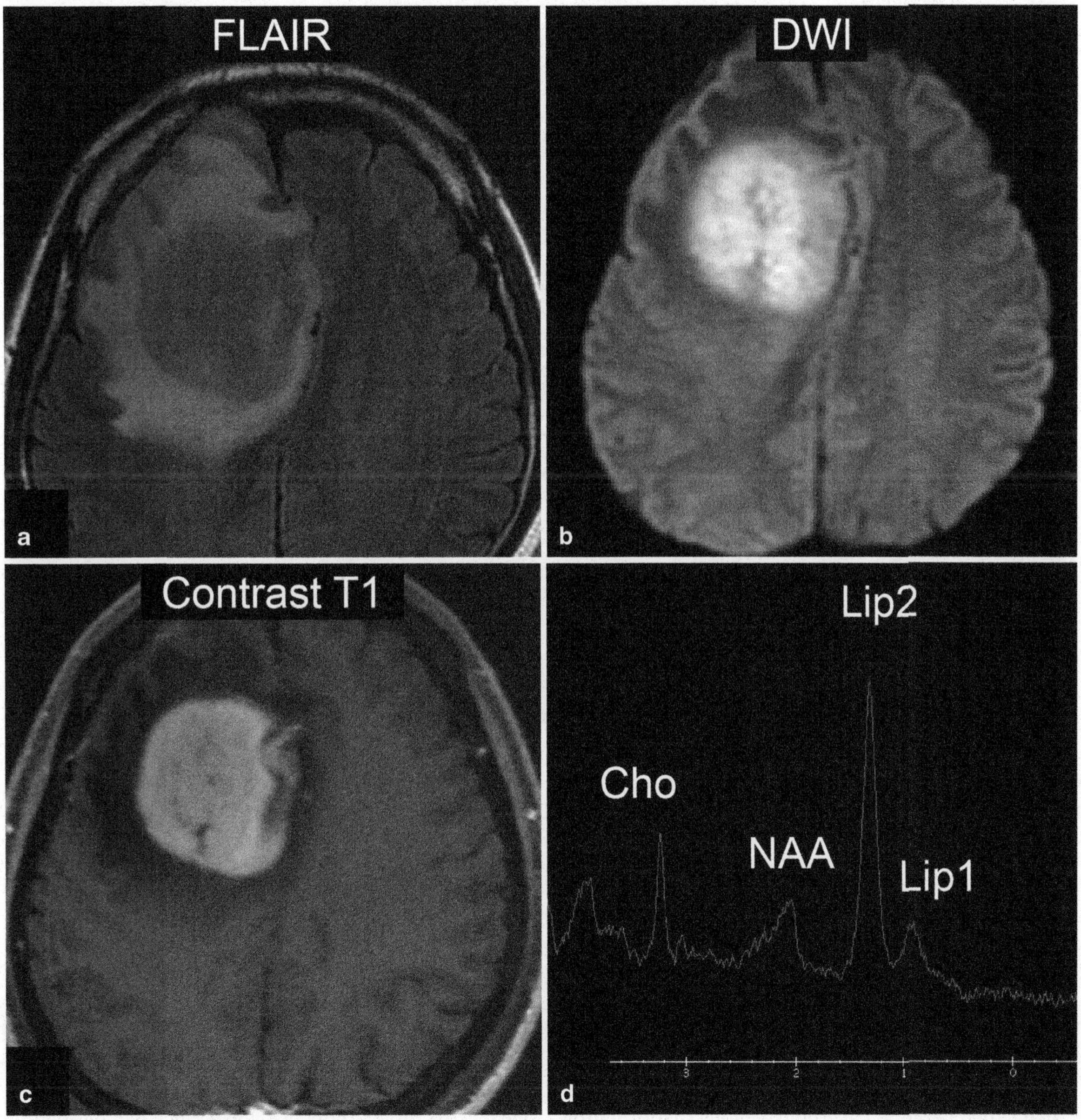

Fig. 6.15 M/61, CNS lymphoma. (**a**) MRI, FLAIR: An intracerebral tumor is observed in the right frontal lobe with peripheral white matter edema. (**b**) DWI: DWI shows that this tumor has a very high signal intensity, thus reflecting hypercellularity. (**c**) Contrast T1WI: The tumor is enhanced without central necrosis. (**d**) MRS (TE 35 ms): No elevation of Cho level and reduction in NAA are observed, indicating that the tumor is from glial cells. The extremely high peak in lipid level (1:0.9 mm and 2:1.3 ppm) is a characteristic sign of lymphoma. The above findings indicate lymphoma rather than a malignant glioma. The tumor was surgically removed and confirmed to be a diffuse large B-cell lymphoma by pathological examination

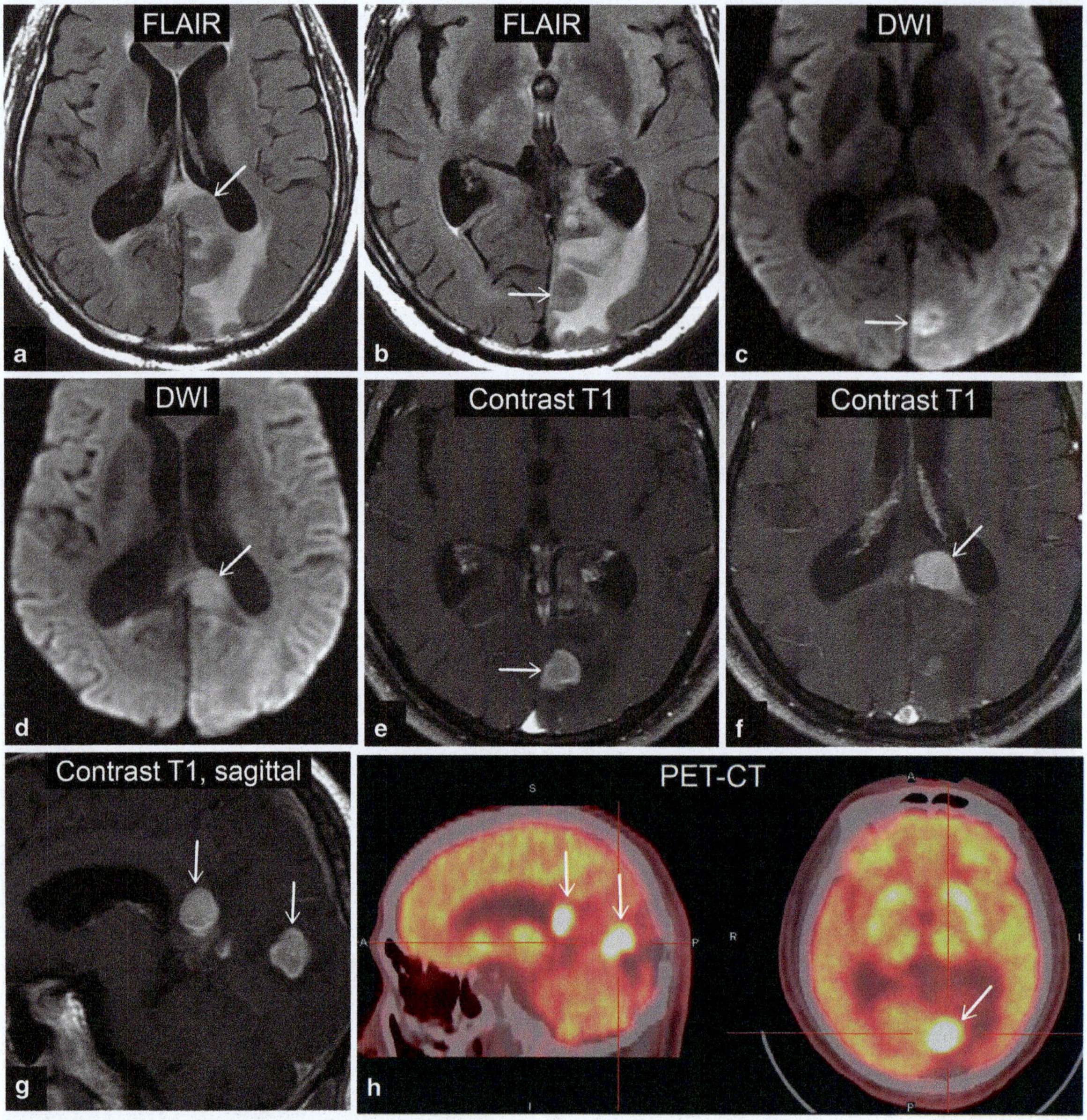

Fig. 6.16 M/76, CNS lymphoma. The patient has mild-degree dementia with increasing severity in the last month. (**a**, **b**) MRI, FLAIR: An area of white matter edema is observed in the left occipital lobe and splenium of the corpus callosum with two suspected tumors (arrows) in the edema area. (**c**, **d**) DWI: The two suspected tumors show hyperintensity (arrows) on DWI, the white matter edema has no signal change. (**e**–**g**) Contrast T1WI: The two tumors have strong enhancement without central necrosis (arrows). (**h**) FDG PET-CT: The two tumors show intense FDG uptake (arrows). The tumor in the occipital lobe was surgically removed, and the pathological findings showed non-GC-type diffuse large B-cell lymphoma

6.4.9 Hemangioma

Cerebral cavernous hemangioma, shortened to cavernoma, develops from blood vessels in the brain (Figs. 6.17 and 6.18). As the cavernous hemangioma is not a true neoplasm, so it is also called cerebral cavernous venous malformation. It is a common intracranial tumor, often observable in MRI examination. In most cases, patients never have symptoms. In some instances, the patient experiences intracerebral hemorrhage, with headache, seizure, or nervous symptoms.

CT: This tumor cannot be seen in CT images unless it is sufficiently large (Fig. 6.17), which appears white (hyperdense) on CT scans. Contrast media cannot enhance the tumor.

MRI: Because the hemangioma contains multiple small cysts, so a typical popcorn appearance can be seen in T2WI and FLAIR. T2*WI and SWI images more clearly show the hemosiderin in the hemangioma (Figs. 6.17 and 6.18).

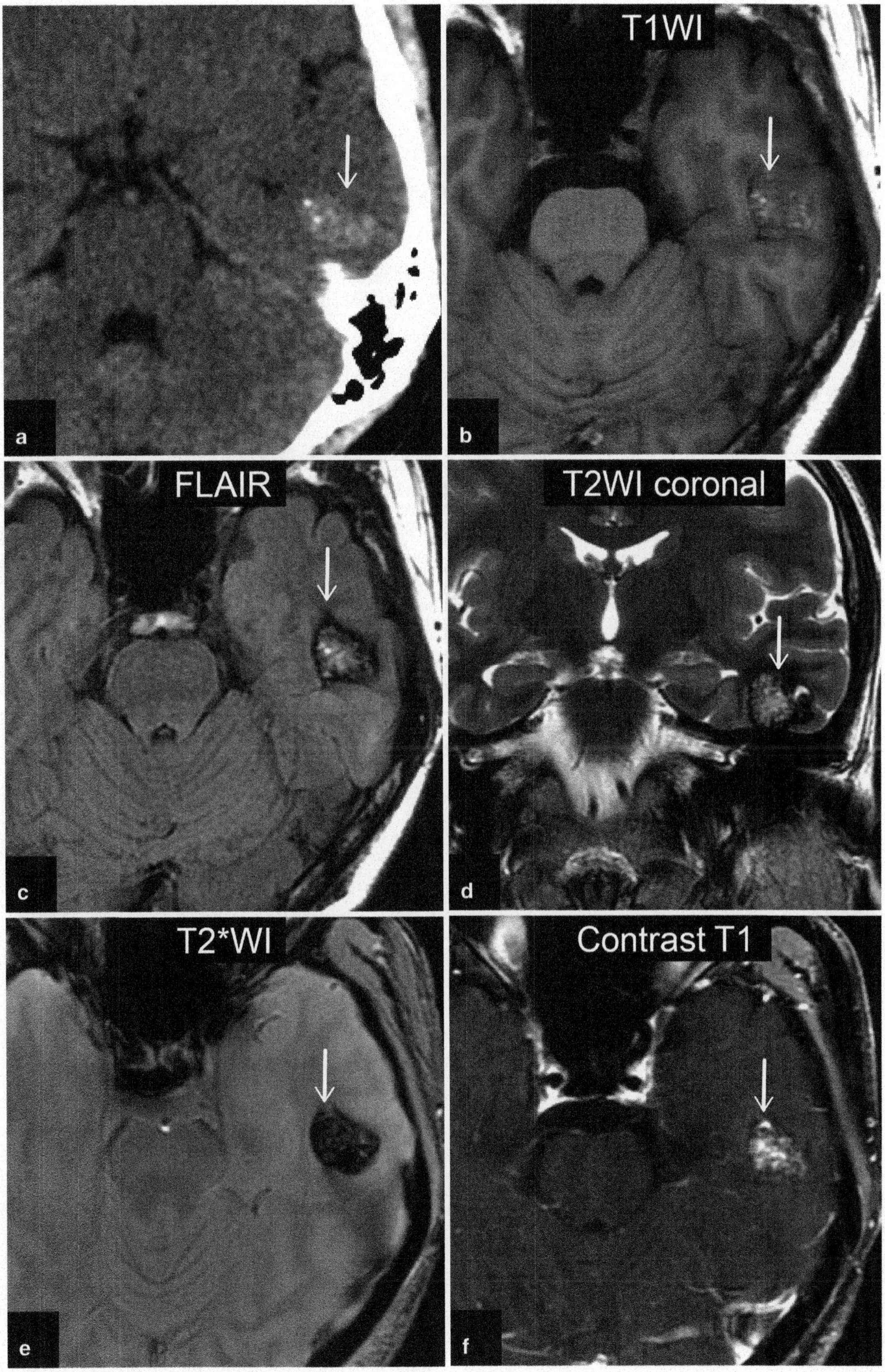

Fig. 6.17 M/26, Cavernous hemangioma. The patient received CT and MRI examinations because of seizures. (**a**) CT: A small mass with calcification (arrow) is observed in the left temporal lobe. (**b**) MRI, T1WI: The mass shows heterogeneous hyperintensity. (**c, d**) FLAIR, T2WI: The rim hypointensity reflects hemosiderin deposition. Many tiny cysts in this mass exhibit a "popcorn appearance." (**e**) T2*WI: The entire mass showing hypointensity reflects hemosiderin deposition. The mass still shows many tiny cysts. (**f**) Contrast T1WI: This mass is enhanced. A mass with numerous tiny cysts and hemosiderin deposition is a characteristic sign of cavernous hemangioma

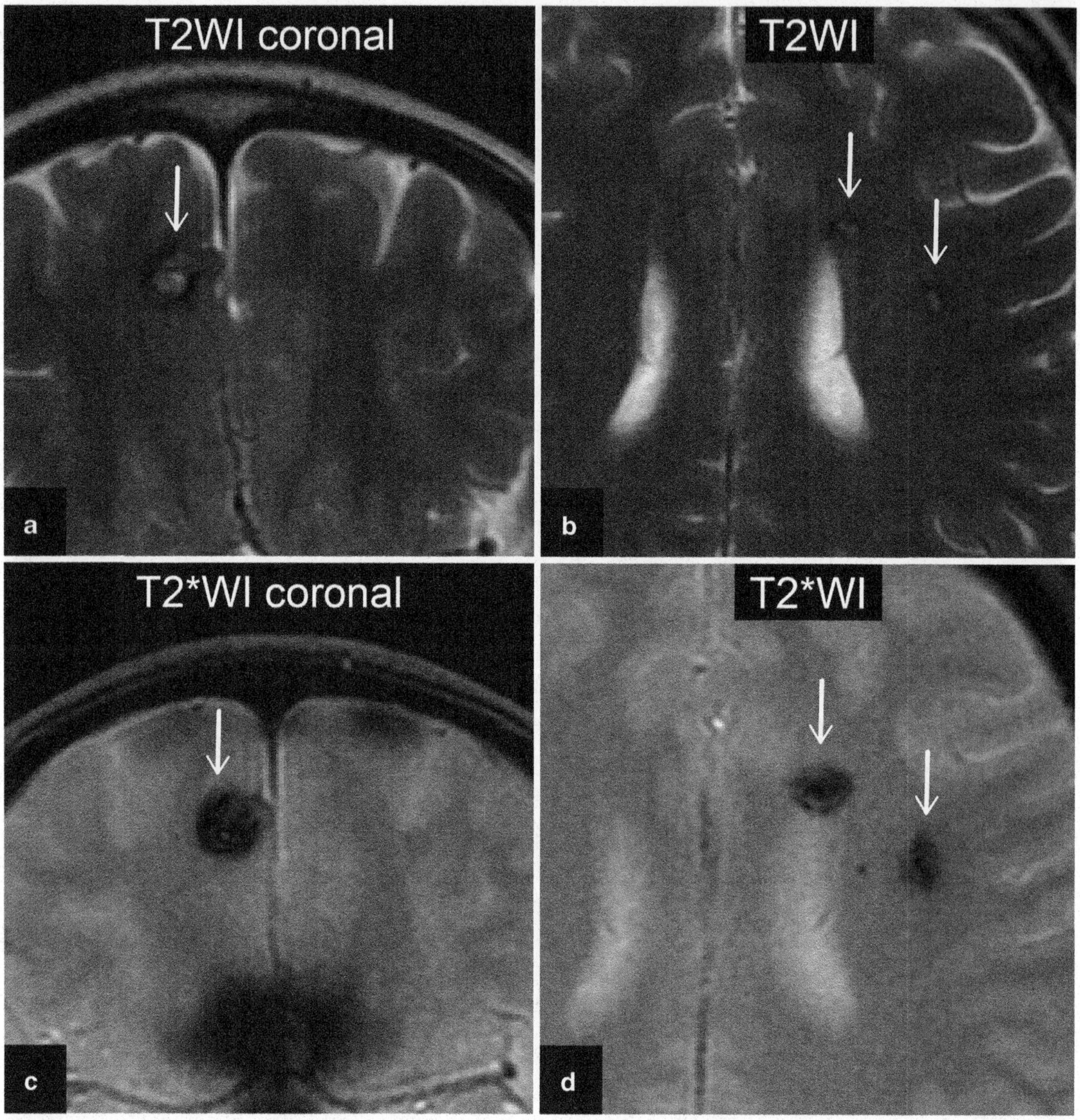

Fig. 6.18 F/25, Cavernous hemangiomas. A healthy lady received an MRI examination. Incidentally, multiple small lesions are present in the bilateral frontal lobes. T2*WI shows that all the masses have hemosiderin deposition, and T2WI presents tiny popcorn-like central cysts in the masses. Hence, all the lesions in the bilateral frontal lobes are small cavernous hemangiomas

6.4.10 Hemangioblastoma

Hemangioblastoma, WHO Gr I.

This tumor develops from blood vessels in the brain and mostly in the cerebellum (Fig. 6.19, 6.20, and 6.21). It can also develop in the spinal cord. Approximately 20% of hemangioblastomas accompany von Hippel-Lindau disease. By contrast, about 40% of patients with von Hippel-Lindau disease develop hemangioblastoma in their lifetime (Fig. 6.20).

Age: Mostly young adults.

CT and MRI: Two types exist:

1. A large cyst with a mural nodule can be identified (Figs. 6.20 and 6.21). This mural nodule can be enhanced by contrast media, whereas the cyst is a pseudocyst, the cyst wall of which cannot be enhanced by contrast medium.
2. Only a single round tumor exists (Figs. 6.19 and 6.20), and it is strongly enhanced by contrast medium.

Both the mural nodule in a cyst and the single round tumor represent the hemangioblastoma itself. During vertebral angiography, these structures contain abundant abnormal vessels and exhibit intense tumor staining.

Hemangioblastoma, either as a cyst with a mural nodule or a single-round tumor, can be enhanced by contrast medium; however, it does not show slightly hyperintense DWI signals as most intracranial tumors do. Hemangioblastoma is hypointense (dark) on DWI (Fig. 6.19) or exhibits no signal change because hemangioblastoma has abundant blood vessels and contains a large volume of blood. This imaging sign is useful in discriminating hemangioblastoma from other cerebellar tumors [6].

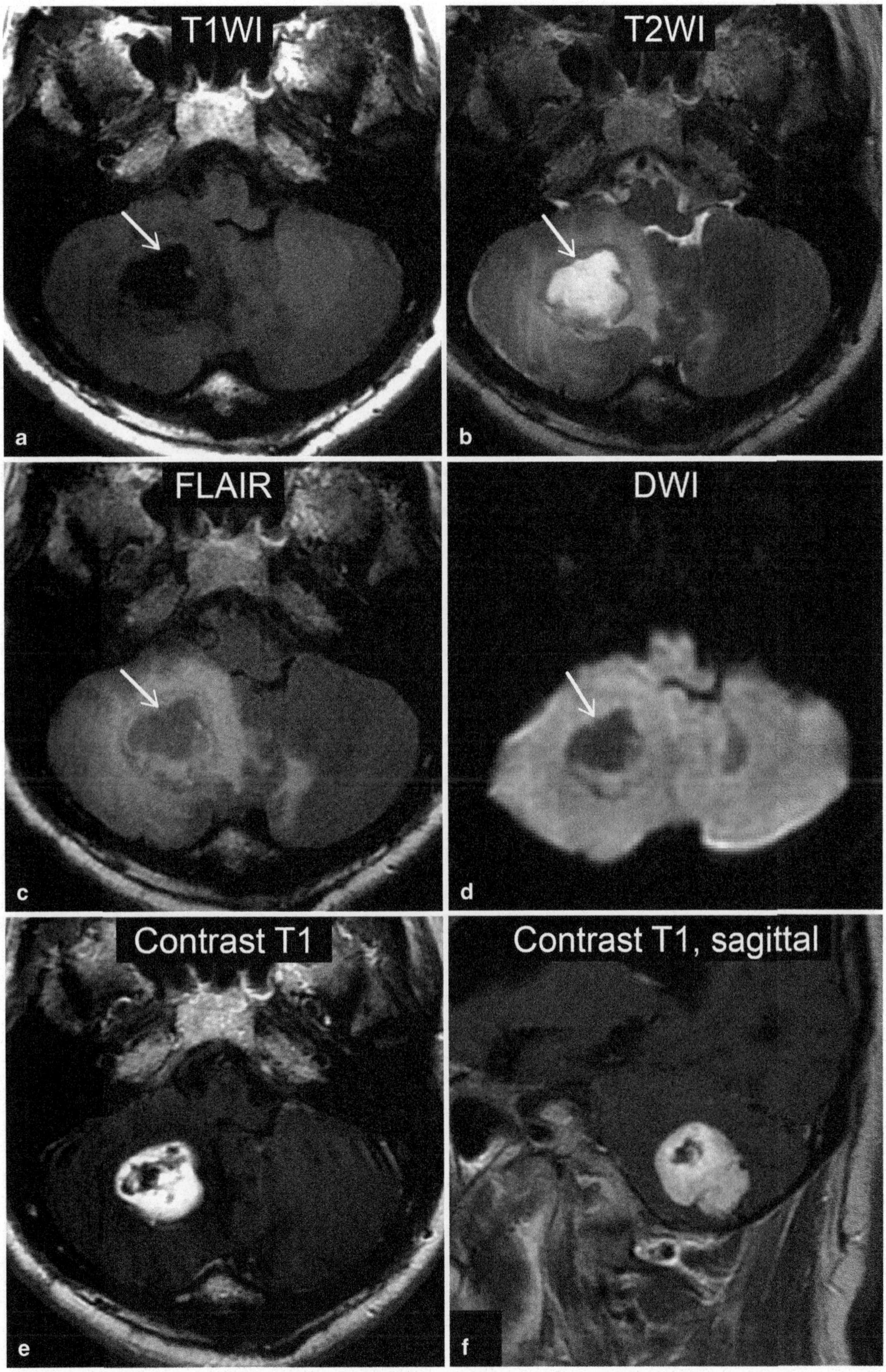

Fig. 6.19 M/51, Hemangioblastoma. This patient suffered from severe headaches for 1 month. (**a–d**) MRI: A tumor (arrows) in the right cerebellum with peripheral white matter edema. The tumor shows hypointensity (dark) on T1WI and hyperintensity (white) on T2WI and is dark gray on FLAIR and dark on DWI. Hence, this tumor likely contains fluid, is a cystic mass. (**e**, **f**) Contrast T1WI: This tumor has strong enhancement by Gd-DTPA, which only has some central necrosis. Hence, the tumor has high vascularity, actually is a solid mass. This tumor was surgically removed and confirmed to be hemangioblastoma (WHO grade I) by pathological examination. Comment: A solid tumor that shows hypointensity on DWI is a characteristic sign for hemangioblastoma

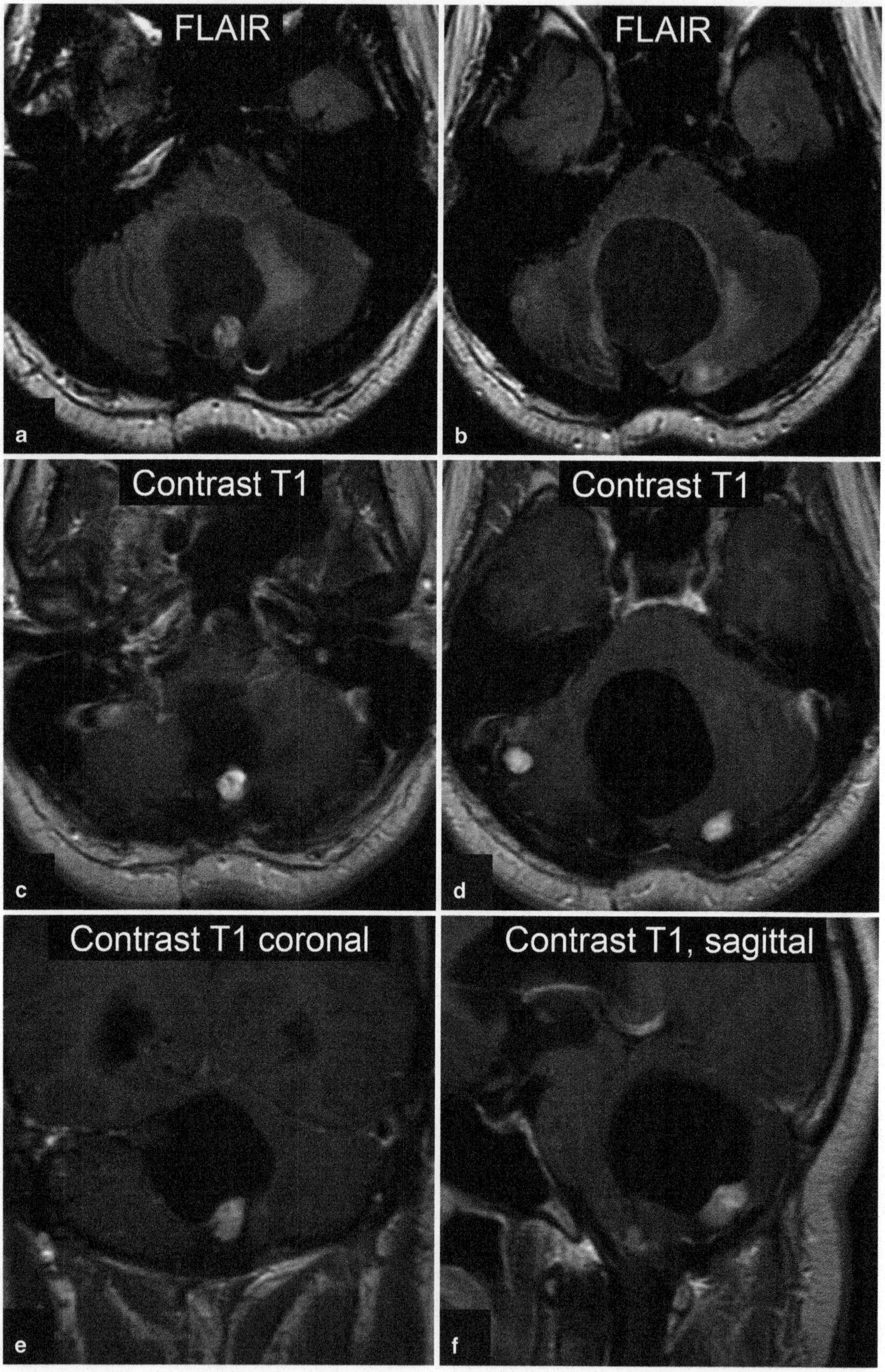

Fig. 6.20 M/40, Hemangioblastoma. This is a patient with von Hippel–Lindau disease and has a history of renal cell carcinoma and adrenal tumor. (**a**, **b**) FLAIR: A large cystic tumor in the middle of the cerebellum, a nodular soft tissue mass with hyperintensity in the posterior wall, and some peripheral white matter edema in the left cerebellum are observed. (**c**–**f**) Contrast T1WI: The nodular mass in the posterior wall of this large cystic mass has strong contrast enhancement but shows no contrast enhancement on the cystic wall. The other two small nodular masses with strong enhancement are observed in the bilateral cerebella. The three tumors were surgically removed and confirmed to be hemangioblastomas by pathological examination. Comment: This patient has three cerebellar hemangioblastomas. One appears as a big cyst with mural nodular mass; the cyst is a pseudocyst, so no enhancement on the wall, this tumor has "mural nodular sign," and it is a characteristic sign of hemangioblastoma. The other two appear as small solid masses

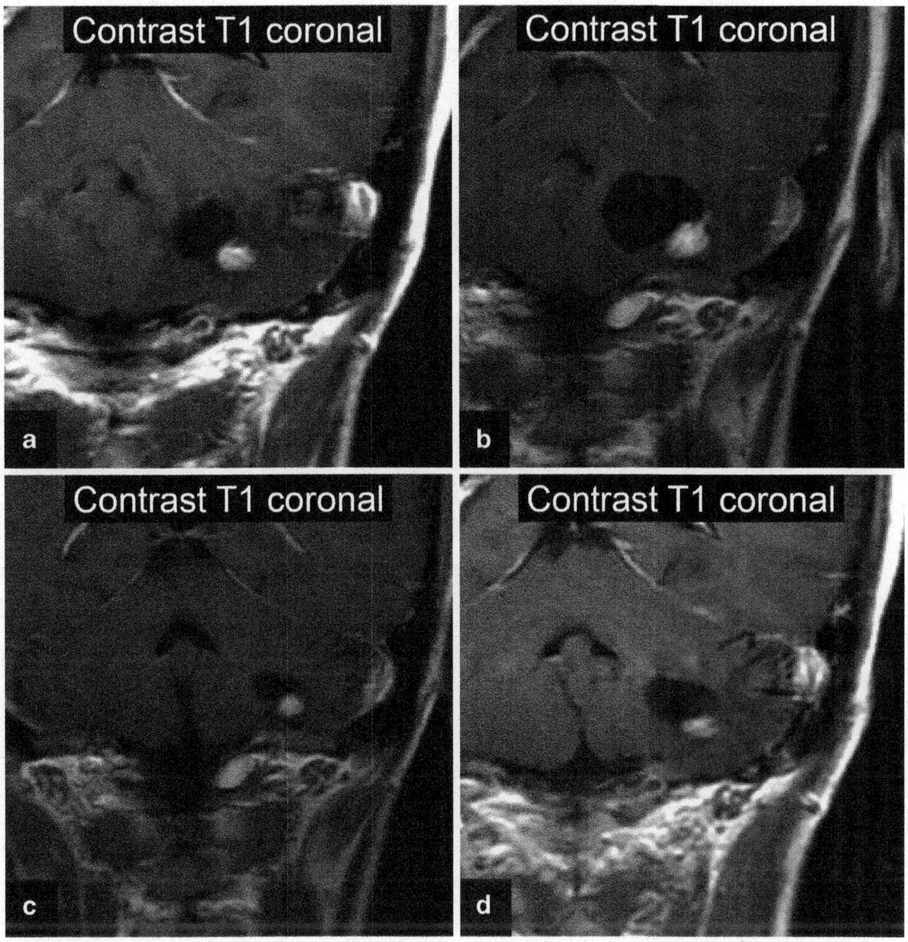

Fig. 6.21 F/53, Hemangioblastoma. The patient complained of dizziness and inability to stand still for 1 month. (**a**) MRI, contrast T1WI: A small nodular mass is associated with the cyst in the left cerebellum. Strong enhancement of the nodular mass, unenhanced the cystic wall. The "mural nodular sign" is a characteristic sign of hemangioblastoma. (**b**) The second follow-up MRI was performed after 6 months. A slight enlargement of the cyst with mural nodular mass is observed. (**c**) Post gamma knife radiation treatment and third follow-up MRI was performed after 9 months. The sizes of the tumor mass decrease. (**d**) Fourth follow-up MRI was performed after 6 years. This tumor remains the same

6.4.11 Metastasis

Metastases include intra-axial cerebral parenchymal metastases (Figs. 6.22, 6.23, 6.24, 6.25, 6.26, 6.27, and 6.28), ventricular wall or intraventricular metastases, and subarachnoid or leptomeningeal metastases (Figs. 6.22, 6.28, and 6.29) as well as extra-axial skull and skull base metastases (Figs. 6.23 and 6.28). Metastasis is mainly hematogenous. Because the brain requires a considerable amount of blood, malignant tumors in any part of the body may metastasize to the brain or skull through blood circulation.

Direct invasion of tumors also occurs. For example, nasopharyngeal carcinoma, paranasal sinus carcinoma, and oral carcinoma can directly invade the skull base and brain.

Brain metastasis can be observed through imaging based on the following signs:

1. Multiple in number.
2. Small in volume.
3. Necrosis often occurs in the center, forming ring enhancement.
4. Disproportional large areas of peritumoral white matter edema.

These are imaging signs of brain parenchymal metastasis; however, they are not absolute standards. Some metastases may exist in solitary form, exhibit large-volume tumors, generate no tumor necrosis, and possibly lack peritumoral white matter edema.

In most patients with a known history of malignant carcinomas in other body parts, once one or multiple intracranial tumors have been identified, metastasis must be considered. Hence, the diagnosis of brain metastasis is not difficult.

In addition to intracranial metastases, combine with leptomeningeal metastases also often occurs (Figs. 6.22, 6.28, and 6.29), resulting in poor CSF circulation and hydrocephalus.

Brain metastases are often complicated with skull or skull base metastases, most of which are osteolytic metastases (Figs. 6.23 and 6.28).

A single metastasis tumor with necrosis in the center, ring enhancement, and peritumoral white matter edema has similar feature to brain abscess in imaging. DWI can then be used for discrimination. Metastasis necrosis often shows no diffusion restriction in DWI, appearing dark in the image (Figs. 6.24, 6.25, 6.26, and 6.27). By contrast, the pus of an abscess has intense diffusion restriction, appearing white in DWI (Chap. 7).

In MRS, the elevation of lactate and lipid is seen in the necrotic part of the metastatic tumor [5] (Figs. 6.24 and 6.25).

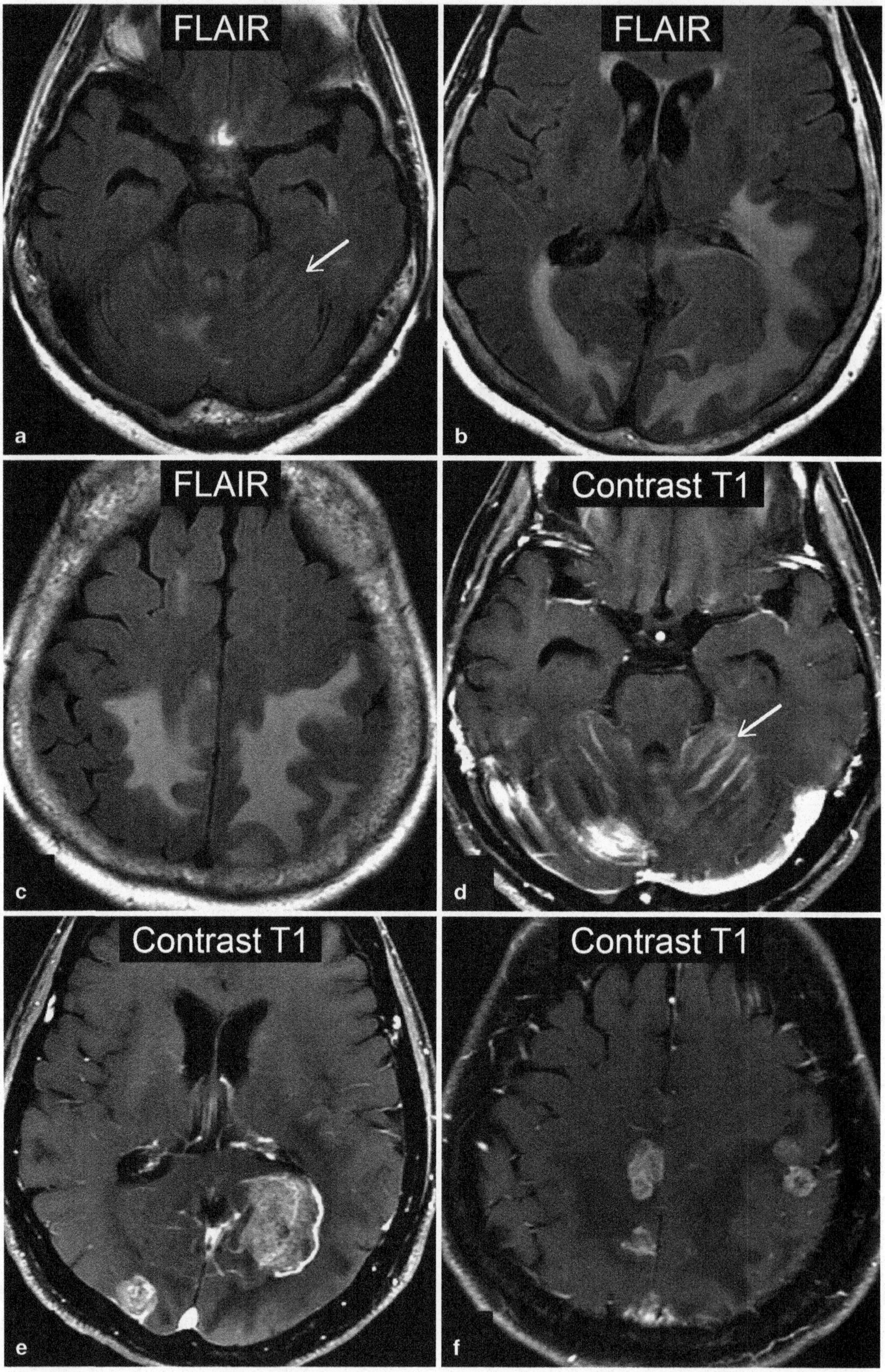

Fig. 6.22 F/62, Breast cancer with brain metastases. (**a–c**) FLAIR: White matter edemas are observed in the right cerebellum and bilateral parieto-occipital lobes. The sulci of bilateral cerebella show linear hyperintensity (arrow). (**d–f**) Contrast-enhanced T1WI: Enhanced tumor masses with variable sizes within or on the margin of white matter edemas indicate brain metastases. The linear enhancement in the sulci of bilateral cerebella indicates leptomeningeal metastases (arrow)

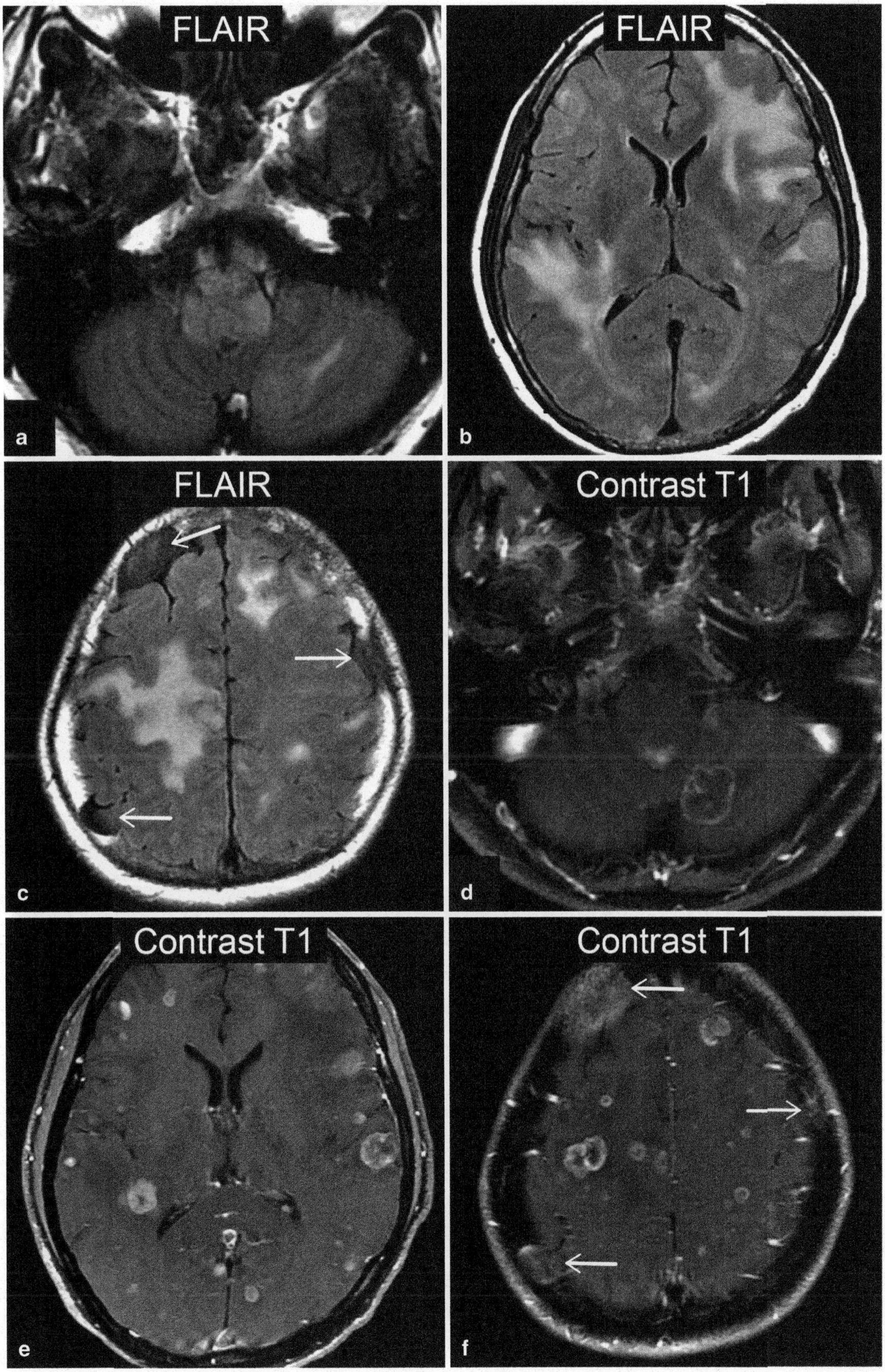

Fig. 6.23 F/42, Lung cancer with the brain and cranial metastases. (**a–c**) MRI, FLAIR: Multiple areas of brain tissue edemas are observed in the brainstem, left cerebellum, and bilateral cerebral hemispheres. The edemas are mainly in the white matter. (**d–f**) Contrast T1WI: Many small tumor masses are enhanced, and most have central necroses that form ring enhancements. The above tumor masses are typical brain metastases. Three areas of bony metastases are observed in the cranium (arrows)

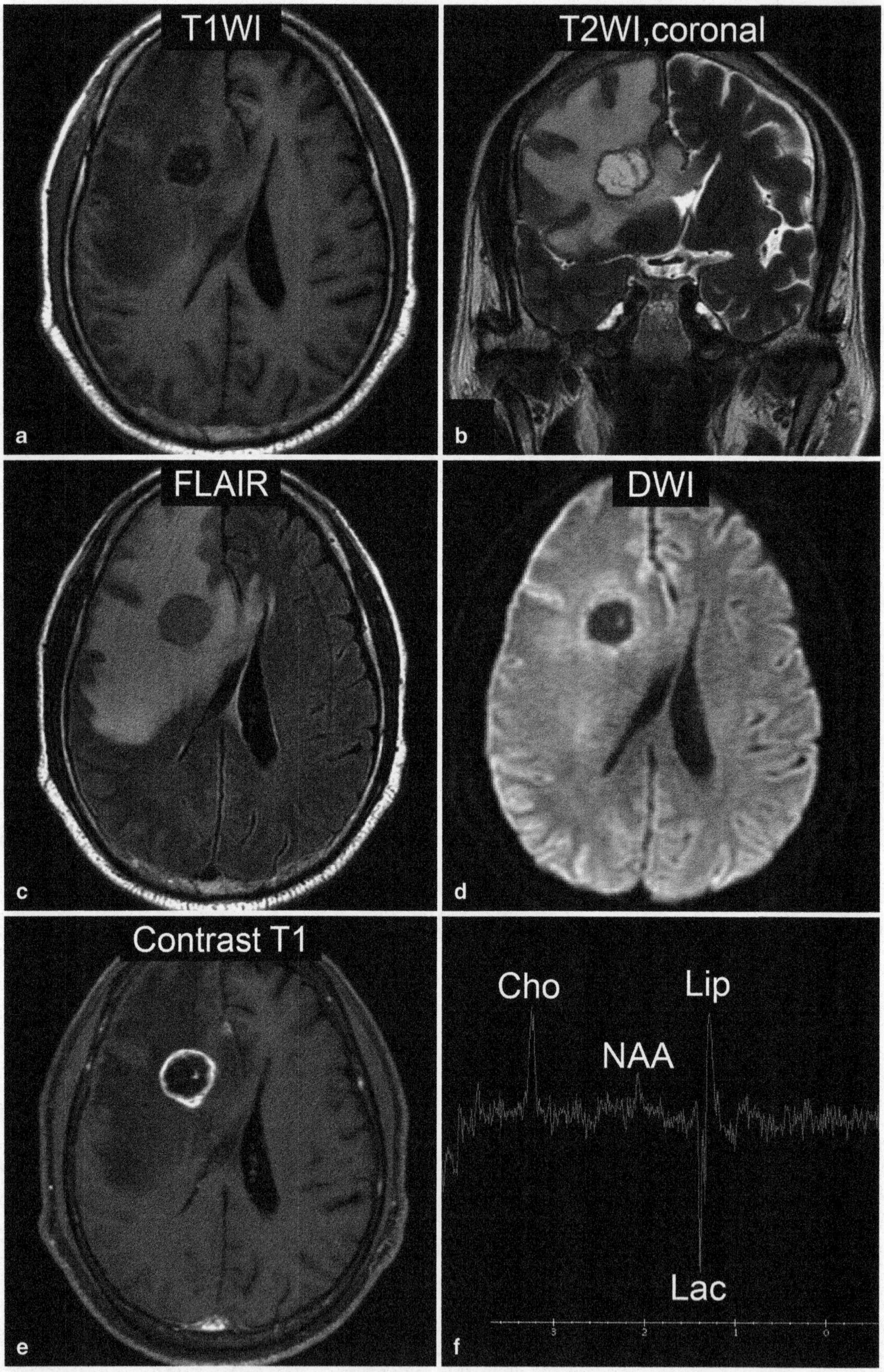

Fig. 6.24 M/51, Solitary metastases from silent lung cancer. The patient suffered from dizziness, headache, and weakness in the left limbs, and was suspected of having suffered a stroke. (**a–e**) MRI: A small mass in the right frontal lobe has a large area of peripheral white matter edema. This mass shows hypointensity on T1WI, hyperintensity on T2WI, intermediate signal intensity on FLAIR, hypointensity on DWI, and ring enhancement after contrast medium administration. Hence, the tumor demonstrates severe central necrosis. (**f**) MRS (TE 144 ms): The extremely low NAA and elevated lactate/lipid levels are the MRS characteristics of metastasis. Pathological examination confirms metastasis from a silent lung small-cell carcinoma

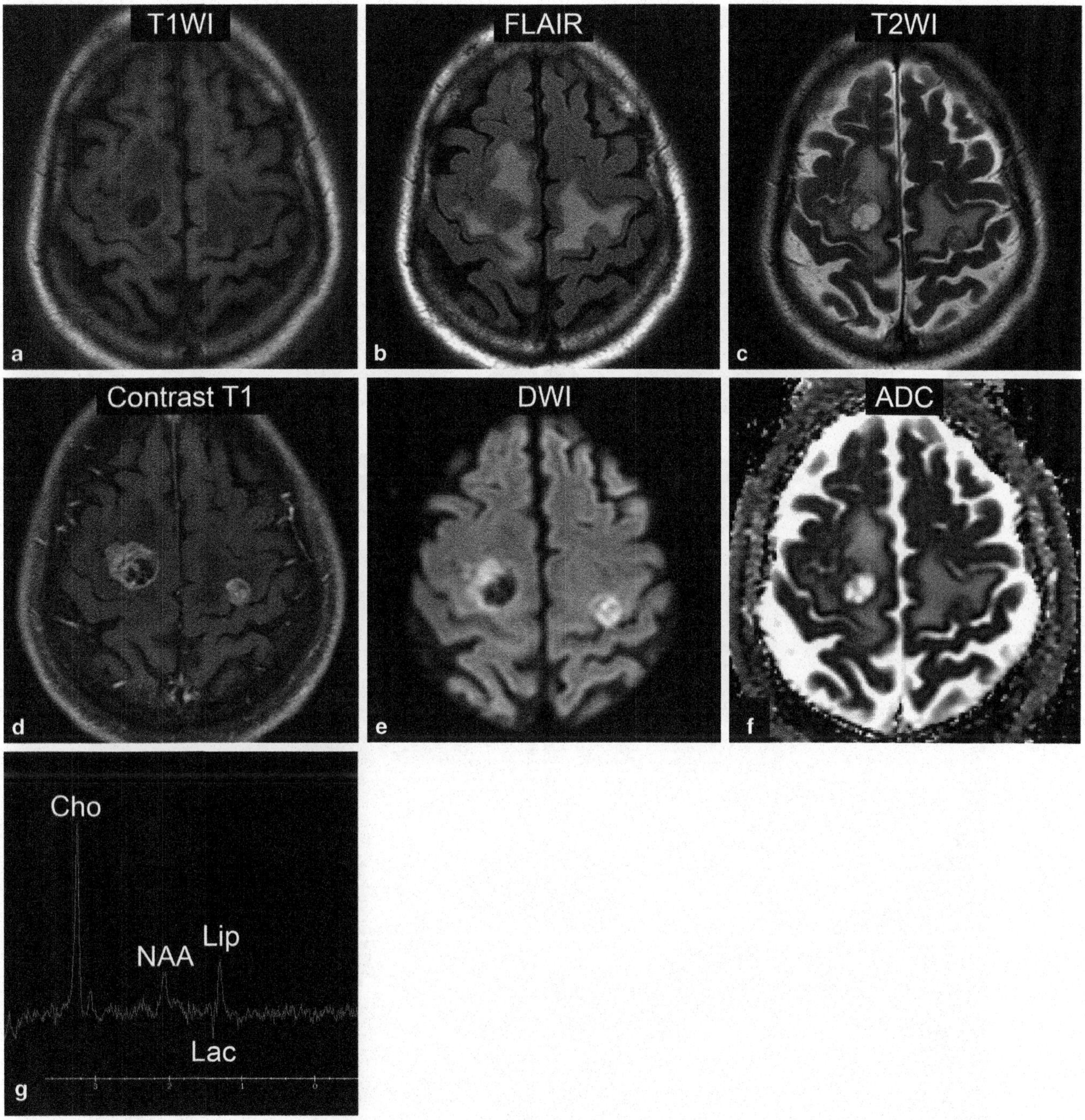

Fig. 6.25 M/79, Lung cancer with brain metastases. (**a–f**) MRI: Two small tumor masses are observed in the deep portions of the bilateral frontal lobes with peripheral white matter edema. Contrast T1WI shows central necrosis in the right tumor with the necrotic part showing hypointensity on T1WI, hyperintensity on T2WI, hypointensity on DWI, and hyperintensity on ADC, which reflects a fluid component. The left tumor is solid, showing mild hyperintensity on DWI, hypointensity on ADC. (**g**) MRS (TE 144 ms): The tumor shows elevated Cho level and reduced NAA level and with lactate/lipid

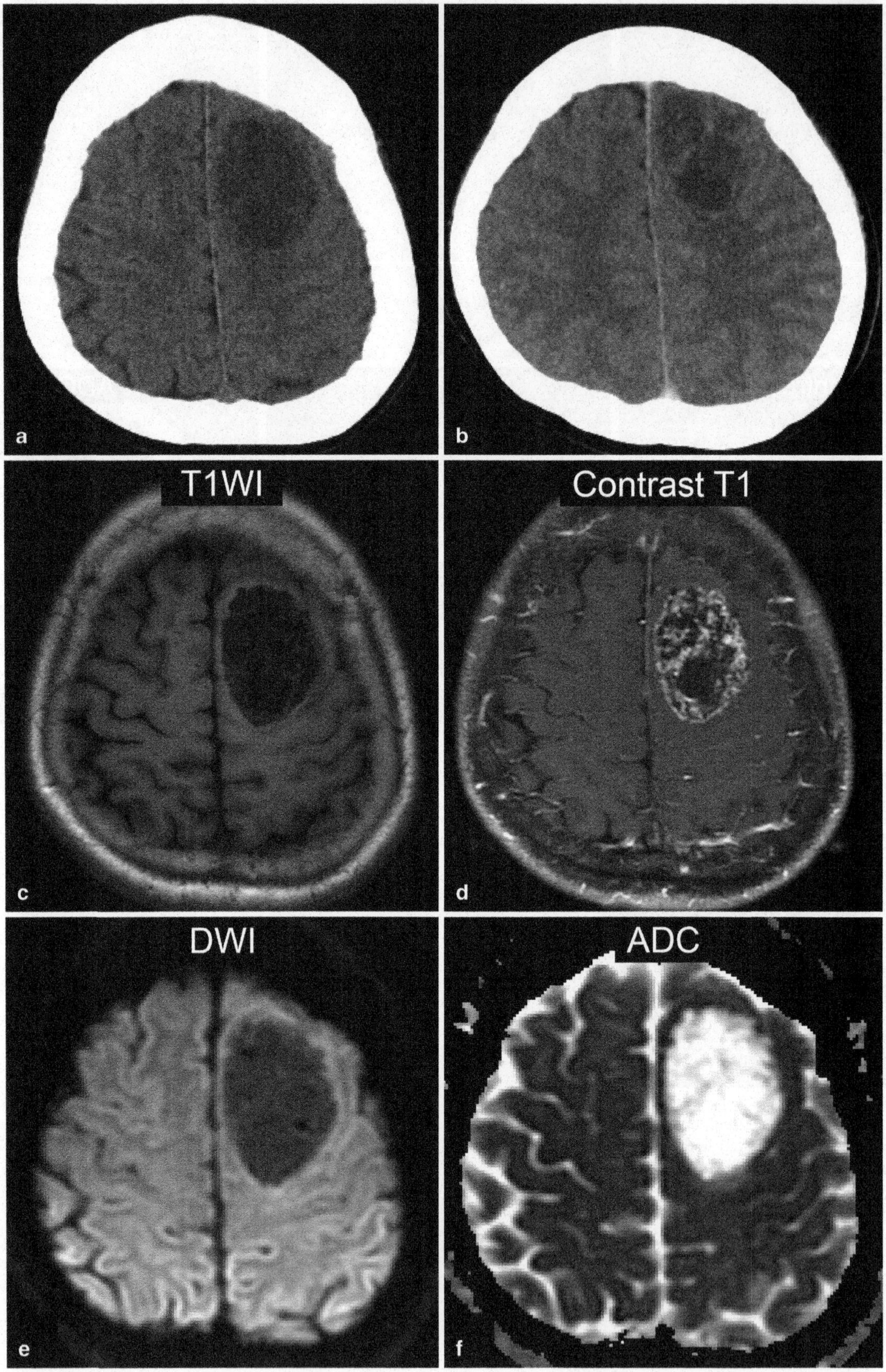

Fig. 6.26 F/57, Solitary metastasis. CT and MRI were performed for a clinical symptom of a seizure. (**a**) CT: A hypodense tumor mass is observed in the left frontal lobe. (**b**) Contrast CT: The tumor exhibits slight enhancement. Hence, the tumor mass possibly has a cystic component or severe central necrosis. (**c, d**) MRI, T1WI, and contrast T1WI: Hypointensity on T1W and heterogeneous enhancement of this tumor reflect irregular central necrosis. (**e, f**) DWI, ADC: Hypointensity on DWI and hyperintensity on ADC of this tumor are characteristic signs of severe tumor necrosis. The tumor was surgically removed and confirmed to be a metastatic adenocarcinoma from lung cancer by pathological examination

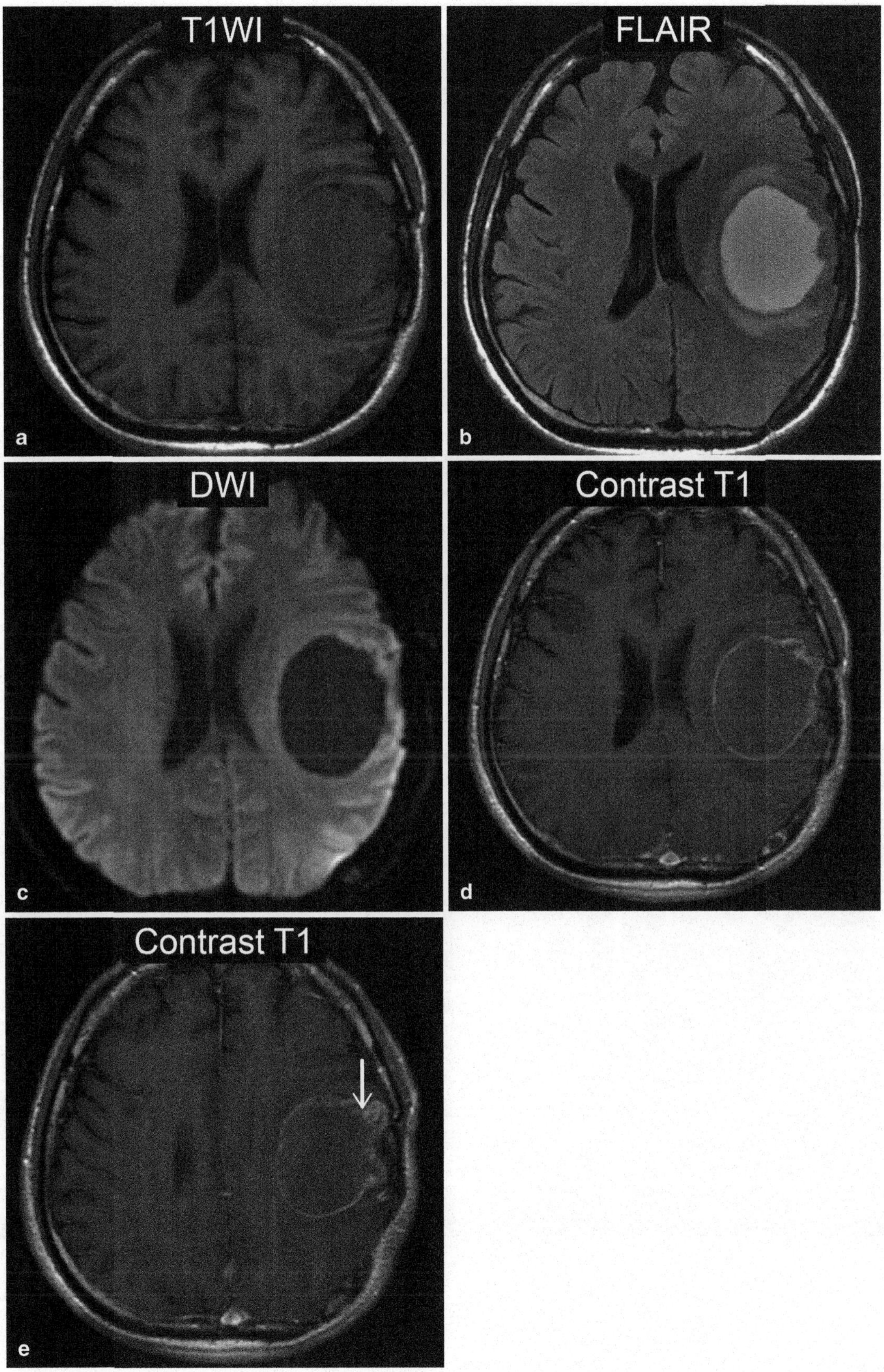

Fig. 6.27 M/51, Solitary metastasis. A thyroid cancer patient complained of weakness in the right limbs for 2 weeks. MRI reveals a large mass in the left frontoparietal lobes that shows intermediate signal intensity on T1WI, hyperintensity on FLAIR. Contrast T1WI shows ring enhancement, which reflects severe central necrosis; the features are like a brain abscess. However, the lateral wall is slightly thick (arrow); this is the portion of soft tissue mass and hypointensity on DWI, hence, this mass is not an abscess. The tumor was surgically removed and confirmed to be a metastatic tumor of thyroid carcinoma by pathological examination

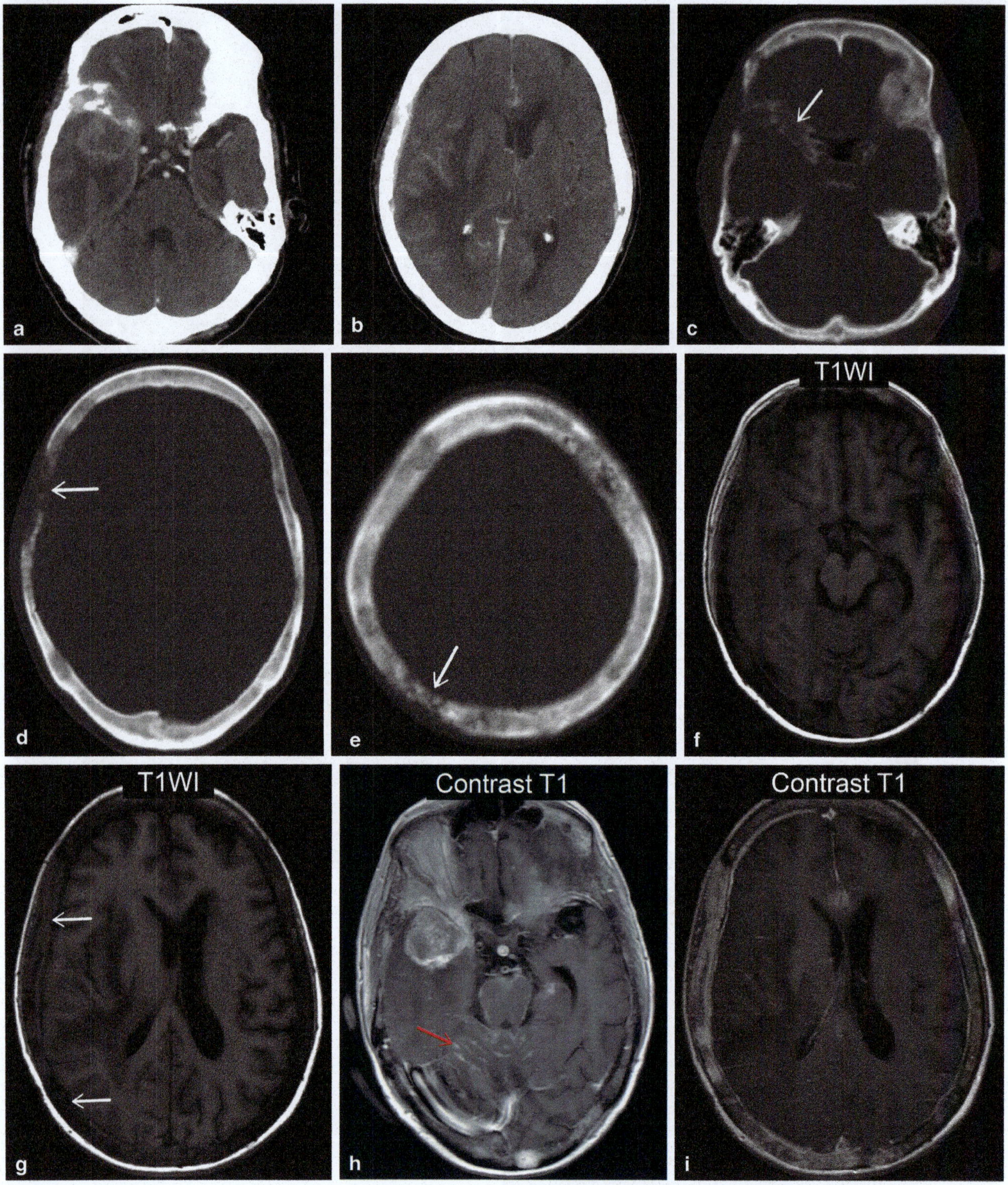

Fig. 6.28 F/62, Breast cancer with the brain and cranial metastases. (**a**, **b**) Contrast CT: A tumor with central necrosis is observed in the right temporal lobe with a large area of peripheral white matter edema that even extends to the right internal and external capsules. (**c–e**) CT, bone window settings: The osteolytic lesions (arrows) in the sphenoid bone and frontal and parietal cranial bones are bony metastases. (**f–i**) MRI, T1WI, and contrast T1WI: The findings are similar to those of CT. The bony metastases (arrows) show contrast enhancement, and leptomeningeal metastasis (red arrow) is observed in the sulci of the superior vermis

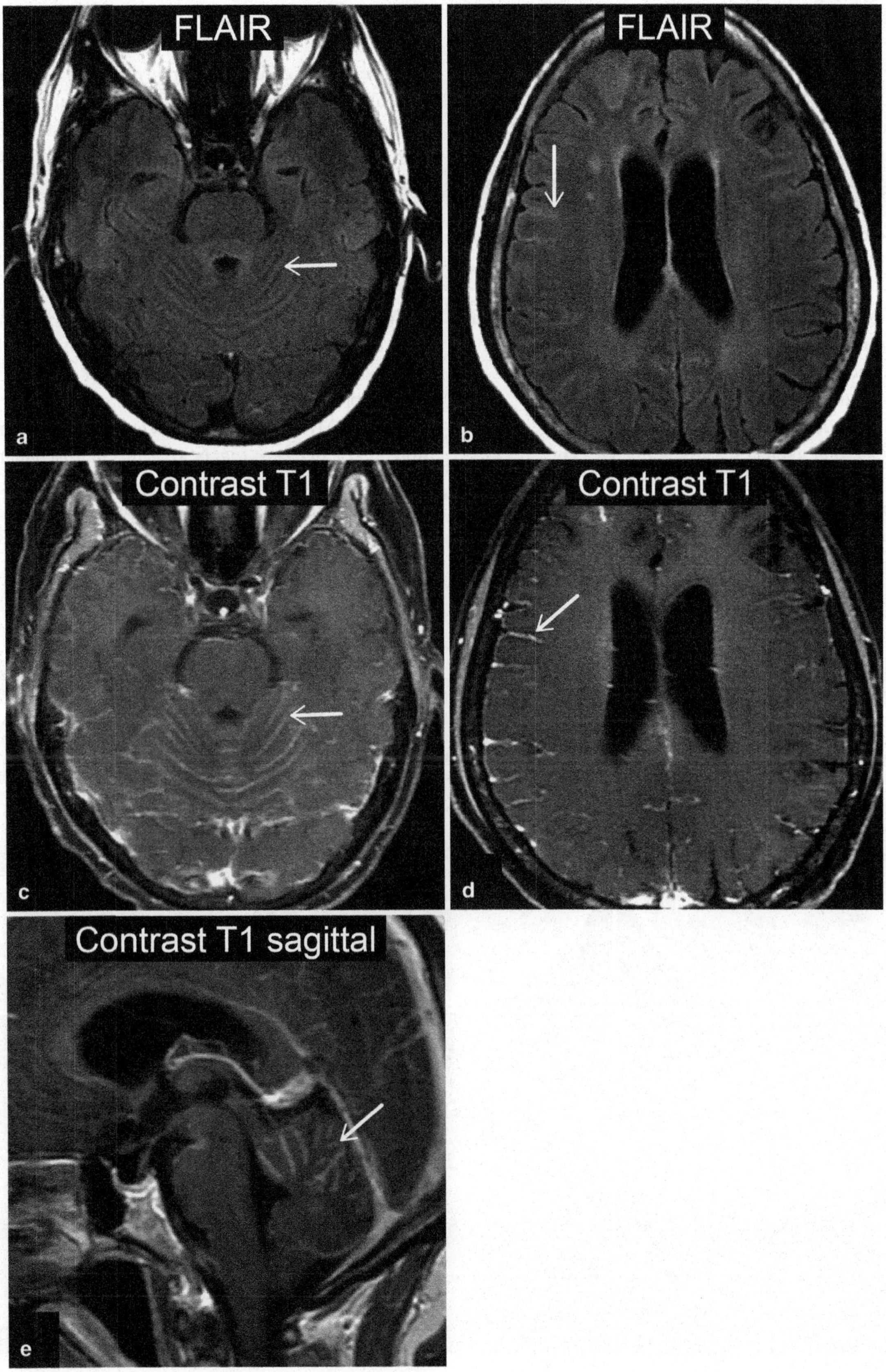

Fig. 6.29 F/55, Leptomeningeal metastasis. A breast cancer patient complained of headache and dizziness. (**a**, **b**) MRI, FLAIR: There are slight widening of cerebellar and cerebral sulci with sulcus hyperintensity sign (arrows) and mild dilatation of the bilateral lateral ventricles. (**c**–**e**) Contrast T1WI: The linear enhancements in the sulci (arrows) of the cerebellum and right cerebral hemisphere indicate leptomeningeal metastases, which is a type of subarachnoid metastasis

6.5 Intraventricular Tumors

Intraventricular tumors have two types. Tumors develop from ventricular walls and the choroid plexus [7]. Ventricular walls contain ependymal cells, glial cells, and neurons. Therefore, ependymoma, astrocytoma, and neurocytoma may develop. The choroid plexus contains neuroepithelial cells, creating CSF and growing papilloma and carcinoma. The choroid plexus also contains arachnoid cap cells that grow meningioma.

Neoplasms of the Ventricular Wall and Septum Pellucidum:

- Ependymoma Gr II, III (Figs. 6.30 and 6.31).
- Subependymoma Gr I.
- Central neurocytoma Gr II (Fig. 6.32).
- Subependymal giant cell astrocytoma Gr I (Fig. 6.11).

Neoplasms of the Choroid Plexus:

- Choroid plexus papilloma Gr I, II (Figs. 6.33 and 6.34), and carcinoma Gr III.
- Meningioma Gr I (Fig. 6.35).

6.5.1 Ependymoma

The ependymal cells are a thin layer of cells on the ventricular wall and in the central canal of the spinal cord. Therefore, ependymoma mostly develops on the ventricular wall or in the spinal cord. It may also develop in the cerebral hemisphere.

Intracranial ependymoma is mostly seen in the fourth ventricle (Fig. 6.31), which accounts for 60% of all cases. It may also develop at the lateral ventricle (Fig. 6.30) and third ventricle.

Age: Both children and adults may develop ependymoma, with more instances in children, especially those between 1 and 5 years. Ependymoma development another peak at the age of approximately 30 years.

CT and MRI: CT can be used to discover tumor calcification in 50% of cases (Fig. 6.30). The contrast enhancement is observable with some cystic change. Calcification cannot be easily identified using MRI. However, the relationship between the tumor and the ventricle is clear in MRI.

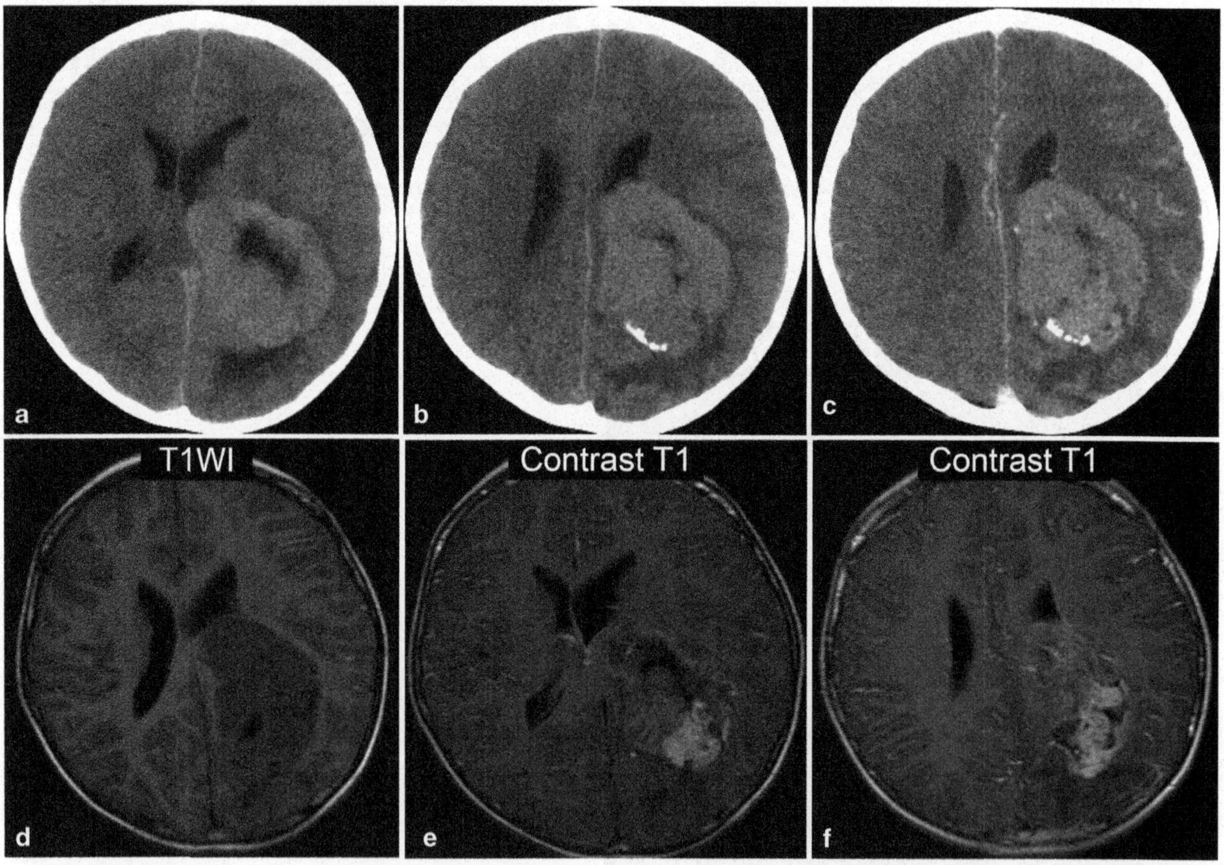

Fig. 6.30 M/6, Ependymoma of the lateral ventricle. (**a–c**) CT: A large tumor is observed in the left lateral ventricle with some marginal linear calcification (**b**) and mild contrast enhancement (**c**). (**d–f**) MRI: The tumor shows hypointensity on T1WI, and its contrast enhancement is more evident in the MRI than CT. The tumor was surgically removed and confirmed to be an anaplastic ependymoma (WHO grade III) by pathological examination

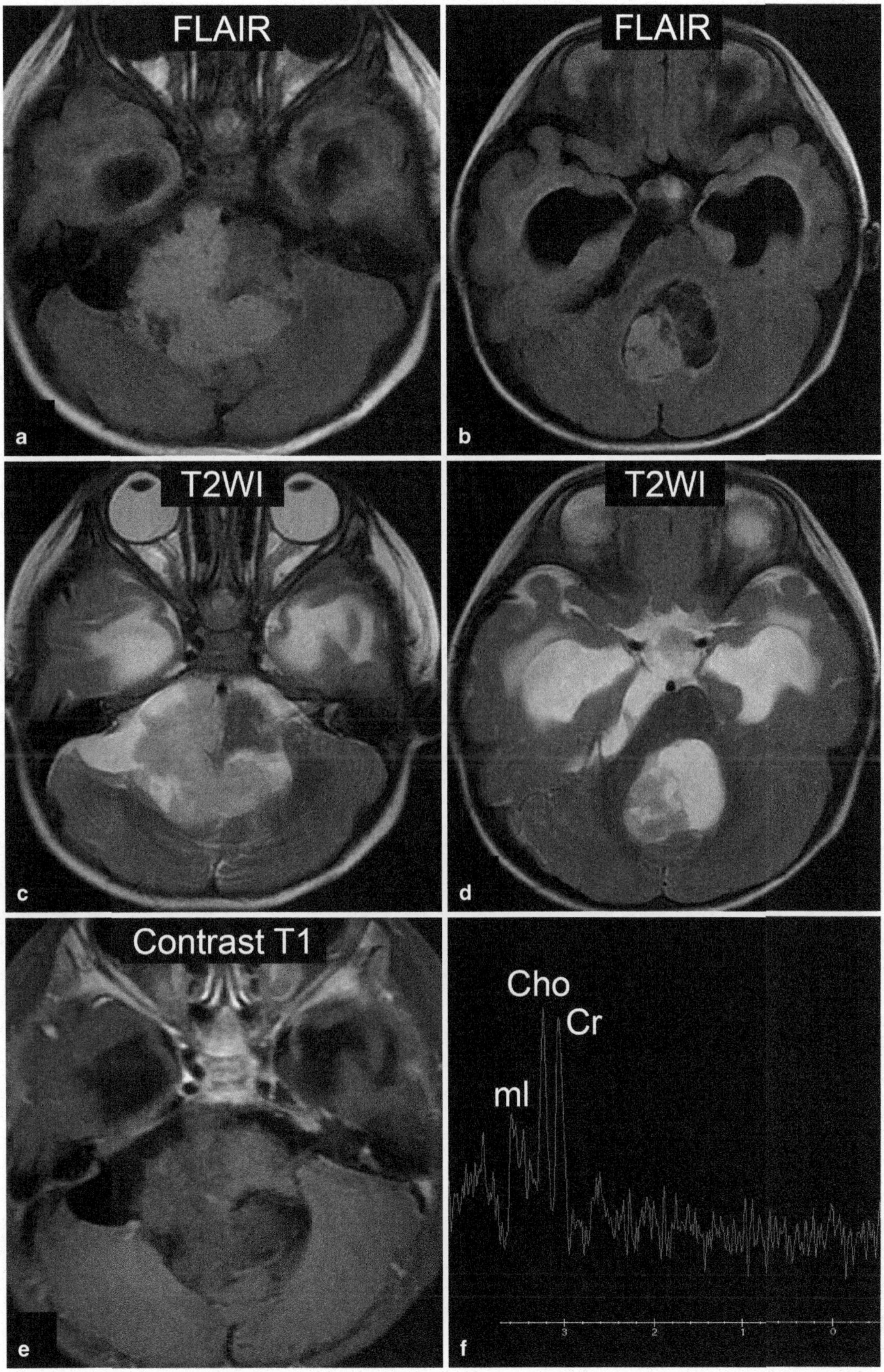

Fig. 6.31 F/16, Ependymoma of the fourth ventricle. (**a–d**) MRI: A tumor in the fourth ventricle anteriorly extends and compresses the right side of the medulla oblongata. (**e**) Contrast T1WI: The tumor shows weak contrast enhancement. (**f**) MRS (TE 144 ms): The tumor shows elevated Cho, Cr, and myoInositol (mI) levels, and NAA is absent. The tumor was surgically removed and confirmed to be an ependymoma, WHO grade II, by pathological examination

6.5.2 Central Neurocytoma

Central neurocytoma is an intraventricular tumor developing from neurons in the foramen of Monro or septum pellucidum (Fig. 6.32). It is a slowly growing, benign tumor.

Age: Young adults; more common in women than men.

CT and MRI: The tumor fully occupies the lateral ventricle with numerous tiny cysts and a moderate level of contrast enhancement. In CT, most tumors can be observed to have certain calcifications. Because most central neurocytomas are large and fully occupy the two lateral ventricles with many tiny cysts, the entire tumor plus the enlarged ventricles looks like a "leopard," which is a characteristic sign of central neurocytoma.

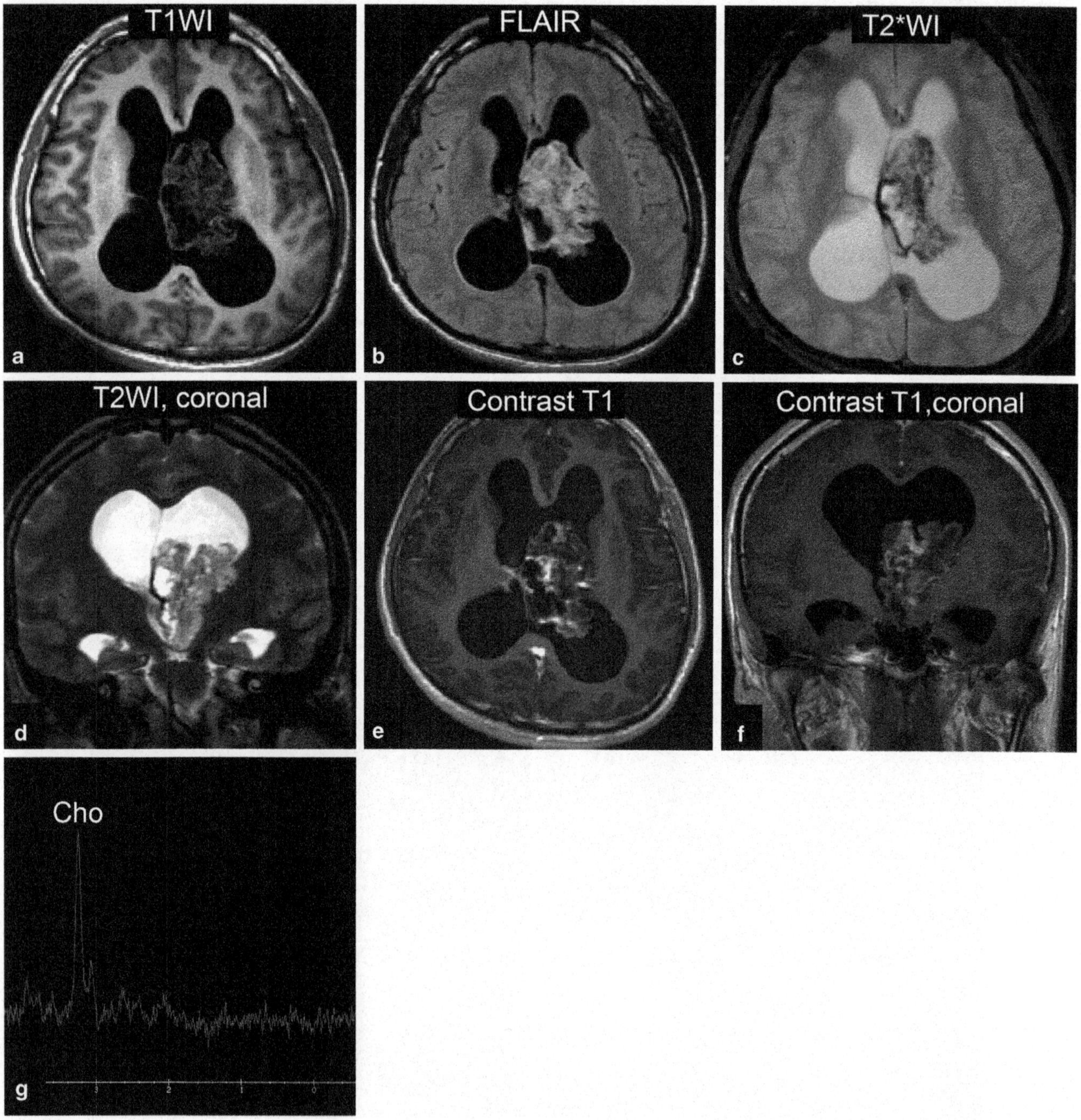

Fig. 6.32 M/35, Central neurocytoma. (**a–d**) MRI: A large tumor is observed in the left lateral and third ventricles with heterogeneous signal intensity and contains numerous small cysts. It causes severe hydrocephalus. Hypointensity on T2*WI indicates calcifications. (**e, f**) Contrast T1WI: This tumor shows heterogeneous contrast enhancement. The entire tumor plus the enlarged ventricles look like a "leopard," which is a characteristic sign of central neurocytoma. (**g**) MRS (TE 144 ms): This tumor exhibits elevated Cho level and absence of NAA. This tumor was surgically removed and confirmed to be a central neurocytoma by pathological examination

6.5.3 Subependymal Giant Cell Astrocytoma

As explained on Sect. 6.4.6 and Fig. 6.11.

6.5.4 Choroid Plexus Papilloma

This tumor develops from the choroid plexus in ventricles (Figs. 6.33 and 6.34). This tumor easily causes hydrocephalus for two reasons: the tumor obstructs the CSF flow path in the ventricle, and if the papilloma secretes CSF, CSF overproduction hydrocephalus may occur.

CT and MRI: Intraventricular tumors have an uneven surface and can be favorably enhanced by contrast media.

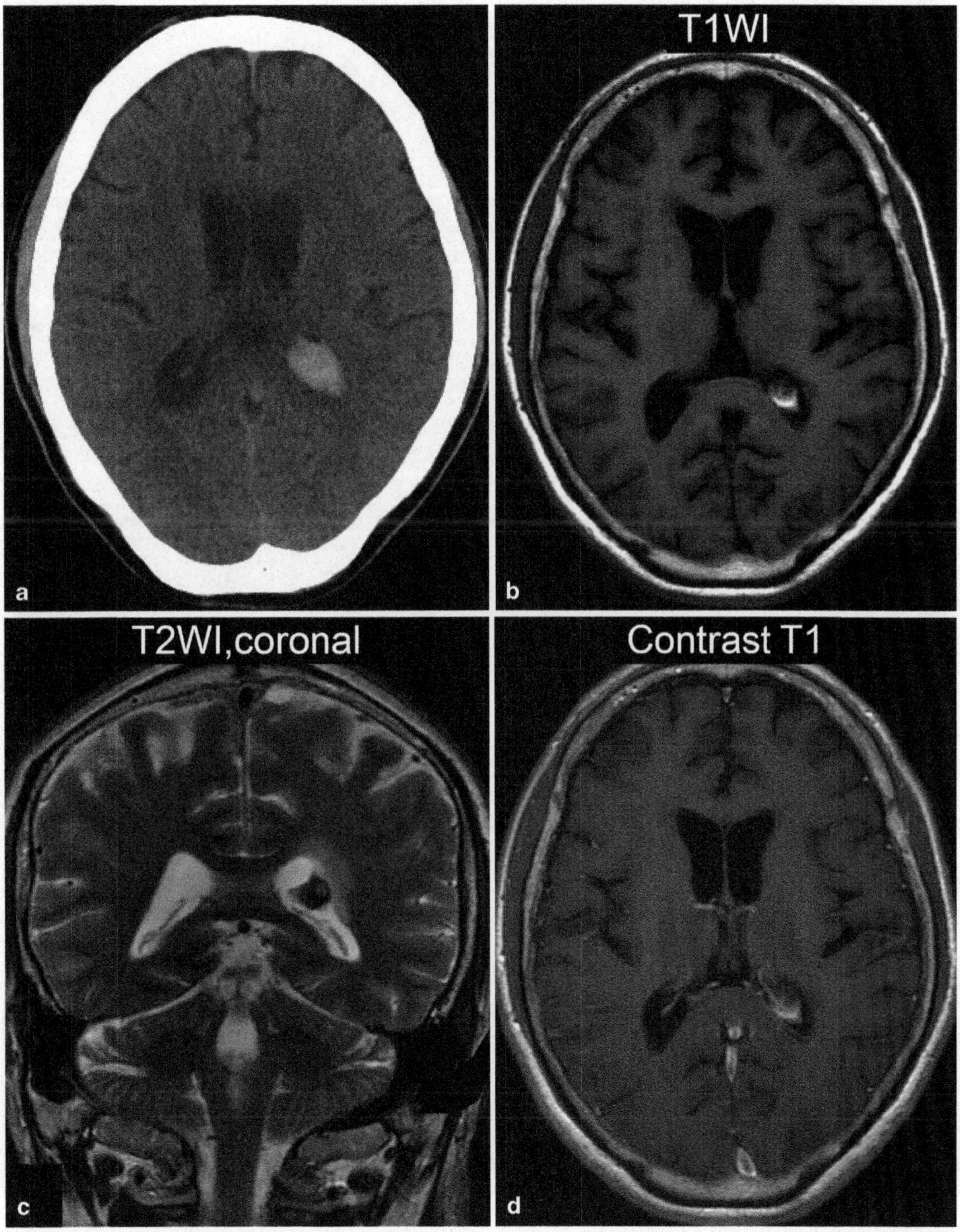

Fig. 6.33 M/55, Choroid papilloma with tumor bleeding. This patient suffered from a sudden onset of severe headache. (**a**) CT: A blood clot is observed in the left lateral ventricle. (**b–d**) MRI: This hyperintensity on T1WI and hypointensity on T2WI of this blood clot reflects acute hematoma. No contrast enhancement is observed. The hematoma was surgically removed and showed a papilloma from choroid plexus with tumor bleeding, as confirmed by pathological examination

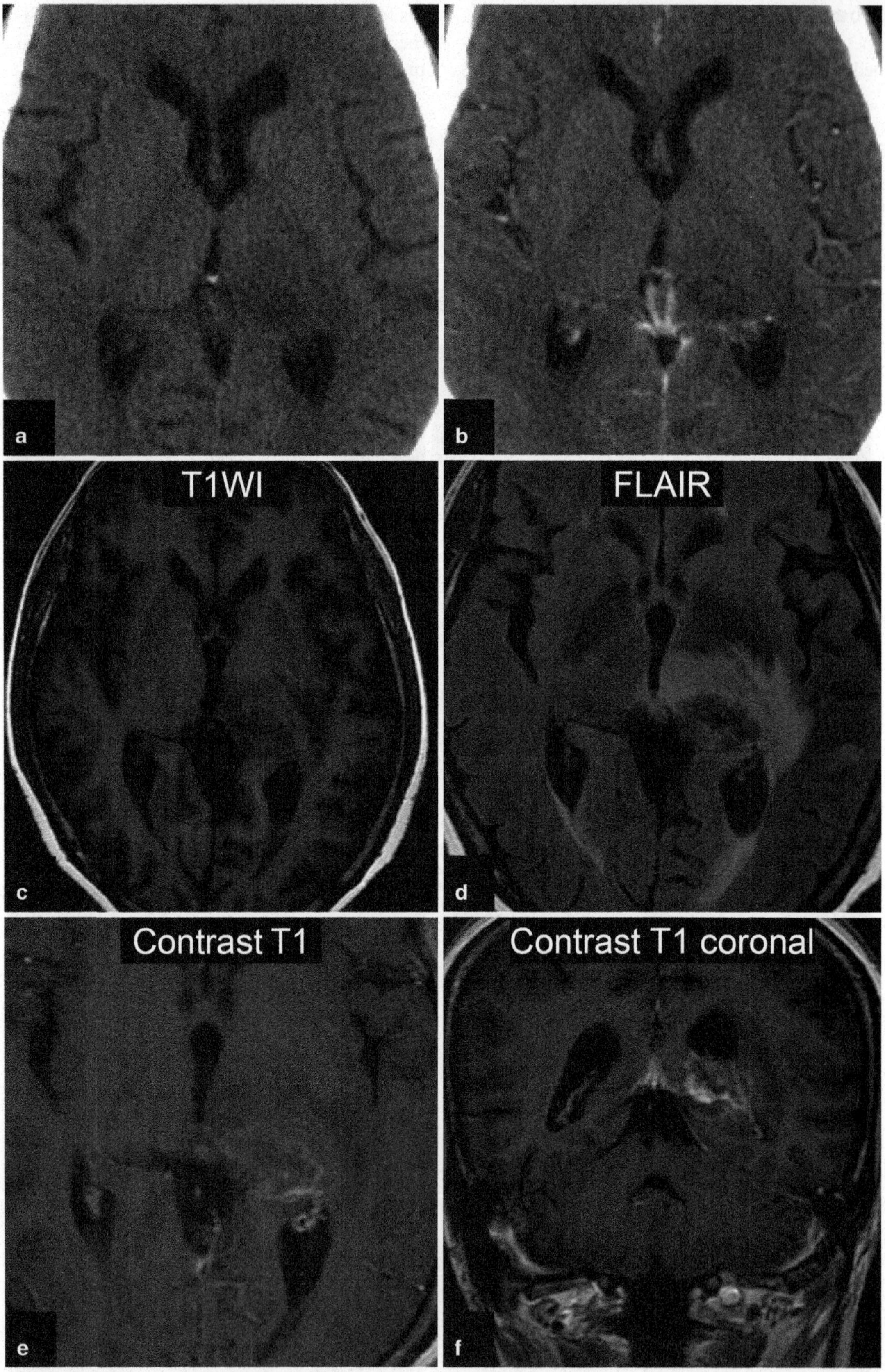

Fig. 6.34 F/50, Choroid papilloma. (**a**) CT: A faint hypodense lesion is observed in the left thalamus. (**b**) Contrast CT: This lesion shows weak contrast enhancement. (**c, d**) MRI: This lesion shows hypointensity on T1WI and FLAIR. FLAIR also shows peripheral white matter edema. (**e, f**) Contrast T1WI: This lesion shows heterogeneous contrast enhancement with irregular central necrosis. The exact location of this tumor is in the left lateral ventricle and not in the thalamus. This tumor was endoscopically removed and confirmed to be a choroid plexus papilloma by pathological examination

6.5.5 Choroid Meningioma

Choroid meningioma develops from the intraventricular choroid plexus (Fig. 6.35). It only accounts for 0.5–2% of all intracranial meningioma cases. However, it is the most common intraventricular tumor among adults aged between 40 and 60 years. Choroid meningioma is more common in women than in men. Approximately 80% of the cases develop at the trigone of the lateral ventricle.

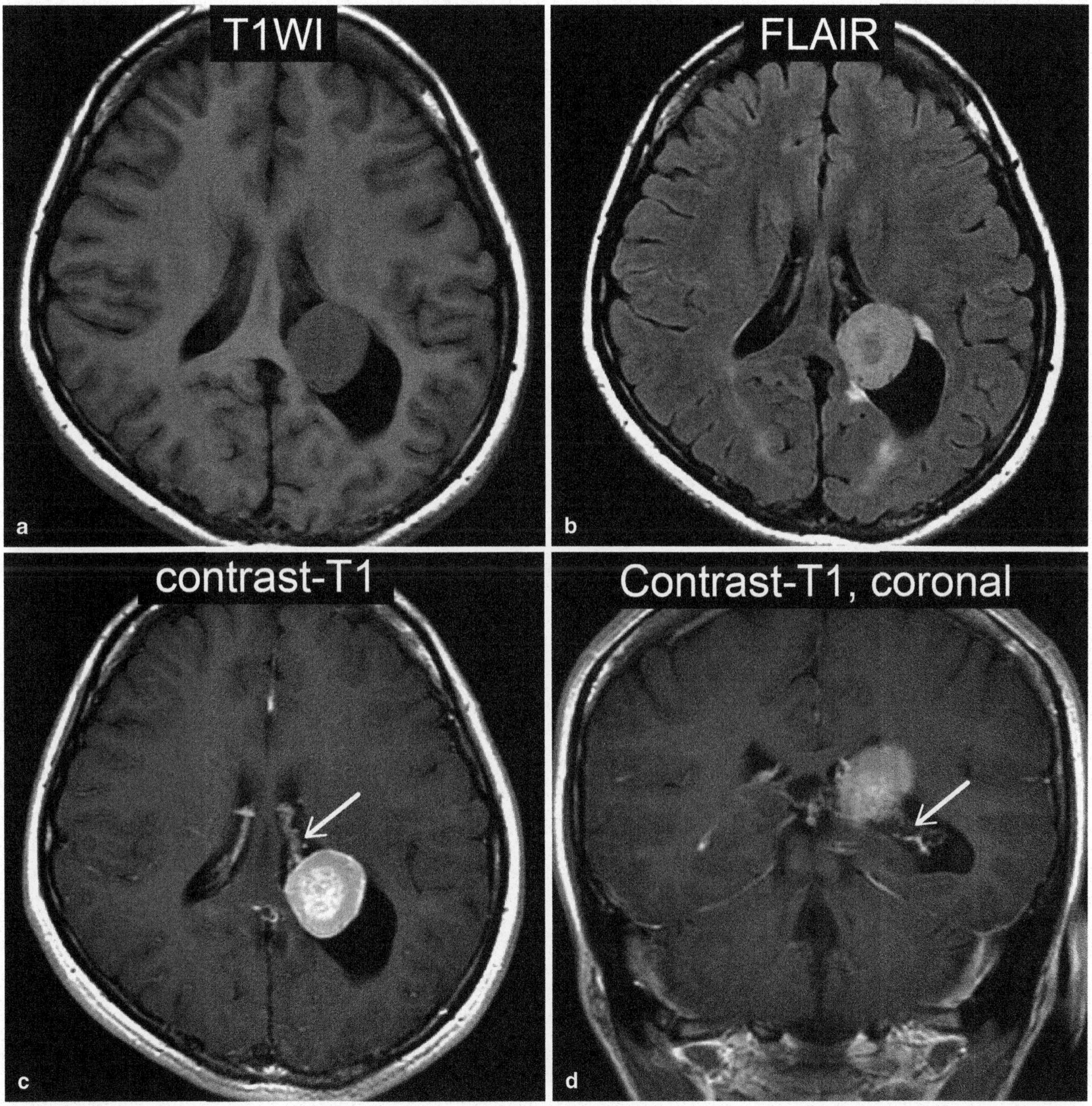

Fig. 6.35 F/29, Intraventricular meningioma. MRI: A tumor mass in the left lateral ventricle shows intermediate signal intensity on T1WI and hyperintensity on FLAIR. It has a well and homogeneous contrast enhancement and arises from the choroid plexus (arrow). This tumor was surgically removed and confirmed to be a choroidal meningioma (transitional-type meningioma) by pathological examination

6.6 Extra-Axial Intracranial Tumors

6.6.1 Meningioma

2016 WHO classification of meningiomas [1]:

Grade I Variants
- Angiomatous meningioma.
- Fibroblastic meningioma.
- Lymphocyte-rich meningioma.
- Meningothelial meningioma.
- Metaplastic meningioma.
- Microcystic meningioma.
- Psammomatous meningioma.
- Secretary meningioma.
- Transitional meningioma.

Grade II Variants
- Atypical meningioma.
- Choroid meningioma.
- Clear cell meningioma.

Grade III Variants
- Anaplastic meningioma.
- Papillary meningioma.
- Rhabdoid meningioma.

Meningioma develops from the meninges.

Age: Middle-aged to older adults; more common in women than men.

Location: Because meninges exist everywhere in the intra-cranium, meningioma develops anywhere that meninges exist, particularly near the parasagittal region (Figs. 6.39, 6.40, and 6.47), cerebral convexity (Figs. 6.36, 6.37, and 6.44), middle cranial fossa (Fig. 6.38), anterior fossa (including olfactory groove and planum sphenoidale; Figs. 6.41 and 6.43), posterior fossa (Fig. 6.42), foramen magnum (Fig. 6.45), falx (Figs. 6.39, 6.46, and 6.47), and tentorium. Meningioma may also develop from the intraventricular choroid plexus (Figs. 6.35 and 6.46).

Clinical symptoms: Meningioma generally causes no symptoms when it is small and causes nonspecific symptoms such as headache and vomiting only when it has grown to a considerable size and increased the intracranial pressure. Meningioma may also generate neurological symptoms when it compresses brain tissue. However, if meningioma develops from the skull base and compresses the cranial nerves or brain stem, specific symptoms may occur even when it is small; these symptoms cause patients to seek medical assistance.

6.6.1.1 CT

1. Calcification is observed in 40% of meningiomas (Figs. 6.36, 6.41, and 6.43) and can be identified in CT, facilitating the diagnosis of meningioma.
2. Hyperostosis occurs in approximately 15% of bones in contact with meningioma (Figs. 6.36 and 6.38). Therefore, the window width must be adjusted to inspect the adjacent bone. If hyperostosis is identified, the diagnosis of meningioma can be confirmed.
3. Although meningioma is an extra-axial tumor, it often causes peritumoral white matter edema (Figs. 6.36, 6.38, 6.40, 6.41, and 6.44).
4. Before contrast medium injection, images are generally isodense or slightly hyperdense.
5. After contrast medium injection, homogeneous enhancement is observed with a clear outline. Central necrosis or cystic change rarely occurs in the meningioma.

6.6.1.2 MRI

Meningioma is a gray-dark (mild hypointensity) in T1WI in some cases and isointense in other cases. T2WI is generally gray-dark. After injection of gadolinium-DTPA, the MRI results are homogeneous with intense contrast enhancement as are those of CT. Moreover, a segment of the dura with meningioma may be enhanced and is called the dural tail sign (Figs. 6.37, 6.38, 6.39, 6.42, 6.43, 6.44, and 6.45). Although some other tumors occasionally exhibit the dural tail sign, the sign is specific to meningioma.

6.6.1.3 Atypical Meningioma and Anaplastic Meningioma

If any of the following situations occur, we should consider the tumor to be atypical meningioma or anaplastic meningioma:

1. Apparent cystic change in the tumor.
2. Irregular outline of the tumor (Fig. 6.44).
3. Osteolysis of the nearby skull (Fig. 6.47) instead of hyperostosis.
4. Tumor development penetrating the skull and reaching the scalp (Fig. 6.47).

6.6.1.4 Multiple Meningiomas

Multiple meningiomas are possible (Fig. 6.46). The diagnosis must be performed carefully, with discernment of whether the patient has neurofibromatosis. If the intracranial meningioma associated with schwannomas or spinal tumors, it is likely to be neurofibromatosis (Fig. 6.66).

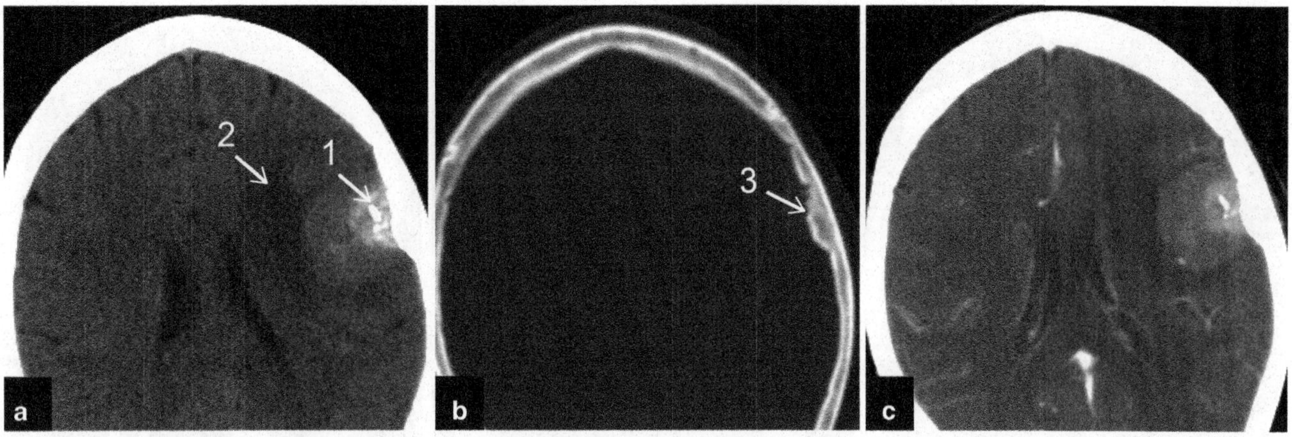

Fig. 6.36 F/57, Meningioma. This patient suffered from convulsions. (**a**) CT: A tumor mass in the left frontal lobe contains calcifications (1) with peripheral white matter edema (2). (**b**) Bone window setting: A focal hyperostosis (3) in the tumor area of the left frontal bone. (**c**) Contrast CT: This tumor has homogeneous contrast enhancement. A tumor contains calcifications, no central necrosis, hyperostosis of the nearby cranium; these are characteristic signs of meningioma. This tumor was surgically removed and confirmed to be a meningioma by pathological examination

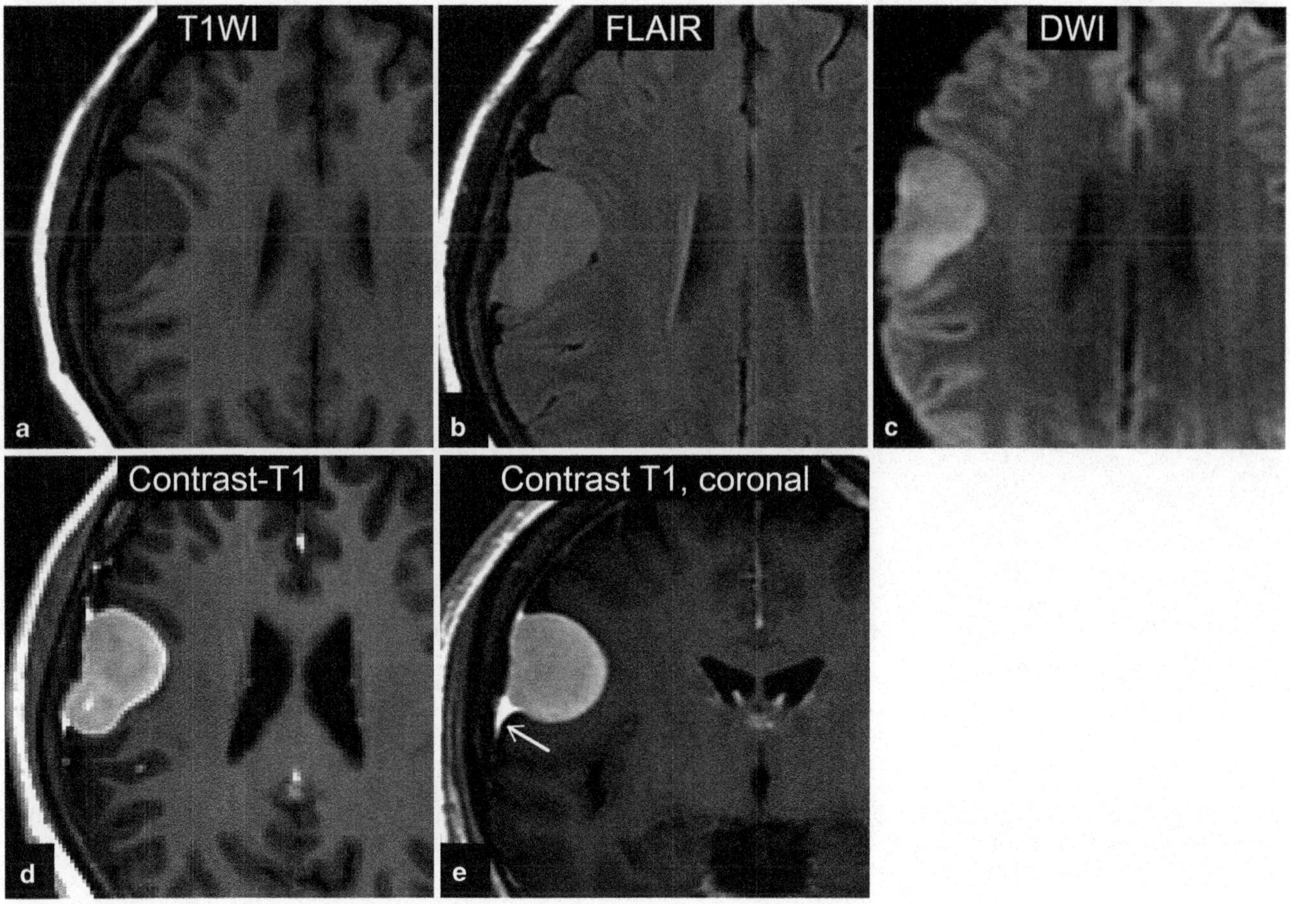

Fig. 6.37 F/44, Meningioma. (**a**, **b**) MRI, T1WI, and FLAIR: A tumor mass is observed in the right frontal lobe with homogeneous signal intensity and smooth outer margin. (**c**) DWI: This tumor demonstrates mild hyperintensity on DWI. (**d**, **e**) Contrast T1WI: This tumor has strong and homogeneous enhancement with a smooth outer margin. The enhancement of the adjacent dura (arrow) is a "dural tail sign." The strong and homogeneous enhancement with a dural tail sign is the characteristic findings of meningioma. This tumor was surgically removed and confirmed to be a transitional-type meningioma by pathological examination

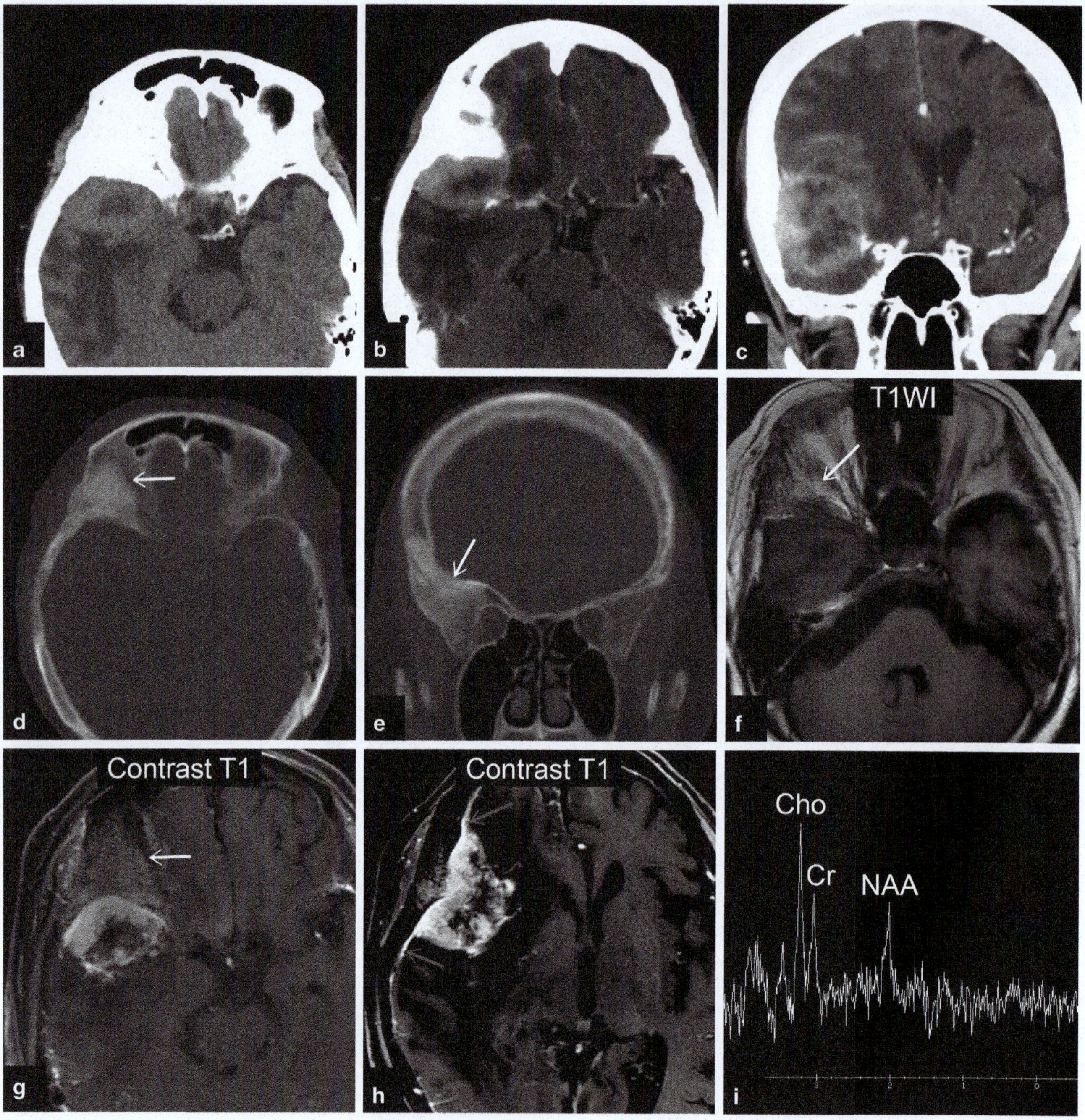

Fig. 6.38 F/74 Meningioma with hyperostosis. This patient exhibited left-side hemiparesis and was considered to have suffered a stroke. (**a**) CT: A tumor mass with peripheral white matter edema is observed in the right temporal lobe. (**b, c**) Contrast CT, axial, and coronal sections: Unlike a typical meningioma, the tumor shows heterogeneous enhancement. (**d, e**) Bone window setting, axial, and coronal sections: Hyperostosis (arrow) in the greater wing of the sphenoid bone. The hyperostosis in the adjacent bone is a characteristic sign of meningioma. (**f–h**) MRI: This tumor mass has strong enhancement and central necrosis with a dural tail sign (red arrows). The dural tail sign is also a characteristic sign of meningioma. The hyperostosis (white arrows) is difficult to recognize in the MRI. (**i**) MRS (144 ms): The tumor has elevated Cho and reduced NAA. This tumor was surgically removed and confirmed to be a meningothelial meningioma (WHO grade I) by pathological examination

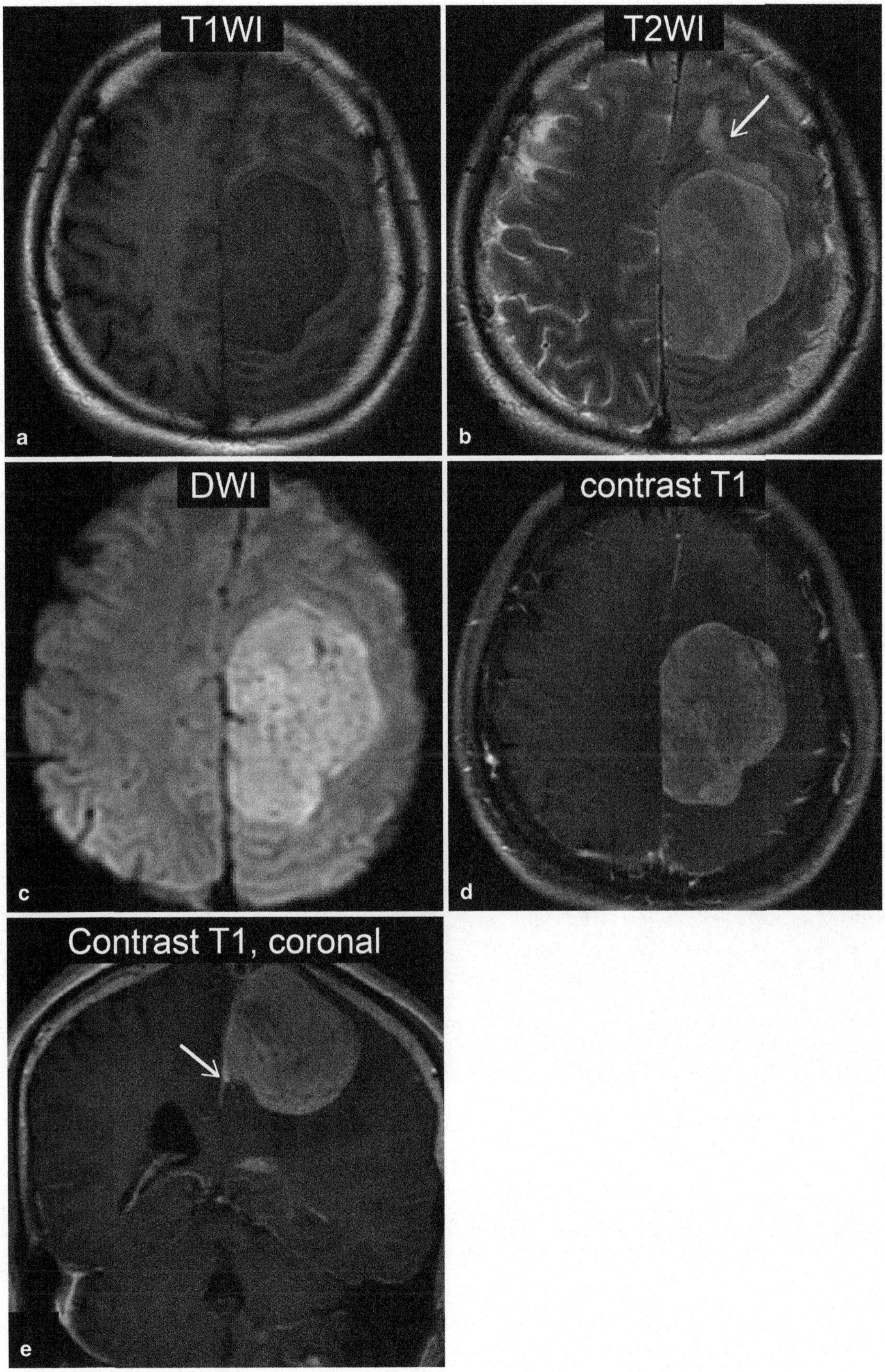

Fig. 6.39 M/37, Meningioma. The right limbs of the patient gradually weakened for more than a month. (**a**) MRI, T1WI: A large tumor mass in the left frontoparietal lobes shows mild hypointensity on T1WI. (**b**) T2WI: This tumor shows mild hyperintensity with some peripheral white matter edema (arrow). (**c**) DWI: This tumor shows hyperintensity on DWI. (**d**, **e**) Contrast T1WI: This tumor has well and homogeneous enhancement with a smooth outer margin. The coronal section clearly shows a dural tail sign (arrow) in the falx. Hence, the tumor is not an intracerebral tumor but an extra-axial tumor, which is a typical meningioma arising from the falx. This tumor was surgically removed, and meningioma of the falx, which was composed of mainly fibroblastic and meningotheliomatous patterns, was confirmed by pathological examination

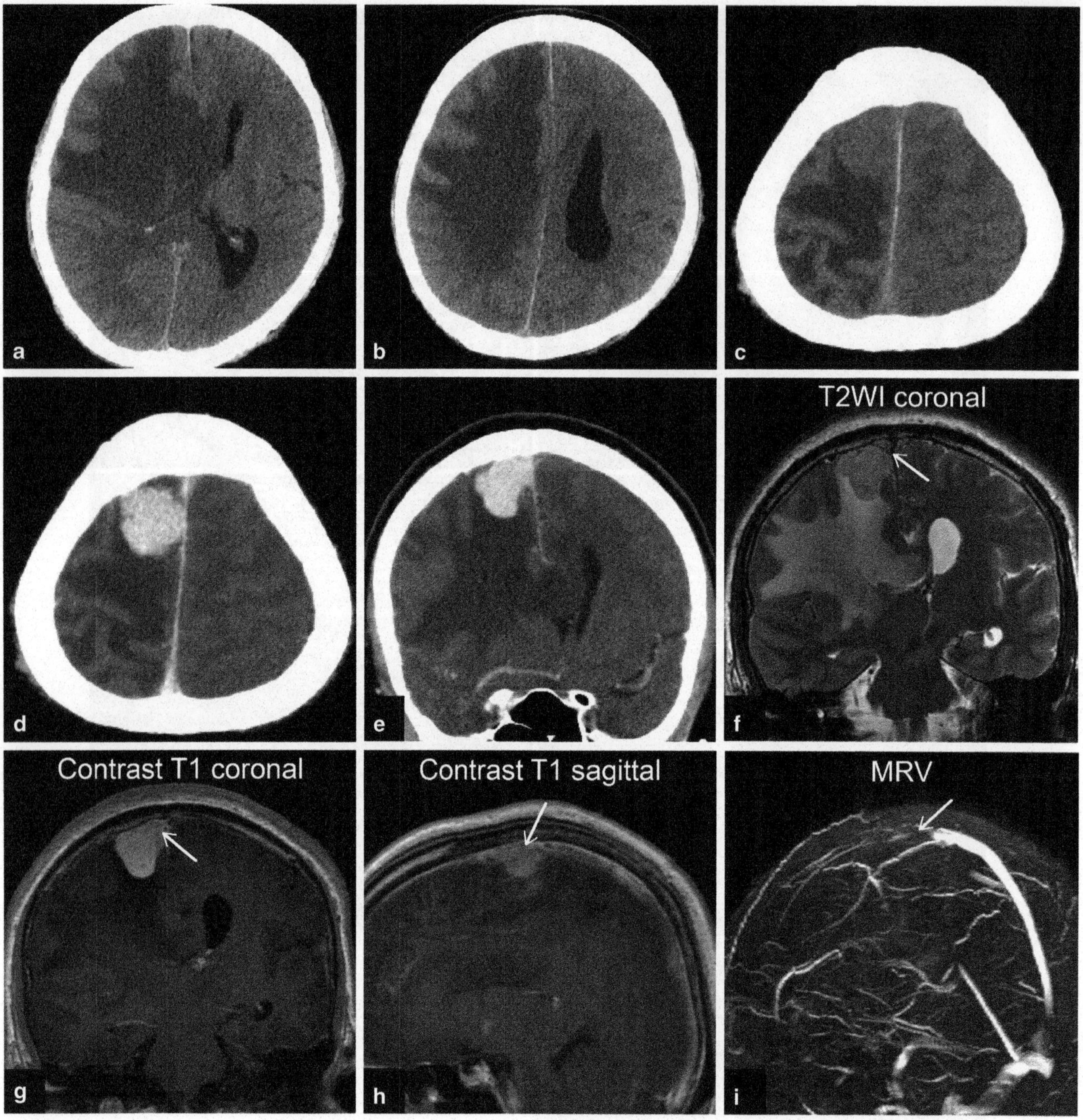

Fig. 6.40 M/54, Small meningioma with a large area of white matter edema and sinus invasion. This patient suffered from weakness of the left lower limb for several months. (**a–c**) CT: A large area of white matter edema is observed in the right frontoparietal lobes. (**d, e**) Contrast CT, axial, and coronal sections: A strong and homogeneous enhanced tumor mass is noted. In the coronal section, this tumor mass adheres to the falx and possibly invades the superior sagittal sinus (SSS). (**f–h**) MRI, T2WI, and contrast T1WI: The findings obtained are similar to those of CT; however, the sagittal section more clearly depicts the invasion of SSS (arrow) by this tumor. (**i**) MR-venogram (MRV): A filling defect in the SSS (arrow) reflects tumor invasion into the SSS. During surgery, the neurosurgeon found that the tumor invaded into the SSS with peripheral brain tissue edema. Meningotheliomatous-type meningioma was confirmed by pathological examination

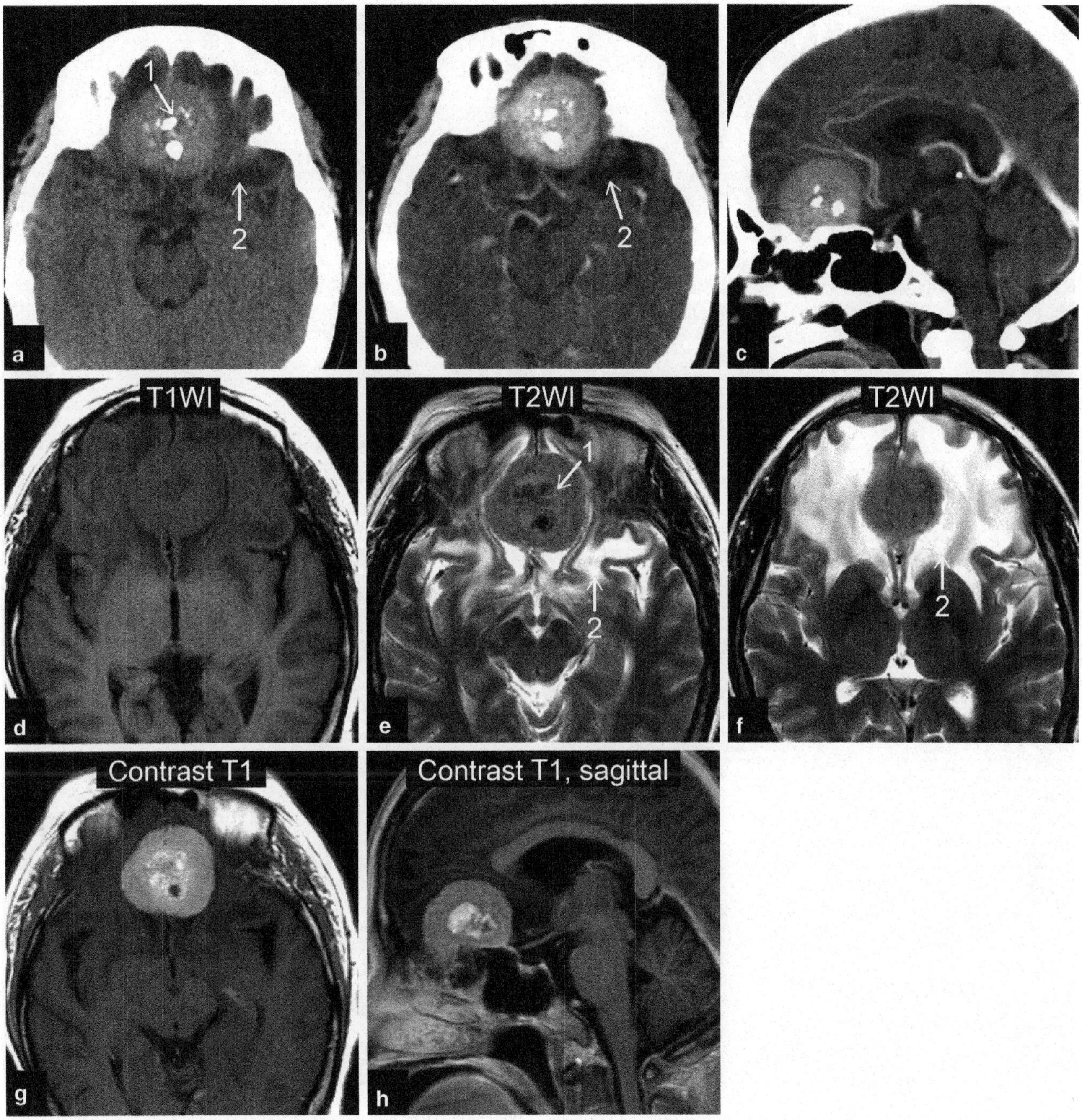

Fig. 6.41 F/53, Olfactory groove meningioma. This patient received CT and MRI examinations because of seizures. (**a**) CT: A large tumor containing calcifications (1) in the middle of the anterior cranial fossa, and with peripheral white matter edema (2) in the bilateral frontal lobes. (**b, c**) Contrast CT, axial, and sagittal: This tumor has homogeneous enhancement. The above features are characteristic signs of meningioma. (**d**) MRI, T1WI: This tumor shows intermediate signal intensity on T1WI, and calcifications are difficult to see. (**e, f**) T2WI: This tumor also shows intermediate signal intensity on T2WI, and T2WI can show calcifications (1) and diffuse white matter edema (2) in the bilateral frontal lobes. (**g, h**) Contrast T1WI: This tumor has homogeneous enhancement. This tumor was surgically removed and found that this meningioma arose from the olfactory nerve. Meningotheliomatous-type meningioma (WHO grade I) was confirmed by pathological examination

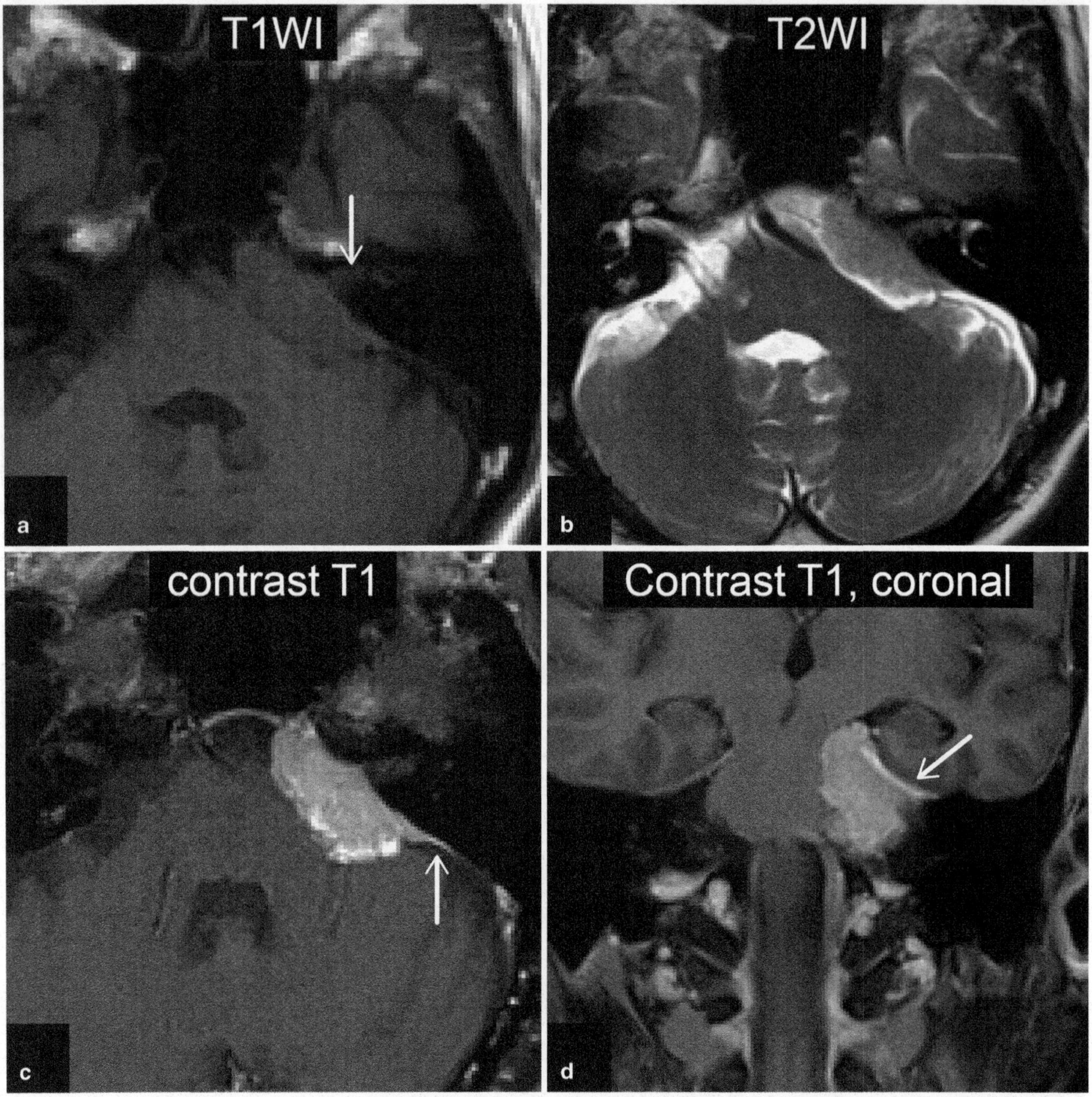

Fig. 6.42 M/73, CP angle meningioma. This patient suffered left-side tinnitus for more than 1 year. (**a, b**) MRI, T1WI, and T2WI: A soft tissue mass is located in the left CP angle cistern, just in the orifice of the left internal auditory canal (IAC) (arrow). A tumor in CP angle cistern near the IAC is always an acoustic schwannoma. (**c, d**) Contrast T1WI: This tumor has homogeneous enhancement with a dural tail sign (arrow) in the adjacent dura. Hence, the tumor is a meningioma and not acoustic schwannoma. This tumor was surgically removed, and meningothelial meningioma from tentorium dura was proven by pathological examination

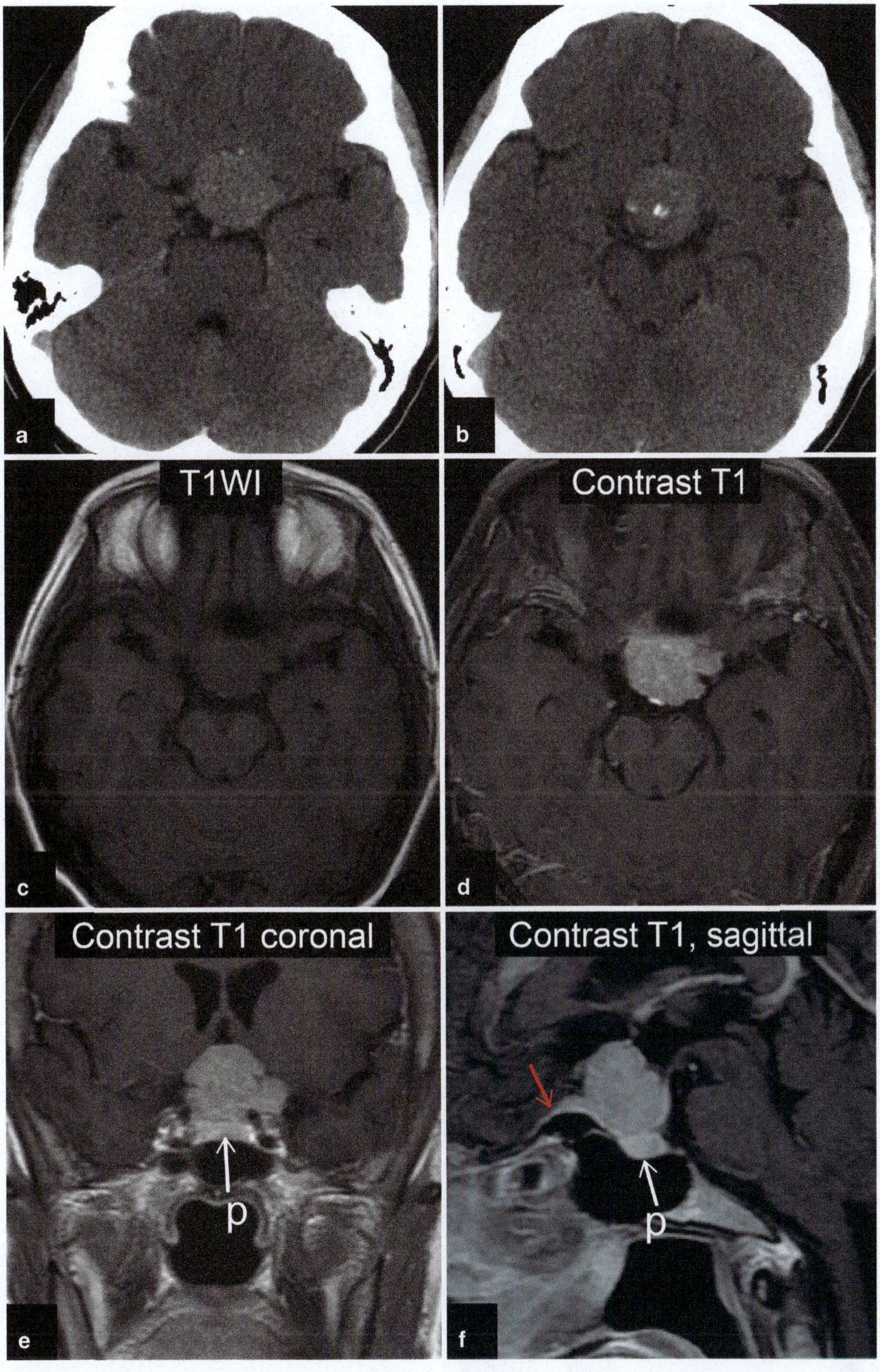

Fig. 6.43 F/65, Planum sphenoidale meningioma. This patient had a visual loss of the left eye and hemianopia of the right eye. (**a**, **b**) CT: A tumor mass with calcifications in the suprasellar cistern is observed. A tumor in the suprasellar cistern is often a pituitary adenoma; however, pituitary adenoma rarely has calcification. (**c**) MRI, T1WI: This tumor shows an intermediate signal intensity on T1WI. (**d**–**f**) Contrast T1WI: This tumor has homogeneous enhancement with the dural tail sign (red arrow in **f**) of dura in the planum sphenoidale. Hence, the tumor is a meningioma of the planum sphenoidale. The normal pituitary gland (p) is seen in the sella turcica. This tumor was surgically removed, and mixed meningotheliomatous and angiomatous meningioma with psammoma bodies were proven by the pathological examination

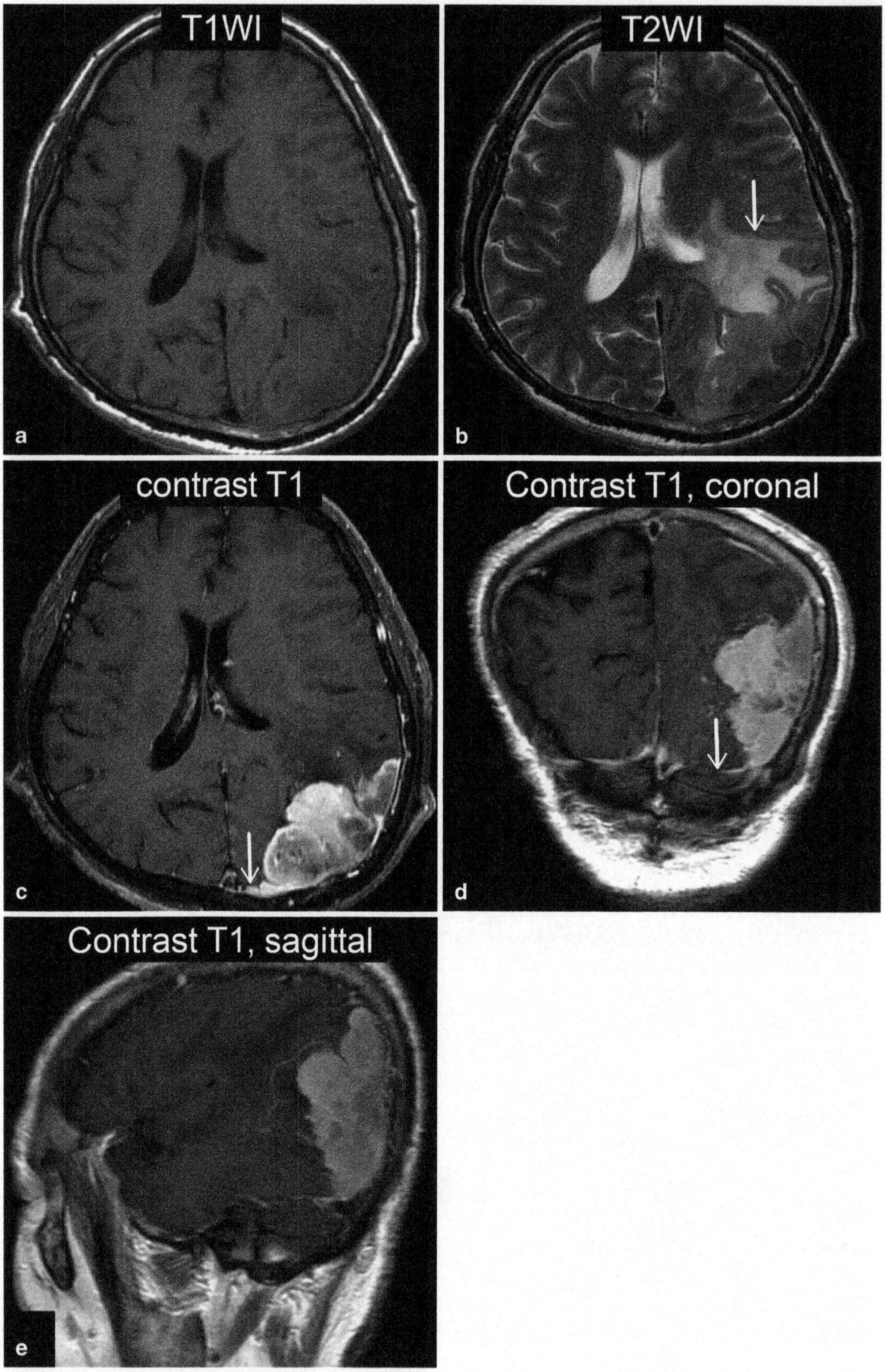

Fig. 6.44 M/67, Atypical meningioma. This patient suffered from severe dizziness, unstable gait, and slow speech for more than a month. (**a**) MRI, T1WI: A soft tissue mass is observed in the left parieto-occipital lobe, and its signal intensity is similar to that of the brain tissue and difficult to see. (**b**) T2WI: Peritumoral white matter edema (arrow) exists in the left parietal lobe. (**c**–**e**) Contrast T1WI: This tumor has strong and homogeneous enhancement with the dural tail sign (arrows). The features of this tumor are similar to those of meningioma; however, unlike ordinary meningioma, which usually shows a smooth outer margin, the outer margin of this tumor is not smooth. This tumor was surgically removed and was an atypical meningioma (WHO grade II) with brain invasion, as confirmed by pathological examination

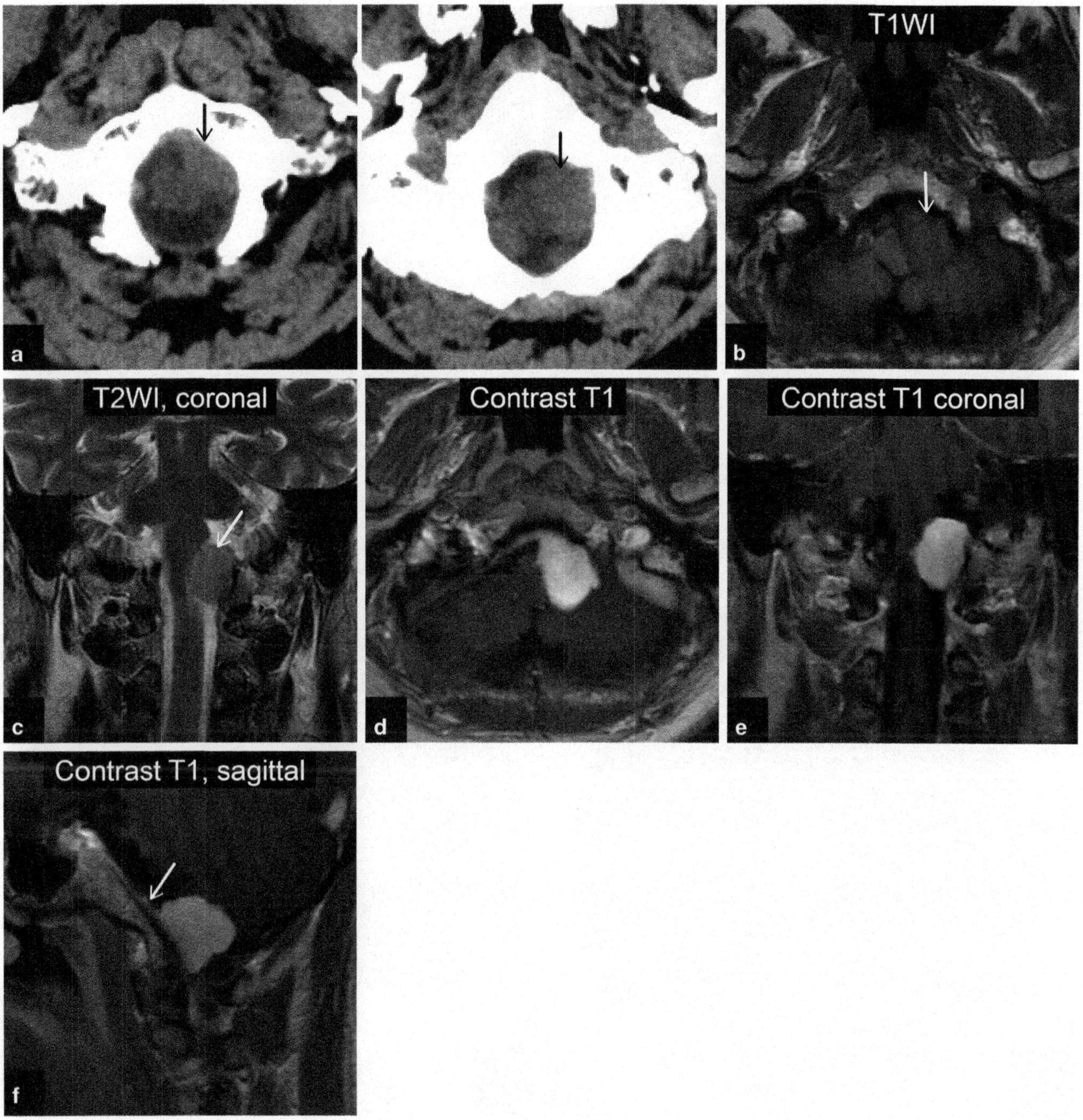

Fig. 6.45 M/52, Foramen magnum meningioma. (**a**) CT: This patient did not have neurological symptoms, such as unsteady gait. In a CT scan of the brain for head trauma, the neuroradiologist sharply found a soft tissue mass (arrows) inside the foramen magnum. Then, an MRI was also performed for further evaluation of this mass. (**b**, **c**) MRI, T1WI, and T2WI: This tumor (arrows) compresses the medulla oblongata. (**d**–**f**) Contrast T1WI: This tumor has strong and homogeneous enhancement with the dural tail sign (arrow). Hence, this tumor is a typical meningioma. This tumor was surgically removed, and meningotheliomatous meningioma was confirmed by pathological examination

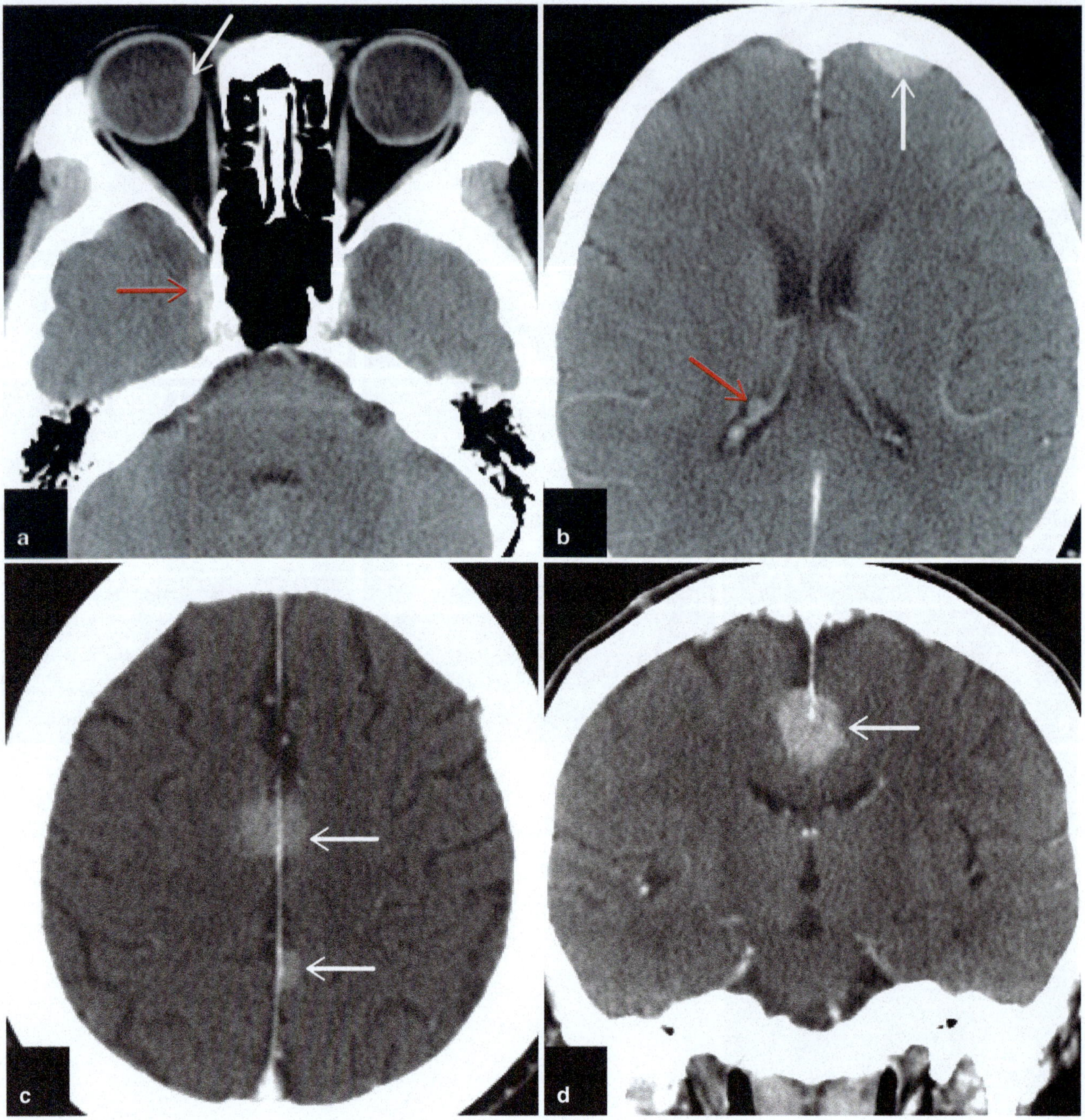

Fig. 6.46 F/58, Multiple meningiomas. The neurofibromatosis patient suffered from gradual deterioration of eyesight; the ophthalmologist found several small tumors in the eye fundus and arranged for a CT examination. (**a**) Contrast CT: The thickening of the retina (white arrow) of the right eyeball reflects a small tumor, which is likely a hamartoma. The prominence of the right cavernous sinus (red arrow) is also due to a small tumor. (**b**) A small mass with homogeneous enhancement (white arrow) outside the left frontal lobe is a typical meningioma. A small mass in the choroid plexus (red arrow) of the right lateral ventricle indicates a small choroidal meningioma. (**c**, **d**) Contras CT, axial, and coronal sections: Two meningiomas (arrows) exist in the falx. Comment: A neurofibromatosis patient may have multiple meningiomas

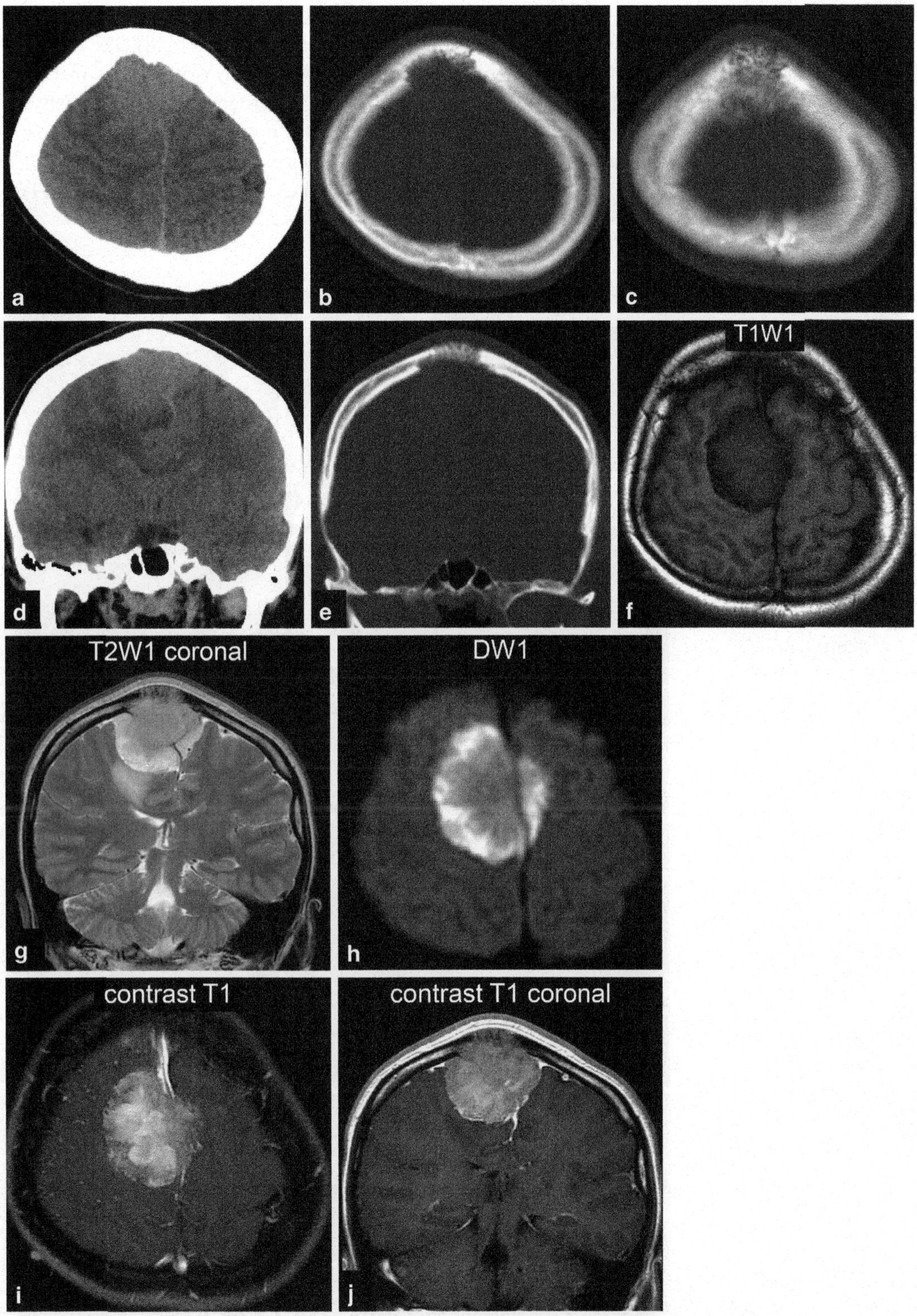

Fig. 6.47 F/28, Atypical meningioma. This patient touched a painful bulging mass on her head by herself. (**a–c**) CT axial and (**d**, **e**) coronal sections: A tumor mass exists between the bilateral frontal lobes. Bone window setting (**b**, **c**, **e**) shows the bony invasion of the adjacent cranial table. (**f–j**) MRI: This tumor shows intermediate signal intensity on T1WI and T2WI and hyperintensity on DWI. It has homogeneous enhancement. This tumor invades and destructs the cranium and extends to the subcutaneous space of the scalp. This tumor was surgically removed and was an atypical meningioma, as confirmed by pathological examination. Comment: Meningioma always causes hyperostosis in the adjacent bone, but the osteolytic invasion, in this case, is atypical

6.6.2 Hemangiopericytoma

Intracranial hemangiopericytoma develops from meninges. This tumor is rare and develops in young adults (aged 30–50 years) and children.

Pathologically hemangiopericytoma is a dural solitary fibrous tumor with WHO Grades I, II, or III.

CT and MRI imaging of hemangiopericytoma is similar to that of meningioma (Fig. 6.48). The dural tail sign is also present; no calcification is observed. In DWI of MRI, the tumor presents heterogeneous hypointensity because of its hypervascularity, not mild hyperintensity as meningioma. The tumor induces bone erosion instead of hyperostosis. Tumor central necrosis is common (Fig. 6.49).

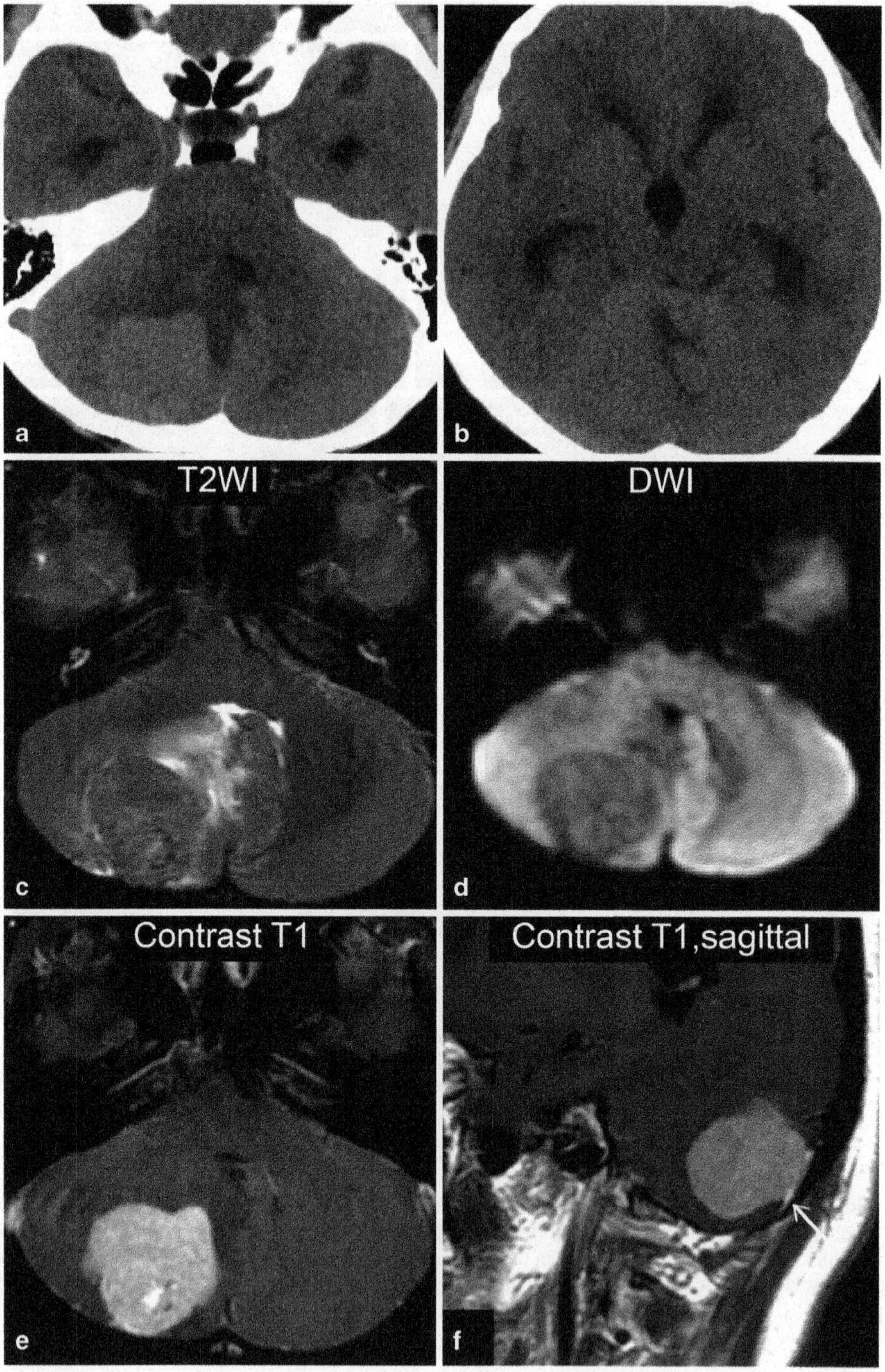

Fig. 6.48 F/42, Hemangiopericytoma. This patient came to the emergency unit because of severe headaches, unsteady gait, and vomiting. (**a**, **b**) CT: A tumor mass is observed in the right cerebellum with peripheral brain tissue edema, compressing the fourth ventricle, and causes hydrocephalus. Dilatation of temporal horns of the bilateral lateral ventricles and third ventricle indicate hydrocephalus. (**c**–**f**) MRI: This tumor shows mild hypointensity on T2WI with peripheral brain tissue edema. Strong and homogeneous enhancement with the dural tail sign (arrow) is observed. Hence, the features of the tumor are similar to those of meningioma. However, unlike meningioma, which always shows hyperintensity on DWI, the tumor presents hypointensity on DWI. This tumor was surgically removed, and the surgeon made sure that this was an extra-axial tumor from the dura. The pathological examination confirmed it to be a hemangiopericytoma

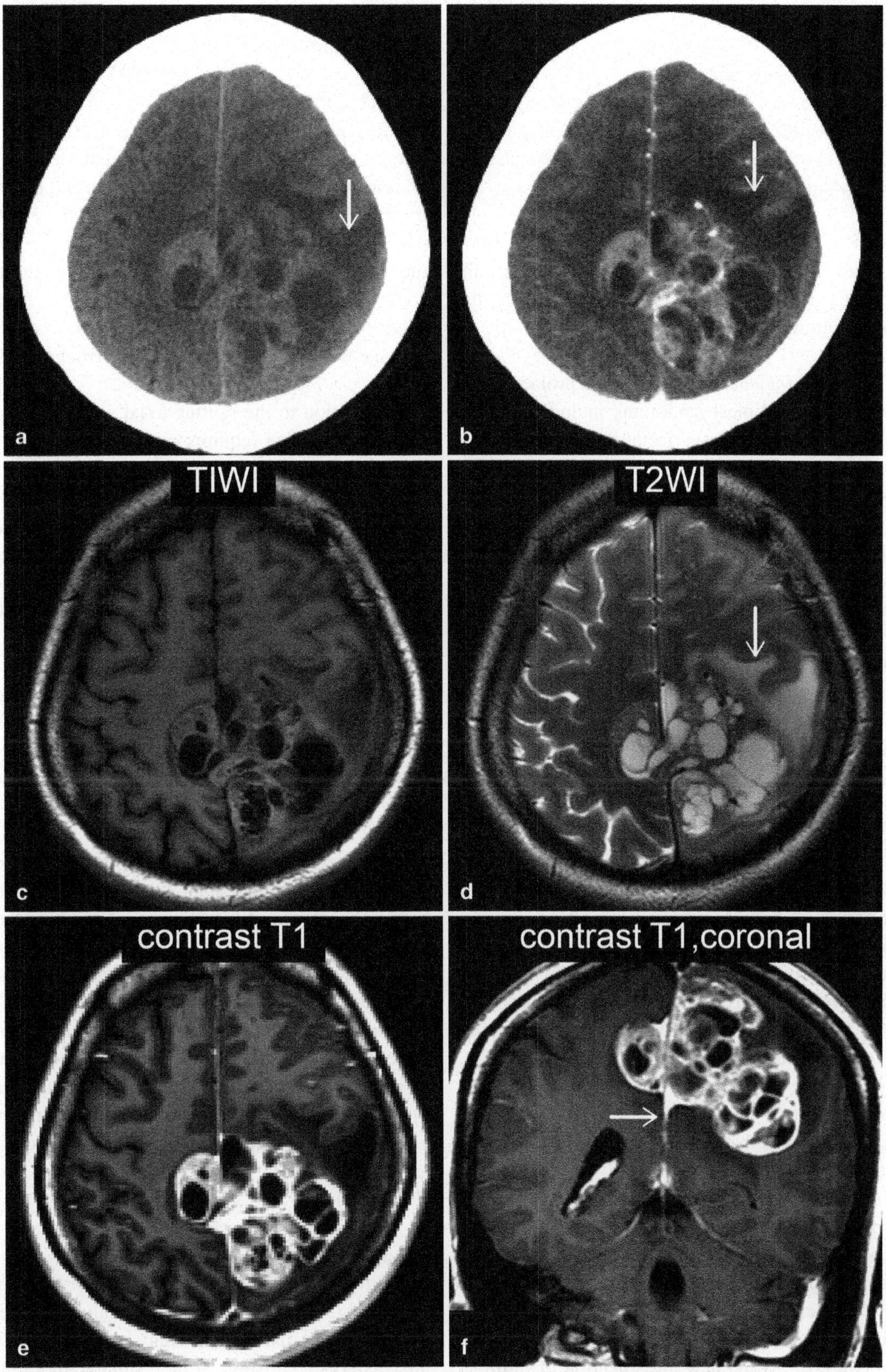

Fig. 6.49 F/36, Hemangiopericytoma. This patient suffered from dizziness, nausea, and vomiting for 2 weeks. (**a**) CT and (**b**) contrast CT: A large tumor mass in the left parietal lobe crosses the falx to the right parietal lobe. This tumor has irregular central necroses and some peripheral white matter edema (arrow). The picture is similar to that of a glioblastoma. (**c, d**) MRI: The findings are the same as those of CT. (**e, f**) Contrast T1WI: Dural tail sign (arrow) is seen on the falx. Hence, this extra-axial tumor comes from the dura of the falx. This tumor was surgically removed and confirmed to be a hemangiopericytoma (grade II) by pathological examination. Comment: Although the shape of this tumor is similar to that of glioblastoma, glioblastoma is an intra-axial tumor, it cannot cross the falx to the other side

6.6.3 Pituitary Adenoma

Age: Young people and general adults.

Position: Sella turcica.

Clinical symptoms: The clinical symptoms of pituitary adenoma are of two types, depending on whether the adenoma secretes hormones.

1. **Functioning:**

   The adenoma secretes hormones and causes symptoms even when the tumor is small. The most common four types are as follows:

   (a) Prolactin

   This type of adenoma is also called prolactinoma. In women, the clinical symptoms include irregular menstruation, menopause, lactation, and infertility (Fig. 6.50). If this adenoma develops in men, it causes impotence.

   (b) Growth hormone

   If a teenager undergoing puberty develops pituitary adenoma and secretes excessive growth hormone, gigantism may occur. In adults, acromegaly may occur (Fig. 6.51), with the front head widened, chin elongated, and palms and knees bulked.

   (c) Adrenocorticotropic hormone (ACTH)

   This hormone may cause Cushing syndrome, including thickened subcutaneous fat, pigmentation, buffalo hump, and moon face.

   (d) Thyroid-stimulating hormone (TSH)

   This hormone induces hyperthyroidism (Fig. 6.52).

Pituitary adenomas that secrete hormones tend to be small in size; some are even microadenomas.

Because pituitary adenoma has the aforementioned particular clinical symptoms, clinical judgment of pituitary adenoma can be made based on symptoms and hormone tests of the blood. If tumors are identified in the sella turcica through CT or MRI, the diagnosis can be confirmed.

2. **Nonfunctioning:**

   Pituitary adenomas that do not secrete hormones grow large enough to induce symptoms (Figs. 6.53, 6.54, 6.55, and 6.56). They may develop upward to the suprasellar region, compress the optic chiasm, and generate bitemporal hemianopsia. Moreover, they may develop further upward and cause a headache. Some even larger tumors compress the third ventricle, but they rarely cause hydrocephalus, this may be because pituitary adenoma grows slowly.

   There is a 2017 WHO new classification of pituitary tumors, emphasizing histopathological and molecular genetics of pituitary neuroendocrine and non-neuroendocrine tumors [8].

6.6.3.1 CT and MRI

Because pituitary adenoma is precisely located at the sella turcica, a tumor identified at the sella turcica, the first consideration is a pituitary adenoma. Before the injection of contrast media, the adenoma and brain tissue exhibit identical density and intensity. After the injection of contrast media, the tumor is enhanced and can be easily identified. Pituitary adenoma often has central necrosis or cystic changes (Figs. 6.54, 6.55, and 6.56). Necrosis and cystic change areas contain water and sometimes hemorrhage (Figs. 6.55 and 6.56).

In addition to the routine axial section, the diagnosis of pituitary adenoma requires coronal and sagittal sections to identify the tumor's compression of the optic chiasm (Figs. 6.53, 6.54, and 6.55) and the third ventricle.

Attention must also be paid to whether the tumor invades the cavernous sinus or encases the internal carotid artery (Fig. 6.56).

At the sella and suprasellar parts, other tumors resembling the pituitary adenoma can exist, including meningioma developing from the planum sphenoidale (Fig. 6.43), craniopharyngioma (Figs. 6.58 and 6.59), Rathke's cleft cyst (Fig. 6.60), and suprasellar germinoma (Fig. 6.69). Therefore, axial, sagittal, and coronal sections must be carefully interpreted.

6.6.3.2 Pituitary Microadenoma

Pituitary adenomas smaller than 10 mm are called microadenomas. Despite their small size, these microadenomas still secrete hormones, if functioning, and induce the aforementioned clinical symptoms, which drive patients to seek medical assistance. Diagnosing microadenomas by using CT and MRI needs careful interpretation of the images. The coronal section is required in combination with contrast medium injection. The content in the sella turcica with low density or intensity is the microadenoma because the contrast enhancement of microadenoma is slower than the normal pituitary gland (Figs. 6.50 and 6.51). The dynamic enhancement technique sometimes is used to visualize microadenoma (Fig. 6.52).

6.6.3.3 Pituitary Apoplexy

The pituitary apoplexy refers to pituitary adenoma hemorrhage (Fig. 6.57), which may result in headache, dizziness, consciousness disorder, and may hemorrhage into suprasellar cisterns, causing some subarachnoid hemorrhage (SAH).

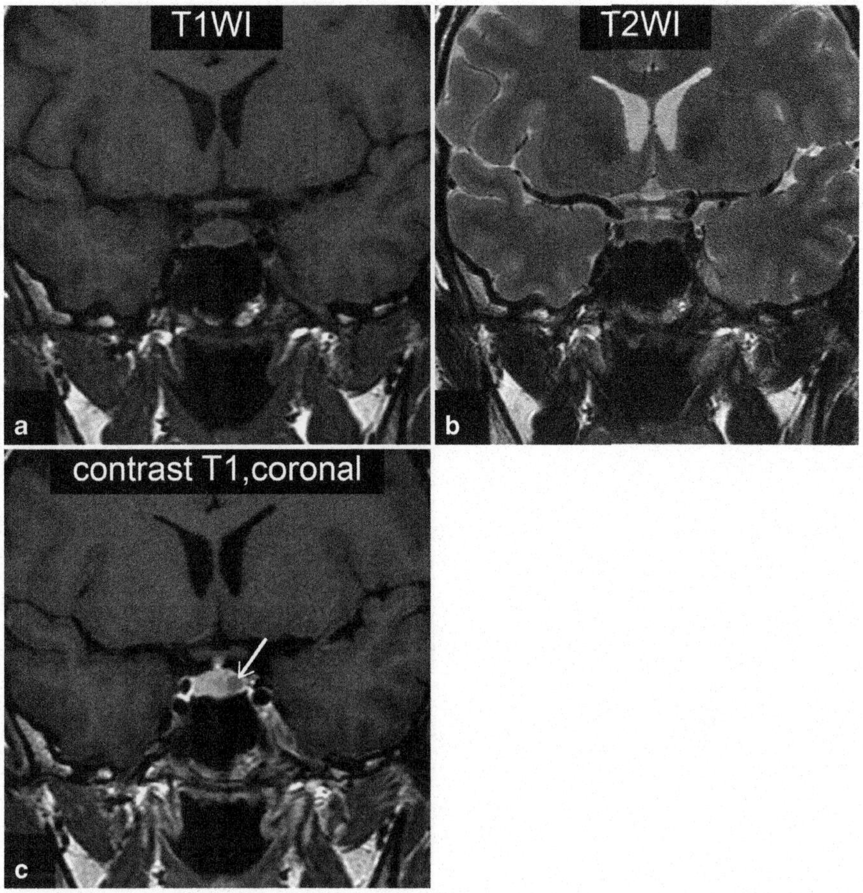

Fig. 6.50 F/22, Pituitary microadenoma. This patient had amenorrhea for 1 year. (**a**, **b**) MRI: The pituitary gland looks normal on T1WI and T2WI. (**c**) Contrast T1WI: A small filling defect (arrow) on the left side of the pituitary gland indicates it is a suspected microadenoma. This tumor is surgically removed and confirmed to be a prolactinoma by pathological examination. Comment: The normal pituitary gland has rapid homogeneous contrast enhancement, whereas an adenoma has delayed enhancement. Hence, adenoma shows a filling defect in the pituitary gland

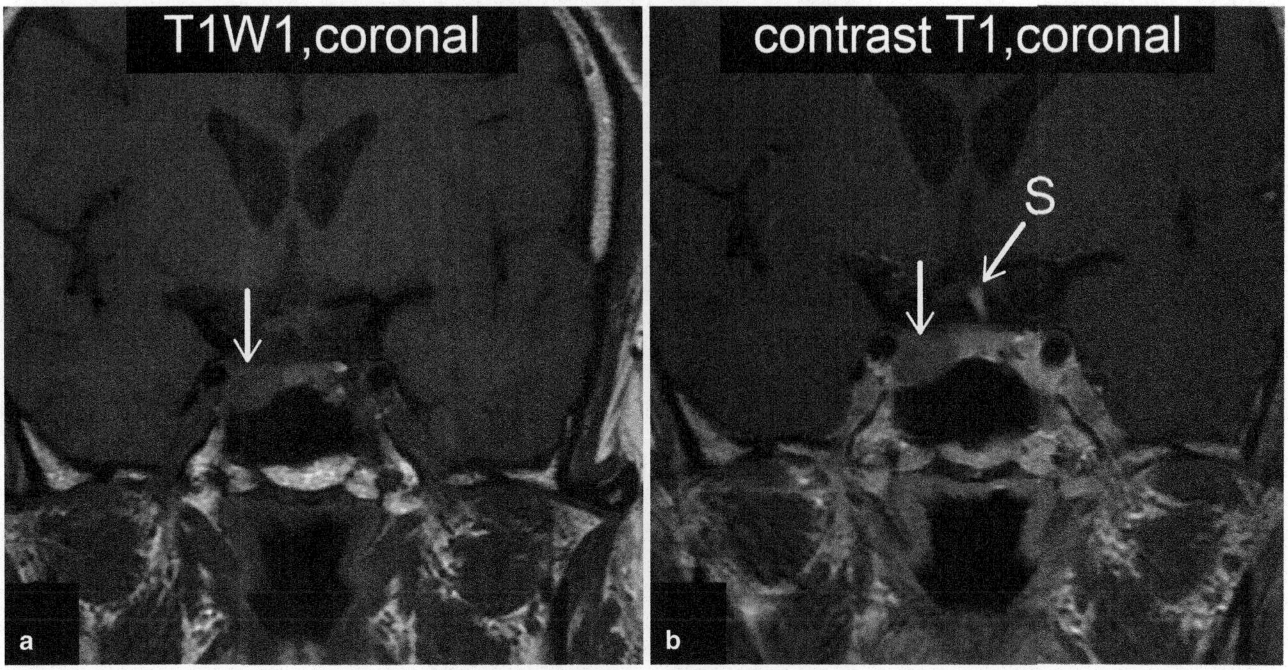

Fig. 6.51 M/55, Pituitary microadenoma. This patient has acromegaly. (**a**) MRI, T1WI: A small tumor mass (arrow) in the right side of the pituitary gland (approximately 8 mm × 7 mm) has a signal intensity lower than the normal pituitary gland, making it easy to distinguish. (**b**) Contrast T1WI: The good enhancement of the normal pituitary gland makes this tumor (arrow) more clearly displayed. Note that the pituitary stalk (s) deviates to the left because of the pressure effect of this microadenoma. This tumor was surgically removed, and a growth hormone-secreting adenoma was confirmed by pathological examination

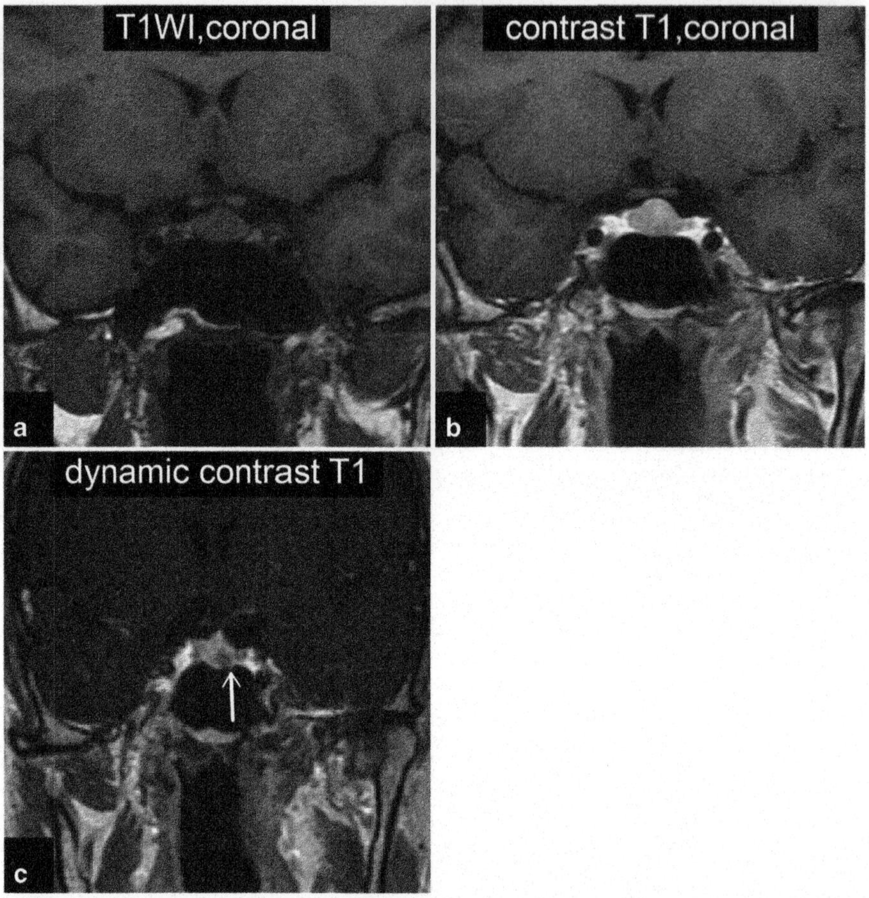

Fig. 6.52 F/39, Pituitary microadenoma. This patient lost a bodyweight of 8 kg in 1 year and was suspected of having hyperthyroidism due to pituitary gland hyperfunction. (**a**) MRI, T1WI: The height of the pituitary gland is 8 mm with convexity in the upper margin. (**b**) Contrast T1WI: The pituitary gland is homogeneously enhanced without abnormality. (**c**) Dynamic contrast T1WI: A small area of slow enhancement (arrow), this is a microadenoma

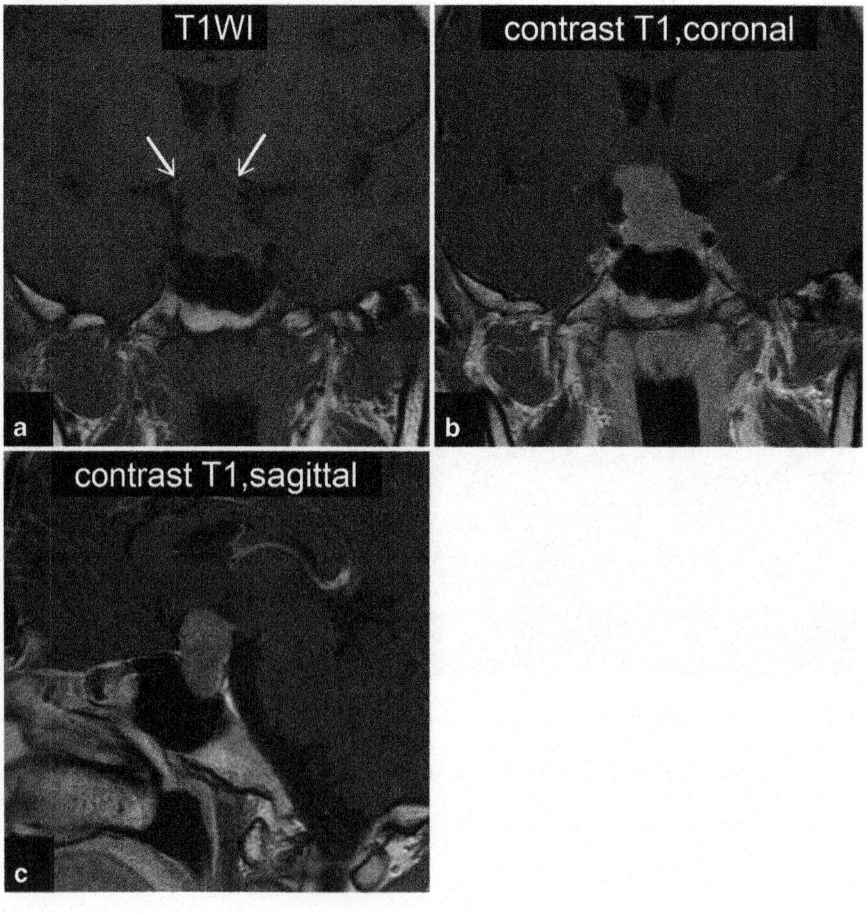

Fig. 6.53 M/30, Pituitary adenoma. This patient complained of blurred vision. The ophthalmologist found that the patient had bitemporal hemianopsia. (**a**–**c**) MRI: A tumor mass in the sella turcica shows intermediate signal intensity on T1WI and homogeneous enhancement by contrast medium. The tumor compresses the optic chiasm (arrows)

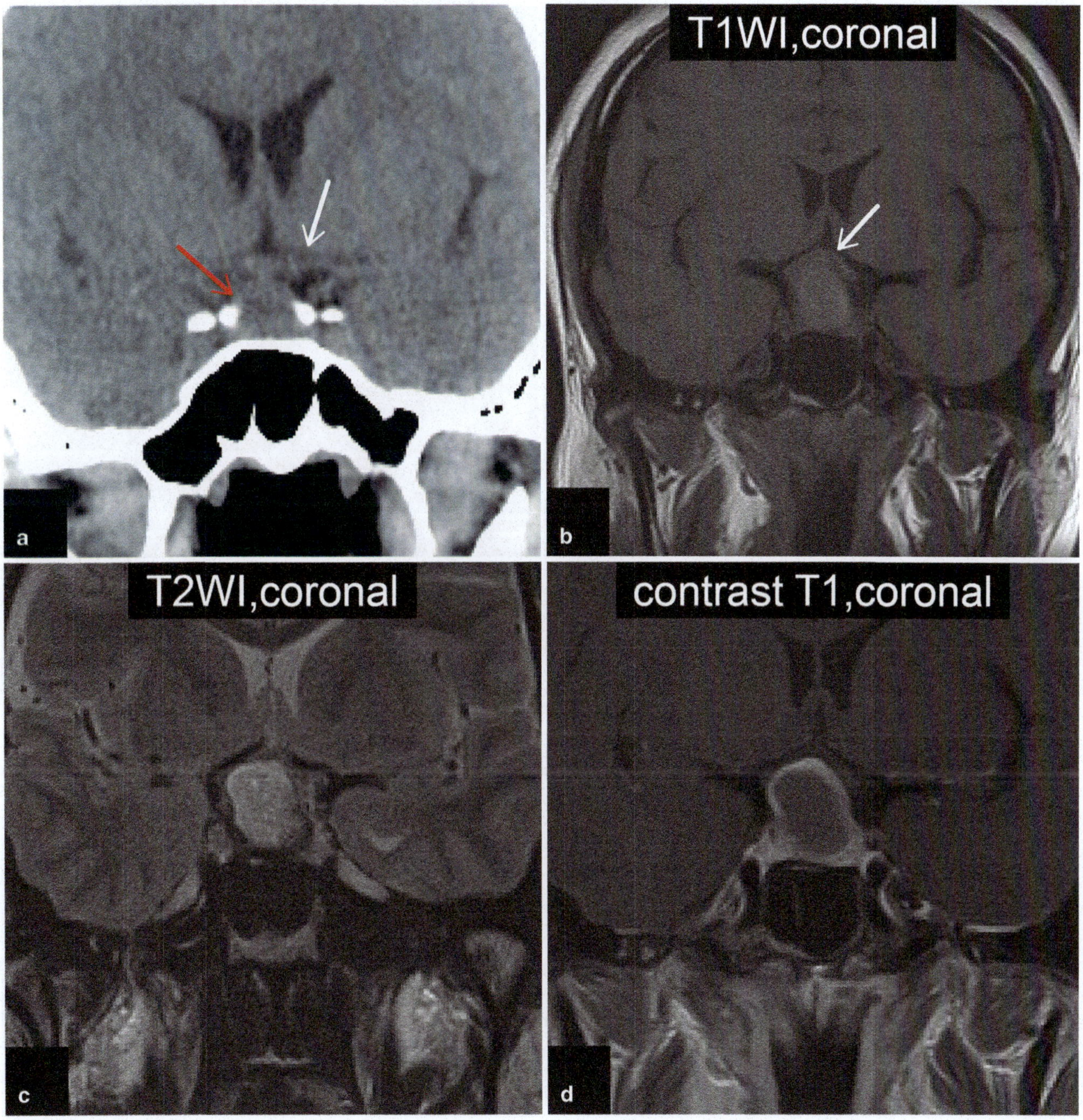

Fig. 6.54 F/33, Pituitary adenoma with cystic change. This patient suffered from headaches and was subjected to a CT examination 3 years ago. (**a**) CT, coronal section: The brain has no abnormal finding. However, the height of the pituitary gland (red arrow) is incidentally found 9 mm, which is abnormal for this age group. The normal height of the pituitary gland in this age is approximately 5–7 mm. The optic chiasm (white arrow) is not compressed. In the last 3 years, the patient suffered from headaches, irregular menstruation, and blurred vision. MRI was performed. (**b–d**) MRI: The height of the pituitary gland is 22 mm with compression on the optic chiasm (arrow), thereby indicating that the tumor is a pituitary adenoma. The tumor shows mild hyperintensity (gray) on T1WI, hyperintensity on T2WI, and marginal enhancement, thus indicating a severe cystic change. These features are typical in pituitary adenoma. Comment: This tumor grew in 3 years. 3 years ago, when CT showed the abnormal height of the pituitary gland, contrast enhancement CT or MRI should have been performed for a possible diagnosis of pituitary adenoma

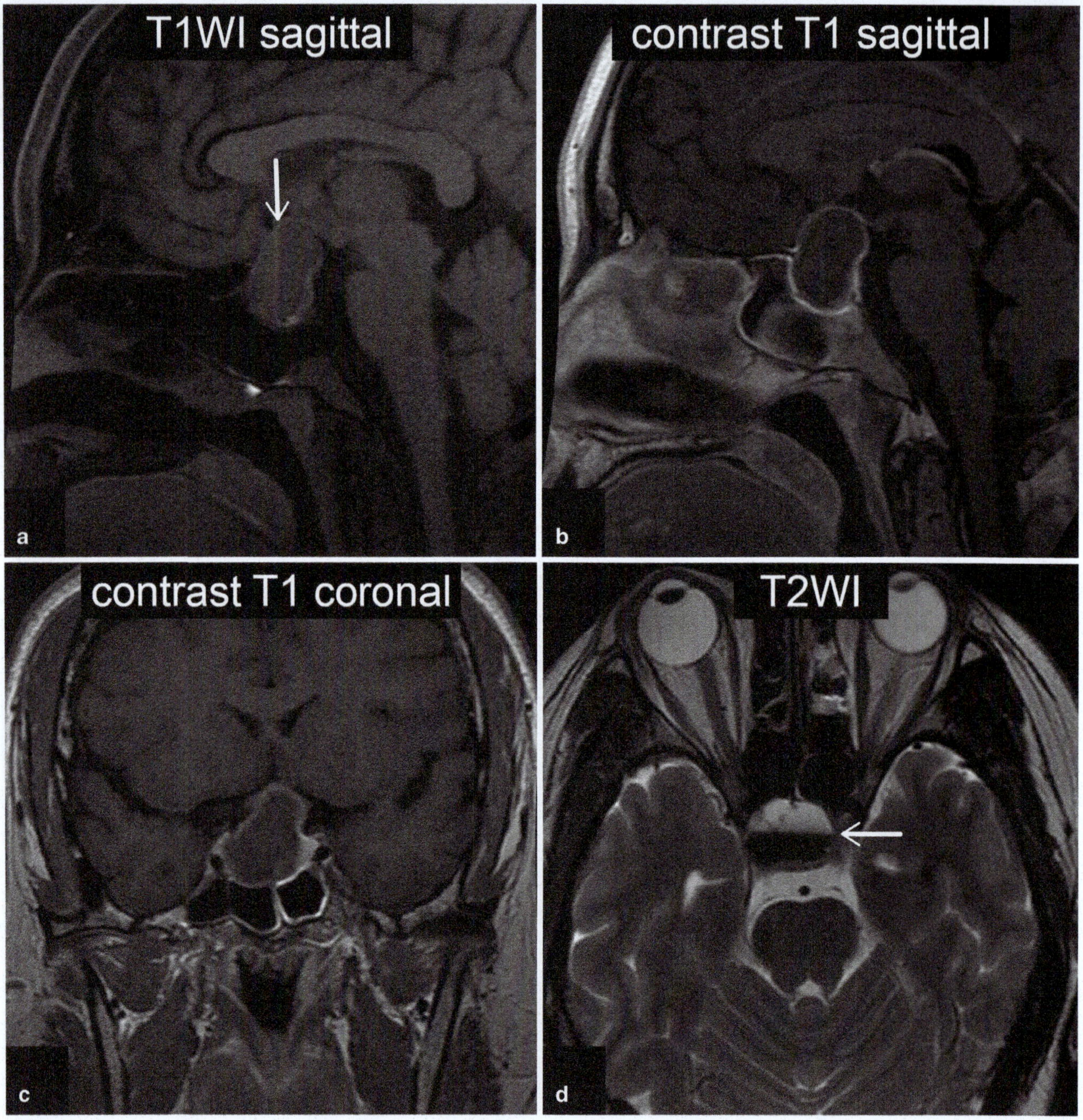

Fig. 6.55 F/36, Pituitary adenoma with cystic change and bleeding. This patient complained of blurred vision and headache and was diagnosed with bitemporal hemianopia. (**a–c**) MRI: A cystic mass is observed in the sella turcica. T1WI shows the fluid-blood level (arrow), and contrast T1WI presents rim enhancement. (**d**) T2WI: Clearly reveals that the upper part of this cystic mass showing hyperintensity is fluid and the lower part showing hypointensity is a blood clot. There is a fluid-blood level (arrow). This mass was surgically removed and confirmed to be a pituitary adenoma with cystic change and bleeding by pathological examination

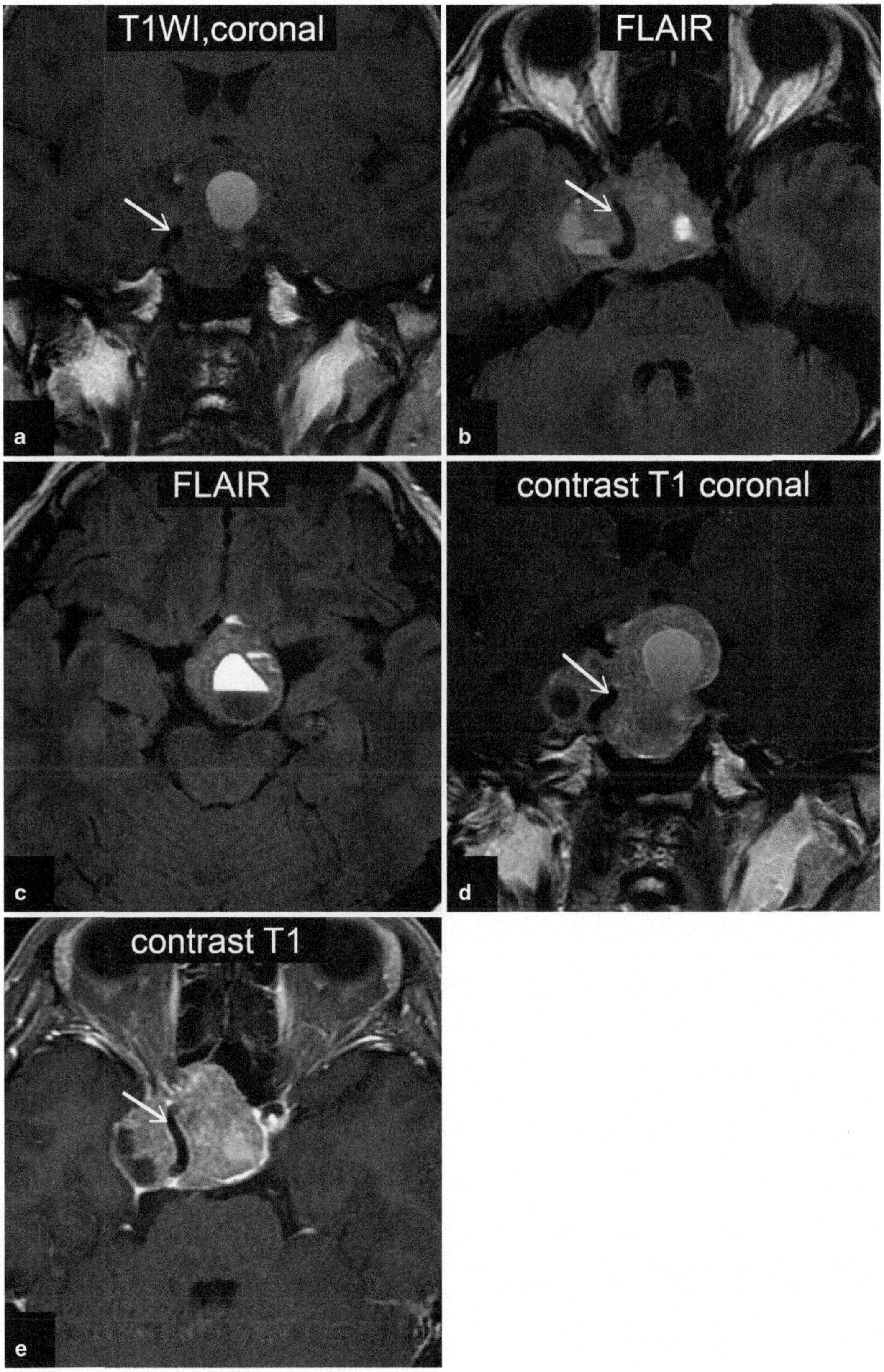

Fig. 6.56 F/52, Pituitary adenoma with cavernous sinus invasion. This patient suffered from blurred vision and was diagnosed with bitemporal hemianopsia. (**a–c**) MRI, T1WI, and FLAIR: A tumor observed in the sella turcica invades into the right cavernous sinus and causes the encasement of the internal carotid artery (ICA) (arrow). A cystic part exists in the superior of this tumor. On T1WI, the cystic part showing hyperintensity, possibly representing protein content. On FLAIR, a fluid level in the cystic part, the upper showing hyperintensity is fluid with protein, and the lower part showing hypointensity is a blood clot. (**d, e**) Contrast T1WI: This tumor mass is well enhanced, extends to the right cavernous sinus, and encases the ICA (arrow)

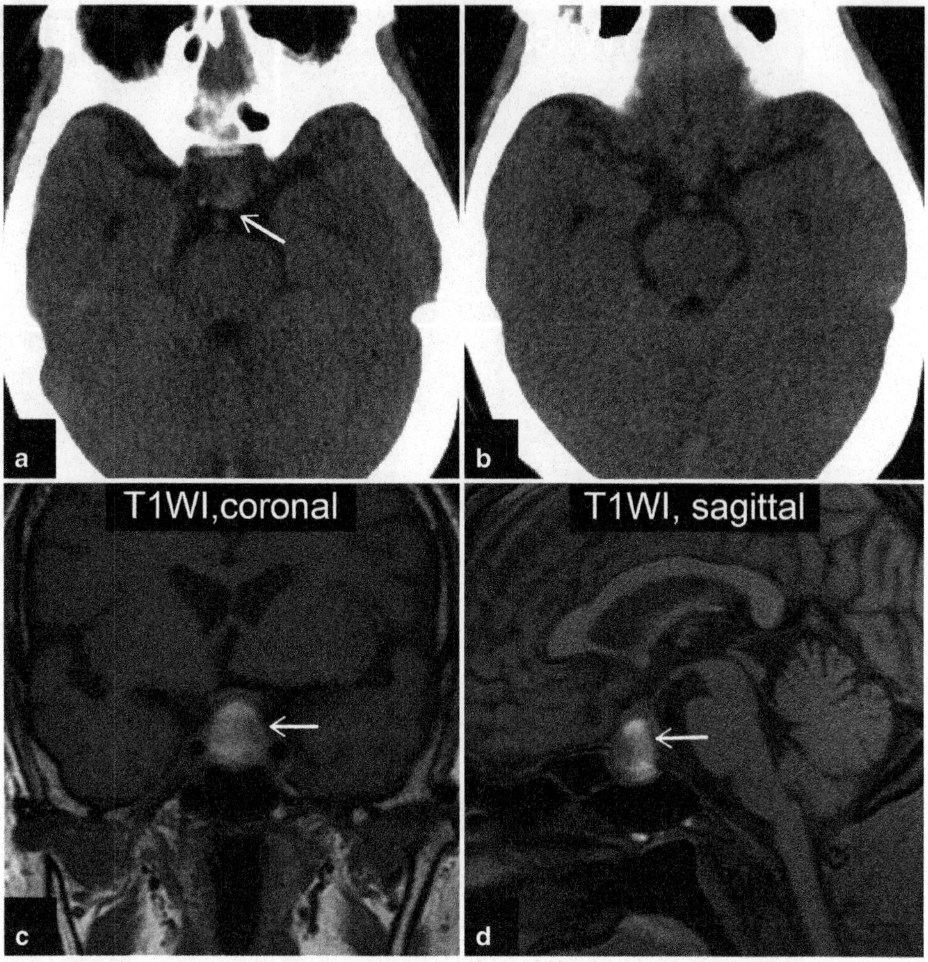

Fig. 6.57 F/61, Pituitary apoplexy. This patient suffered from a sudden onset of severe headache. (**a**, **b**) CT: A small tumor mass (arrow) in the sella turcica showing mild hyperdensity indicates the possibility of a bleeding tumor. (**c**, **d**) MRI, T1WI: The entire tumor mass showing hyperintensity on T1WI represents a bleeding tumor. This tumor was surgically removed, and pathological examination confirmed pituitary adenoma, necrosis, and hemorrhage. A bleeding pituitary adenoma with severe headache is called pituitary apoplexy

6.6.4 Craniopharyngioma

Craniopharyngioma, WHO Gr I

Location: Craniopharyngiomas develop from embryonic remnants of Rathke's pouch. They are mostly located in the suprasellar region, with few of them inside the sella turcica.

Age: The tumor has generally grown large enough to cause symptoms by the ages of 6–20 years (Fig. 6.58). However, the incidence rate amazingly increases in another age range of 50–60 years (Fig. 6.59). Development in other age periods is also possible.

Clinical symptoms: Compression of the optic nerve causes problems in visual acuity. Compression of the pituitary gland generates hormone abnormality similar to that induced by a pituitary adenoma. The tumor may cause diabetes insipidus. It may also compress the foramen of Monro or third ventricle to produce hydrocephalus and cause increased intracranial pressure.

CT: Most craniopharyngiomas have three parts that can be completely shown in CT:

1. Calcifications: In children, craniopharyngiomas exhibit almost 100% have calcifications.
2. Cystic part: Craniopharyngioma is a cystic tumor based on multiple cysts, and each cyst may not be interconnected and can contain diverse components. Therefore, the CT density may vary depending on the protein content.
3. Soft tissue mass part: This part is small in size and can be enhanced using contrast media.

MRI: Because additional sagittal and coronal sections can be obtained using MRI, the diagnosis of craniopharyngioma can be more meticulous when using this technique. Cysts in a craniopharyngioma can contain different signal intensities of protein. Hypointensity, isointensity, and hyperintensity of signals may be present in T1WI. In T2WI and FLAIR, the liquid content results in hyperintensity from all cysts. The disadvantage of MRI is that its identification of calcification is inferior to that of CT. The significant calcification exhibits darker signals in MRI, whereas low calcification is invisible in MRI.

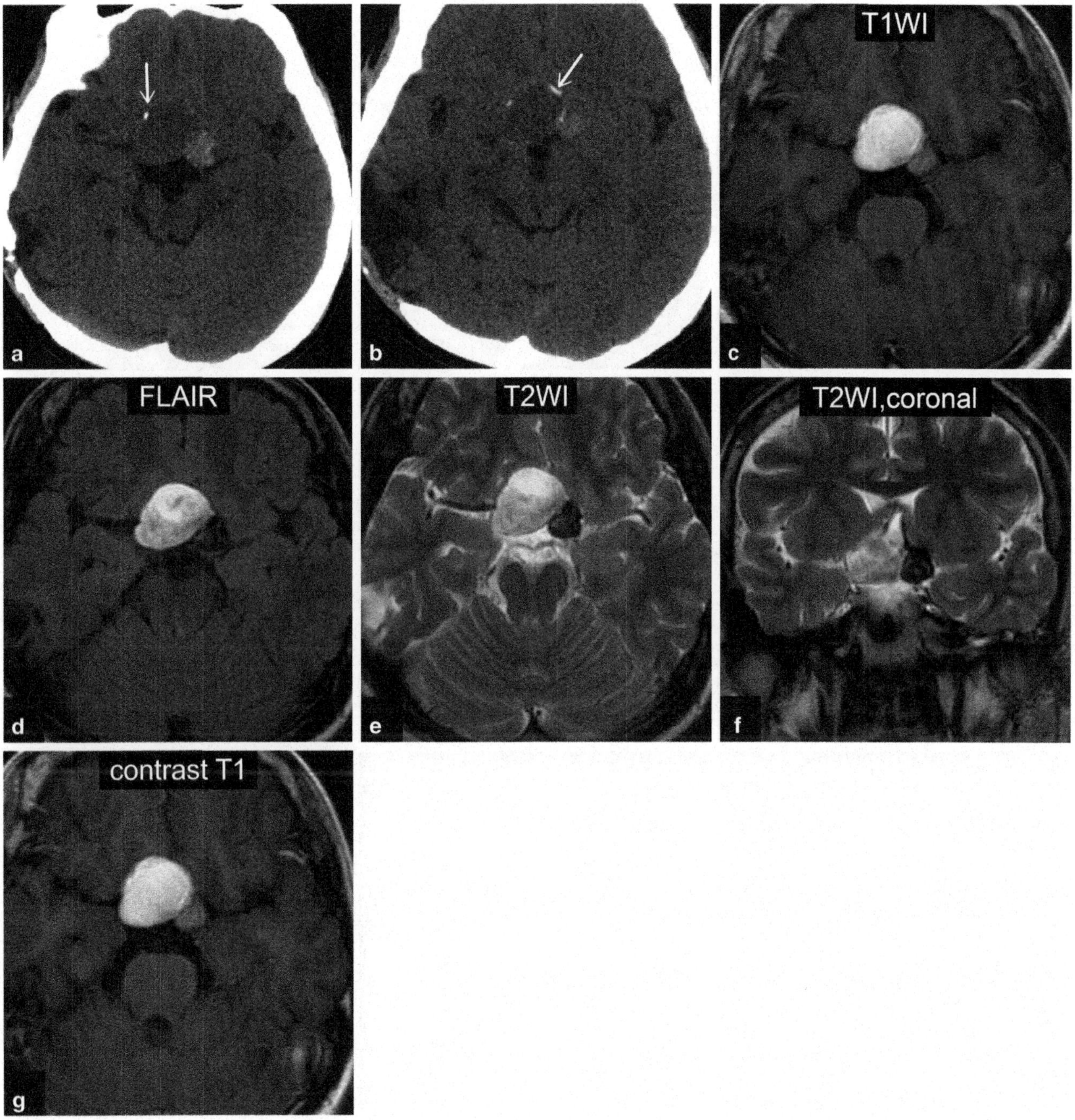

Fig. 6.58 M/20, Craniopharyngioma. (**a**, **b**) CT: A mass in the suprasellar region showing mild hypodensity with marginal calcifications (arrows) is a cystic mass. Another white part exists in the left posterior, which may be another cyst with a high protein component or a calcified soft tissue mass. (**c**–**g**) MRI: This tumor has two components. The larger one is a cyst with high-signal substance showing hyperintensity on T1WI, FLAIR, and T2WI. The left posterior one shows mild hypointensity on T1WI, dark (hypointensity) on FLAIR and T2WI, and no contrast enhancement; this is a calcified soft tissue mass. The above CT and MRI findings are the characteristic features of craniopharyngioma. This tumor was surgically removed and confirmed to be a craniopharyngioma by pathological examination

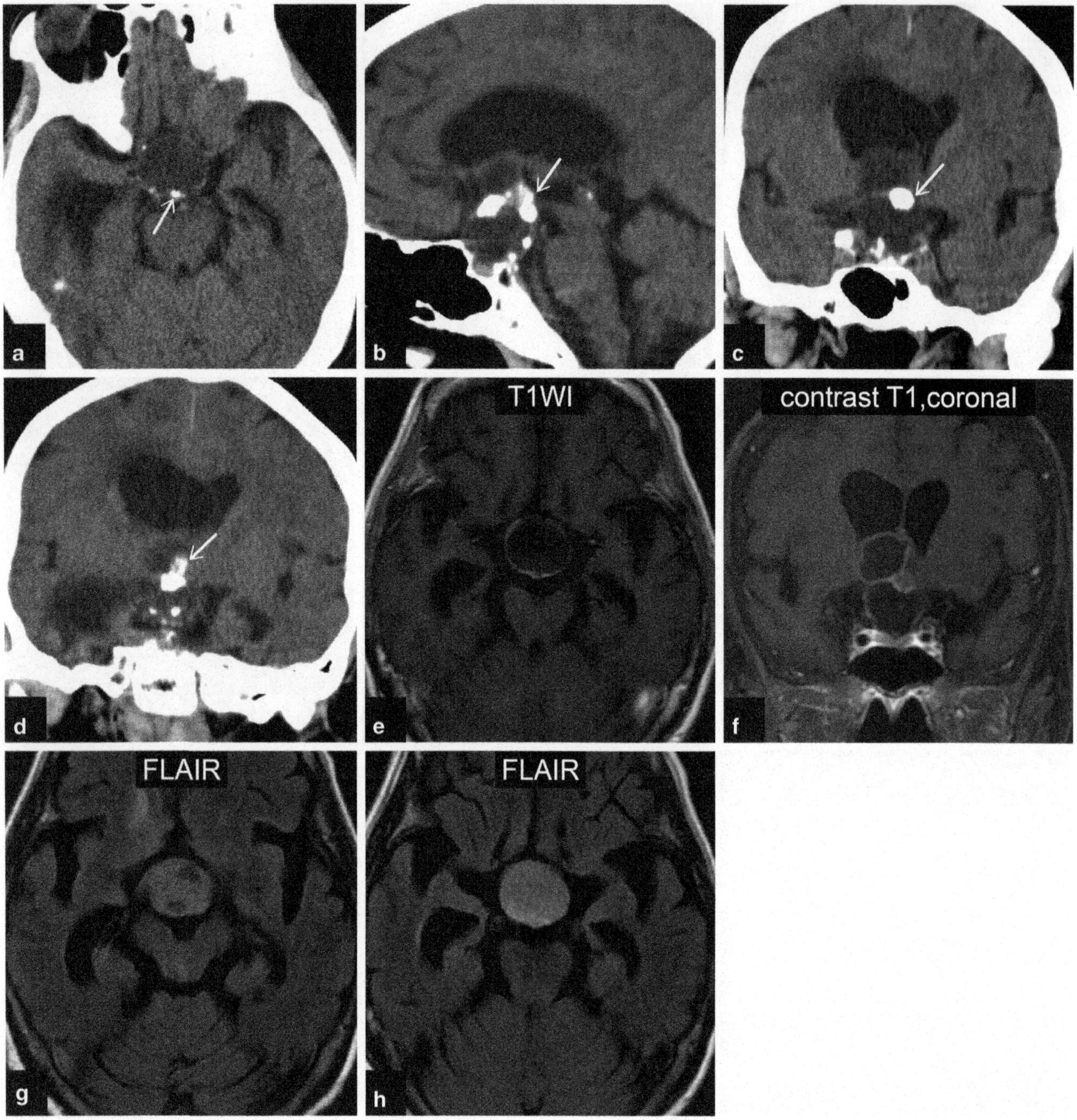

Fig. 6.59 F/66, Craniopharyngioma. This patient complained of blurred vision for several months. (**a**) CT, axial, (**b**) CT, sagittal, (**c**, **d**) CT coronal: The feature of a cystic mass with calcifications (arrows) in the suprasellar region indicates a typical craniopharyngioma. (**e**–**h**) MRI: MRI has difficulty in showing the calcifications. The content of this cystic mass presents hypointensity on T1WI and mild hyperintensity on FLAIR, which indicates a thicker liquid and may contain a protein component. This tumor was surgically removed and confirmed to be a craniopharyngioma by pathological examination

6.6.5 Rathke's Cleft Cyst

The Rathke's cleft cysts develop from sella or suprasellar location with reasonably high incidence. Generally, no symptoms occur. Therefore, most of these cysts are discovered accidentally during an MRI examination of the brain (Fig. 6.60).

The cysts develop from the pituitary embryonic remnant of Rathke's pouch. They are rarely discovered in children. In adults, they must grow large enough to be found in CT and MRI.

CT: Cysts with CSF density are observed in the sellar and suprasellar region.

MRI: The signal is identical to that of CSF, similar to CT. However, some cysts contain mucoid or serous components, which exhibit strong signals in T1WIs and T2WIs.

Injection of contrast media does not enhance the cysts.

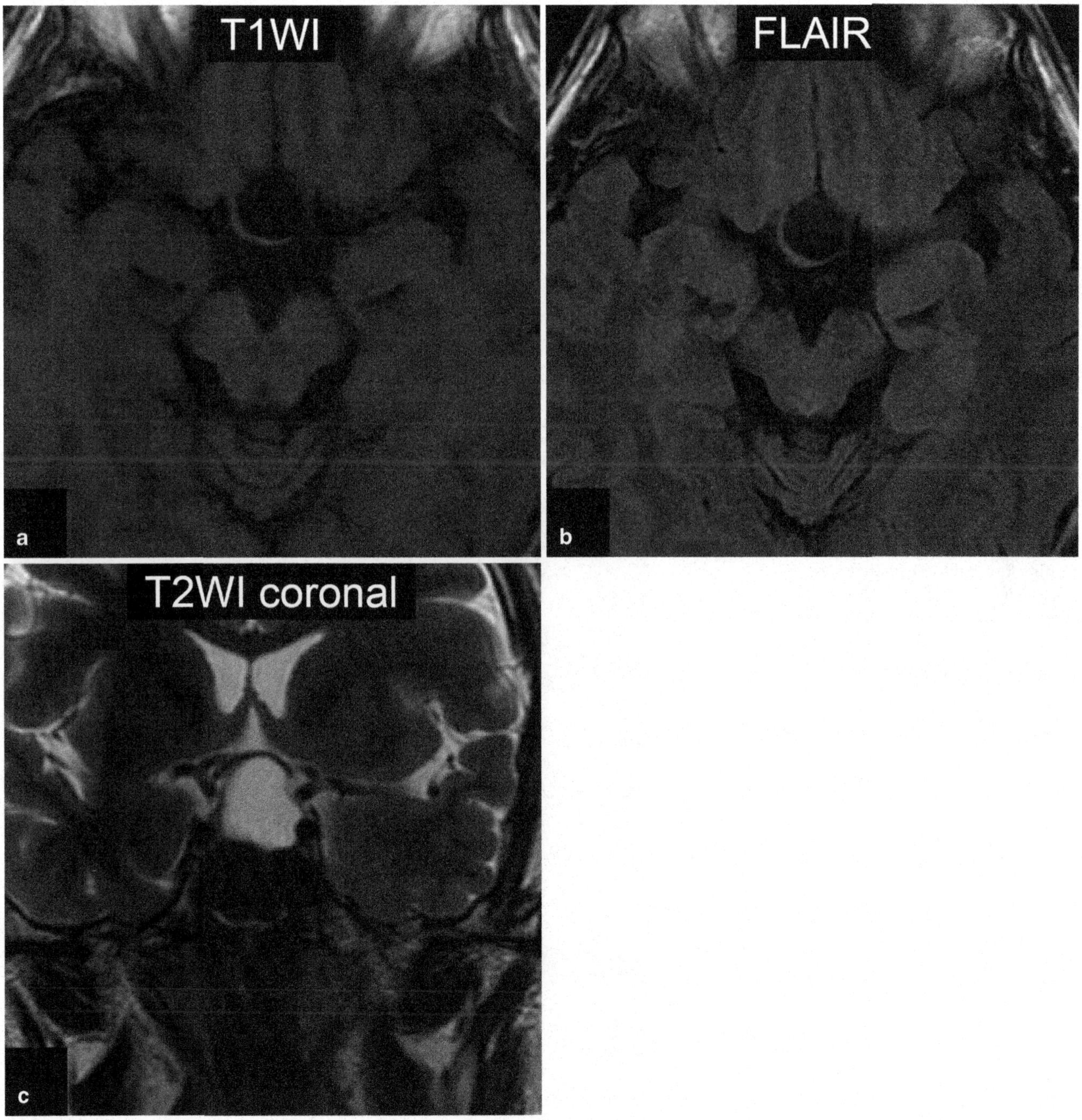

Fig. 6.60 M/47, Rathke's cleft cyst. No clinical symptom. (**a**–**c**) MRI for healthy examination: A cystic mass is incidentally found in the sellar region. The signal intensity of this cystic content is consistent with that of CSF. This mass was surgically removed and confirmed to be a Rathke's cleft cyst by pathological examination

6.6.6 Schwannomas

Intracranial schwannomas, WHO Gr I.

All 12 pairs of cranial nerves may develop tumors. The optic nerve is unique because it mostly develops glioma, with its nerve sheath developing meningioma at an extremely low incidence. The most common tumor at the third to twelfth cranial nerves is schwannoma growing from Schwann cells outside the nerve sheath. The incidence is highest in the eighth cranial nerve (acoustic nerve), followed by the fifth cranial nerve (Fig. 6.67). The incidence in other cranial nerves (Fig. 6.66) is low.

6.6.6.1 Acoustic Schwannoma

Age: Adults.

Location: The internal auditory canal and the middle one-third location of the cerebellopontine (CP) angle cistern. Because the acoustic nerve extending from the brain stem has only a small segment immersed in the CP angle cistern before entering the internal auditory canal, tumors can develop inside and outside the internal auditory canal (Figs. 6.61, 6.62, 6.63, 6.64, 6.65, and 6.66).

Clinical symptoms: Even when an acoustic schwannoma is small, it can cause tinnitus, hearing impairment, and eventually deafness. If the tumor grows larger, it can compress the nearby facial nerve (seventh cranial nerve) or other nerves to generate symptoms. The tumor can also compress the brain stem to cause related symptoms. In a few cases, the tumor even compresses the fourth ventricle or cerebral aqueduct, thereby inducing hydrocephalus and increased intracranial pressure.

CT and MRI: If a tumor develops at the middle one-third of the CP angle cistern, diagnosis of acoustic schwannoma should be considered, especially when the internal auditory canal widening with bony erosion (clearer in CT) (Fig. 6.62). After injection of contrast media, CT and MRI both show favorable contrast enhancement of the tumor. However, acoustic schwannoma can easily exhibit cystic changes (Figs. 6.64 and 6.65). In MRI, the "fruit stalk sign" shows that the tumor has entered the internal auditory canal (Figs. 6.63, 6.64, and 6.65). This is a useful sign of acoustic schwannoma diagnosis.

Small Acoustic Schwannoma

This is also called intracanalicular schwannoma (Figs. 6.61, 6.62, and 6.66).

MRI with Gd-DTPA injection is necessary to reveal this type of small tumor.

Bilateral Acoustic Schwannomas

If acoustic schwannoma occurs on bilateral acoustic nerves or associated with other cranial nerve schwannomas or meningioma, it should be suspected to be neurofibromatosis (Fig. 6.66).

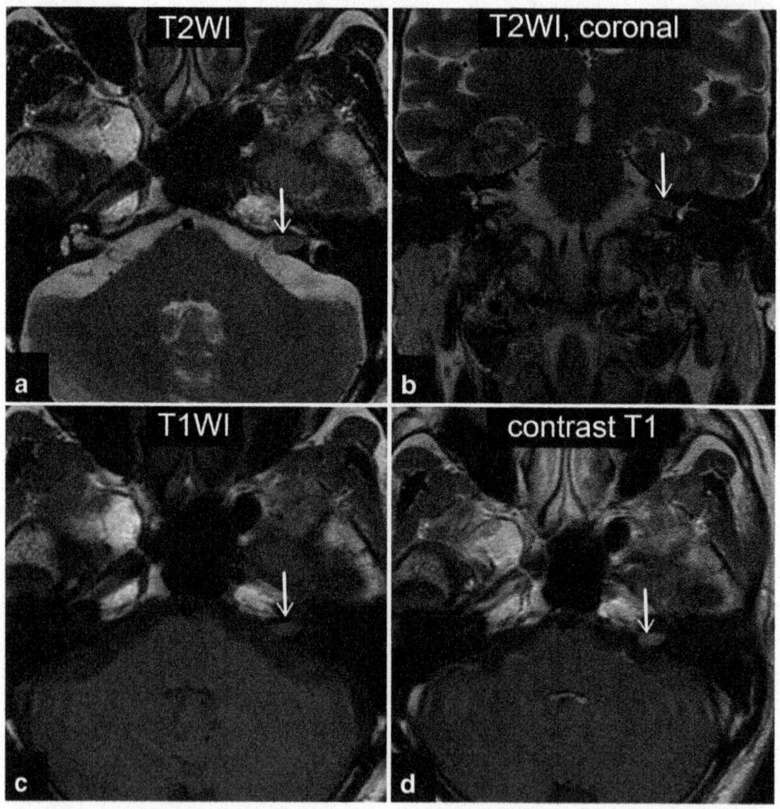

Fig. 6.61 M/59, Intracanalicular acoustic schwannoma. This patient suffered from tinnitus and gradual hearing loss in the left ear in the last one and half years. (**a**, **b**) MR, T2WI: A small tumor (arrow) is observed in the left internal auditory canal. (**c**, **d**) T1WI and contrast T1WI: This mass has mild contrast enhancement (arrow). This is a typical intracanalicular acoustic schwannoma

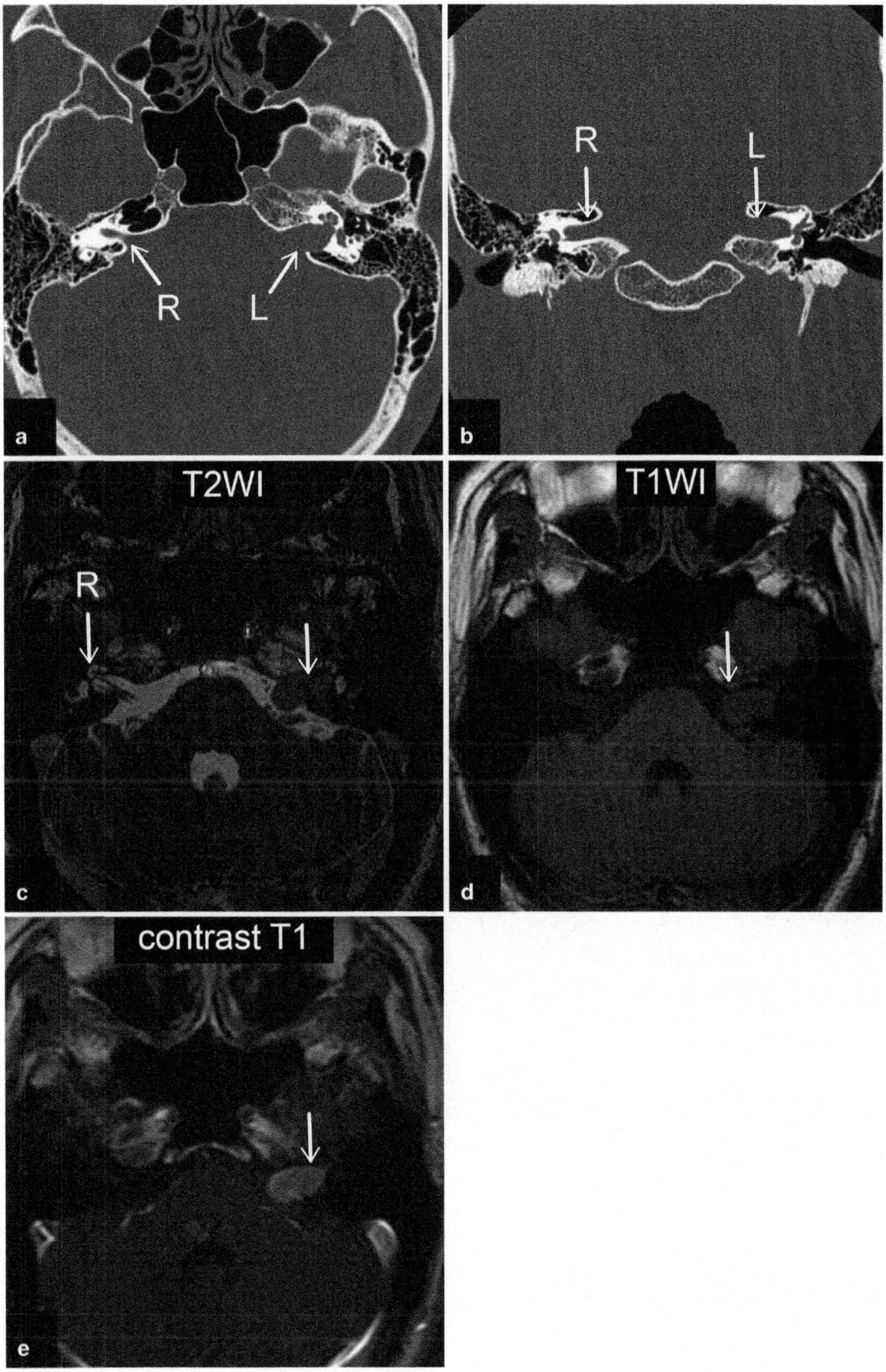

Fig. 6.62 M/29, Small acoustic schwannoma. This patient suffered from tinnitus and gradual hearing loss of the left ear for several months. (**a**, **b**) Mastoid CT, axial, and coronal sections: Compared with the normal right internal auditory canal (R) IAC, the left (L) IAC is slightly widened. This finding indicates the possibility of acoustic schwannoma in the left IAC. (**c**, **d**) MRI, T2WI, and T1WI: A small tumor is observed in the orifice and left IAC (arrow), and the R IAC is normal. (**e**) Contrast T1WI: This tumor is slightly enhanced (arrow). The small tumor is a typical acoustic schwannoma

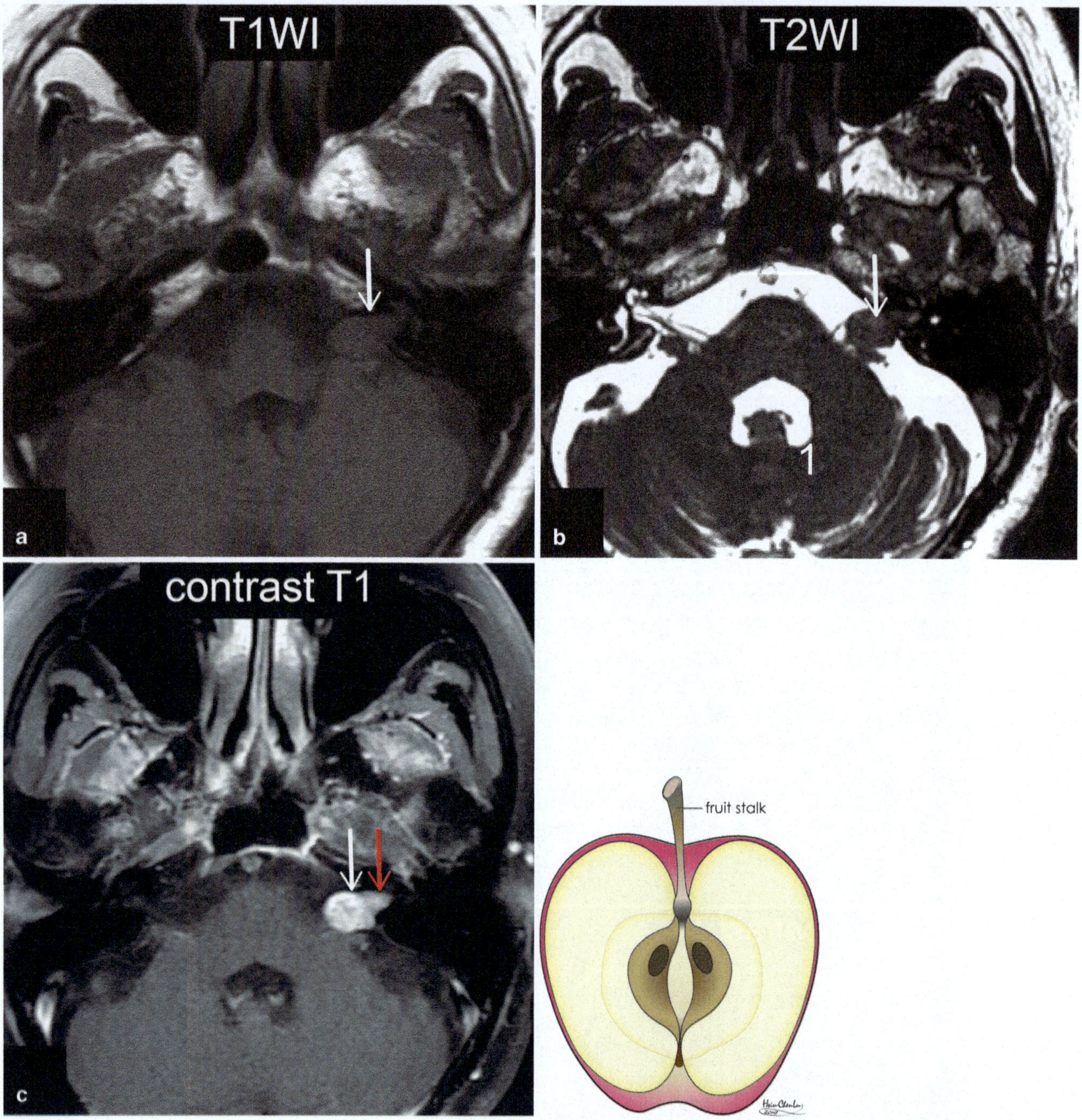

Fig. 6.63 F/70, Acoustic schwannoma. (**a**, **b**) MRI, T1WI, and T2WI: A tumor mass (arrow) is observed in the left CP angle cistern, just in the orifice of left IAC. (**c**) Contrast T1WI: This tumor (arrow) has well enhancement and shows that a fruit stalk (red arrow) extends into the IAC. This feature is a typical sign of acoustic schwannoma

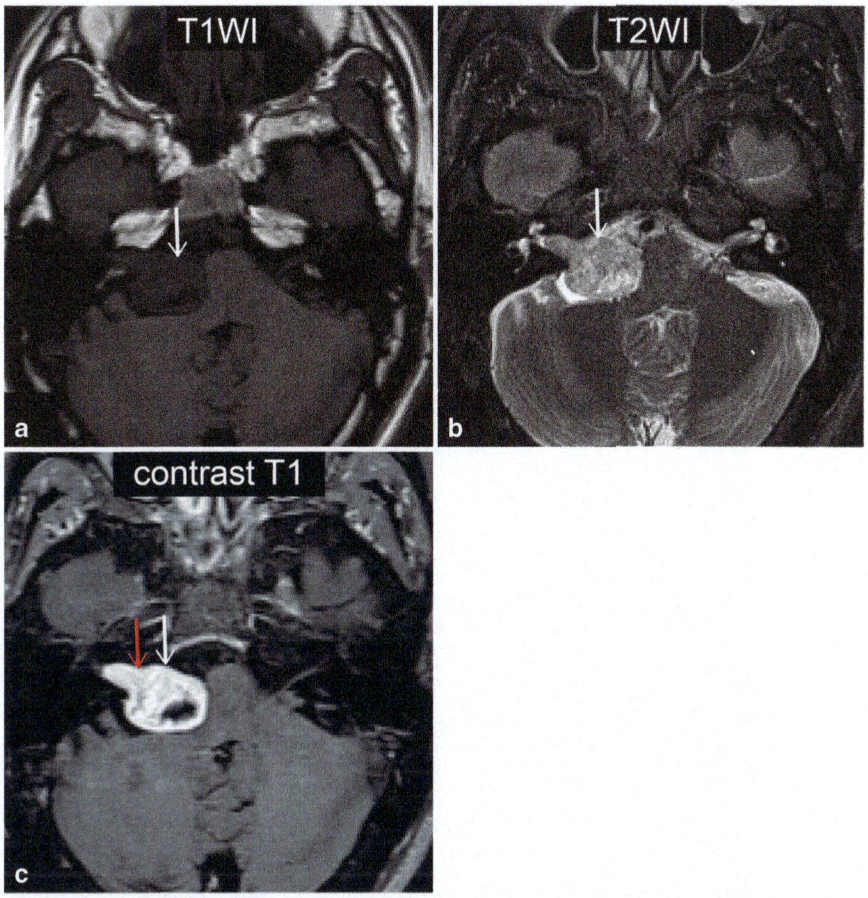

Fig. 6.64 M/47, Large acoustic schwannoma compressing the brainstem. (**a**, **b**) MRI, T1WI, and T2WI: A large tumor mass (arrow) exists in the right CP angle cistern. (**c**) Contrast T1WI: This tumor has well enhancement (arrow), a small cystic part, and a fruit stalk (red arrow) extends into the right internal auditory canal. This tumor is a typical acoustic schwannoma and compresses the right side of the pons

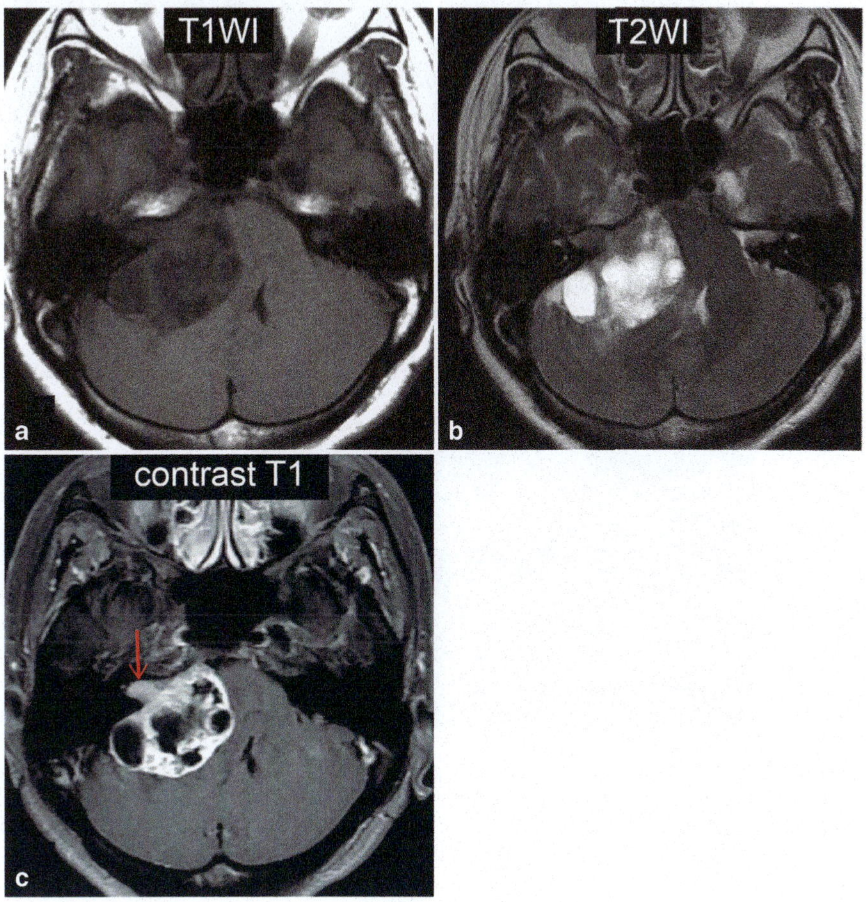

Fig. 6.65 F/44, Large acoustic schwannoma compressing the brainstem. This patient suffered from dizziness and unsteady gait for several months. (**a**, **b**) MRI, T1WI, and T2WI: A large tumor in the right side of the posterior fossa with cystic change severely compresses the pons. (**c**) Contrast T1WI: This tumor has heterogeneous enhancement because of cystic change. A fruit stalk (red arrow) extending into the right IAC is a sign of acoustic schwannoma. Given that acoustic neuroma will first have symptoms of tinnitus and progressive hearing loss, the patient will seek medical treatment. It is rare that an acoustic schwannoma grows to very large to compress the brainstem, such as this patient

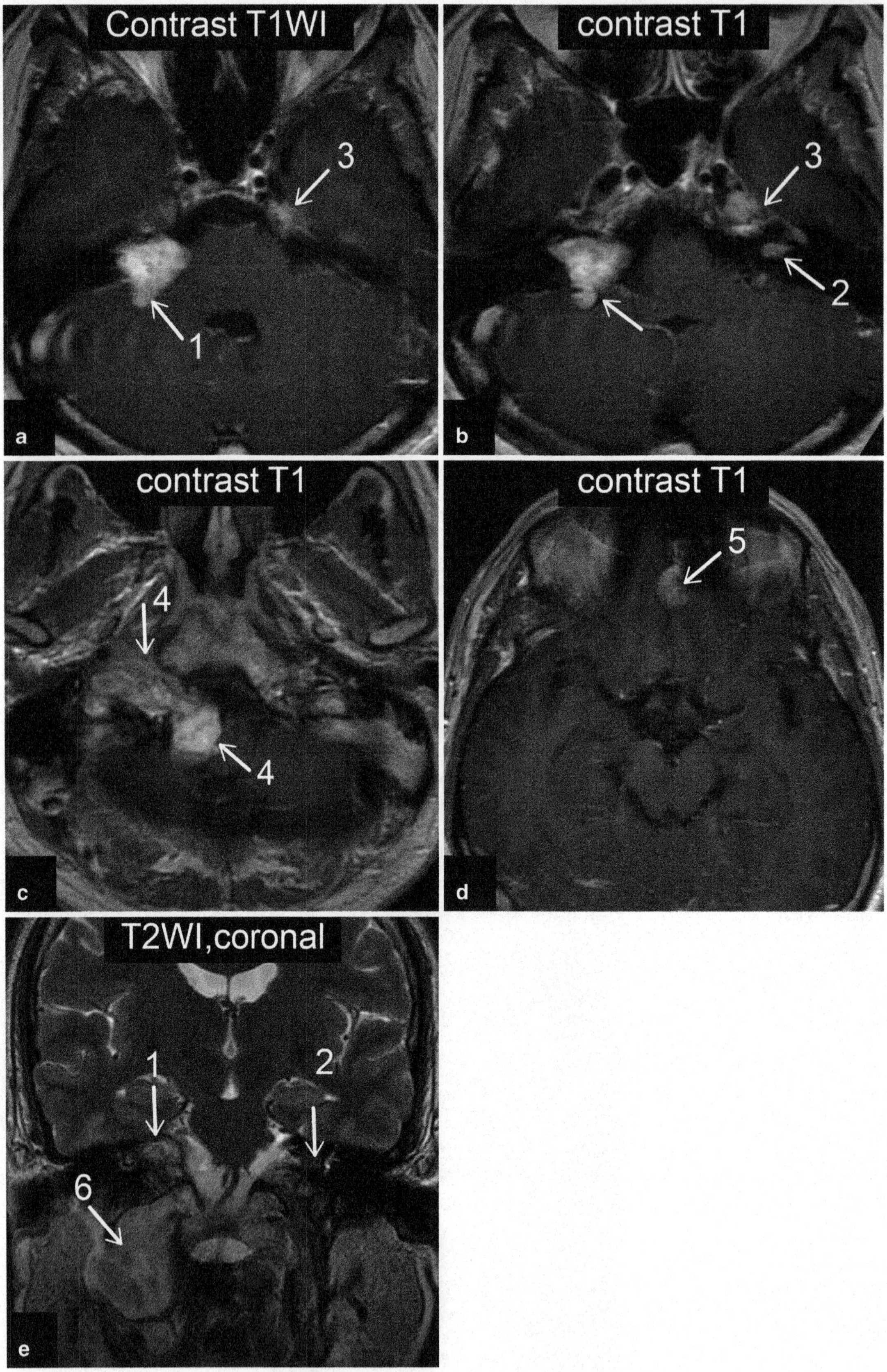

Fig. 6.66 M/32, Multiple schwannomas. A type 2 neurofibromatosis patient. (**a**–**d**) Contrast T1WI: Multiple tumors, including the right-side acoustic schwannoma (1), left intracanalicular acoustic schwannoma (2), left trigeminal schwannoma (3), right hypoglossal nerve schwannoma (4), and a small tumor in the anterior cranial fossa (5), is a meningioma. (**e**) T2WI: A large tumor (6) in the right parapharyngeal space is a neurofibroma of the cervical nerve. Only neurofibromatosis patients may have multiple schwannomas, neurofibroma, and associated with meningioma

6.6.6.2 Trigeminal Schwannoma

The fifth cranial nerve (trigeminal nerve) is extended from the pons, passes through the most anterior portion of the CP angle cistern, and enters the cavernous sinus. If a tumor develops in the trigeminal nerve, its position is at the front of the posterior fossa, or inside the cavernous sinus, or across the petrous bone, forming a dumbbell-shaped tumor between the cavernous sinus and posterior fossa (Fig. 6.67).

The resultant clinical symptoms are nonspecific. A tumor in the cavernous sinus may paralyze the fifth, third, fourth, and sixth cranial nerves. When it is located in the posterior fossa, it may compress the brain stem and causes brain-stem-related symptoms.

The CT and MRI imaging features are similar to those of acoustic schwannoma.

6.6.6.3 Other Schwannomas

Other schwannomas have extremely low incidence rates. If any (Fig. 6.66), the CT and MRI results resemble those of acoustic schwannoma, with favorable contrast enhancement and easily have cystic changes. If a tumor develops in multiple cranial nerves, the diagnosis of neurofibromatosis should be considered.

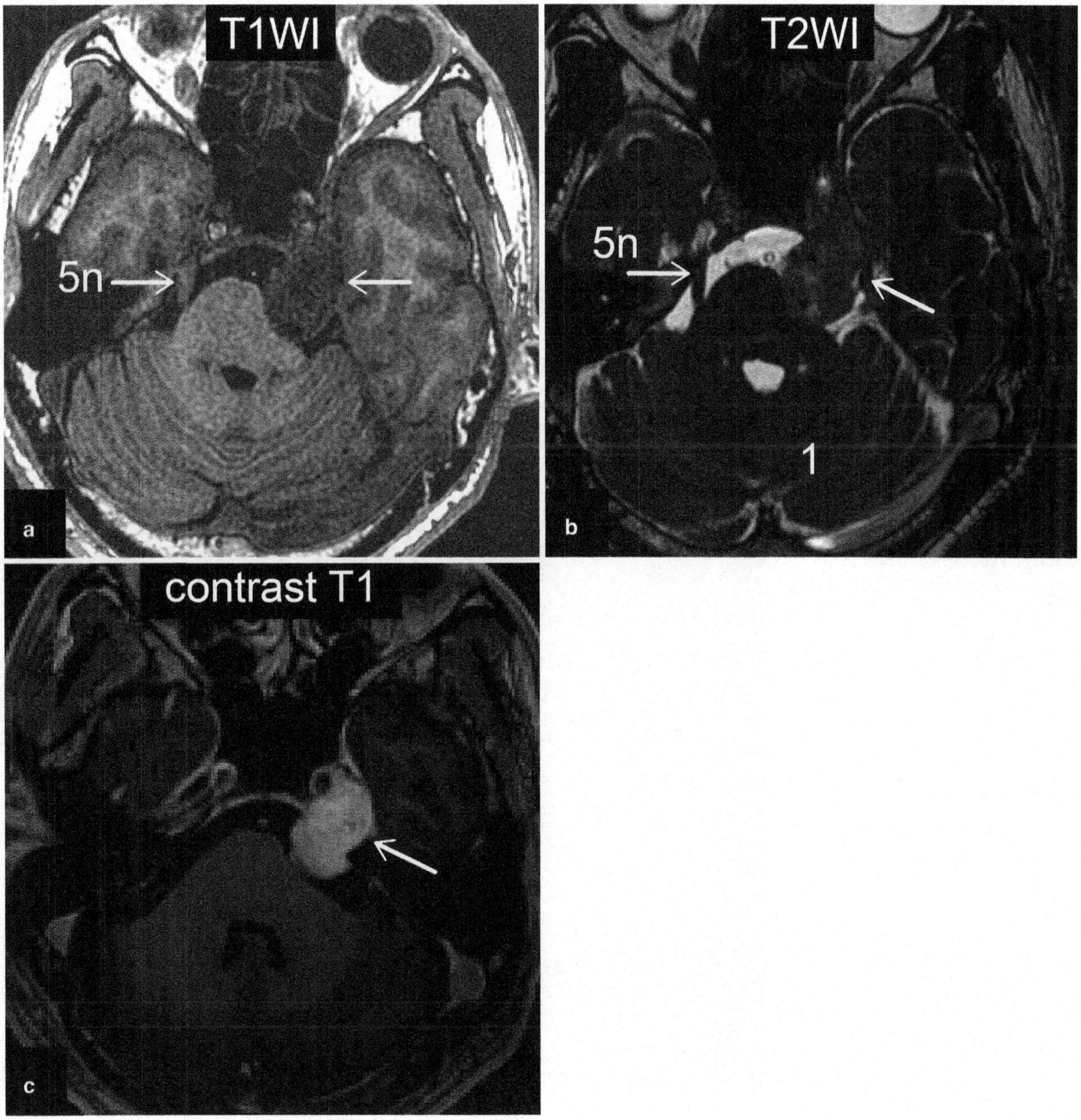

Fig. 6.67 M/57, Trigeminal nerve schwannoma. (**a**, **b**) MRI, T1WI, and T2WI: A tumor mass (arrow) is observed in the front of the left side of the pons, slightly compressing the pons. As compared with the right trigeminal nerve (5 n), these features indicate that the tumor came from the left trigeminal nerve. (**c**) Contrast T1WI: This tumor (arrow) has well enhancement and extends into the cavernous sinus. A tumor in the anterior portion of the cerebellopontine cistern and extends into the cavernous sinus is a typical trigeminal nerve schwannoma

6.6.7 Germ Cell Tumors

Tumors of this type are composed of germ cell derivatives and are of the following five subtypes:

1. Germinoma (Figs. 6.68 and 6.69): the highest incidence and response most favorably to radiation therapy and chemotherapy.
2. Teratoma (Fig. 6.70): including immature and malignant teratomas.
3. Embryonal carcinoma.
4. Yolk sac tumor.
5. Choriocarcinoma.

These germ cell tumors develop in midline locations of the human body, such as the reproductive organs, sacrum, retroperitoneum, and mediastinum. If the tumors develop in intracranial positions, they are also in the midline locations, namely the pineal region (Fig. 6.68), suprasellar region (Figs. 6.69 and 6.70), and thalamus. Few develop in the basal ganglia. Sometimes, two or more tumors may develop simultaneously in different positions. However, they are principally located in the midline.

Germ cell tumors easily spread across the intracranial regions through the CSF. They may even flow into the spinal canal through the CSF and metastasize to the spine. Diagnosis of germ cell tumors can be made through not only CT and MRI but also check tumor markers in the blood or CSF, including α-fetoprotein, ß-HCG, and carcinoembryonic antigen (CEA).

CT and MRI: Germ cell tumors have no unique shape, some tumors exhibit clear outlines, whereas others infiltrate the ventricular wall, and distinction among the five subtypes as mentioned above is difficult. In young adults and children, if the CT and MRI results show any tumor in intracranial midline locations, the tumor should be suspected to be a germ cell tumor (Figs. 6.68 and 6.69). A blood test for tumor markers can be conducted to serve as a reference for diagnosis. The correct diagnosis is reliant on pathology reports.

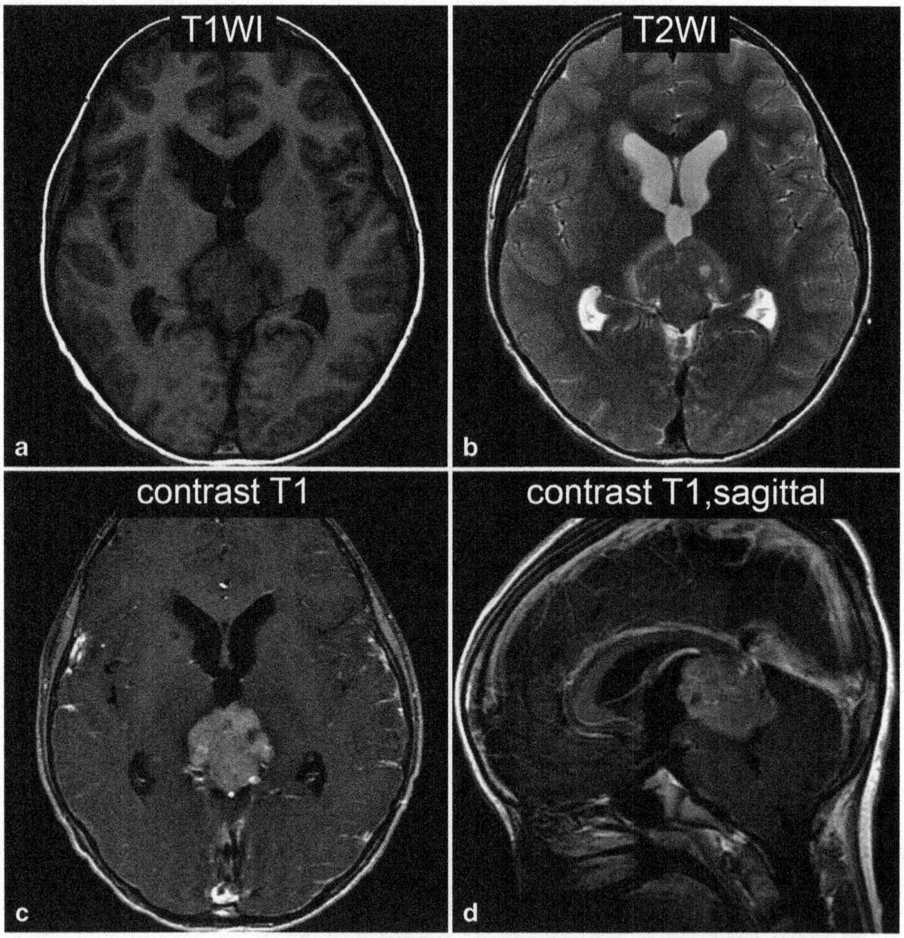

Fig. 6.68 M/8, Germinoma, pineal region. This patient suffered from dizziness and vomiting. (**a–d**) MRI: A tumor mass in the pineal region with strong enhancement and compresses the third ventricle causes mild hydrocephalus. The blood biochemical examination on ß-HCG and α-FTP is normal. This tumor was surgically removed and confirmed to be germinoma by pathological examination

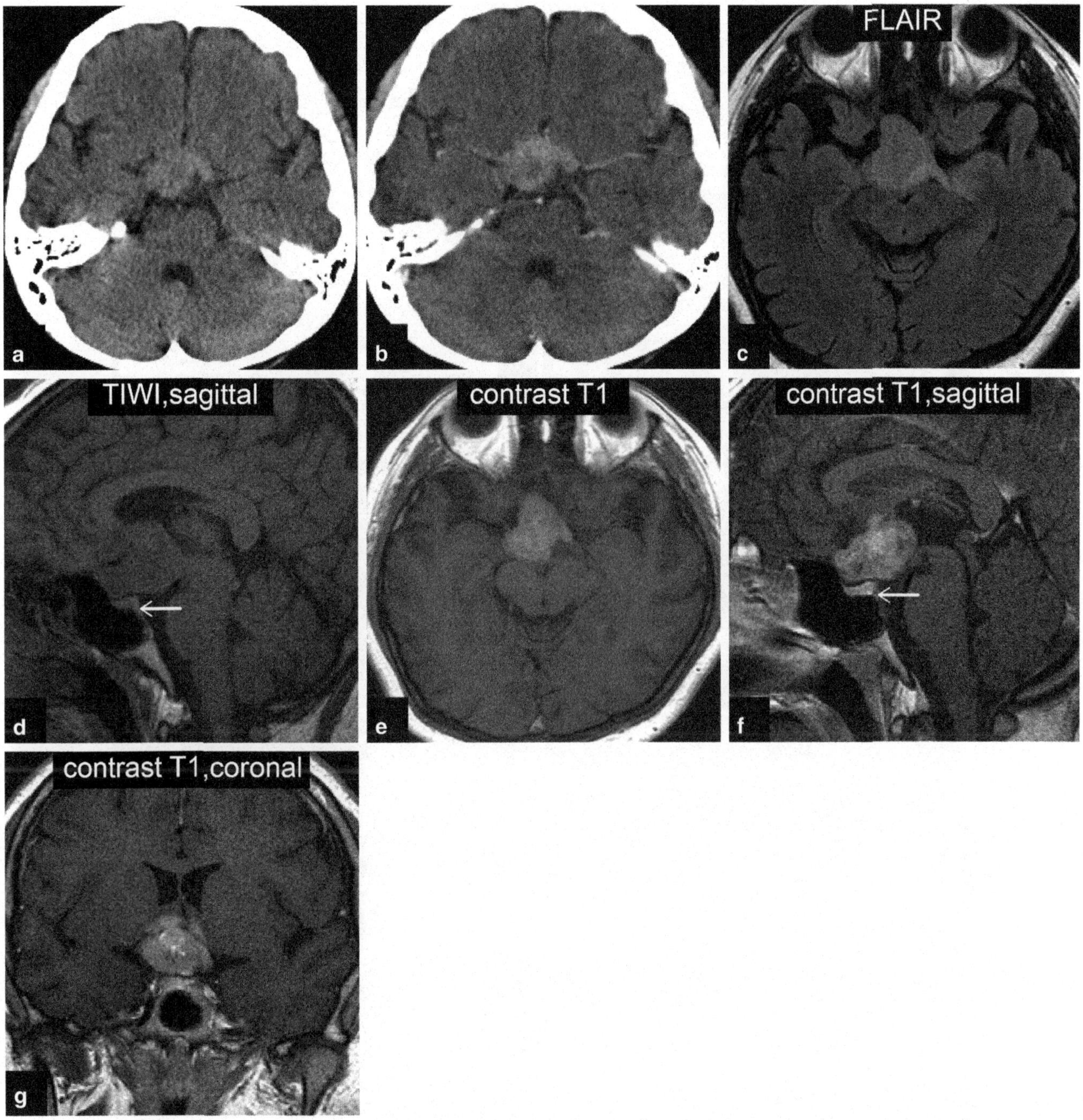

Fig. 6.69 F/20, Suprasellar germinoma. This patient suffered from blurred vision for several months. (**a**) CT (**b**) contrast CT: A tumor mass is observed in the suprasellar region with faint contrast enhancement. (**c–g**) MRI: more clearly to see this tumor, it compresses the optic chiasm. The normal pituitary gland (arrows) is beneath this tumor. This tumor was surgically removed and confirmed to be a germinoma by pathological examination

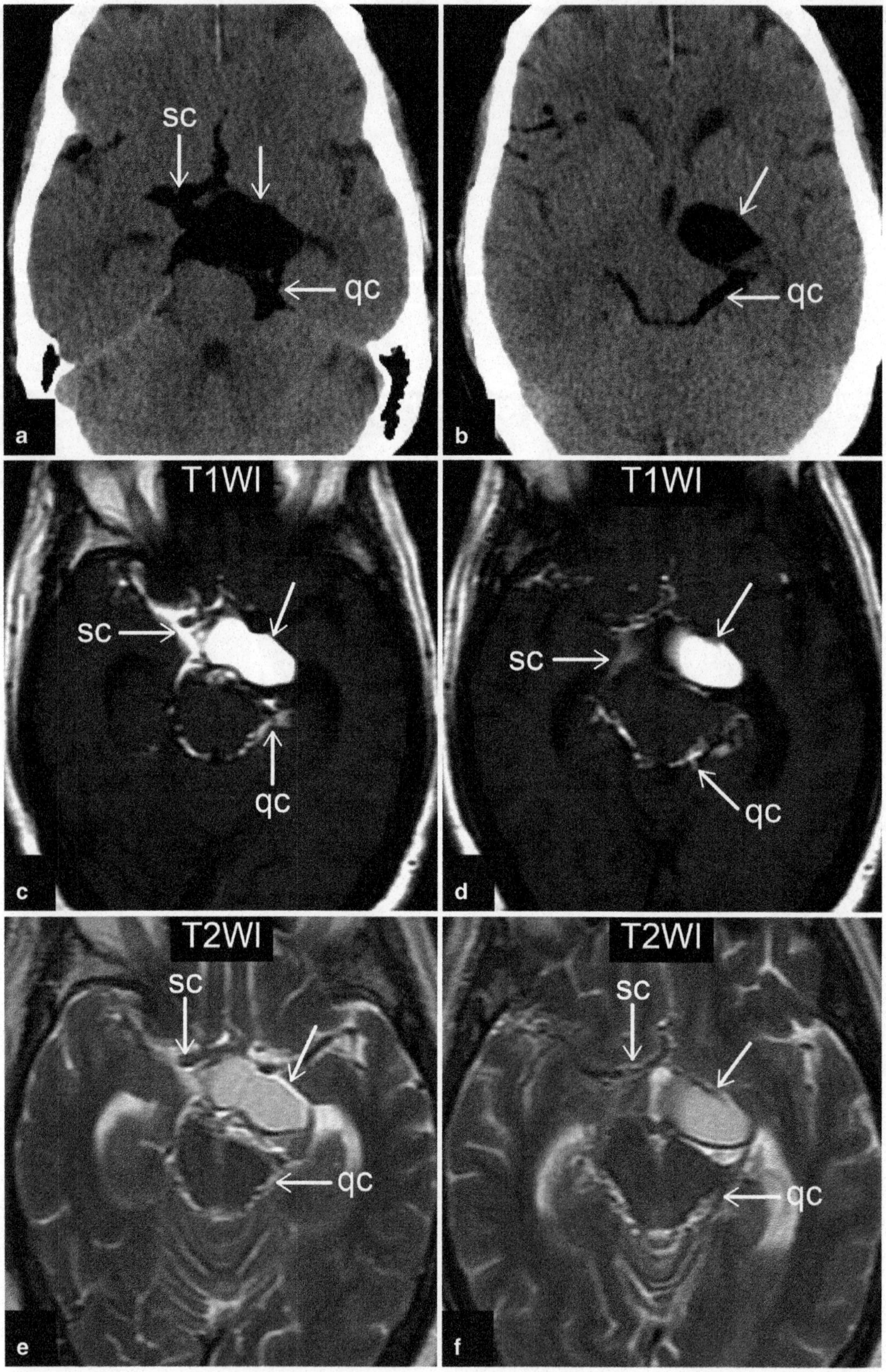

Fig. 6.70 M/76, Suprasellar teratoma. (**a**, **b**) CT: A dark cystic mass (arrows) exists in the sella and suprasellar regions. The darkening of the suprasellar cistern (sc) and quadrigeminal cistern (qc) is also observed. (**c**, **d**) MRI, T1WI: The significant hyperintensity of this mass (arrows) indicates the fatty signal intensity. Hence, this mass contains fatty material. The suprasellar and quadrigeminal cisterns (sc and qc) also contain hyperintensity material, thereby indicating that leakage of the oily substance occurred. (**e**, **f**) T2WI: The hyperintense fat content of this mass (arrows) cannot be distinguished from that of CSF. This tumor was surgically removed, and the neurosurgeon aspirated a considerable amount of fatty material. The pathological microscopic inspection of the skin, respiratory tract epidermis, and fatty tissue indicate that the mass is a mature teratoma

6.6.8 Tumors of the Pineal Region

These tumors include those developing from the pineal gland:

Pineocytoma Gr I.

Pineal parenchymal tumors of intermediate differentiation Gr II or III (Fig. 6.71).

Pineoblastoma Gr IV.

Papillary tumor of the pineal region Gr II or III.

Besides, this region is prone to developing germinomas (Fig. 6.68). The types are as detailed previously in Sect. 6.6.7.

The tectum of the midbrain is easily compressed by tumors of the pineal region, causing Parinaud syndrome, and also may compress the cerebral aqueduct, thereby resulting in obstructive hydrocephalus.

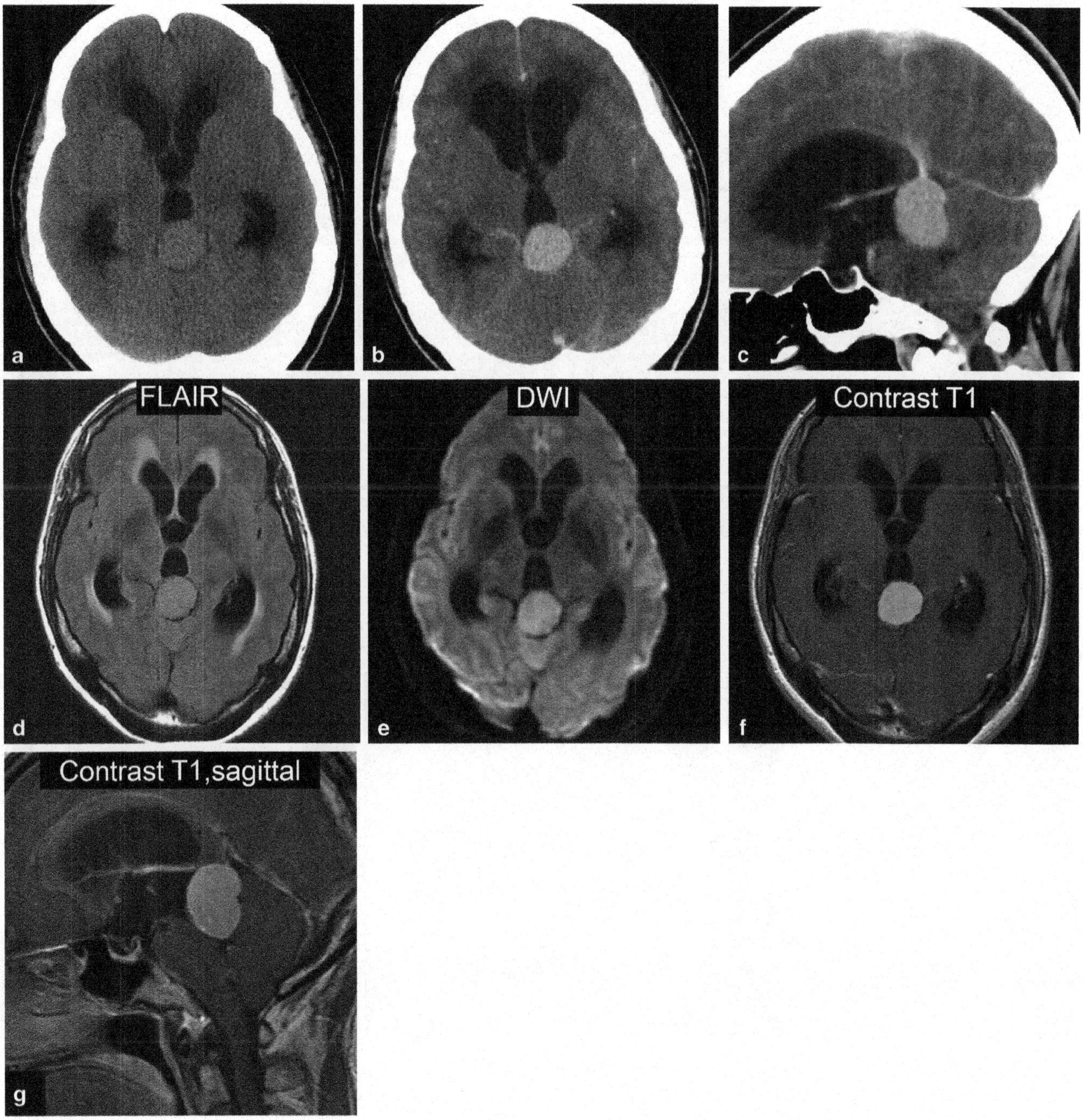

Fig. 6.71 F/53, Pineal gland tumor. This patient suffered from severe headaches and diplopia. (**a**) CT (**b**, **c**) contrast CT in axial and sagittal sections: A well-defined soft tissue mass with good contrast enhancement in the pineal region compressing the aqueduct causes obstructive hydrocephalus. (**d–g**) MRI: The findings are similar to those of CT. This tumor was surgically removed and confirmed to be a pineal parenchymal tumor with intermediate differentiation by pathological examination

6.6.9 Arachnoid Cyst

Arachnoid cysts are common intracranial benign cysts without symptoms. They are located in the subarachnoid space and contain CSF. They are also observed in the spinal canal.

Arachnoid cysts are most often located in the middle cranial fossa (Figs. 6.72 and 6.73) and posterior cranial fossa.

In CT and MRI, an arachnoid cyst has smooth outlines and density identical to that of CSF.

In young people, arachnoid cysts may induce chronic subdural hematoma (Figs. 3.24 and 6.73) and cause severe symptoms.

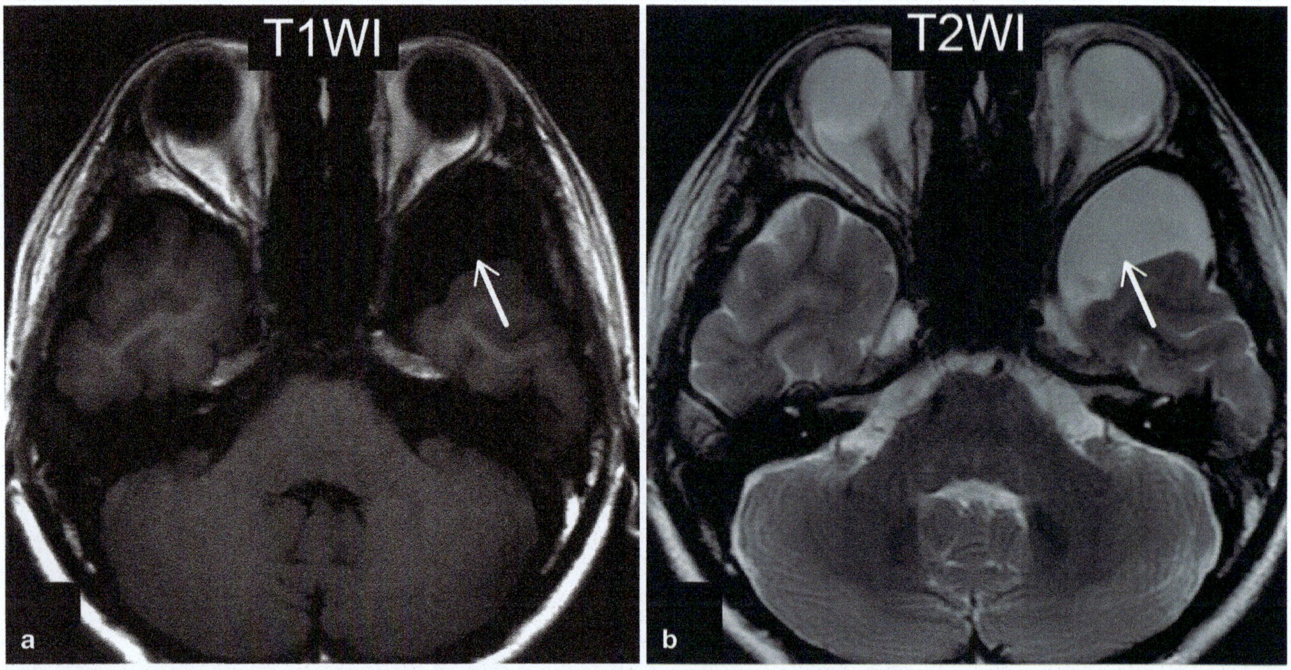

Fig. 6.72 F/41, Arachnoid cyst. No symptoms. In a healthy examination, the MRI incidentally found a cystic mass in the left middle cranial fossa with signal intensity consistent with that of CSF. Hence, the mass is a typical arachnoid cyst

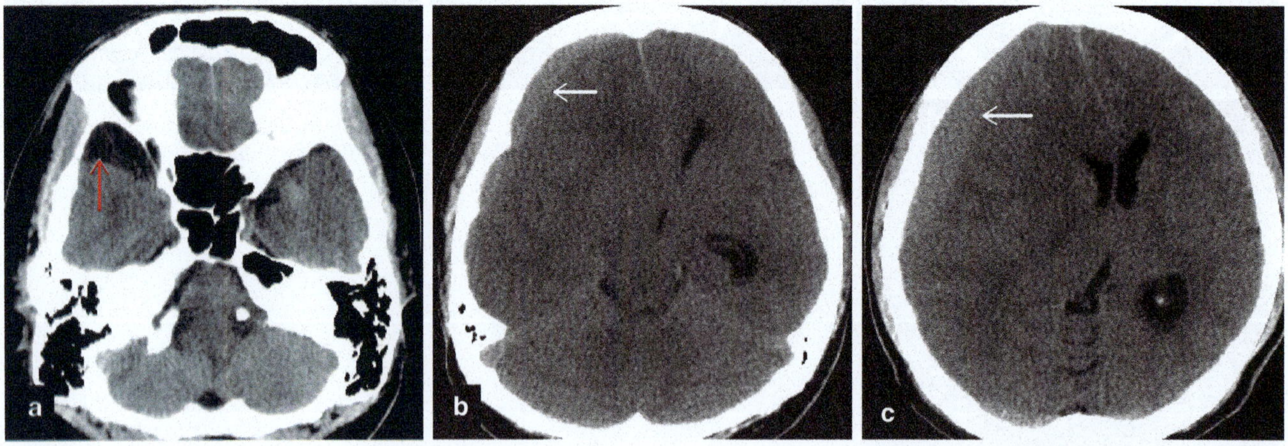

Fig. 6.73 M/31, Arachnoid cyst caused chronic subdural hematoma (SDH). This patient complained of severe headaches and vomiting for 2 days. CT: A chronic SDH (arrow) in the right frontotemporal region causes a strong mass effect, the right lateral ventricle is compressed, and the midline shifts to the left side. An arachnoid cyst (red arrow) is observed in the right middle cranial fossa. This chronic SDH was surgically drained, and neurosurgeon found an arachnoid cyst in the right middle cranial fossa. Comment: Young adults rarely have chronic SDH. If chronic SDH occurs, it is always caused by an arachnoid cyst

6.6.10 Epidermoid Cyst

Epidermoid cysts have a smooth and shiny appearance. Surgeons also refer to such cysts as "pearly tumors." The cysts develop from the epithelium encased in the cranium during neural tube closure in the third to fifth weeks of embryonic development. However, the cysts generate symptoms only when they grow sufficiently large to exert pressure on the patient, which is generally during middle age.

The cysts tend to develop in the center of the posterior cranial fossa (Fig. 6.74), CP angle cistern, foramen magnum (Fig. 6.75), and suprasellar cistern.

The main components of epidermoid cysts are cholesterol and keratinous matter. Cholesterol is a lipid; however, epidermoid cysts do not exhibit lipid density or signal intensity in either CT or MRI. Conversely, they show density and signals identical to those of the CSF, namely appearing dark in CT, dark in MRI T1WI, and white in T2WI. These results are similar to those of arachnoid cysts. However, the FLAIR and DWI results demonstrate that the cysts do not contain CSF; instead, they have non-water content (Figs. 6.74 and 6.75); this finding makes MRI can distinguish the epidermoid cyst with arachnoid cyst.

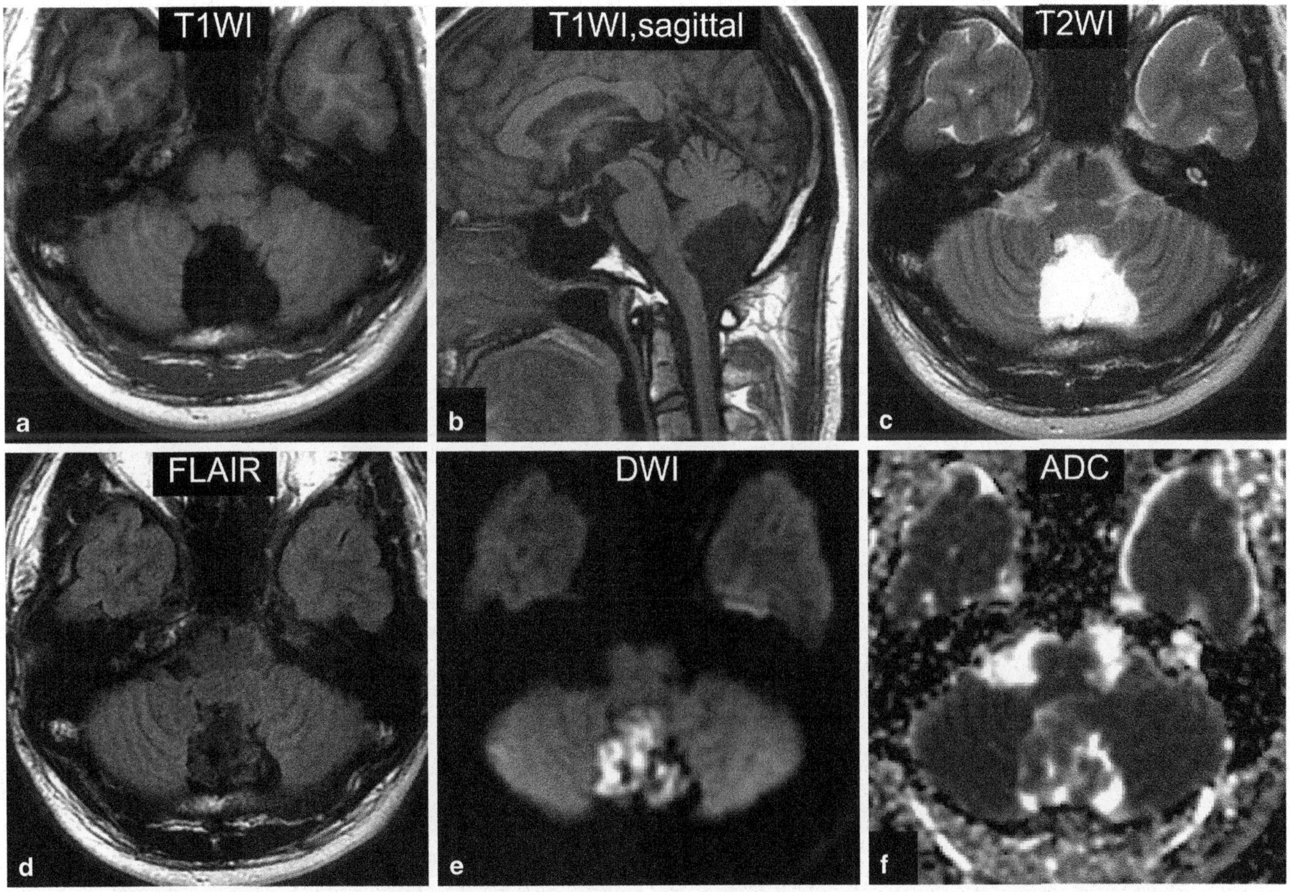

Fig. 6.74 M/36, Epidermoid cyst. This patient suffered from headaches and tinnitus for half a year. (**a–c**) MRI: A mass is observed in the middle of the posterior fossa between the bilateral cerebella. The mass shows hypointensity on T1WI and hyperintensity on T2WI. The signal intensity is consistent with that of CSF. Hence, this mass is like an arachnoid cyst. (**d**) FLAIR: Unlike CSF, FLAIR shows signal intensity in this mass. (**e, f**) Unlike CSF, hyperintensity on DWI reflects the diffusion restriction in mass content. A heterogeneous signal intensity exists on ADC. This mass was surgically removed, and the neurosurgeon found that it contained an oily substance. The pathological examination confirms that the mass is an epidermoid cyst

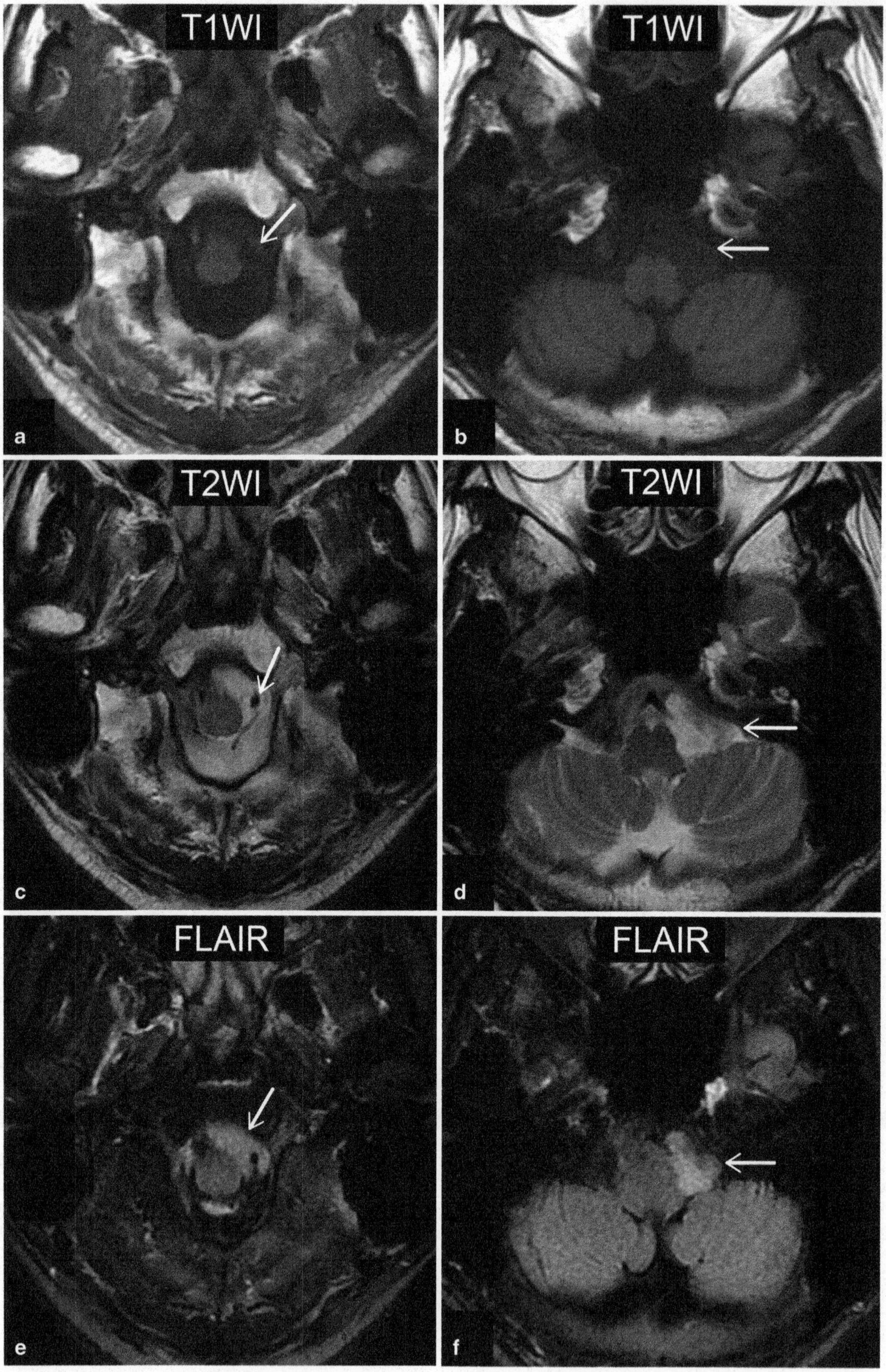

Fig. 6.75 M/62, Epidermoid cyst. No clinical symptom. During a healthy MRI examination, a mass was incidentally found in the foramen magnum. (**a–d**) MRI: This mass (arrows) shows hypointensity on T1WI and hyperintensity on T2WI. These findings are consistent with the signal intensity of CSF, making it difficult to distinguish. However, the medulla oblongata slightly shifts to the right side. (**e, f**) FLAIR: This mass shows hyperintensity (arrow) and is easily recognized. This mass was surgically removed and confirmed to be an epidermoid cyst by pathological examination

6.6.11 Lipoma

The intracranial lipoma is not rare, but it generally does not produce symptoms.

Location: Pericallosal lipomas account for 45% of intracranial lipomas. Half of the pericallosal lipomas are complicated with corpus callosum development dysplasia (Fig. 6.76).

Lipoma may also exist in the quadrigeminal cistern and suprasellar cistern and other locations (Fig. 6.77).

Lipomas exhibit lipid density and signals in both CT and MRI, facilitating diagnosis. In MRI T1WI, in particular, the signals are identical to those of subcutaneous fat.

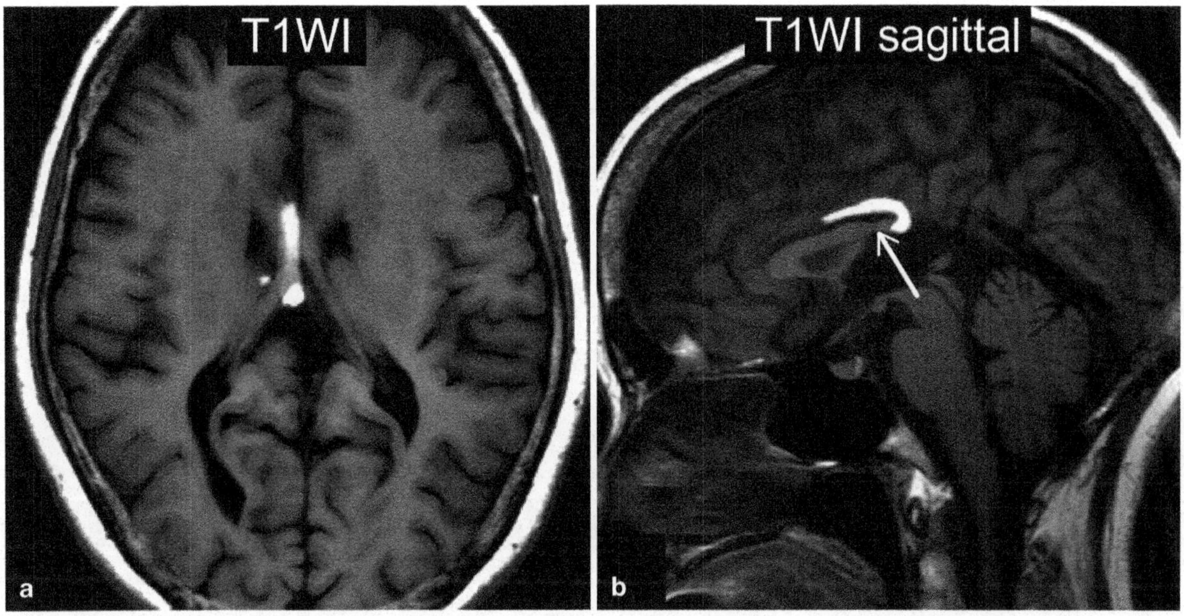

Fig. 6.76 F/64, Lipoma. (**a**, **b**) MRI, T1WI: There is hypoplasia of the corpus callosum (arrow), and a curved knife-shaped tumor above it. This tumor is white, which is the signal intensity of fat, thereby indicating that the tumor is a lipoma. Hypoplasia of corpus callosum is a congenital anomaly and often associated with lipoma

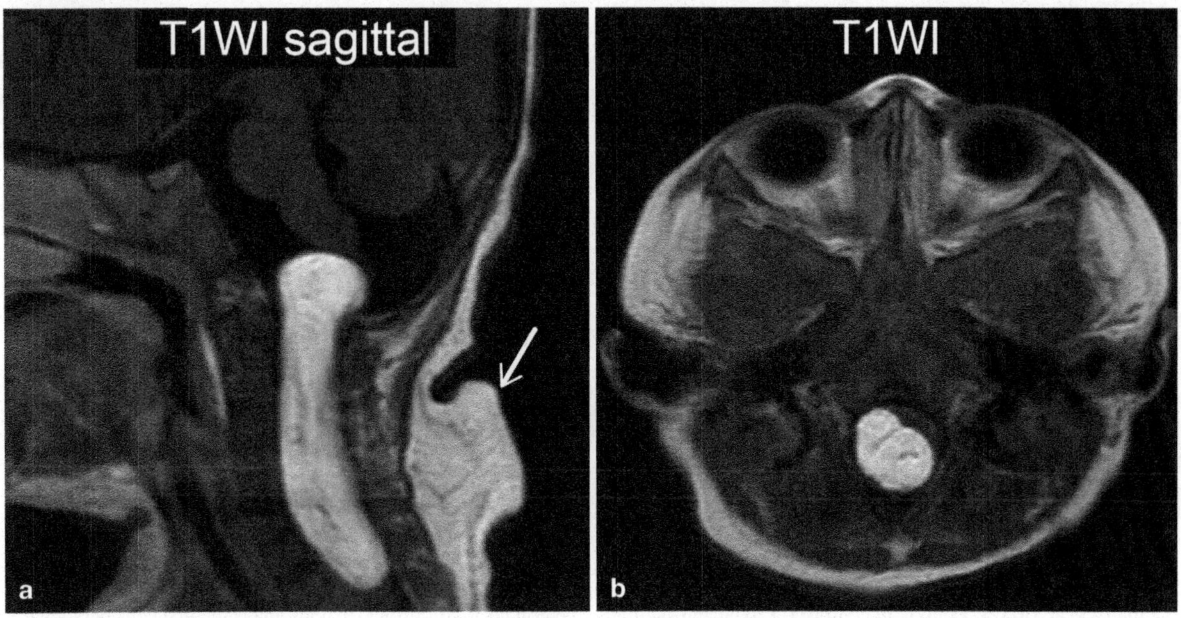

Fig. 6.77 M/2, Lipoma. This boy suffered from unsteady gait and right-side hemiparesis and rigidity. (**a**, **b**) MRI, T1WI: A large- and long-shaped tumor mass is observed in the foramen magnum and cervical spinal canal. Its signal intensity is as white as the subcutaneous fat (arrow), thereby indicating that the mass is a lipoma. This tumor was surgically removed and confirmed to be a lipoma by pathological examination

6.6.12 Chordoma

Chordoma is uncommon. It derives from embryonic primitive notochord remnants, which encompass Rathke's pouch in the suprasellar portion and the top of the coccyx at the bottom. Therefore, chordomas mostly develop in spheno-occipital (clivus) (Fig. 6.78) and sacrococcygeal portions (Fig. 8.68), especially at the clivus and sacrum. Some develop on vertebral bodies.

Intracranial chordoma mostly develops in adults aged between 20 and 40 years.

The diagnosis of chordoma is not difficult. CT images show clivus with osteolysis and replacement by soft tissues. Inside the tumors, osteolytic bone fragments remain.

MRI findings of chordoma are similar to CT results. Besides, irregular contrast enhancement can be observed.

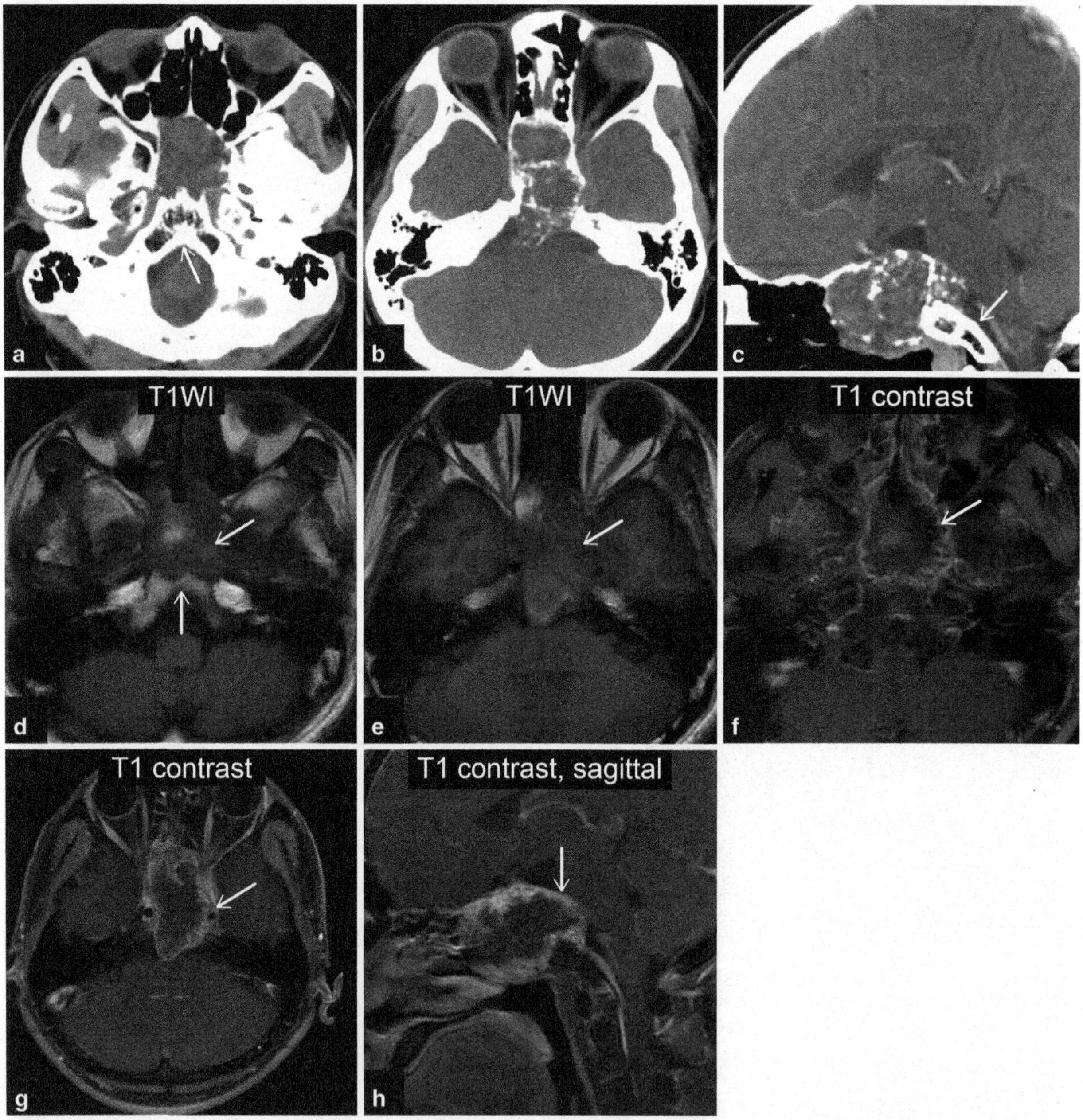

Fig. 6.78 M/35, Chordoma of clivus. This patient suffered headaches for more than a year. (**a**) CT, axial (**b**, **c**) contrast CT axial and sagittal: The inferior portion of clivus (arrows) is normal, the superior portion has osteolysis and is replaced by soft tissue mass containing many tiny bony fragments. This feature is similar to those of a malignant bony tumor. (**d**–**h**) MRI, T1WI, and contrast T1WI: This tumor has severe central necrosis (arrows). Chordoma is the first consideration if a tumor exists in the clivus with osteolysis. The pathological examination confirms that the tumor is a chordoma

References

1. Louis DN, et al. The 2016 World Health Organization classification of tumors of the central nervous system: a summary. Acta Neuropathol. 2016;131:803–20.
2. Komori T. The 2016 WHO classification of tumours of the central nervous system: the major points of revision. Neurol Med Chir. 2017;57:301–11.
3. Al-Okaili RN, et al. Advanced MR imaging techniques in the diagnosis of intraaxial brain tumors in adults. Radiographics. 2006;26:S173–89.
4. Oz G, et al. Clinical proton MR spectroscopy in central nervous system disorders. Radiology. 2014;270:658–79.
5. Lai PH, et al. Brain abscess and necrotic brain tumors: discrimination with proton MR spectroscopy and diffusion-weighted imaging. AJNR Am J Neuroradiol. 2002;23:1369–77.
6. Quadery FA, Okamoto K. Diffusion-weighted MRI of haemangioblastomas and other cerebellar tumors. Neuroradiology. 2003;45:212–9.
7. Koeller KK, et al. Cerebral intraventricular neoplasms: radiologic-pathologic correlation. Radiographics. 2002;22:1473–505.
8. Mete O, Lopes MB. Overview of the 2017 WHO classification of pituitary tumors. Endocr Pathol. 2017;28:228–43.

Medical Imaging of CNS Infection

7

Abstract

For mild meningitis, CT and MRI often have no finding or only show mild hydrocephalus. For bacterial meningitis, CT and MRI may show leptomeningeal enhancement and mild hydrocephalus. Some cases have exudate in the basal cistern, and some cases are associated with arterial or venous infarctions. Some cases are also associated with brain abscess or subdural empyema. CT and MRI can clearly show these complications. Brain abscesses reveal ring enhancement with severe peripheral white matter edema in CT and MRI. DWI and MRS are helpful for differential diagnosis of brain abscess with tumor necrosis. MRI is better than CT to detect encephalitis, showing hyperintensity on T2WI and FLAIR. In some instances, the affected brain tissue has diffusion restriction, indicating hyperintensity on DWI, and some have contrast enhancement because of BBB disruption.

Central nervous system (CNS) infections include meningitis (Figs. 7.1–7.10), brain abscess (Figs. 7.7, 7.11–7.17), epidural and subdural empyema (Fig. 7.7), encephalitis (Figs. 7.18–7.25), and meningoencephalitis (Figs. 7.6, 7.9, and 7.25). Besides, CNS infections may involve the spinal cord and spinal canal, namely encephalomyelitis and meningoencephalomyelitis.

CNS infection pathogenesis includes the virus, bacteria, fungus (Figs. 7.3 and 7.6), and parasites (Fig. 7.17). Some cases of CNS infections involve post-infectious encephalitis, such as acute disseminated encephalomyelitis (ADEM) (Figs. 7.26 and 7.27). However, the pathogen of numerous CNS infection cases has yet to be revealed (Fig. 7.5).

7.1 Meningitis

7.1.1 Purulent Meningitis

Purulent meningitis commonly has the following pathogeneses: (1) Bacteria: tuberculosis (Tb) (Figs. 7.1 and 7.2), streptococcus (Fig. 7.7), enterococcus (Fig. 7.8), *Escherichia coli*, and Hemophilus influenza; (2) Fungus: cryptococcus (Figs. 7.3 and 7.6) and aspergillus; and (3) Parasites: toxoplasma [1].

Clinical symptoms, biochemistry exams, and cerebrospinal fluid (CSF) bacterial culturing are crucial for diagnosing meningitis. Furthermore, medical imaging (e.g., computed tomography (CT)) and magnetic resonance imaging (MRI) can provide essential evidence to support the diagnosis and are critical for follow-up on complications.

7.1.1.1 CT and MRI

The CT and MRI of mild meningitis yield unremarkable results (Fig. 7.5), and these modalities can only detect mild hydrocephalus during the early stages of meningitis (Figs. 7.1, 7.2, and 7.6).

In the cases of severe meningitis, the surface of sulci in the infected area becomes effaced. MRI FLAIR image displays sulcal hyperintensity (Fig. 7.7) [2].

After the injection of contrast agent, the affected area may have leptomeningeal enhancement of the subarachnoid spaces, which are linear enhancement of cortical sulci, and the surfaces of the brain stem, cerebrum, and cerebellum (Figs. 7.2, 7.3, 7.4, 7.5, 7.6, 7.8, and 7.9).

Furthermore, the suprasellar cisterns and other basal cisterns may demonstrate significant contrast enhancements due to the accumulation of inflammatory exudate (Fig. 7.1).

W.-C. Shen, *Diagnostic Neuroradiology*, https://doi.org/10.1007/978-981-15-4051-6_7

Complications

1. Communicating hydrocephalus is caused by subarachnoid space (CSF space) inflammation and adhesion, which lead to disturbances of CSF circulation (Figs. 7.1, 7.2, and 7.6).
2. Cerebral ischemic edema. Bacterial meningitis may have exudate in the subarachnoid space of skull base (basal cisterns); the exudate irritates the small blood vessels which pass through the basal cisterns, and cause vasculitis, blood vessels spasm and constrict, resulting in ischemic infarction [3]. This type of infarction includes arterial infarction, which appears hyperintensity in T2WI and FLAIR and has a high signal intensity in diffusion-weighted imaging (DWI), similar to that exhibited by general acute infarction (Fig. 7.2). However, DWI cannot detect high intensity in some regions due to the infraction being a venous ischemic infarction (Figs. 7.1 and 7.2). Venous ischemic infractions appear hyperintensity in T2WI and FLAIR but no signal change in DWI (see Chap. 5).
3. About 30% of patients exhibit ventriculitis, which shows ventricle walls enhancement in contrast-enhanced CT and MRI (Fig. 7.8); the infected CSF in the ventricles may demonstrate hyperintensity in DWI (Figs. 7.8 and 7.14).
4. Subdural effusion (SDE) (Fig. 7.4) is a common complication of bacterial meningitis, particularly among children. Most SDE occurrences disappear after self-absorption. In the CT and T1W1 and T2W1 imaging of MRI, SDE has a similar density and signal intensity as CSF. However, in FLAIR, the signal intensity of SDE is slightly higher than that of CSF, thereby indicating that the effusion is not pure as CSF but is dirty. But only 20% of SDE cases develop into subdural empyema.
5. Epidural or subdural empyema generally occurs in the cerebral surface or interhemispheric fissures. Under CT and MRI imaging, the empyema membrane is enhanced by the contrast agent (Fig. 7.7). The empyema content exhibits hypodensity on CT, and CSF signal intensity in T1W1, T2W1, and FLAIR MRI imaging. However, under DWI, empyema presents hyperintensity due to high diffusion restriction similar to the brain abscess.
6. Cerebritis and abscess: 10–20% of bacterial meningitis cases may develop into brain abscess (Fig. 7.7).

7.1.2 Viral Meningitis

Viral meningitis, also known as aseptic meningitis, is not rare in clinical cases. The diagnosis of viral meningitis is mainly reliant on clinical symptoms and CSF examinations. Because most viral meningitis cases show negative findings in CT and MRI, so the processes of CT and MRI imaging are commonly excluded when inspecting viral meningitis, except for severe cases or cases in which encephalitis comorbidity is suspected.

7.1.3 Meningoencephalitis

In addition to inflammation of CSF spaces, the bacterial and viral meningitis may also associate with inflammation of brain parenchyma (encephalitis), named encephalomyelitis (Figs. 7.6 and 7.25).

7.1.4 Pachymeningitis

Idiopathic hypertrophic pachymeningitis (Fig. 7.10) is a rare type of meningitis. Symptoms include headache, cranial neuropathies, eye pain, and unsteady gait. Contrast-enhanced CT and MRI show the linear enhancement of the dura in the cerebral and cerebellar surface, the falx and tentorium, but no enhancement in the cortical sulci. This is called pachymeningeal enhancement [4].

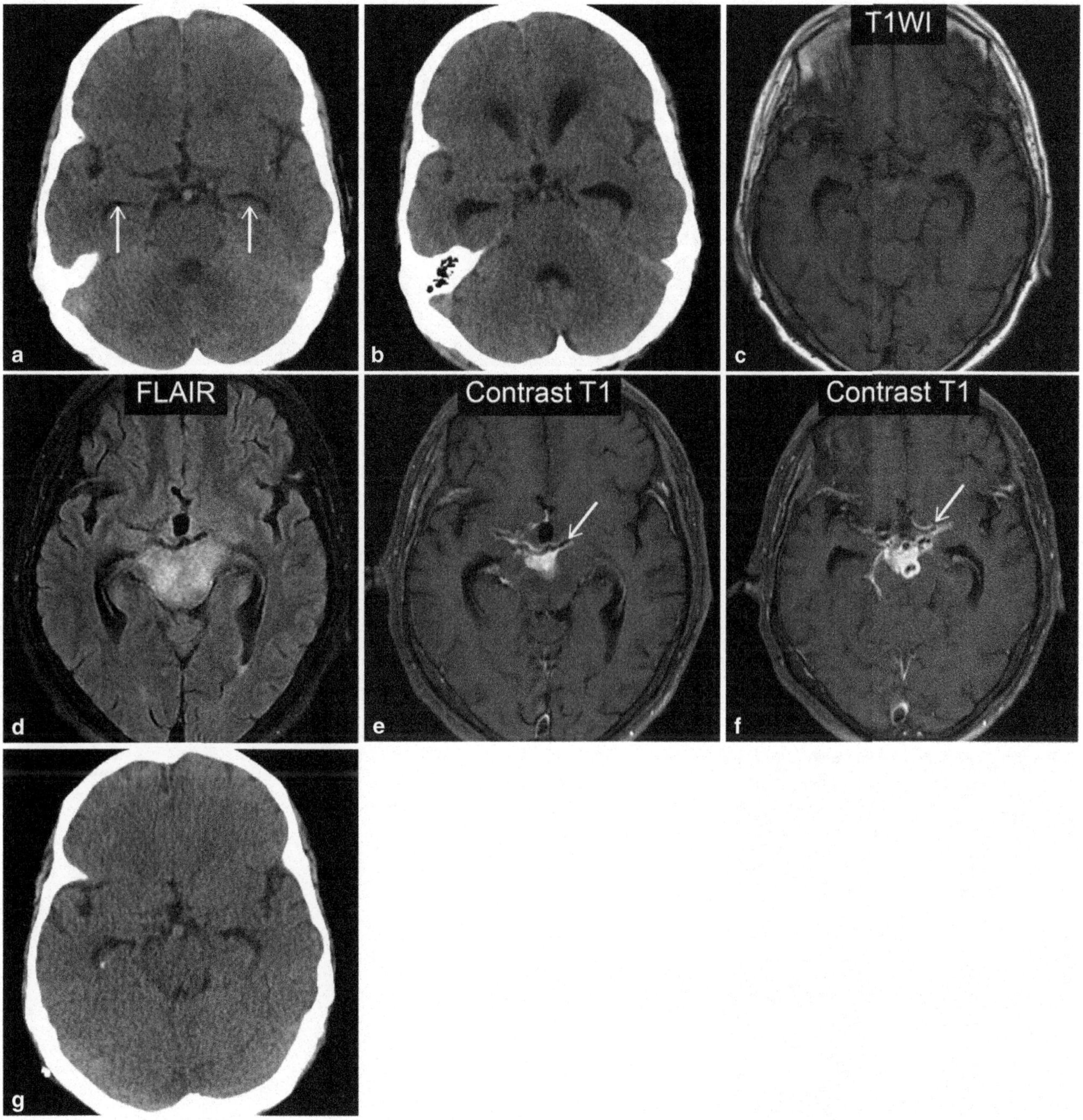

Fig. 7.1 M/50, TB meningitis. This patient suffered a severe headache and mild fever. (**a**) CT: Bilateral temporal horns (arrows) are slightly dilated, indicating mild hydrocephalus. (**b**) CT 3 weeks later: Hydrocephalus is worse than that in (**a**). (**c, d**) MRI 1 week after the last CT, T1WI, FLAIR: Hydrocephalus persists. The midbrain shows hyperintensity on FLAIR, but no signal change is observed on DWI (not shown). These findings represent venous infarction due to the impairment of venous return. (**e, f**) Contrast T1WI: The suprasellar cistern (arrows) is enhanced, indicating the adhesion by inflammatory exudate. CSF culture cultivated tuberculosis (TB) , the patient responded well to the anti-TB medical treatment and gradually returned to a healthy condition. (**g**) CT 6 months later: Hydrocephalus is relieved

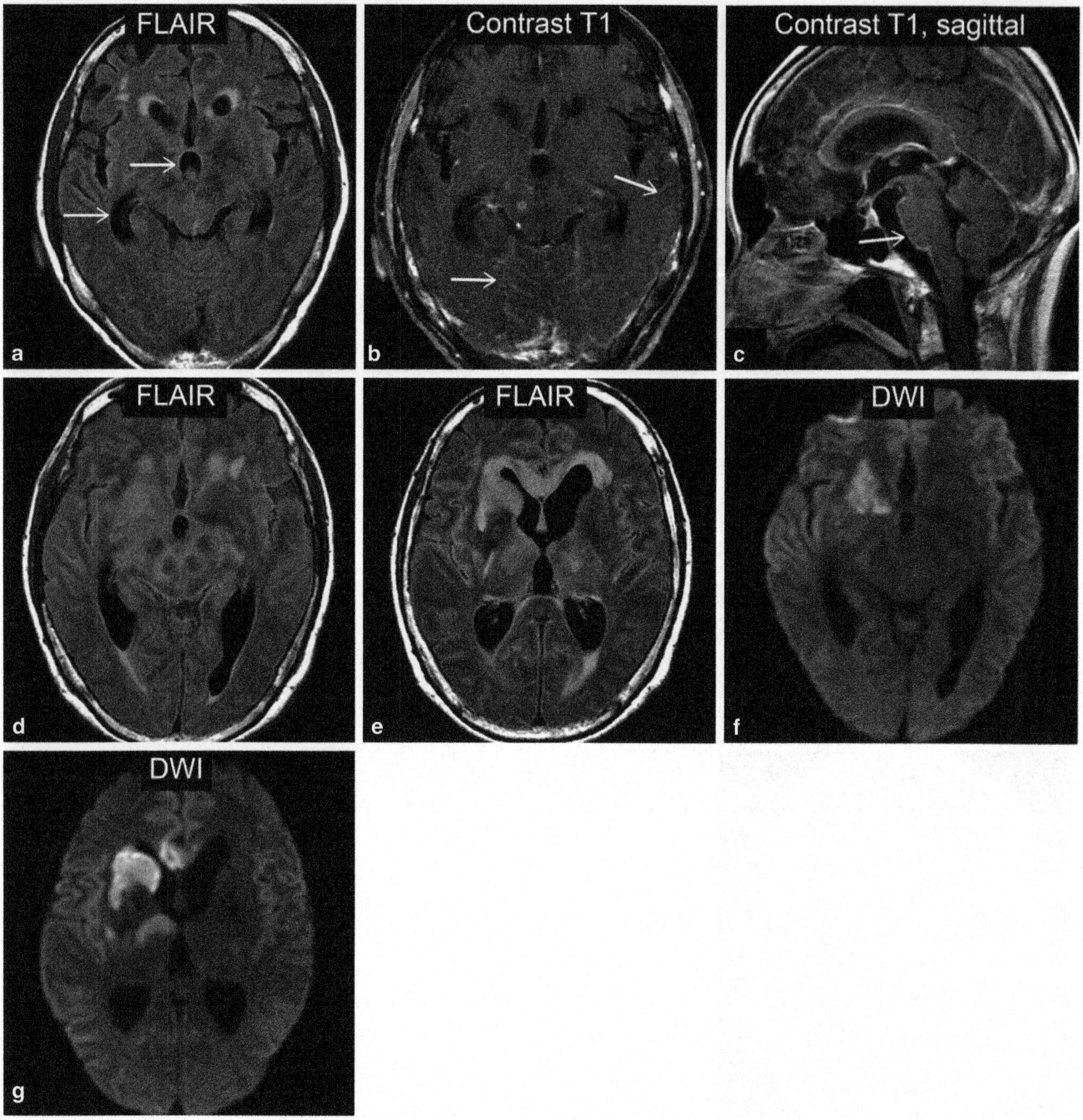

Fig. 7.2 F/59, TB meningitis with infarctions. The patient suffered headaches and consciousness disturbance. (**a**) MRI, FLAIR: bilateral lateral ventricles and third ventricle (arrows) are dilated, indicating hydrocephalus. (**b**) Contrast T1WI: Leptomeningeal enhancement (arrows) is identified in the cortical sulci of the cerebellar vermis and the left temporal lobe. (**c**) Contrast T1WI, sagittal: Linear enhancement found on the anterior surface of the brainstem (arrow). The above findings are indicative of bacterial meningitis. CSF tested tuberculosis acid-fast stain was positive, and TB bacteria were cultured. Follow-up MRI 2 weeks later (**d**, **e**) FLAIR: Hyperintensity is identified in the entire midbrain, right corpus striatum, bilateral thalami, and genu of the corpus callosum. (**f**, **g**) DWI: In the above areas, the right corpus striatum, the anterior portion of the right thalamus, and the genu of the corpus callosum exhibit diffusion restrictions (hyperintensity), such as acute arterial infarctions that are a common complication of TB meningitis. The other areas without diffusion restriction may be venous infarctions caused by impairment of venous return

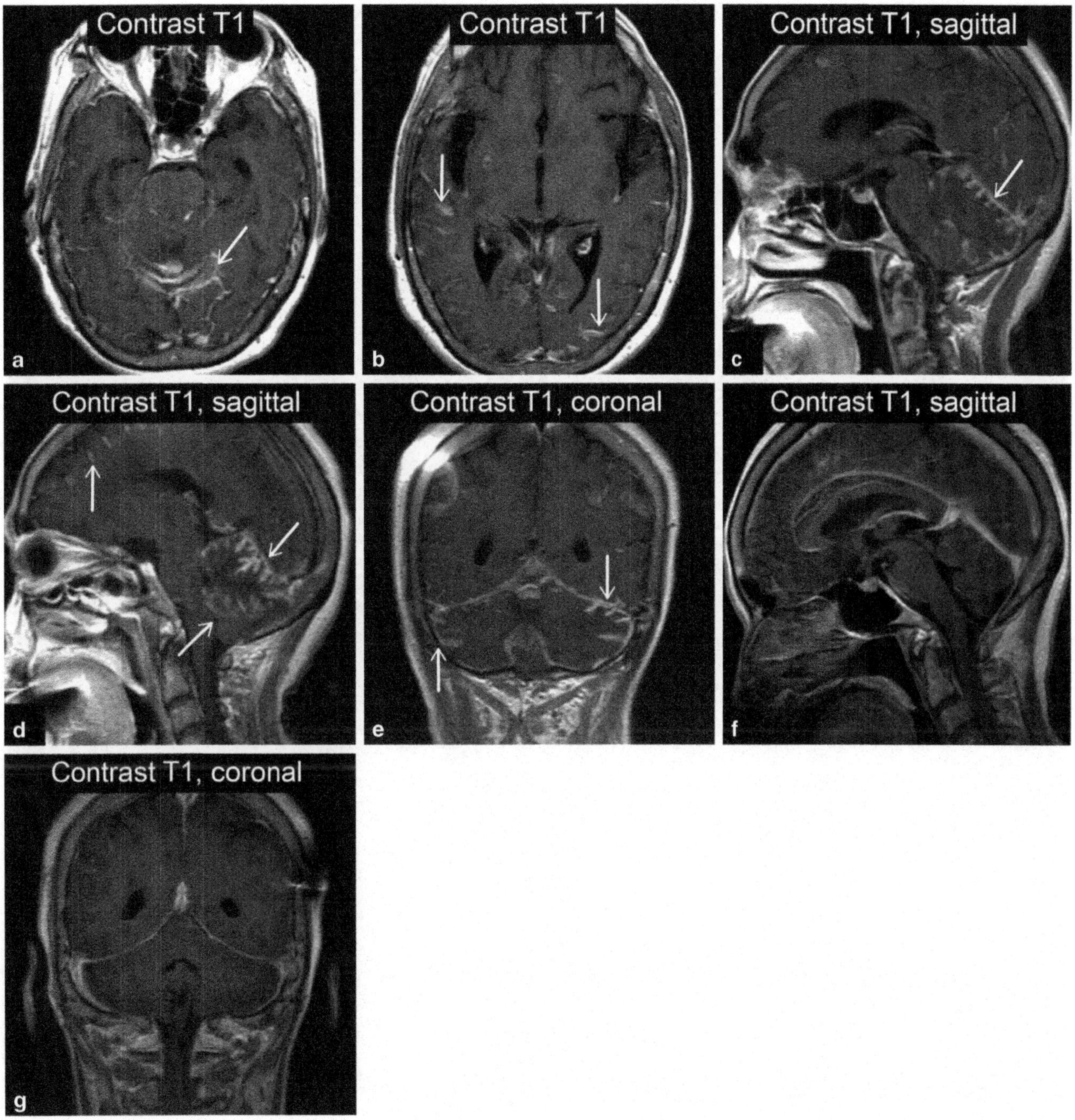

Fig. 7.3 F/66, Cryptococcal meningitis. (**a**–**e**) MRI, T1WI contrast: Leptomeningeal enhancement (arrows) observed in the cerebral and cerebellar sulci and the tentorium, this is a typical sign of meningitis. CSF culture showed cryptococcus. This patient recovered well after antibiotic treatment. (**f**, **g**) Follow-up MRI, 6 months later: No more leptomeningeal enhancement is observed

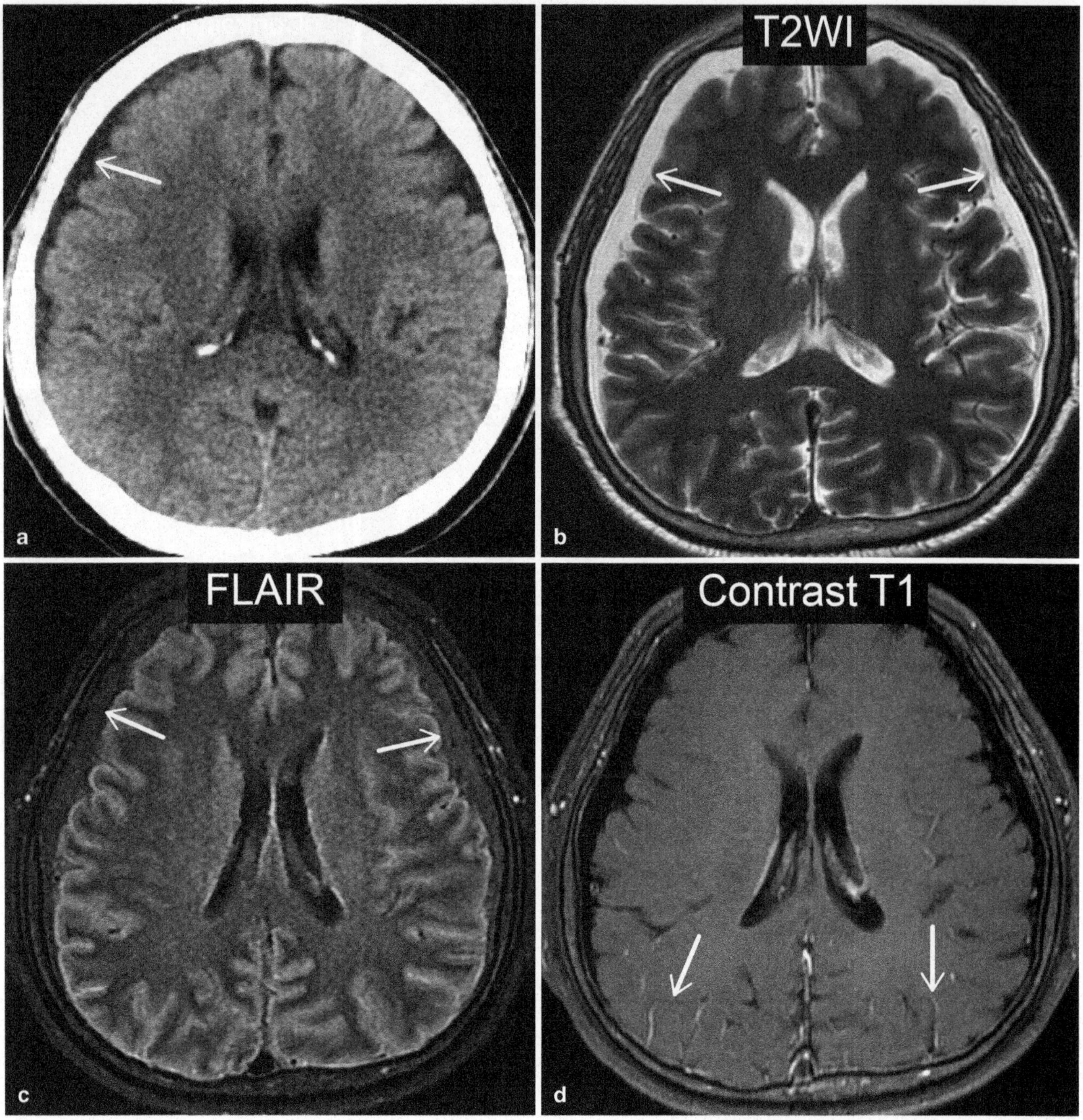

Fig. 7.4 M/58, Subdural effusion caused by meningitis. Right otitis media patient presented with recent right ear pain, fever, unsteady gait, and gradual poor response. CT of the first day showed no significant abnormalities are identified (not shown). (**a**) CT, 1 day later: Subdural effusion (SDE) (arrow) is seen outside the right frontal lobe. MRI examination was performed on the fourth day. (**b**) T2WI: SDEs (arrows) are seen outside the bilateral cerebral hemispheres. The signal intensity is as white as the CSF of the ventricles. (**c**) FLAIR: The signal intensity of the bilateral SDEs (arrows) is not as dark as the CSF; this is indicating that the fluid is not pure CSF but is contaminated due to bacterial infection. (**d**) Contrast T1WI: Slight sulcus leptomeningeal enhancement (arrows), which is a sign of meningitis

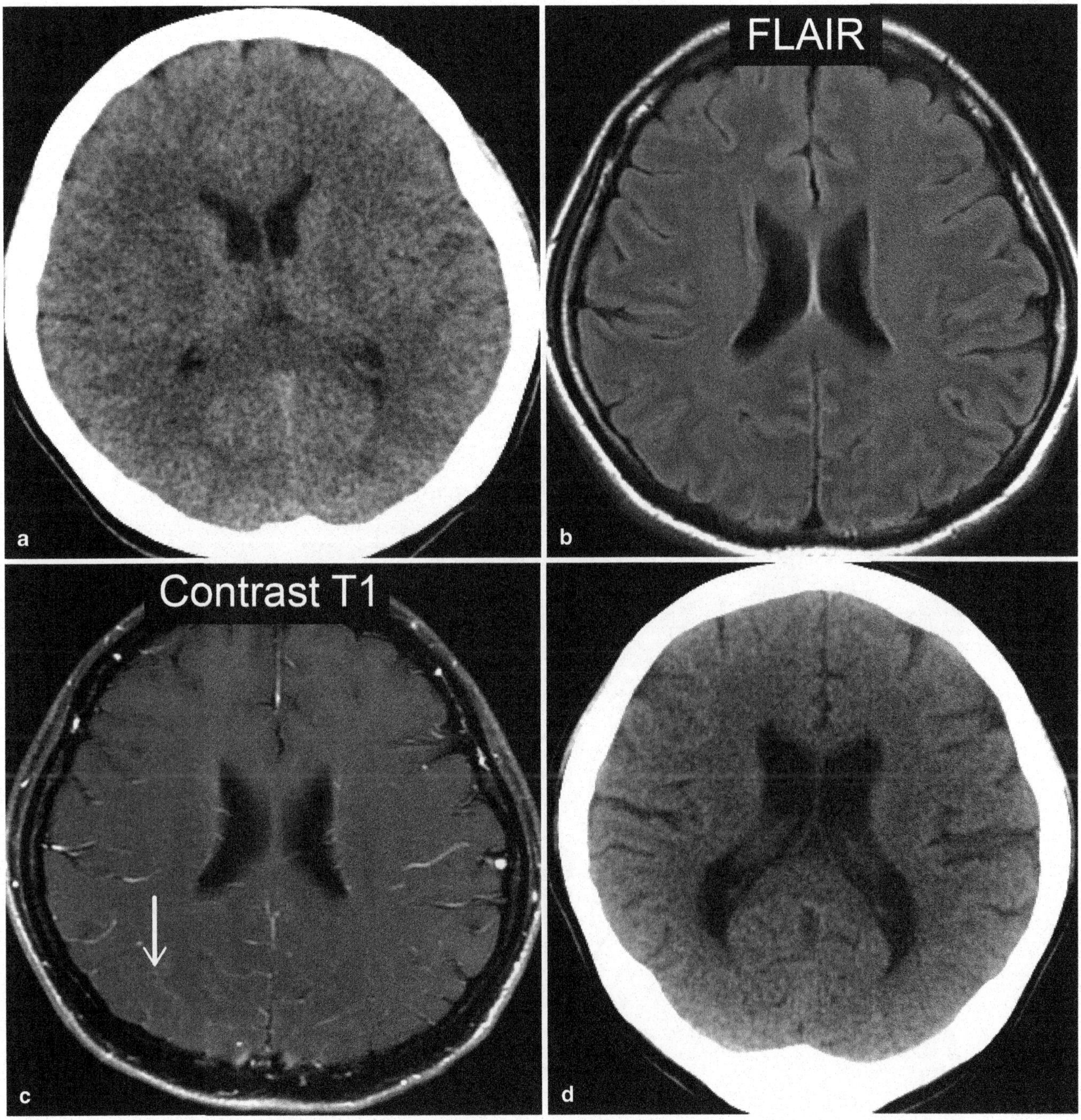

Fig. 7.5 F/37, Brain atrophy due to meningitis. The patient had CT and MRI examinations due to headache and fever and underwent a CSF test, which showed increased protein and white blood cells. Such high levels indicate infection, but bacteria and viruses were not detected. (**a**) CT: No abnormalities exist. (**b**) MRI, FLAIR: No signal change is seen. (**c**) Contrast T1WI: Minimal linear enhancement (arrow) identified in the sulci of the bilateral temporo-occipital lobes may indicate meningitis. The patient showed slightly impaired intelligence and a symptom of epilepsy after recovering from this acute symptom. (**d**) CT, 18 months later: The ventricles are slightly dilated, and the sulci are widened. These conditions reflect diffuse brain atrophy, which is a sequela of meningitis

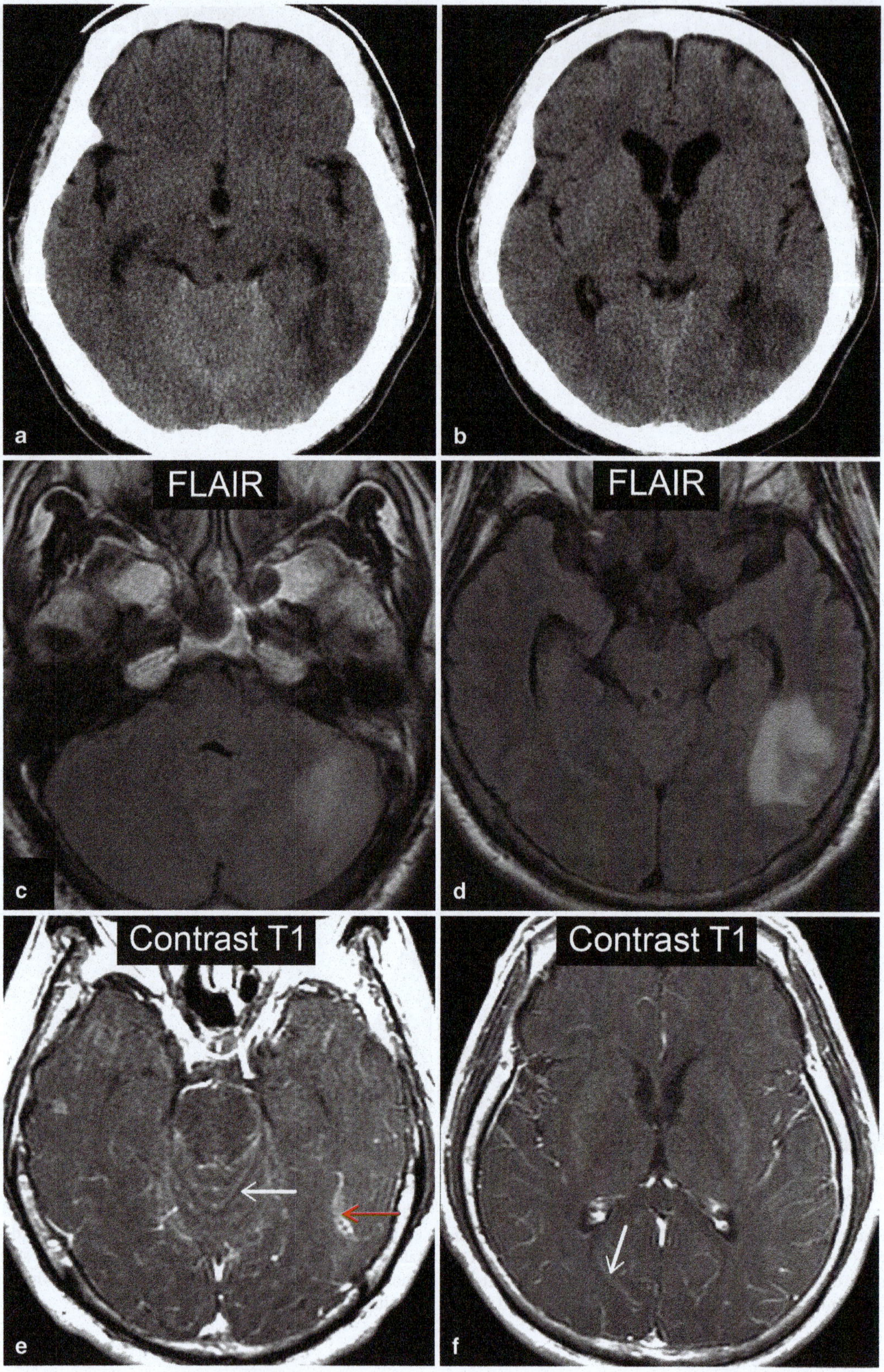

Fig. 7.6 M/56 Cryptococcal meningoencephalitis. This patient suffered fever, severe headache, loss of consciousness, clinically suspected meningitis, and CSF-cultured cryptococcus. (**a**, **b**) CT: The temporal horns of the bilateral lateral ventricles and the third ventricle are slightly dilated, indicating mild hydrocephalus. Edema is observed in some brain tissues in the left temporal lobe. (**c**, **d**) MRI, FLAIR: In addition to the temporal lobe, the left cerebellum has a high-signal lesion with no signal changes in DWI (not shown). Thus, these lesions are not infarctions, possibly are encephalitis. (**e**, **f**) Contrast T1WI: Leptomeningeal enhancement observed in the sulci of the occipital lobe and the superior vermis (white arrows) is indicative of meningitis. Some enhancement is identified in the lesion in the left temporal lobe (red arrow), which reflects encephalitis. Therefore, this case is identified as cryptococcal meningoencephalitis

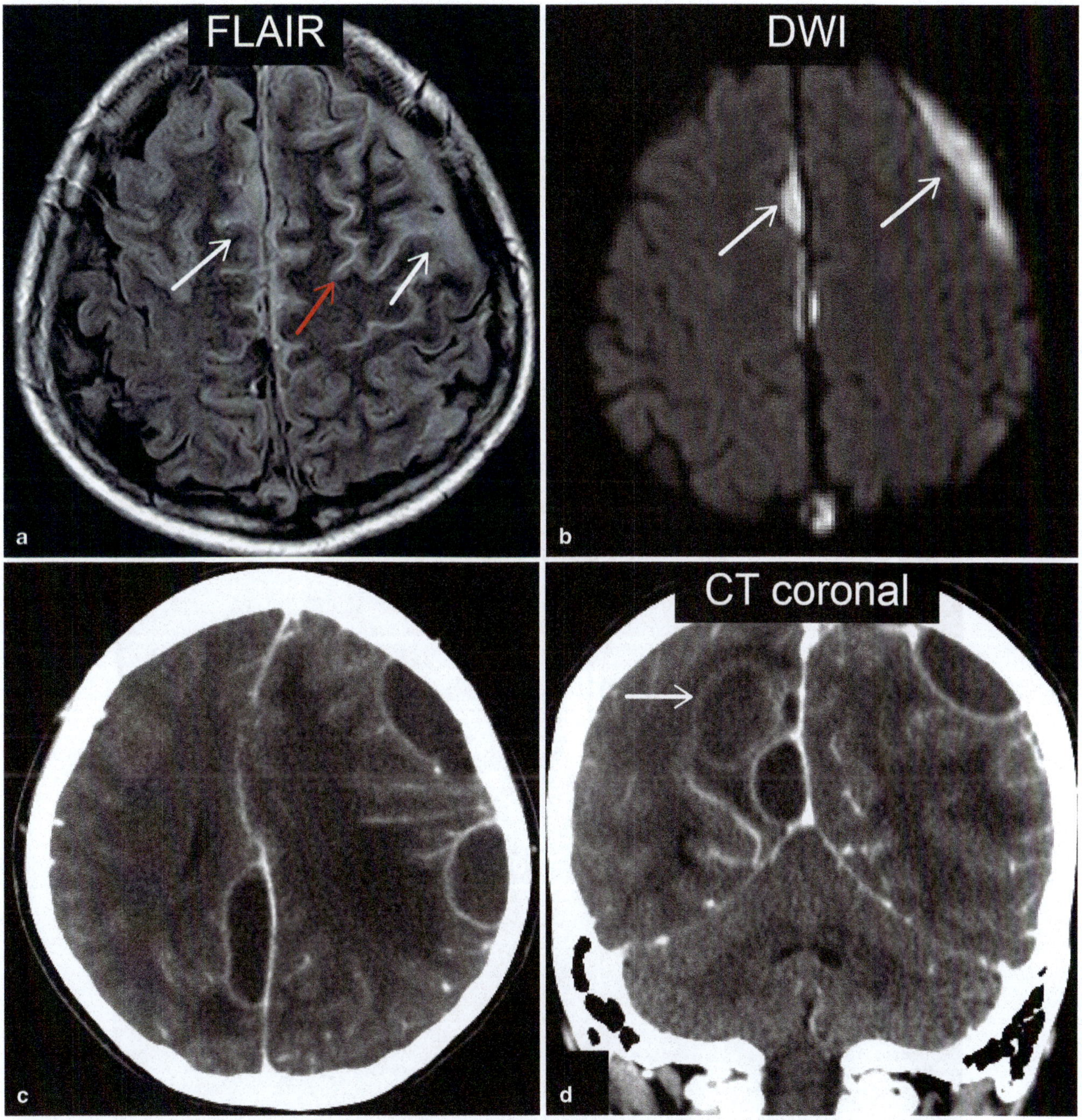

Fig. 7.7 F/17, Meningitis with empyema and brain abscess. The patient suffered a high fever, headache, and consciousness disturbance. (**a**, **b**) MRI, FLAIR, DWI: The sulcus of the left frontal lobe has sulcal hyperintensity (red arrow), which indicates meningitis. There are also subdural effusions outside the left frontal lobe and in the interhemispheric fissure (white arrows). In DWI, these effusions are white, indicating a strong diffusion restriction. Therefore, these effusions are pus, and the pus outside the brain is empyema. Streptococcus is cultured in CSF and blood, and the condition worsens after 2 weeks of antibiotic treatment. (**c**, **d**) contrast CT, 2weeks later, axial and coronal: The empyemas are relatively large, and the right parietal lobe has a brain abscess (arrow). The patient underwent surgery to drain these extracerebral empyemas and intracerebral abscess. Antibiotic treatment was also applied, and the patient's condition improved

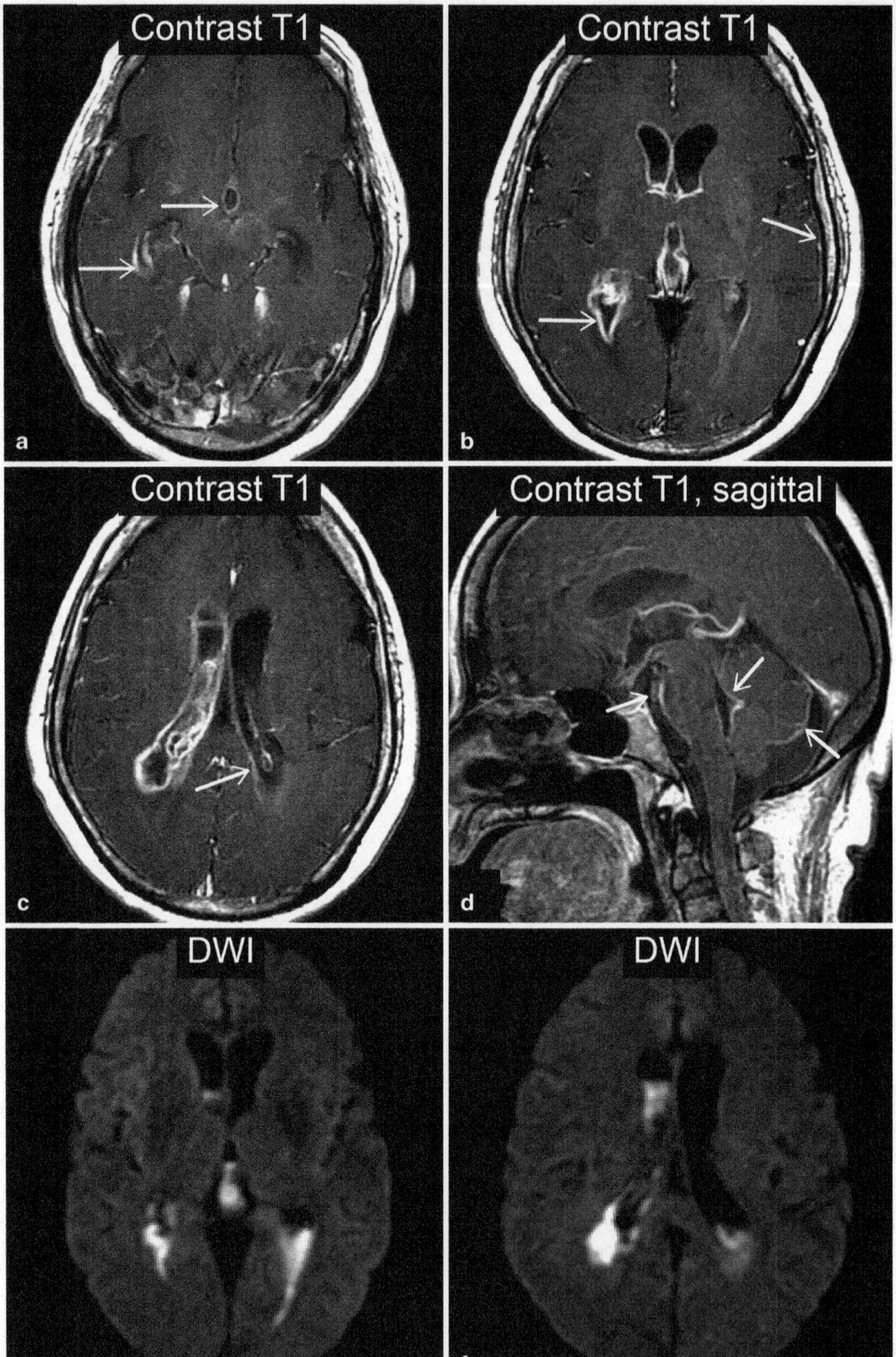

Fig. 7.8 F/61, Meningitis with ventriculitis. (**a–d**) Contrast T1WI: Linear leptomeningeal enhancement (arrows) is observed on the surfaces of the brainstem and the cerebellum and in the sulci. Ependymal enhancement is also identified in the ventricular walls. This condition is typically identified as meningitis combined with ventriculitis. (**e**, **f**) DWI: Hyperintensities are seen in the bilateral lateral ventricles and the third ventricle. This condition reflects the infection of the CSF in these ventricles. The hyperintensity is pus, which has strong diffusion restriction. CSF culture showed *Enterococcus faecium*

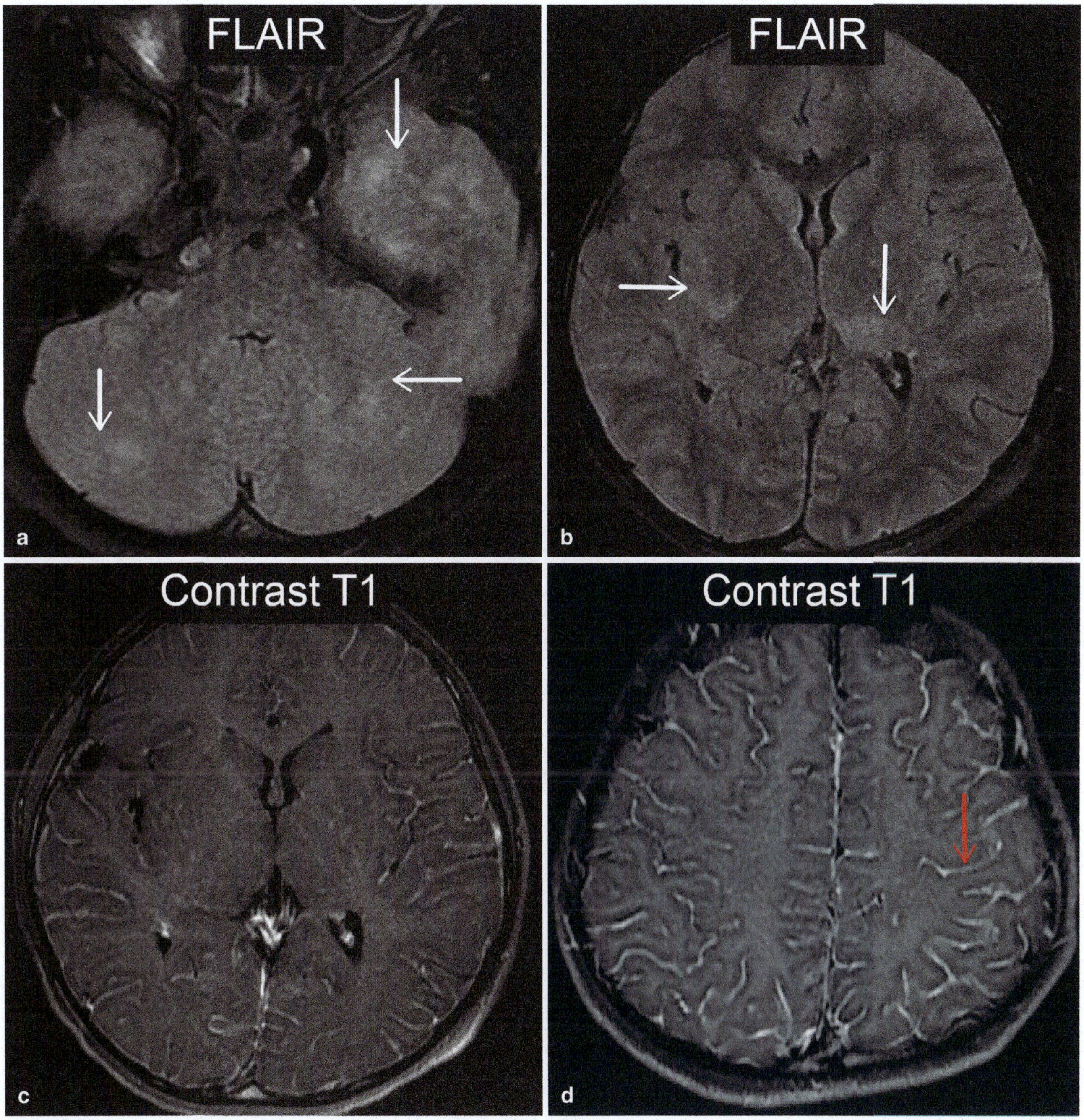

Fig. 7.9 M/8, Viral meningoencephalitis. The patient suffered high fever, followed by status epilepticus and then combined with acute hepatitis and renal function decline. (**a**, **b**) MRI, FLAIR: Multiple hyperintense lesions (arrows) are observed in the bilateral cerebella, left temporal lobe, left thalamus, and posterior part of the right putamen. These lesions indicate encephalitis. (**c**, **d**) Contrast T1WI: Diffuse leptomeningeal enhancement is identified in the sulci of the bilateral cerebral hemispheres, indicating meningitis. The hyperintense lesions mentioned above in brain parenchyma seen in FLAIR are not enhanced. The brain parenchyma and CSF spaces all exhibit pathological changes. Therefore, the condition is meningoencephalitis

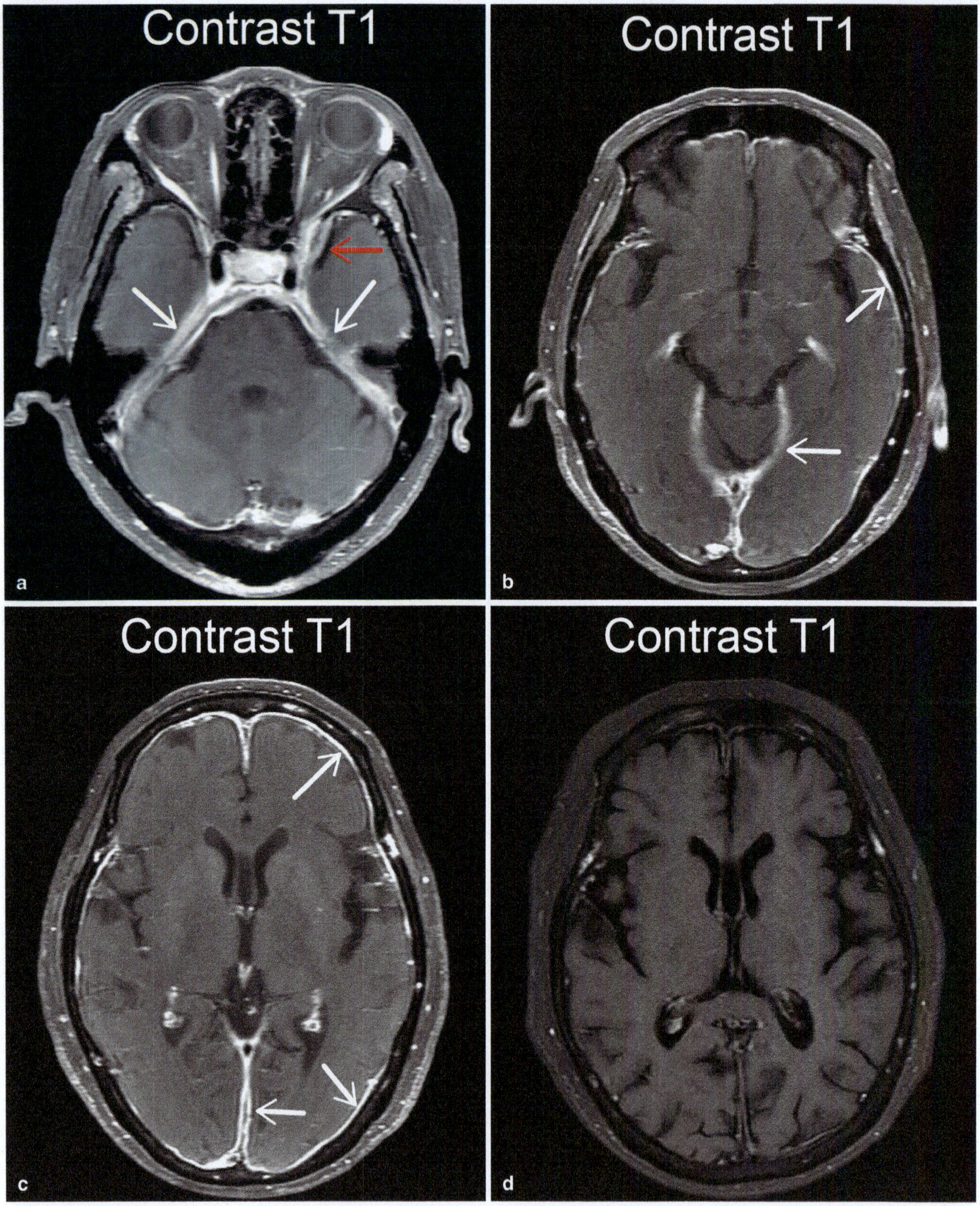

Fig. 7.10 F/74, Idiopathic hypertrophic pachymeningitis. The patient suffered a headache, left eye pain, and ptosis. (**a**–**c**) MRI contrast T1WI: Linear enhancement (arrows) is observed for the tentorium, falx, and dura of the bilateral cerebral surfaces but not for the cortical sulci. These findings suggest this case as typical pachymeningeal meningitis. Dura hypertrophy (red arrow in **a**) is seen beside the left cavernous sinus. Thus, the left eye pain and ptosis are caused by pachymeningitis. This condition is regarded as Tolosa Hunt syndrome. No findings were obtained from CSF and blood culture. The patient received steroid treatment and exhibited an effective response. (**d**) Follow-up MRI after 6 years: no more abnormal dural enhancement

7.2 Brain abscess

Similar to purulent meningitis, common causes of brain abscess include the following: (1) bacteria: Tb (Fig. 7.16), streptococcus (Figs. 7.7 and 7.13), and enterococcus (Fig. 7.12); (2) fungus: cryptococcus and aspergillus; and (3) parasites: toxoplasma (Fig. 7.17).

Brain abscess occurs in the cerebrum, cerebellum, and basal ganglion. In general, only one brain abscess occurs, with few cases of multiple brain abscesses (Fig. 7.16). Recurrent brain abscesses are more common in patients with immune system deficiency (Fig. 7.17).

7.2.1 CT Imaging

The classic CT image of brain abscess is a circular cystic lesion surrounded by a capsule enhanced by contrast agent that constitutes ring enhancement (Figs. 7.7, 7.11, 7.12, 7.13, and 7.15). The capsule is thin and has even thickness. In some cases, the brain abscess may extrude, forming another smaller abscess, which may or may not is connected to the original abscess. In certain CT sections, this recalls the appearance of a mother and daughter (Fig. 7.11).

Brain abscess generally causes severe perifocal white matter edema.

7.2.2 MRI imaging

The MRI images of brain abscess are similar to CT image, the abscess is hypointensity on T1WI, hyperintensity on T2WI and FLAIR, with ring enhancement of the capsule, and severe peripheral white matter edema. The MRI image for brain abscess is much more precise than CT.

A metastatic tumor (Fig. 2.9) and glioblastoma (Fig. 7.15) easily have tumor necrosis and associated with severe peritumoral white matter edema, and the appearance is similar to brain abscess. Because CT imaging and conventional MRI imaging produce similar images for brain abscess and tumor necrosis, the new MRI techniques, DWI and magnetic resonance spectroscopy (MRS) can be of assistance for differential diagnosis [5, 6].

1. *DWI: The pus within the brain abscess exhibits strong diffusion restriction. Therefore, the pus is bright on DWI, is dark on the ADC map (Figs. 2.10, 7.11–7.16). By contrast, metastasis and glioblastoma tumors contain necrotic brain tissues in liquid form. In most cases, these liquids appear hypointensity (dark) on DWI and hyperintensity (white) on ADC, respectively. Because these necrotic tissues do not exhibit diffusion restriction (please refer to Chaps. 2 and 6). Therefore, differentiating abscess and tumor necrosis on DWI and ADC images is easy.*
2. *MRS: In MRS, brain abscess exhibits unique values of lactate and lipid (1.3 ppm), amino acid (valine, leucine; 0.9 ppm), alanine (1.5 ppm), acetate (1.9 ppm), and succinate (2.4 ppm) (Figs. 2.10, 7.11, 7.12, and 7.15)* [5].

   MRS of tumor necrosis only exhibits higher lactate/lipid values (please refer to Chaps. 2 and 6).

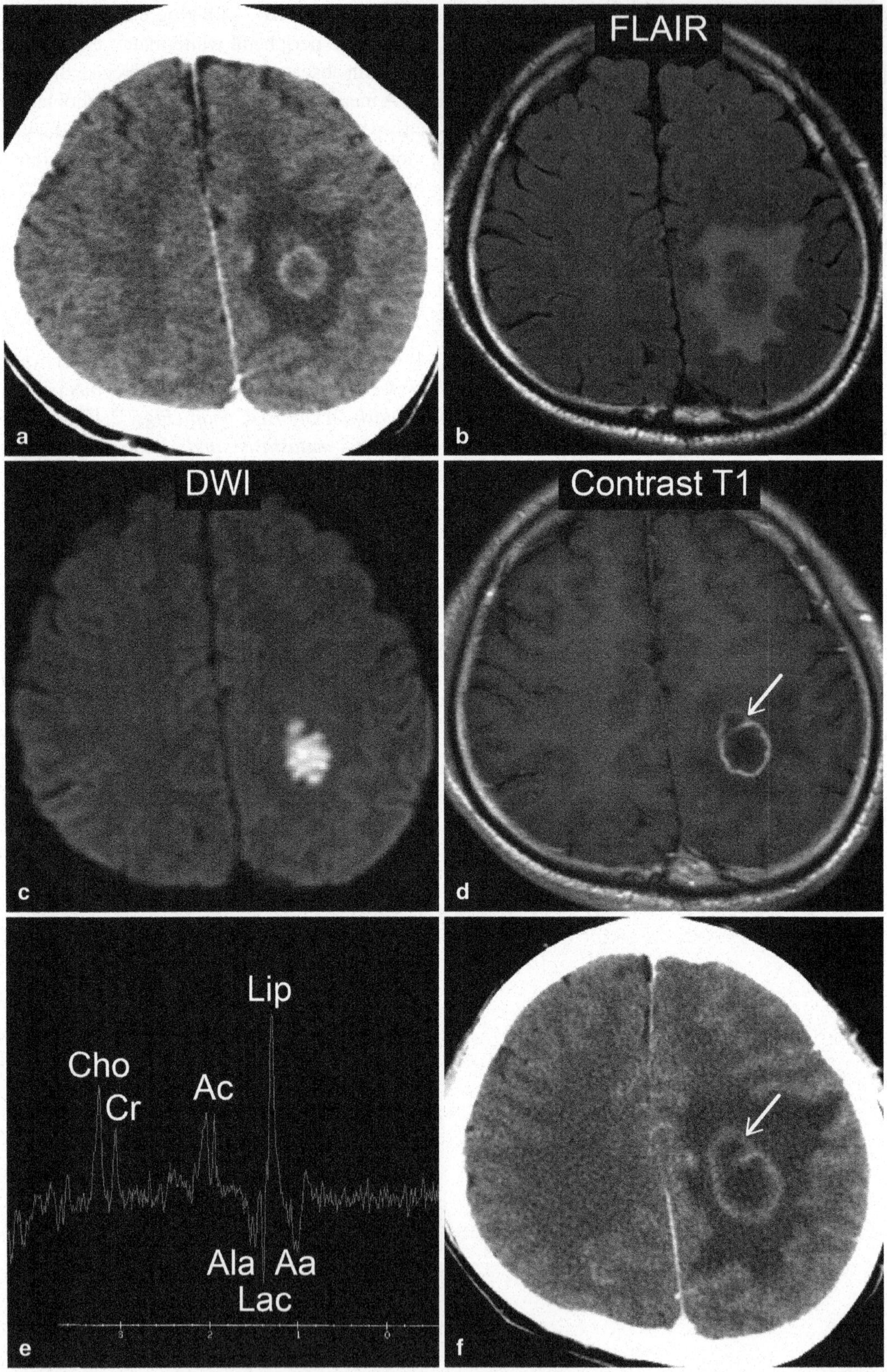

Fig. 7.11 M/53, Brain abscess in the left parietal lobe. (**a**) Contrast CT: A small cystic lesion is observed in the left centrum semiovale with peripheral white matter edema. (**b–d**) MRI: MRI was performed 2 days later. This cystic mass is clarified, and a small lesion (arrow) is seen next to the main cyst (mother-and-daughter sign). The content of this cyst appears bright on DWI, suggesting strong diffusion restriction that is characteristic of pus. In DWI, the peripheral white matter edema shows no signal change, thus it is invisible because this edema is vasogenic edema; that is, no diffusion restriction occurs. (**e**) MRS (TE 144 ms): Acetate (1.99 ppm) (Ac), alanine (1.5 ppm) (Ala), lactate/lipid (1.3 ppm) (Lac/Lip), and amino acid (0.9 ppm) (Aa) are observed. The choline (Cho) and creatine (Cr) are normal brain tissue components. The MRS findings are characteristic of a brain abscess. (**f**) Follow-up contrast CT, another 3 days later: The abscess is larger than before (arrow). The neurosurgeon performed surgery to drain the pus after this CT

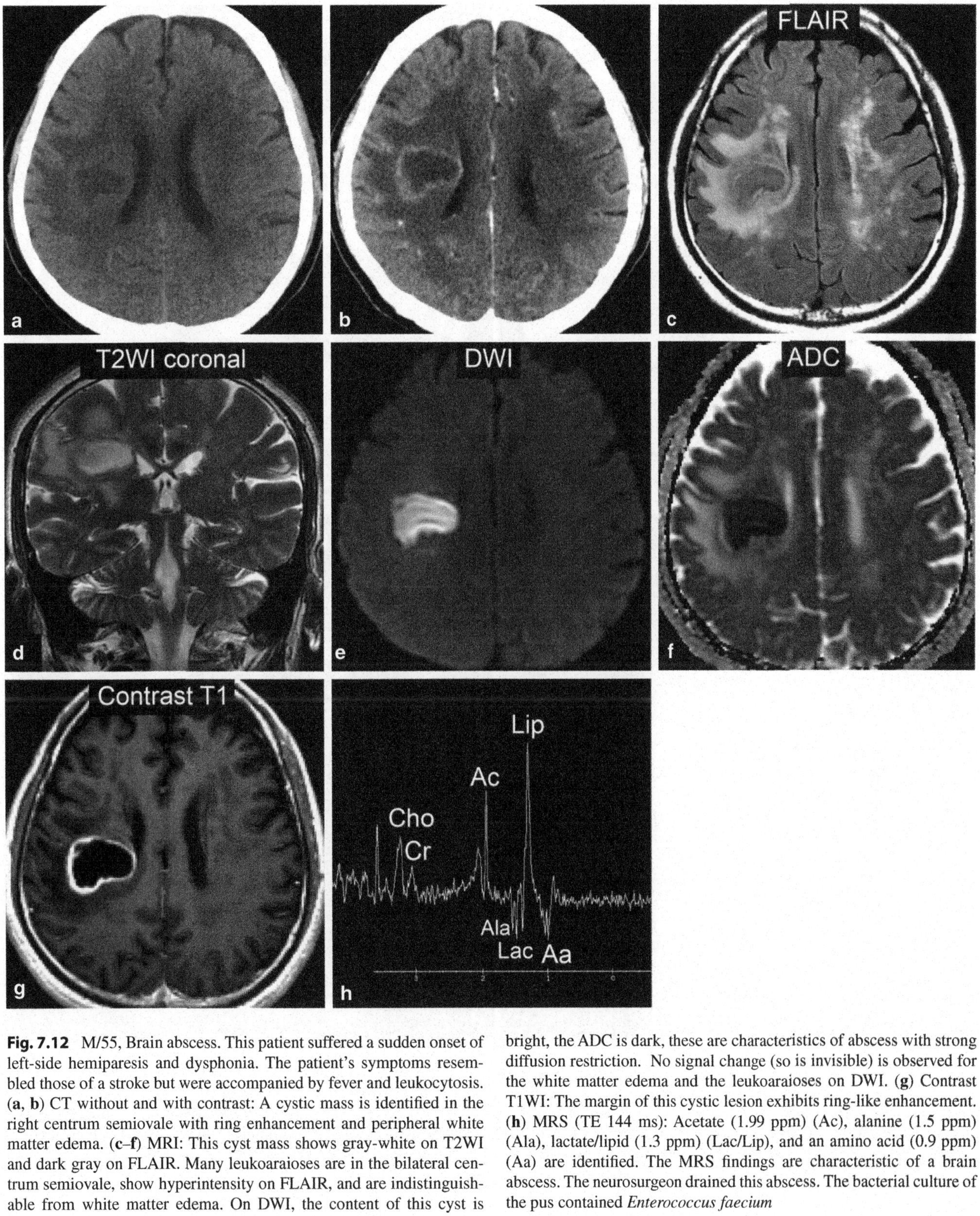

Fig. 7.12 M/55, Brain abscess. This patient suffered a sudden onset of left-side hemiparesis and dysphonia. The patient's symptoms resembled those of a stroke but were accompanied by fever and leukocytosis. (**a**, **b**) CT without and with contrast: A cystic mass is identified in the right centrum semiovale with ring enhancement and peripheral white matter edema. (**c**–**f**) MRI: This cyst mass shows gray-white on T2WI and dark gray on FLAIR. Many leukoaraioses are in the bilateral centrum semiovale, show hyperintensity on FLAIR, and are indistinguishable from white matter edema. On DWI, the content of this cyst is bright, the ADC is dark, these are characteristics of abscess with strong diffusion restriction. No signal change (so is invisible) is observed for the white matter edema and the leukoaraioses on DWI. (**g**) Contrast T1WI: The margin of this cystic lesion exhibits ring-like enhancement. (**h**) MRS (TE 144 ms): Acetate (1.99 ppm) (Ac), alanine (1.5 ppm) (Ala), lactate/lipid (1.3 ppm) (Lac/Lip), and an amino acid (0.9 ppm) (Aa) are identified. The MRS findings are characteristic of a brain abscess. The neurosurgeon drained this abscess. The bacterial culture of the pus contained *Enterococcus faecium*

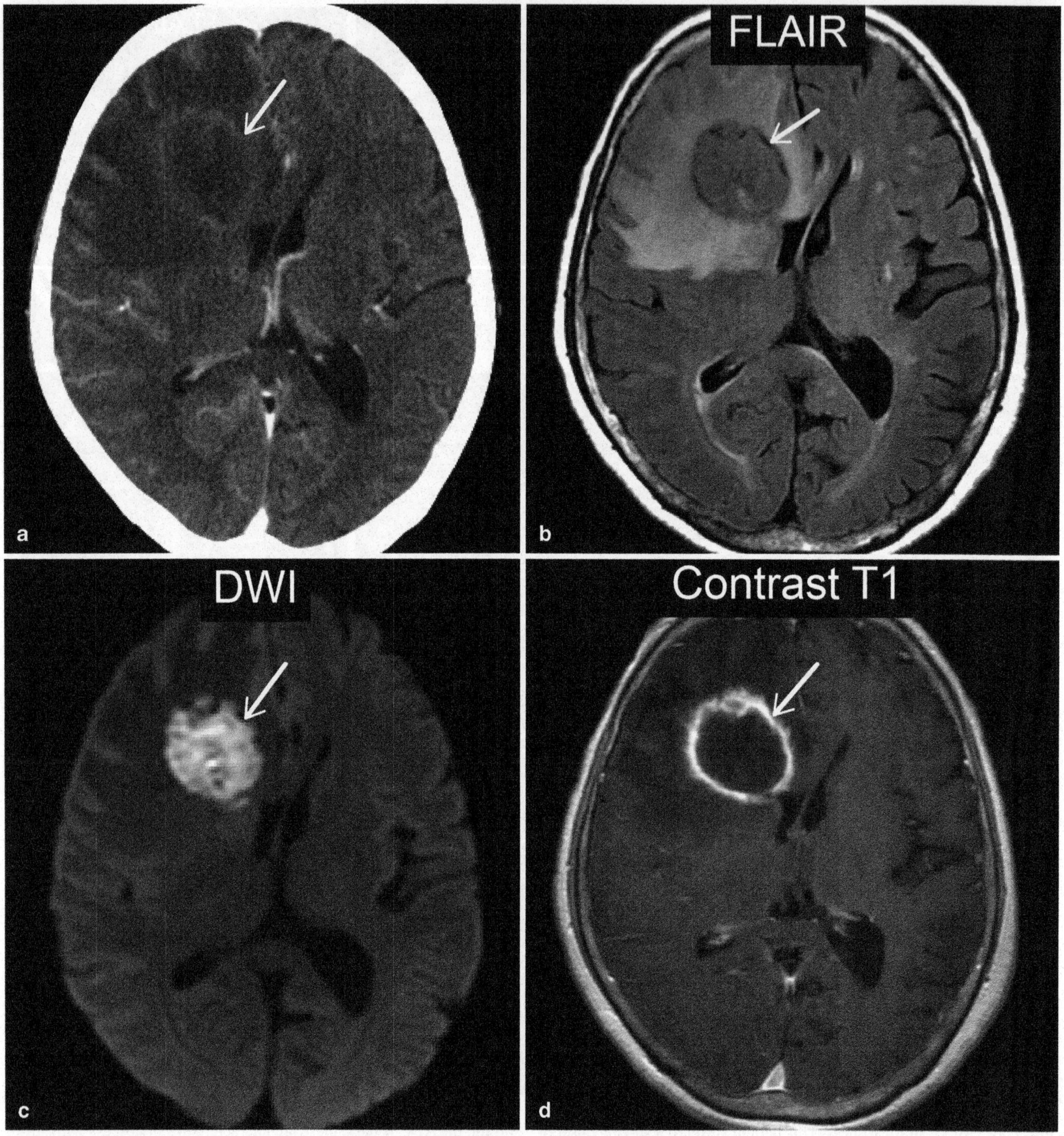

Fig. 7.13 F/71, Brain abscess. The patient suffered a headache and fever for a week. (**a**) Contrast CT: Brain tissue edema is observed in the right frontal lobe, and a ring-enhanced lesion (arrow) is found within the edema. (**b**) MRI, FLAIR: A lesion with peripheral white matter edema is observed in the subcortex of the right frontal lobe. The contents of this lesion show gray-dark (arrow) on FLAIR. (**c**) DWI: The content of this lesion shows bright (arrow) on DWI, indicating strong diffusion restriction that is characteristic of an abscess. (**d**) Contrast T1WI: This lesion has ring-like enhancement (arrow) and thus has a thin capsule. The abscess was surgically drained, and bacteria culture of the pus found *Streptococcus viridans*

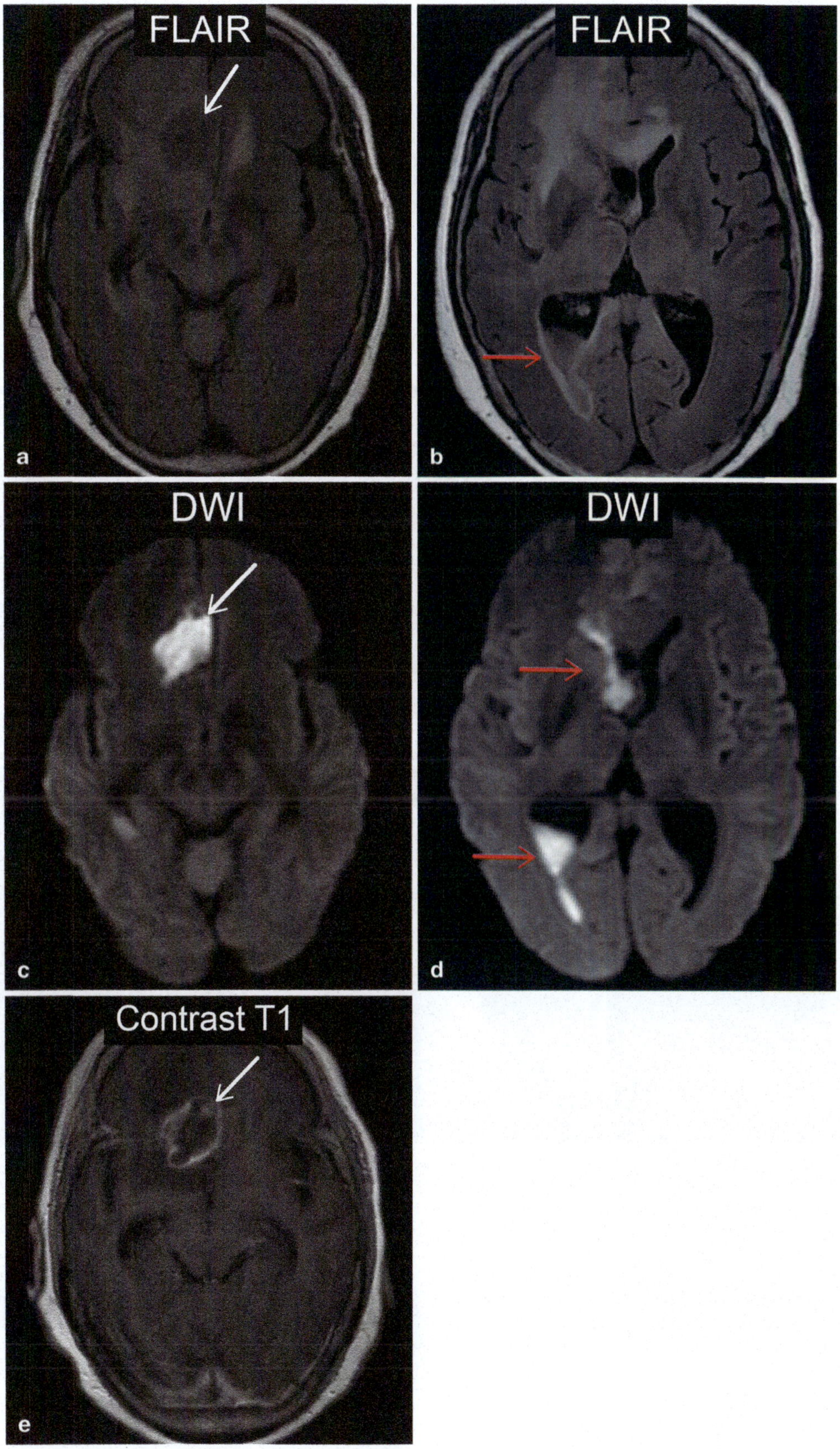

Fig. 7.14 F/70, Brain abscess ruptured into the ventricle. (**a**, **b**) MRI, FLAIR: The right frontal lobe has a lesion (arrow) and peripheral white matter edema. Some CSF with mild hyperintensity (red arrow) is observed in the right lateral ventricle. (**c**, **d**) DWI: This lesion has bright content (white arrow), which indicates a strong diffusion restriction. Thus, this lesion is an abscess. The right lateral ventricle also has the same high-signal substance (red arrows), which is the pus flowing into the ventricle. (**e**) Contrast T1WI: The lesion in the right frontal lobe has marginal enhancement. Therefore, this is a cystic lesion contains pus and is thus an abscess

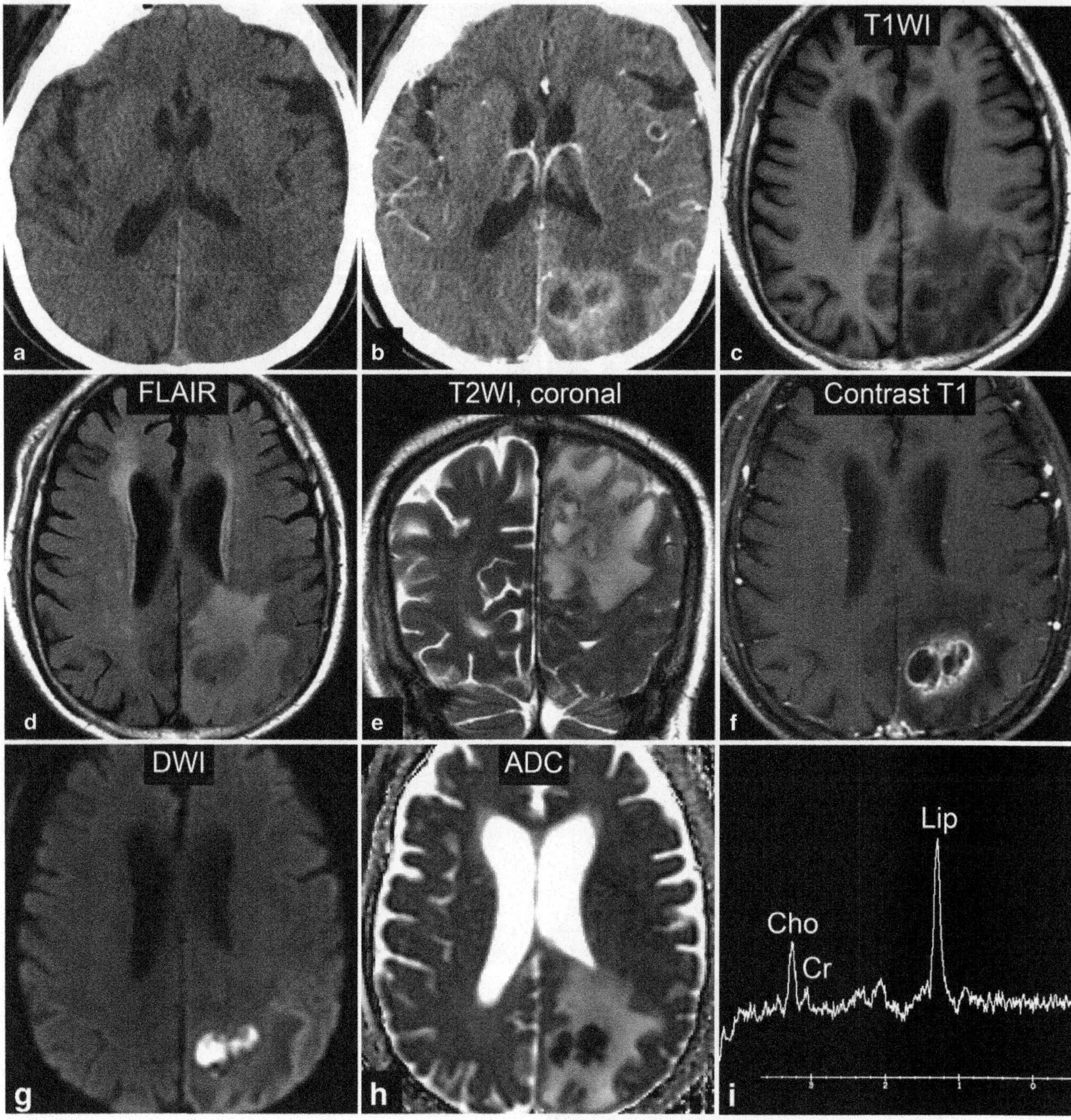

Fig. 7.15 M/70, Brain abscess resembling a glioblastoma. The patient suffered right-side hemiparesis, possibly experienced a stroke, and was sent to the emergency department. (**a**) CT, (**b**) contrast CT: Brain tissue edema is observed in the left occipital lobe, and an irregular enhancement lesion resembling a glioblastoma is found in the edema area. (**c–f**) MRI: An enhanced mass lesion with irregular cystic contents and peripheral white matter edema is identified. The feature resembles a glioblastoma with irregular central necrosis. (**g, h**) DWI: The content of the "necrotic area" is bright, and noticeably indicates diffusion restriction. The ADC coefficient is extremely low (hypointense). Tumor necrosis is unlikely, but the feature resembles an abscess. (**i**) MRS (TE 144 ms): The choline amount is small, the NAA disappears, and the lipid is elevated. Because no appearance of acetate, alanine, and amino acid, thus, the MRS is favoring tumor necrosis not brain abscess. However, finally, surgery and pathology confirmed this lesion as brain abscess

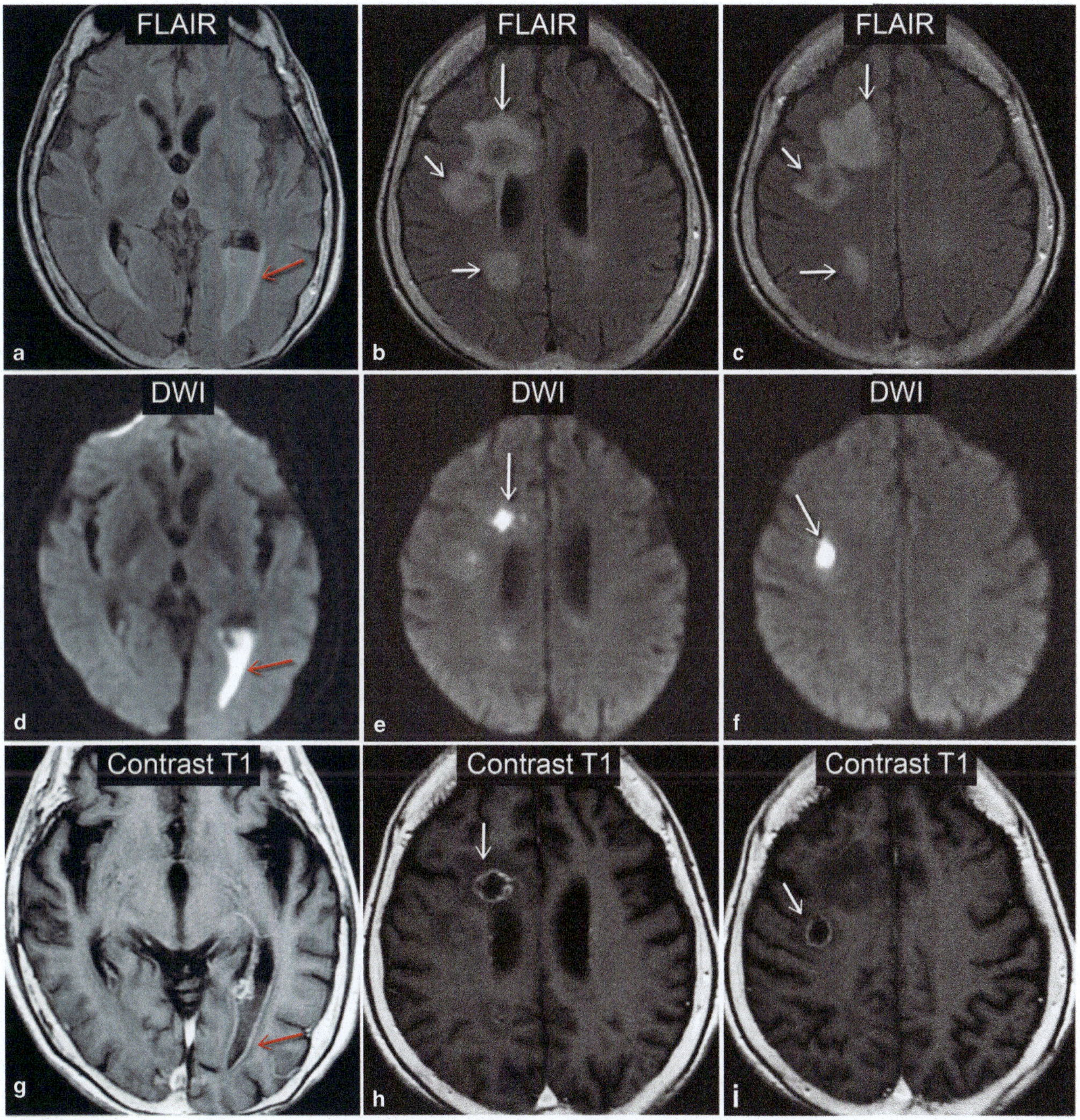

Fig. 7.16 F/80, TB abscesses with ventriculitis. A patient with pulmonary TB had left-side weakness and fever. (**a–c**) MRI, FLAIR: Three hyperintense lesions (white arrows) are observed in the right cerebral hemisphere; they may be brain tissue edemas. The cerebrospinal fluid in the left lateral ventricle is also hyperintense (red arrow). (**d–f**) DWI: The middle of the above lesions is bright (white arrows) on DWI, indicating diffusion restriction. The peripheral edema has no signal on DWI, so is vasogenic edema. Therefore, the features are similar to brain abscesses with peripheral white matter edemas. The content of the left lateral ventricle appears bright (red arrow) and thus may be pus flowing into the lateral ventricle. (**g–i**) Contrast T1WI: Ring-enhanced lesions (white arrows) are identified within the three edema areas. Thus, these lesions are typical brain abscesses with peripheral white matter edemas. The left lateral ventricular wall (red arrow) exhibits linear enhancement, reflecting ventriculitis

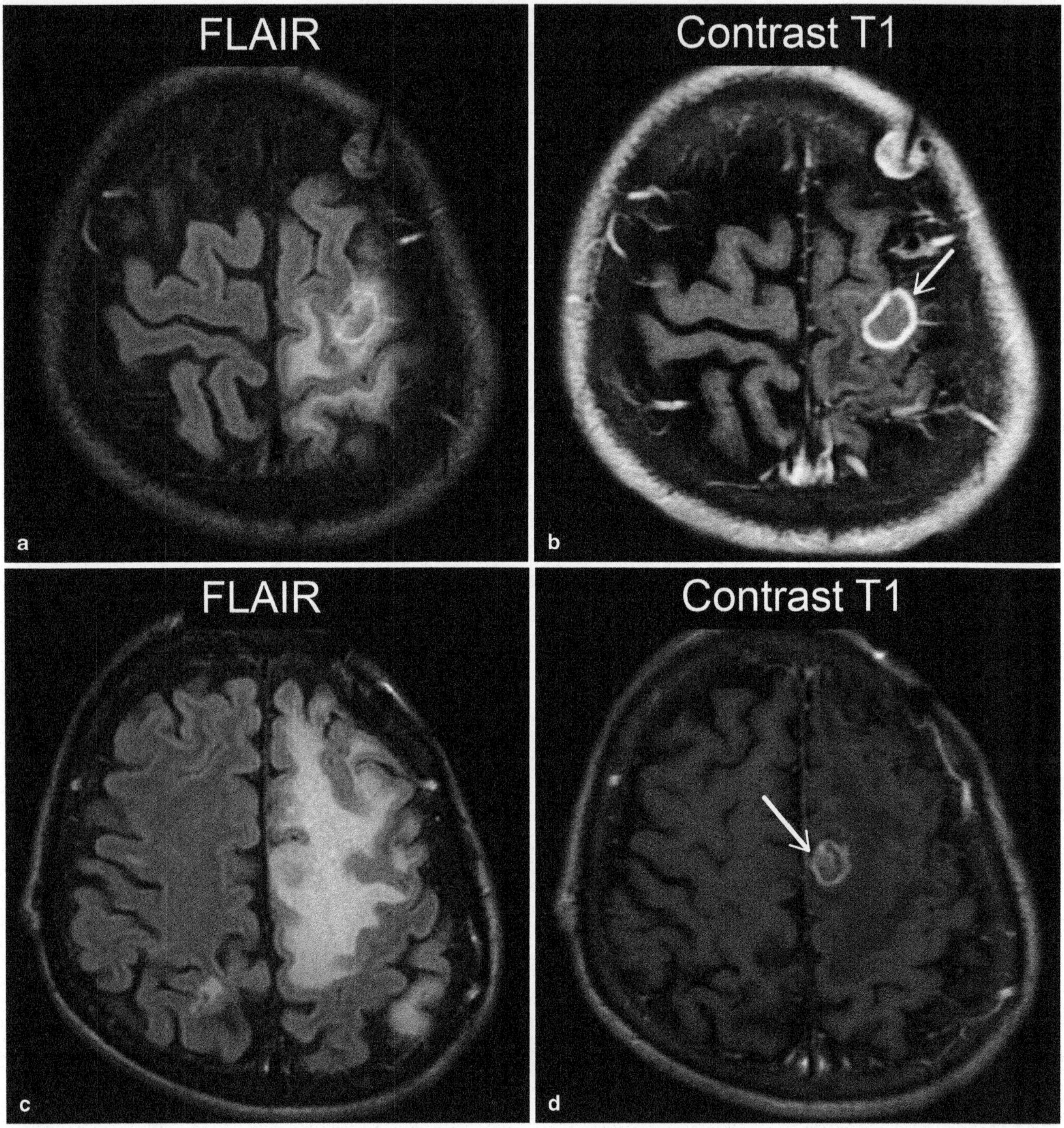

Fig. 7.17 M/37, HIV with toxoplasmosis. AIDS patient experienced repeated CNS infection. (**a**, **b**) MRI: A cystic lesion with ring-like enhancement and some peripheral white matter edema is found in the left frontal lobe (arrow). This lesion is an abscess. Toxoplasma is detected in blood culture. (**c**) The patient was infected again. MRI, 3 years later, FLAIR: A large area of brain tissue edema is identified in the left frontoparietal lobes. (**d**) Contrast T1WI: A small, ring-enhanced cystic mass is observed within the above edematous region, is identified as an abscess (arrow). Surgery found that this mass had central necrosis, and pathology confirmed that this is encephalitis caused by toxoplasma

7.3 Viral Encephalitis

7.3.1 Encephalitis Types

1. Viral encephalitis is caused by direct viral infection of brain tissues. The most common form of viral encephalitis is herpes simplex encephalitis (Figs. 7.18 and 7.19). Other viruses—including enterovirus (Figs. 7.20 and 7.21), Japanese encephalitis virus (Fig. 7.23), influenza (Fig. 7.24), varicella, and measles—can also cause encephalitis. In some cases, the pathogenesis virus cannot be determined (Figs. 7.22 and 7.25). In some instances, encephalitis may be comorbid with meningitis, called meningoencephalitis (Fig. 7.25) [6–9].
2. Chronic viral encephalitis includes subacute sclerosing panencephalitis, Epstein–Barr virus encephalitis, and Rasmussen encephalitis.
3. Post-infectious encephalitis refers to encephalitis caused by the autoimmune system due to past viral infection. This category includes ADEM (Figs. 7.26 and 7.27), acute hemorrhagic leukoencephalitis, and acute necrotizing encephalitis [7].

7.3.1.1 CT and MRI Imaging of Encephalitis

CT: In some cases, the lesion is undetectable. Injuries are observable through the abnormally low density of brain tissues (Fig. 7.19). Sometimes, irregular contrast enhancement in the involving area is observed.

MRI: Lesions are more easily detected using MRI than CT [6–9], particularly for T2WI and FLAIR images, where the encephalitis areas are bright (hyperintense). Some cases show no signal change on DWI in encephalitis regions (Fig. 7.22). In some cases, the encephalitis regions have diffusion restrictions and show hyperintensity on DWI, but not as bright as cytotoxic edema of acute infarction (Figs. 7.18, 7.19, and 7.24).Some encephalitis may have irregular enhancement by contrast media (Figs. 7.22 and 7.25).MRS: The encephalitis areas may show elevation of choline and the appearance of lactate (Figs. 7.19 and 7.22).

7.3.2 Herpes Simplex Encephalitis

Pathogen: HSV2 for infants and HSV1 for children and adults.

Infection location: HSV2 encephalitis does not have a specific infection location for infants. However, HSV1 encephalitis mainly occurs in the limbic system, including the temporal lobe, insular cortex, subfrontal area, and cingulate gyri. The infection first occurs on one side and then develops to both sides (Figs. 7.18 and 7.19) [7].

7.3.3 Enteroviral Encephalitis

Enteroviral encephalitis may be caused by 68–71 types of enterovirus, coxsackie A, and echovirus. Clinically, enteroviruses cause hand–foot–mouth disease. Enterovirus 71 may infect the brain or spinal cord, causing encephalitis or encephalomyelitis or myelitis, respectively.Enteroviral encephalitis generally infects the brain stem, specifically the middle and posterior parts of the medulla oblongata, the posterior part of the pons (pontine tegmentum), the middle of the midbrain, and the dentate nucleus of the cerebellum (Figs. 7.20 and 7.21) [10, 11].

7.4 ADEM

ADEM is a type of encephalitis caused by the autoimmune response after a patient has been infected by a virus or bacteria (e.g., common upper respiratory tract infection, gastroenteritis, or musculoskeletal inflammation) or has received a preventative injection (e.g., measles and chickenpox vaccines). Within 1–3 weeks of being infected or receiving the dose of vaccine, the patient may suddenly develop fever, headaches, lethargy, convulsions, psychological symptoms, or even enter a coma or die.

MRI: T2WI and FLAIR imaging in MRI is more capable of revealing ADEM pathogeneses than CT scanning. Numerous asymmetrical hyperintense lesions can be discovered in the cerebral deep white matter, brain stem, and the cerebellum (Figs. 7.26 and 7.27). Furthermore, some involving areas show moderate diffusion restriction (moderate hyperintense) on DWI, and some areas have abnormal contrast enhancement [7].

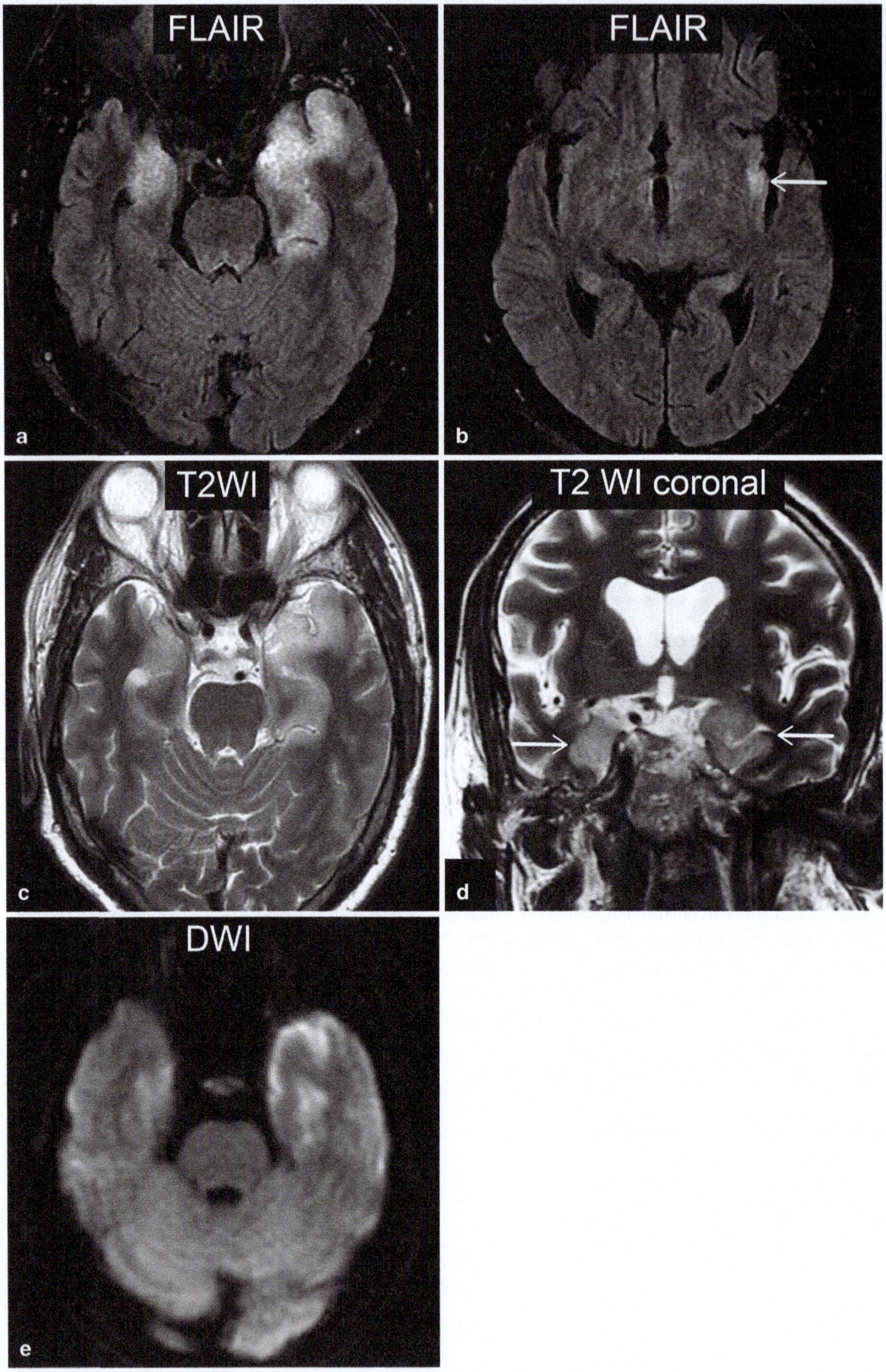

Fig. 7.18 M/65, Herpes simplex encephalitis. The patient suffered consciousness disturbance, fever, and vomiting. (**a–d**) MRI: The brain tissue in the mesial parts of the bilateral temporal lobes, including the hippocampus and the insular cortex, show hyperintensity on FLAIR and T2WI (arrows). This pattern is typical of herpes simplex (HSV) encephalitis. (**e**) DWI: Some parts of the above areas show hyperintensity on DWI; only these areas have diffusion restriction

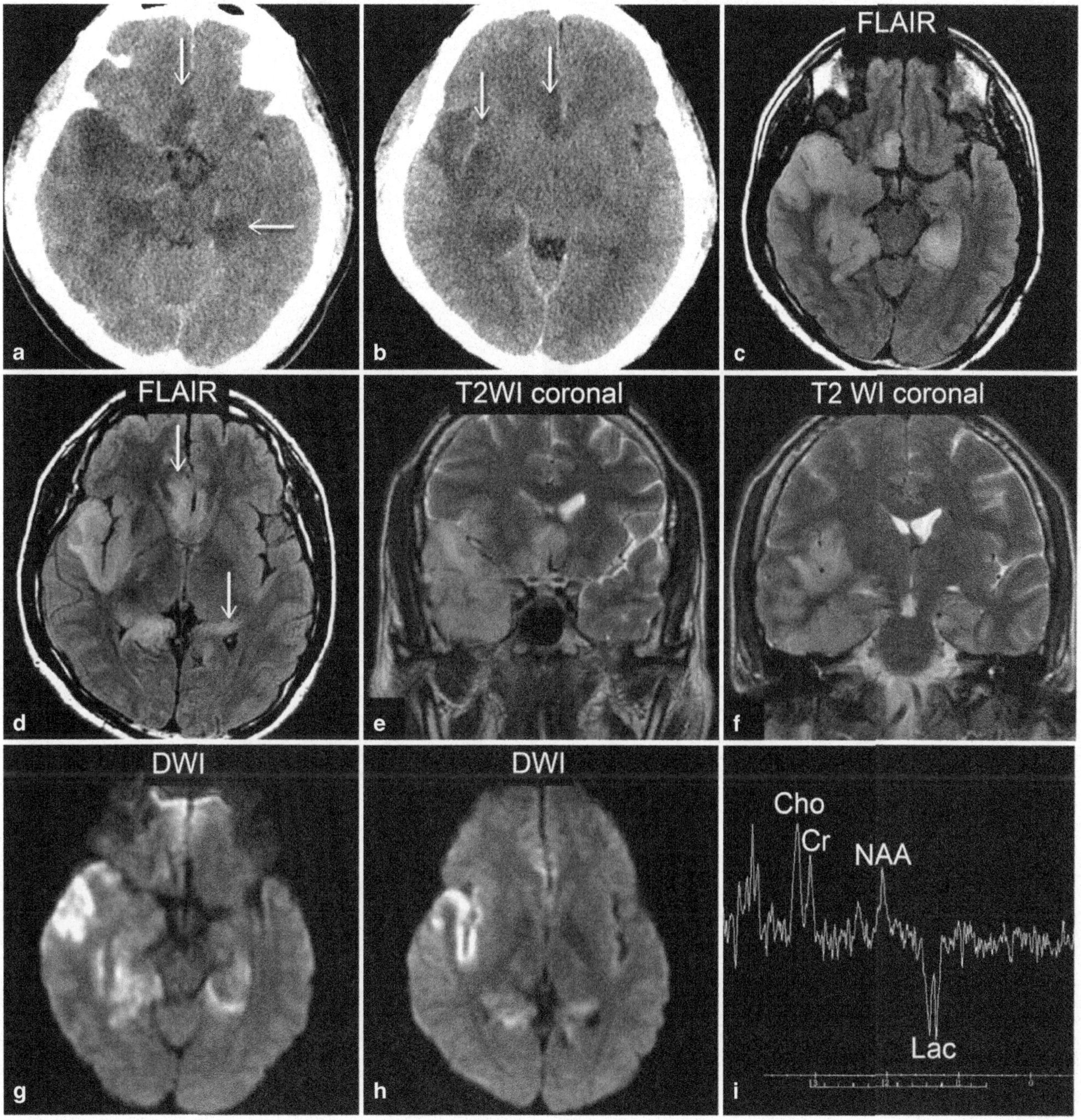

Fig. 7.19 M/44, Herpes simplex encephalitis. The patient suffered consciousness disturbance, fever, and vomiting. (**a**, **b**) Contrast CT: Hypodense lesions (arrows) are found in the right temporal lobe, including the hippocampus and the insular cortex. There is also a hypodense lesion in the left temporal lobe. (**c**–**f**) MRI: The above areas show hyperintensity on FLAIR and T2WI, a typical feature of HSV encephalitis. (**g**, **h**) Most of the above lesion areas are hyperintense on DWI, reflecting diffusion restriction. (**i**) MRS (TE 144 ms): Elevation of lactate (Lac) and mild elevation of choline, the NAA is slightly decreased. Please note, this MRS was performed on TE 144 ms; the lactate is inverted and showing doublet peak

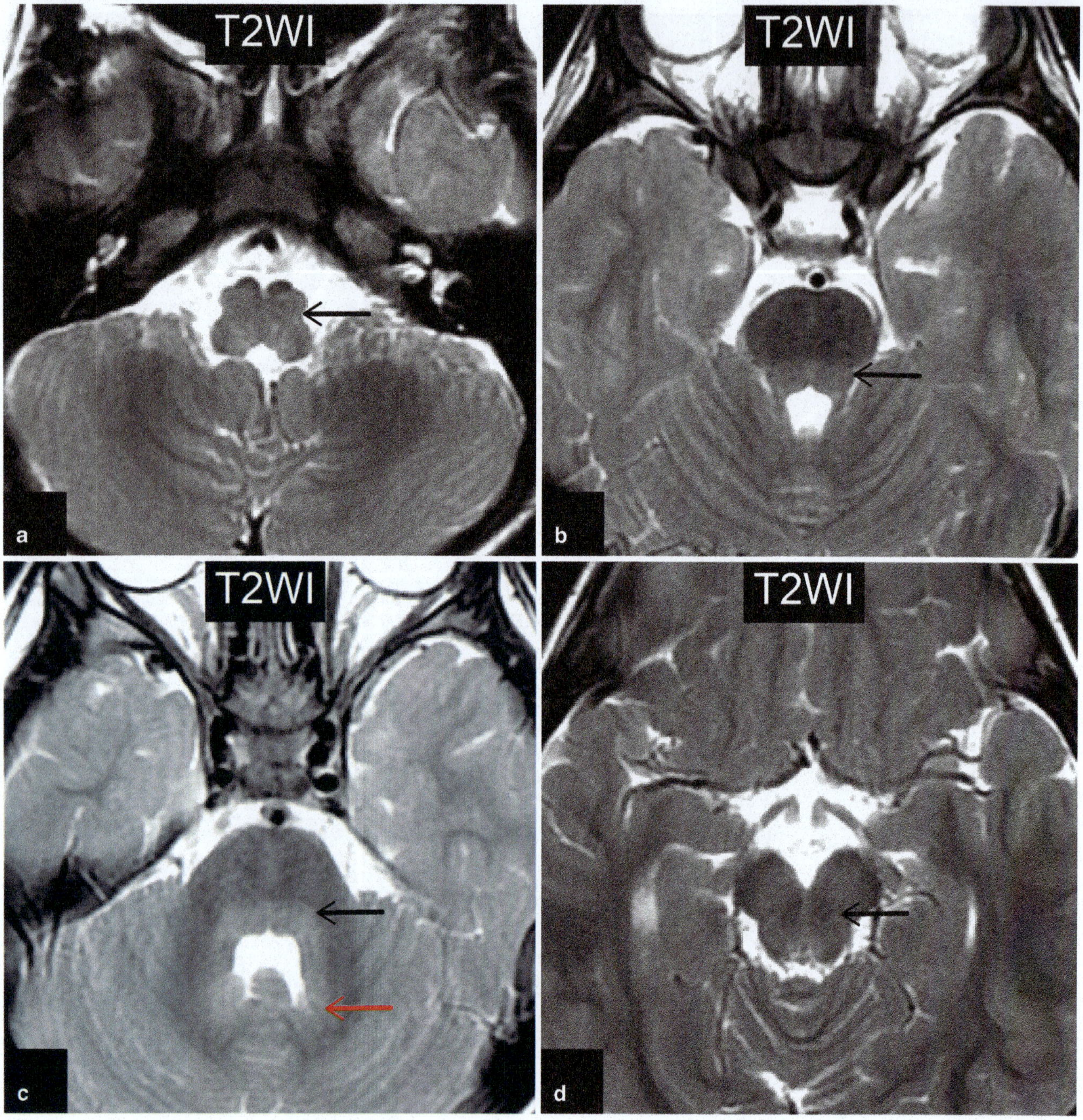

Fig. 7.20 M/27 months, Enteroviral encephalitis. The boy suffered high fever, mouth ulcers, and vesicles in the skin of the hands and feet; these features indicate a typical hand-foot-mouth disease caused by enterovirus 71. The symptoms were associated with gait instability and myoclonic jerk. Thus, CNS involvement was suspected. (**a**) MRI T2WI: Hyperintensity is observed in the entire medulla oblongata (arrow) except for the pyramids. (**b**, **c**) T2WI: Hyperintensity is found in the posterior of the pons (black arrow) and extends to the bilateral dentate nuclei (red arrow) of the cerebellum. (**d**) The middle part of the midbrain presents hyperintensity (arrow). These image features are characteristic of enteroviral encephalitis. The patient recovers well after intensive care and treatment

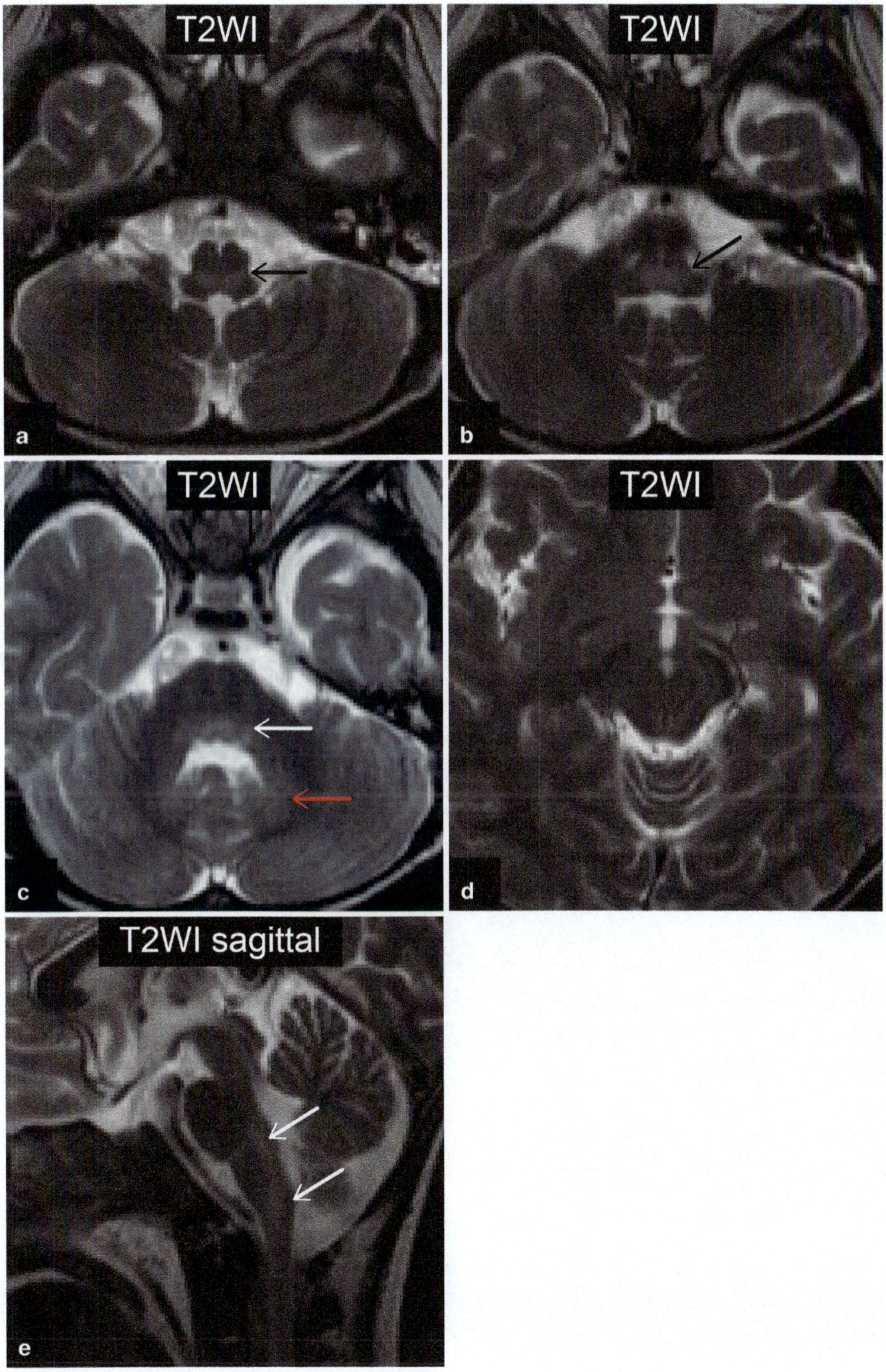

Fig. 7.21 F/24 months, Enteroviral encephalitis. The girl suffered high fever, mouth ulcers, and vesicles in the skin of the hands and feet; these symptoms indicate a typical hand-foot-mouth disease caused by enterovirus 71. Gait instability is also observed. Hence, CNS involvement is suspected. (**a**, **b**) MRI, T2WI: The posterior of the medulla oblongata shows hyperintensity (arrow). (**c**) T2WI: Hyperintensity is identified in the posterior of the pons (white arrow) and extends to the bilateral dentate nuclei (red arrow) of the cerebellum. (**d**) T2WI: No abnormal signal intensity is found in the midbrain. (**e**) T2WI, sagittal: Hyperintensity is observed in the posterior of the medulla oblongata and the pons (arrows). These findings are characteristic imaging signs of enteroviral encephalitis

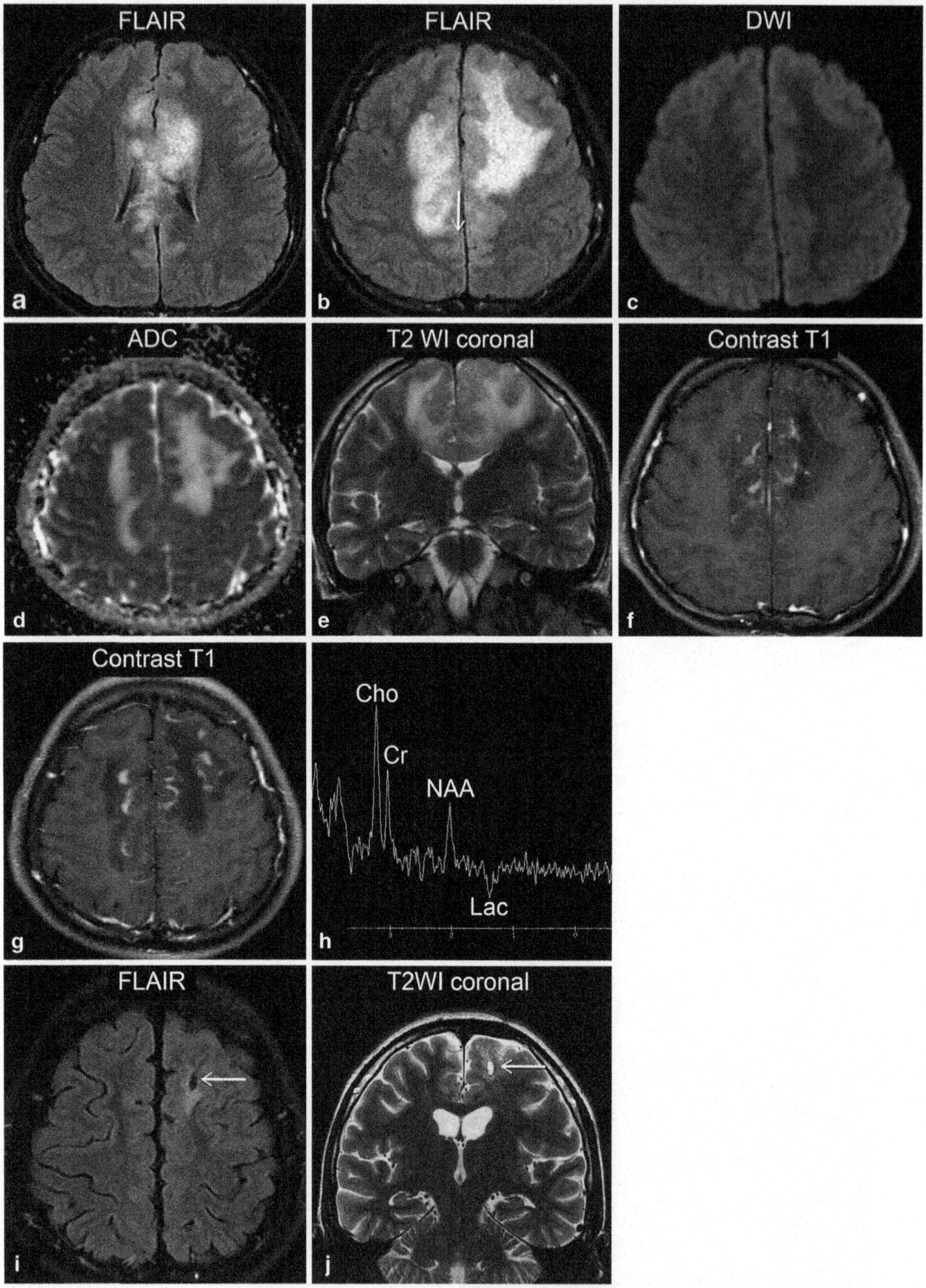

Fig. 7.22 M/16, Viral encephalitis. The patient suffered a seizure and became unconscious. He was clinically considered to have CNS infection. (**a**–**e**) MRI: A large area of brain tissue in the corpus callosum, bilateral cingula, and bilateral frontoparietal lobes shows hyperintensity on FLAIR and T2WI. However, no signal change on DWI and hyperintensity is observed on ADC. These findings indicate a high diffusion coefficient, different from that in infarction edema or astrocytoma. (**f**, **g**) Contrast T1WI: Irregular enhancement is seen in this area. Therefore, the BBB is broken. (**h**) MRS (TE 144 ms): Choline elevates, NAA falls, and some lactate appears. (**i**, **j**) The patient recovered well and had a follow-up MRI after 3 months. Only a small part of brain tissue damage has remained (arrows)

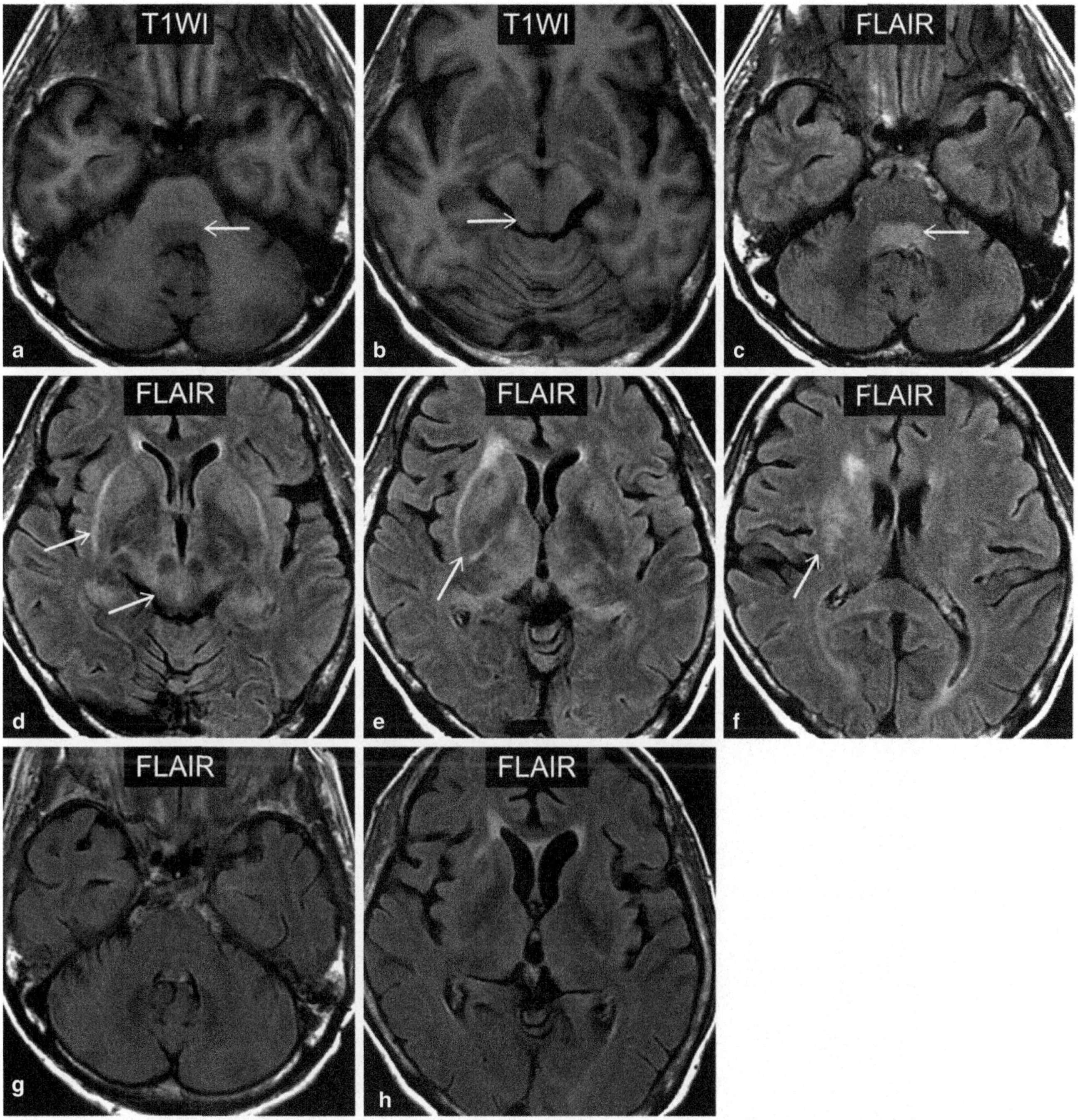

Fig. 7.23 F/50, Japanese encephalitis. The patient experienced chills, high fever, left limb weakness, and dysphonia. (**a, b**) T1WI: Hypointensity (arrows) is identified in the posterior of the pons and the midbrain. (**c–f**) FLAIR: Hyperintensity (arrows) is observed in the posterior of the pons and the midbrain. Hyperintensity (arrows) is also seen in the bilateral putamina, especially the putaminal capsules, the bilateral thalami, and the posterior limb of the right internal capsule. These findings represent a kind of encephalitis. The virus reaction test confirmed Japanese encephalitis. (**g, h**) This patient recovered well and had a follow-up MRI after 1 month. No abnormal signal intensity was found in the above areas

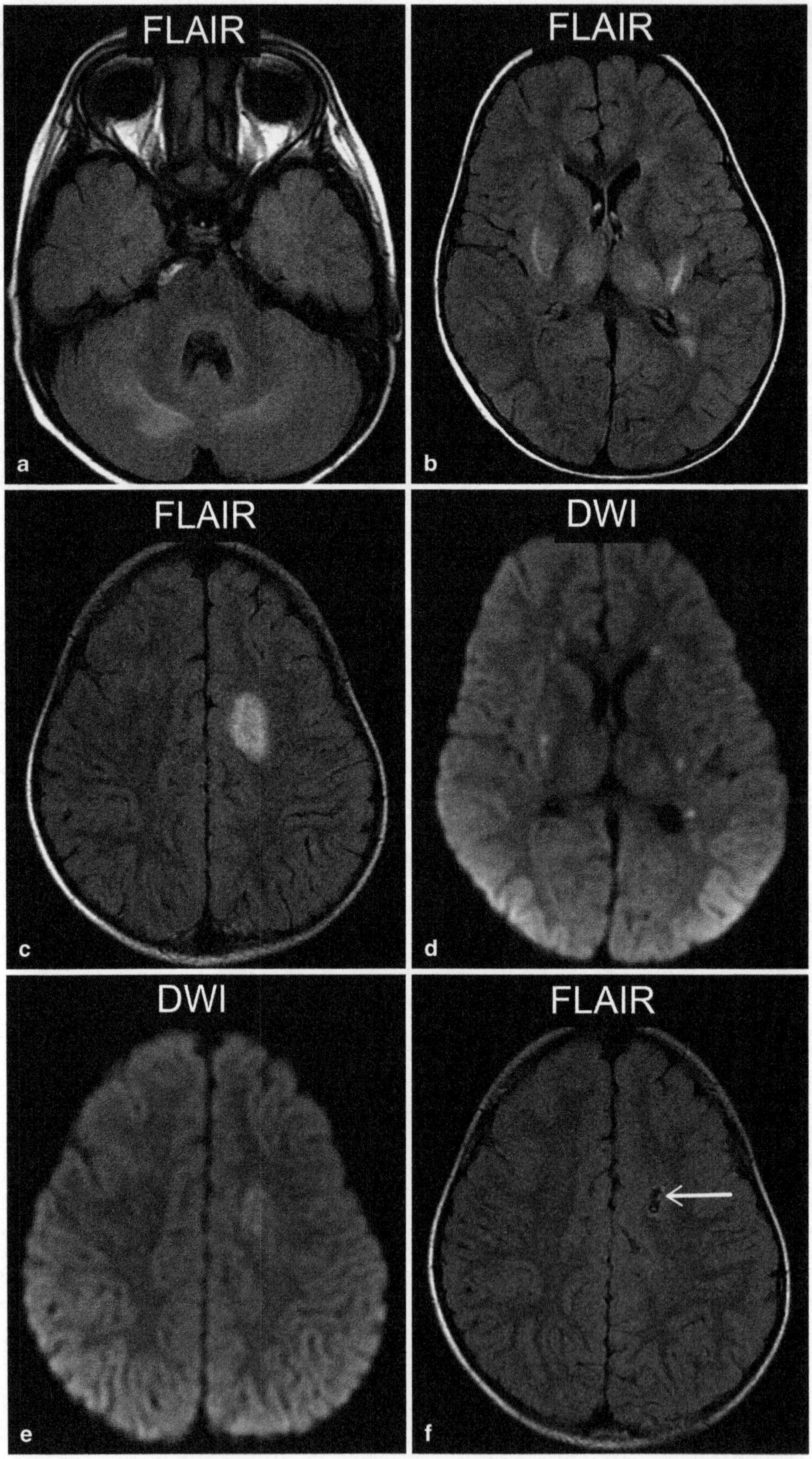

Fig. 7.24 M/25, Influenza encephalitis. (**a–c**) FLAIR: Hyperintense lesions are found in the deep portions of the bilateral cerebella, the bilateral thalami, and parts of the bilateral putamina and the left corona radiata. (**d**, **e**) DWI: Only small punctate hyperintensities within the above lesions. (**f**) The patient recovered well and had a follow-up MRI 2 months later. Most of the above lesions had disappeared. Only small residual necrosis (arrow) in the left corona radiata remained

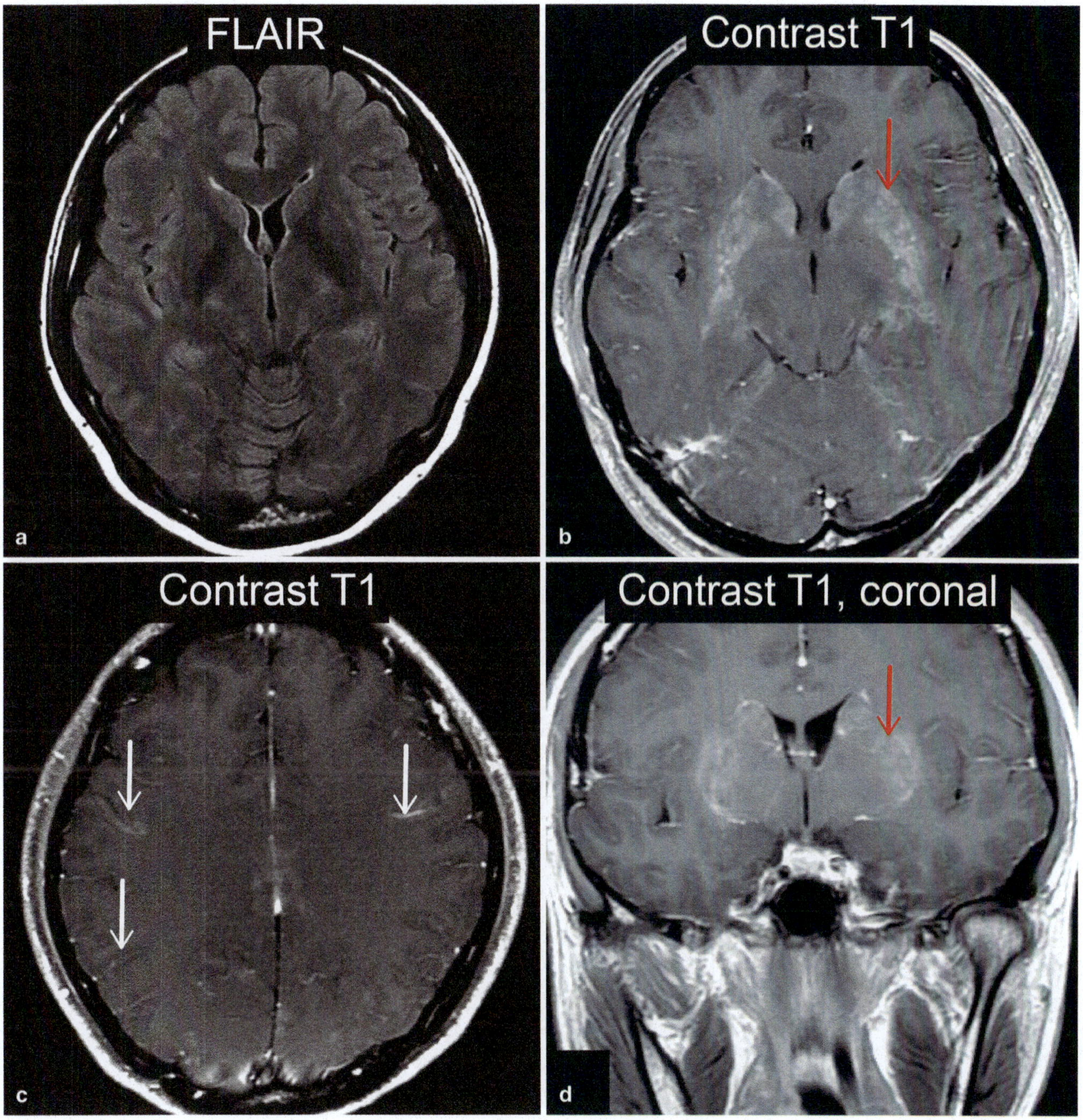

Fig. 7.25 F/38, Meningoencephalitis. The patient suffered fever, headache, seizure, and loss of consciousness. Her condition was clinically considered to be CNS infection. CSF study also showed elevation of protein and some white blood cells. Meningitis or encephalitis was confirmed. (**a**) MRI, FLAIR: No visible abnormal signal intensity is identified. (**b–d**) Contrast T1WI: Enhancement in the bilateral corpus striatum (putamen and caudate nucleus) (red arrow) indicates BBB disruption in the brain tissue of these areas. Leptomeningeal enhancement (white arrows) seen in the sulci suggests the involvement of meningitis. Thus, this condition is meningoencephalitis

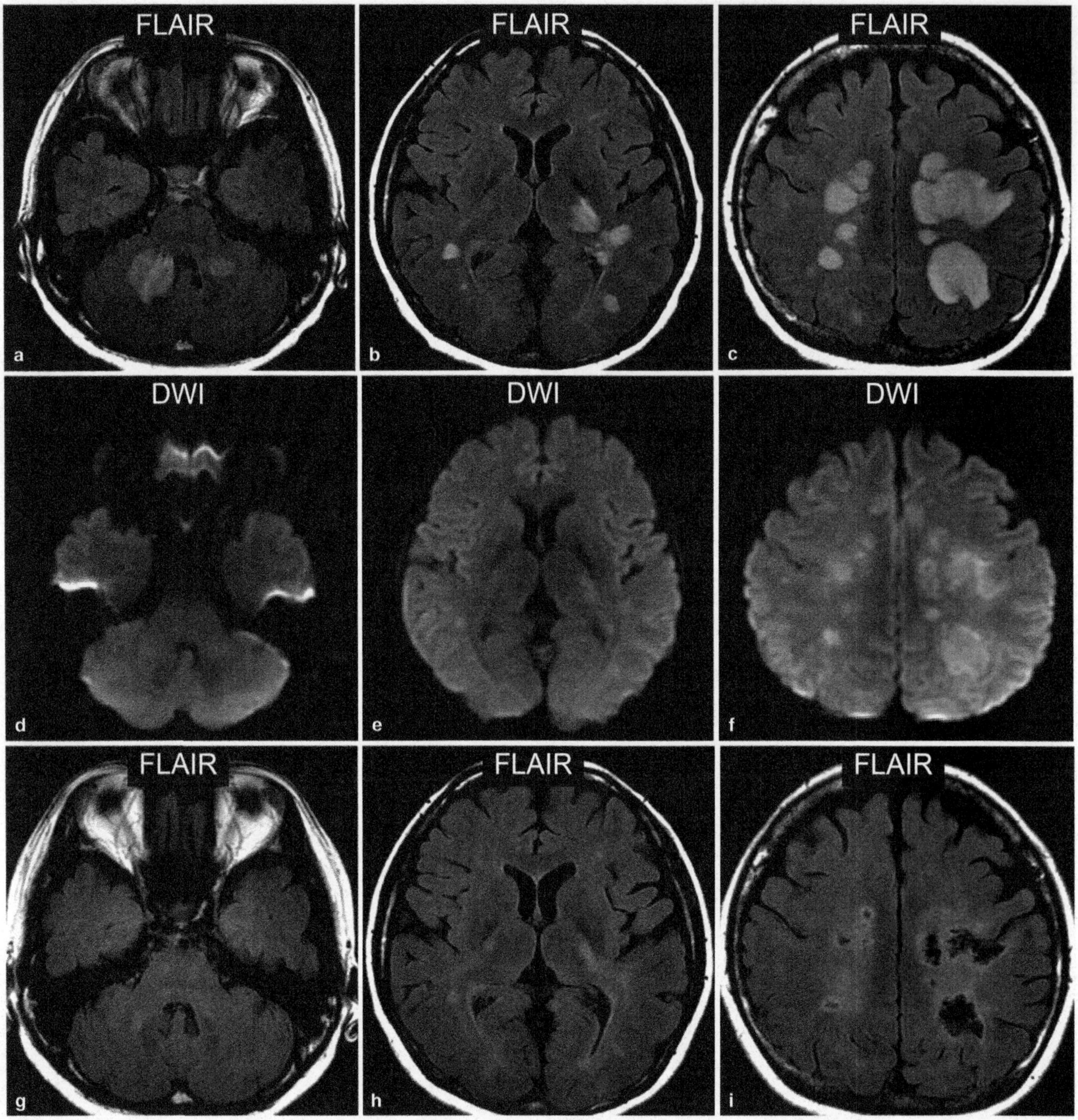

Fig. 7.26 F/44, Acute disseminated encephalomyelitis (ADEM). The patient complained of fever, vomiting, and diarrhea. Her condition was initially suspected to be acute gastroenteritis. After 3 days, she had right limb weakness, mild alteration of consciousness, and then coma and convulsions. (**a–c**) MRI, FLAIR: Multiple hyperintense lesions are found in the bilateral cerebella, the left thalamus, and the bilateral centrum semiovale. (**d–f**) DWI: These lesions show only a slight increase in signal intensity on DWI, reflecting mild diffusion restriction. (**g–i**) The patient was later stabilized, but the right limb remained weak. Follow-up MRI was performed 9 months later. Part of the lesions remained mildly hyperintense on FLAIR. The lesions in the centrum semiovale showed necrosis and cavitary change. The above course on a 44-year-old adult with pre-infection. After 3 days, she developed symptoms of encephalopathy. MRI showed multiple hyperintense lesions, which are typical of ADEM

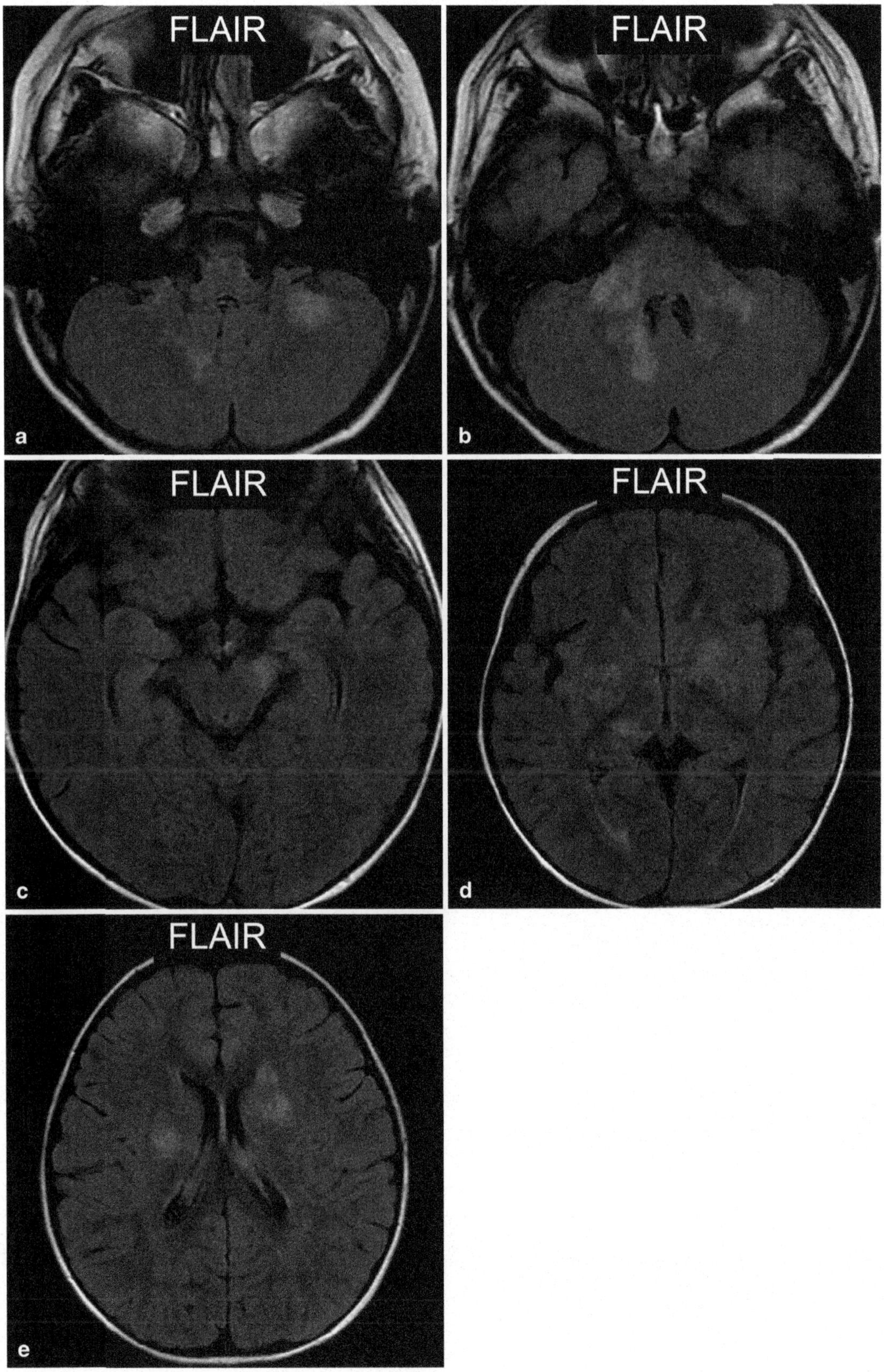

Fig. 7.27 F/3, Acute disseminated encephalomyelitis (ADEM). The 3-year-old girl had a high fever 25 days before her visit. Her fever was possibly due to acute otitis media. After 15 days, she started to have an unsteady gait and hand tremor. (**a**–**e**) MRI, FLAIR: Multiple hyperintense lesions are found in the bilateral cerebella, pons, left cerebral peduncle of the midbrain, bilateral basal ganglia, and the right thalamus. All these lesions have no signal change on DWI and no enhancement after contrast medium administration (not shown). The patient recovered well and had a follow-up MRI 3 months later. Only two small residual lesions remained (not shown). The above course, a 3-year-old child, experienced pre-infection. She began experiencing ataxia and tremor, which are symptoms of encephalopathy, 15 days later. MRI showed multiple high-signal lesions, which are typical of ADEM

References

1. Oliveira CR, et al. Brain magnetic resonance imaging of infants with bacterial meningitis. J Pediatr. 2014;165:134–9.
2. Stuckey SL, et al. Hyperintensity in the subarachnoid space on FLAIR MRI. AJR. 2007;189:913–21.
3. Hsieh FY, et al. Locations of cerebral infarctions in tuberculous meningitis. Neuroradiology. 1992;34:197–9.
4. Lee YC, et al. Idiopathic hypertrophic cranial pachymeningitis: case report with 7 years of imaging follow-up. AJNR Am J Neuroradiol. 2003;24:119–23.
5. Lai PH, et al. Brain abscess and necrotic brain tumor: discrimination with proton MR spectroscopy and diffusion-weighted imaging. AJNR Am J Neuroradiol. 2002;23:1369–77.
6. Tsuchiya K, et al. Diffusion-weighted MR imaging of encephalitis. AJR. 1999;173:1097–9.
7. Lo CP, Chen CY. Neuroimaging of viral infections in infants and young children. Neuroimaging Clin N Am. 2008;18:119–32.
8. Bykowski J, et al. Acute pediatric encephalitis neuroimaging: single-institution series as part of the California Encephalitis Project. Pediatric Neurology. 2015;52:606–14.
9. Takanashi J, et al. Influenza-associated encephalitis/encephalopathy with a reversible lesion in the splenium of the corpus callosum: a case report and literature review. AJNR Am J Neuroradiol. 2004;25:798–802.
10. Shen WC, et al. MR imaging findings of enteroviral encephalitis: an outbreak in Taiwan. AJNR Am J Neuroradiol. 1999;20:1889–95.
11. Chen CY, et al. Acute flaccid paralysis in infants and young children with enterovirus 71 infection: MR imaging findings and clinical correlates. AJNR Am J Neuroradiol. 2001;22:200–5.

8 Medical Imaging of Spinal Diseases

Abstract

For the diagnosis of spinal diseases, X-rays are the first line of a routine inspection. You can first understand the spinal bony structures, but the information is limited. CT shows the spinal bony changes, the spinal canal, and neuroforamina, but CT cannot evaluate the spinal cord. MRI is the most important tool for the diagnosis of spinal diseases because MRI can see the spinal bony structures and intervertebral discs, and only MRI can see the spinal cord. Degenerative spondylosis is the most common spinal disease; however, the clinical symptoms have significant variations; many persons have degenerative spinal changes but do not have significant symptoms. X-rays can be routinely examined. You can see spine osteophytes, spondylolisthesis, scoliosis, compression fracture, etc. through X-ray. For more severe patients, we consider CT or MRI. CT can look at the degenerations of vertebral bodies, discs, facet joints and ligaments, and spinal canal stenosis in detail. MRI is especially indicated for the evaluation of cervical and thoracic degeneration because of the need to see the spinal cord. For spinal injury, CT can evaluate the fractures, subluxation. Sagittal and coronal reconstructions of spine CT images are vital for spinal injury. MRI surpasses CT for spinal trauma. T1WI is sensitive to vertebral fractures. Combine T1WI and T2 STIR, MRI can distinguish new and old fractures and detect whether there is edema or bleeding in the spinal cord. For the diagnosis of a spinal tumors, MRI is the most important modality. For intramedullary tumors, only MRI can see the tumor mass and associated syringomyelia. There is a CSF space-widening sign for MRI to distinguish the intradural extramedullary tumor and spinal cord. For spinal metastases, MRI is more sensitive than CT. Osteomyelitis often combines with discitis, called spondylodiscitis. Myelitis may present linear hyperintensity in the spinal cord seen in T2WI, sagittal section. The enteroviral myelitis shows symmetrical hyperintensity in the bilateral ventral horns of the spinal cord seen in axial section.

8.1 Imaging of the Spine and Spinal Anatomy

The human spine comprises the cervical spine (C1–7), thoracic spine (T1–12), lumbar spine (L1–5), and downward connects with the sacrum (S1–5) and coccyx (Figs. 8.1, 8.2, 8.3, 8.4, and 8.5).

The following diagnostic tools can be used to examine spinal diseases. The appropriate diagnostic tool depends on clinical symptoms and the clinically suspected disease.

1. **X-ray:** Used for the routine examination of all spinal diseases, X-rays are typically the first to be performed. However, computed tomography (CT) scan and magnetic resonance imaging (MRI) can be administered directly to young adults with sciatica. In X-ray tests, the anteroposterior (AP) and lateral views of the spine are routinely imaged, along with oblique views of the spine, if necessary (Fig. 8.1).
2. **CT:** As a primary tool for the examination of spinal disease, CT yields the most explicit images of bony structures. However, the spinal cord cannot be viewed clearly with CT. CT has been replaced by MRI in the examination of the cervical and thoracic spines. CT is used for only the axial section. However, current multislice CT can quickly reconstruct images in the sagittal and coronal planes. Such reconstructions must be included as a routine procedure (Fig. 8.2).
3. **MRI:** MRI provides a direct view of the spinal structures, such as the spinal cord, spinal canal, the vertebral bodies, and intervertebral discs. MRI has surpassed CT as the foremost imaging instrument for the diagnosis of spinal diseases. MRI offers a wide scope of examination, even in instances of inaccurate clinical positioning; thus, pathologies are rarely missed in MRI.

   The sequences for spinal MRI are T1-weighted (T1WI), T2-weighted (T2WI), and T2-short-tau inversion recovery (STIR) for sagittal sectioning, followed by T2WI or T2 STIR for transverse sectioning (Figs. 8.3, 8.4, and 8.5). If a tumor or inflammatory disease is suspected, an intravenous injection containing gadolinium contrast media is required.

W.-C. Shen, *Diagnostic Neuroradiology*, https://doi.org/10.1007/978-981-15-4051-6_8

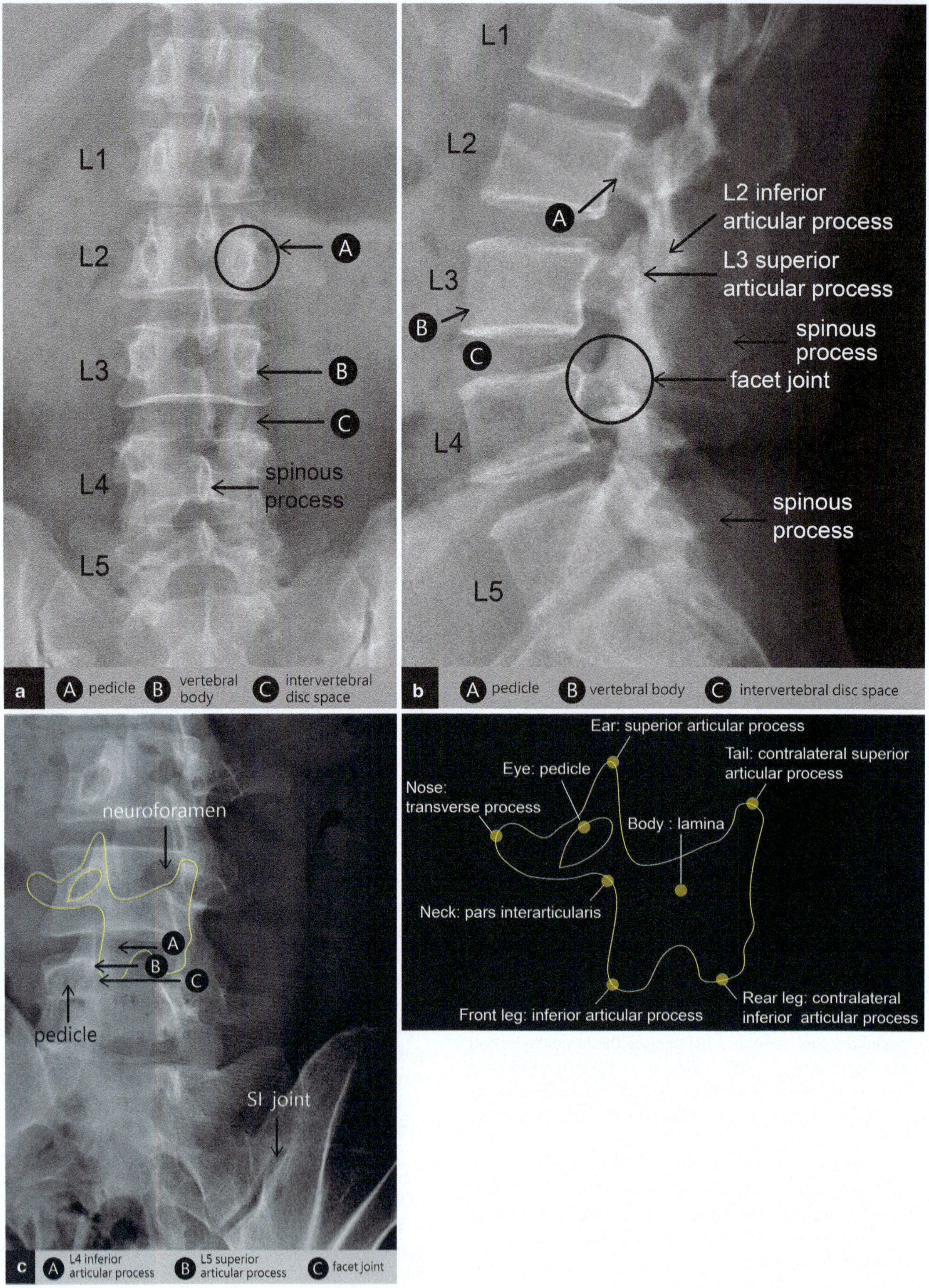

Fig. 8.1 X-ray of the normal lumbar spine. (**a**) AP view, (**b**) lateral view, (**c**) oblique view: The posterior component of the spine appears similar to a Scotland dog

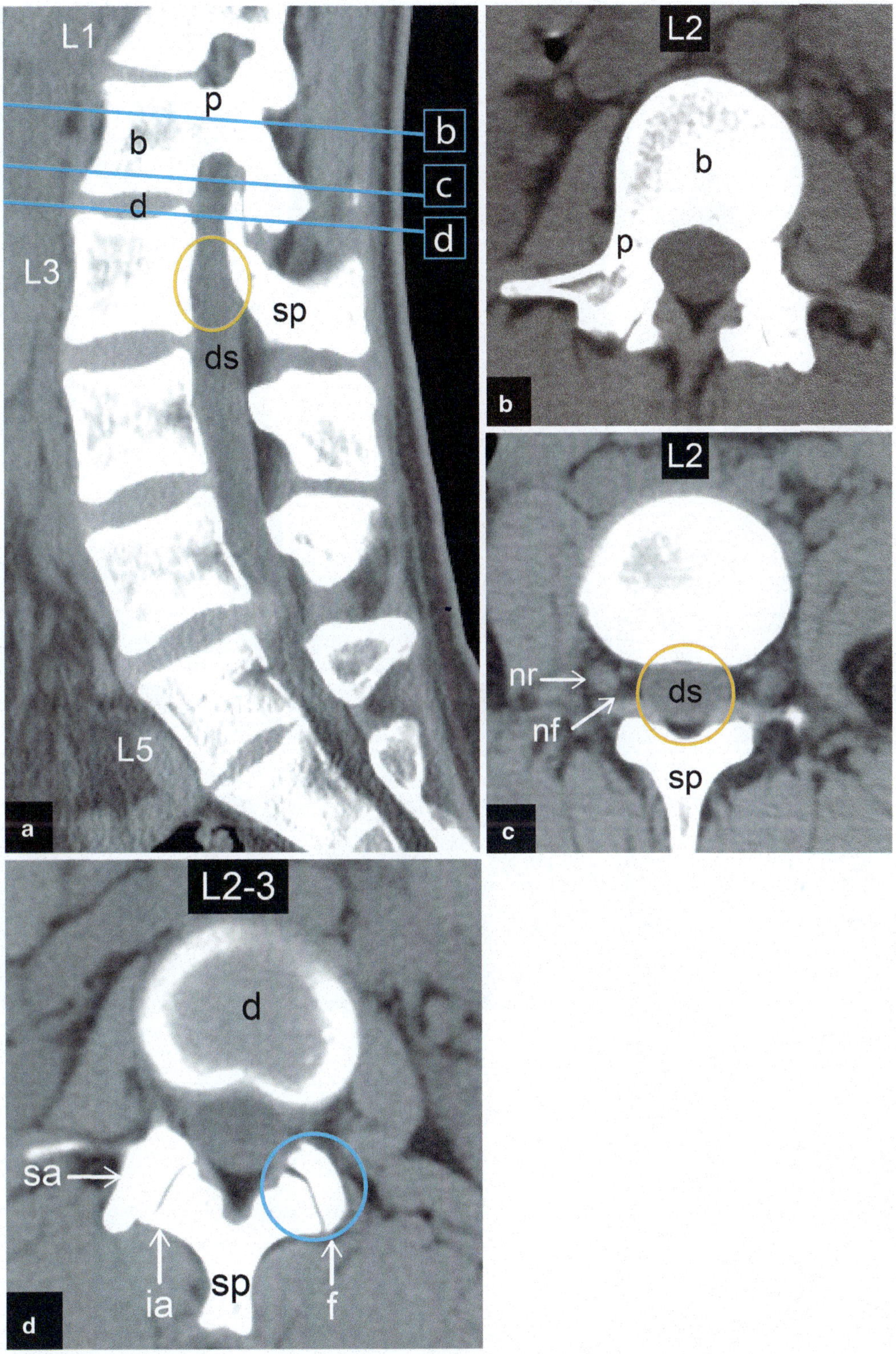

Fig. 8.2 CT of the normal lumbar spine
(**a**) Sagittal reconstruction; (**b–d**) axial sections
b: L2 vertebral body
p: pedicle
d: L2–3 intervertebral disc
Yellow circle: spinal canal
ds: dural sac (thecal sac), contains CSF
nf: neuroforamen
nr: L2 nerve root
Blue circle, f: facet joint
sp: spinous process
ia: L2 inferior articular process
sa: L3 superior articular process
** CT does not show the cauda equina nerves in the dural sac and cannot distinguish the nucleus pulposus and annulus fibrosus of the intervertebral disc

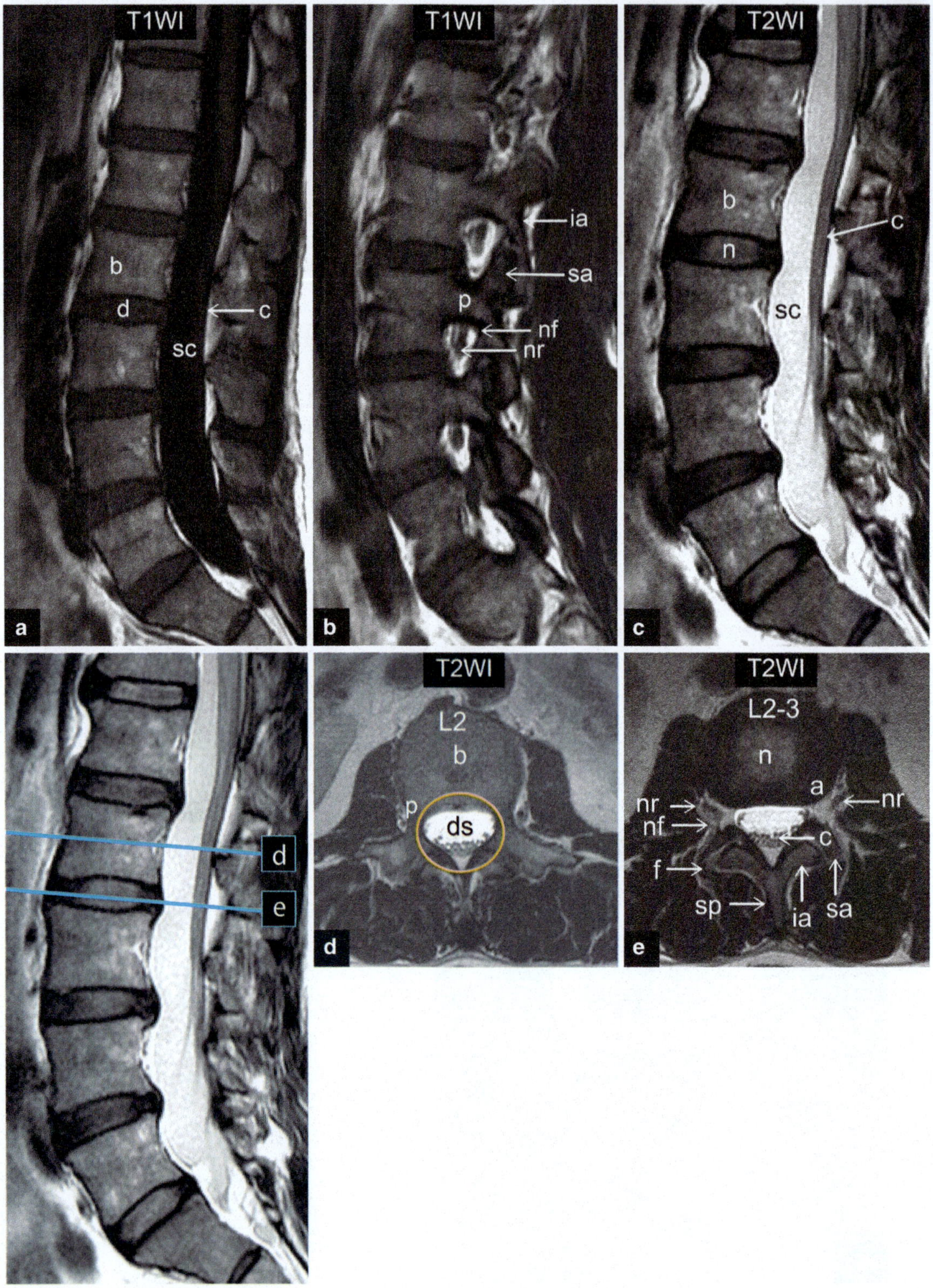

Fig. 8.3 MRI of the normal lumbar spine
(**a**, **b**) T1WI sagittal, (**c**) T2WI sagittal, (**d**, **e**) T2WI axial sections
b: vertebral body
p: pedicle
d: intervertebral disc
yellow circle: spinal canal (sc)
ds: dural sac (thecal sac), contains CSF and cauda equina nerves
nf: neuroforamen
nr: nerve root
c: cauda equina nerves
n: nucleus pulposus
a: annulus fibrosus
f: facet joint
sp: spinous process
ia: L2 inferior articular process
sa: L3 superior articular process

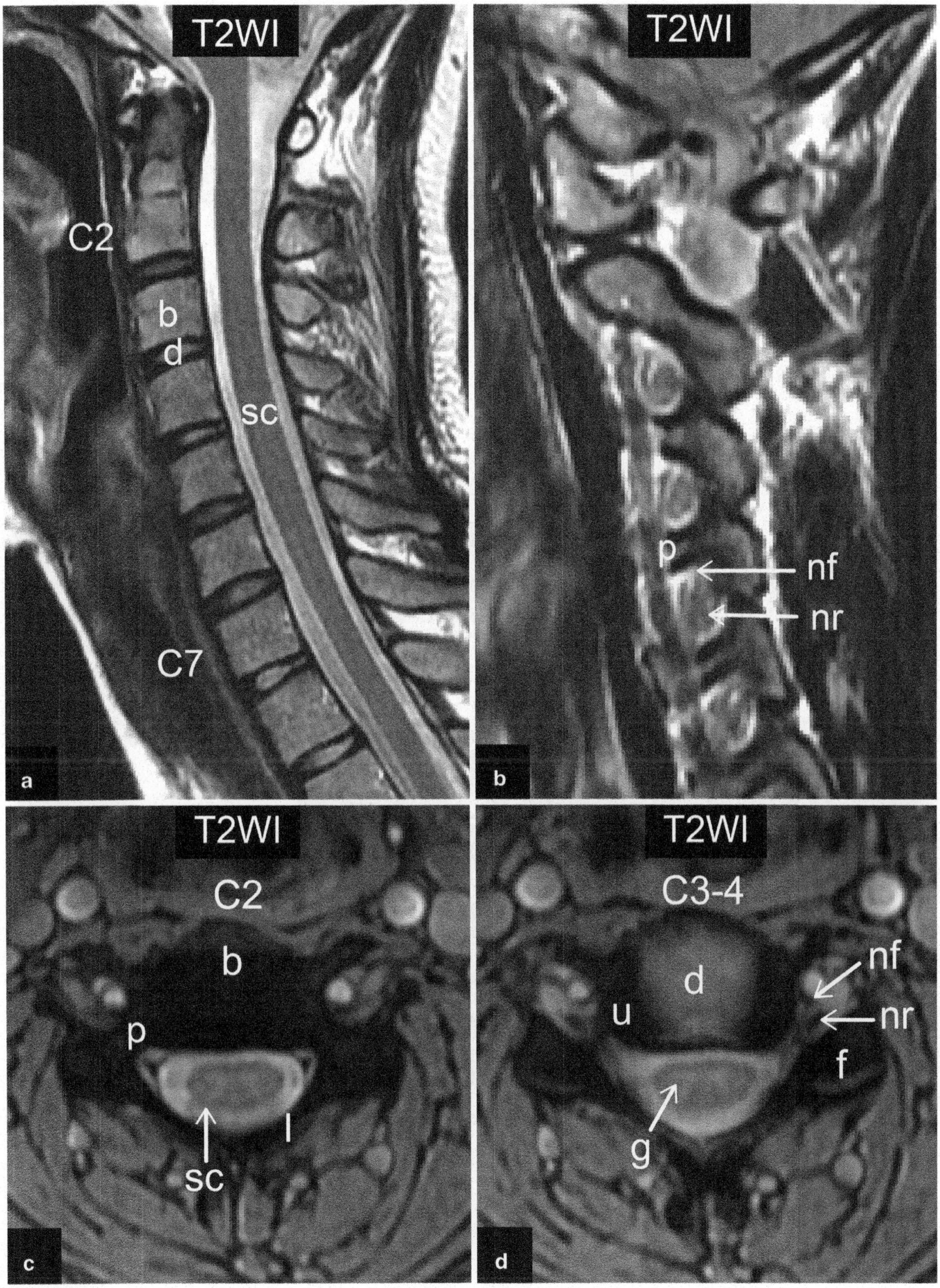

Fig. 8.4 MRI of the normal cervical spine
b: C3 vertebral body
p: pedicle
u: uncinate process
d: C3–4 intervertebral disc
nf: neuroforamen
nr: nerve root
f: facet joint
l: lamina
sc: spinal cord
g: gray matter of spinal cord

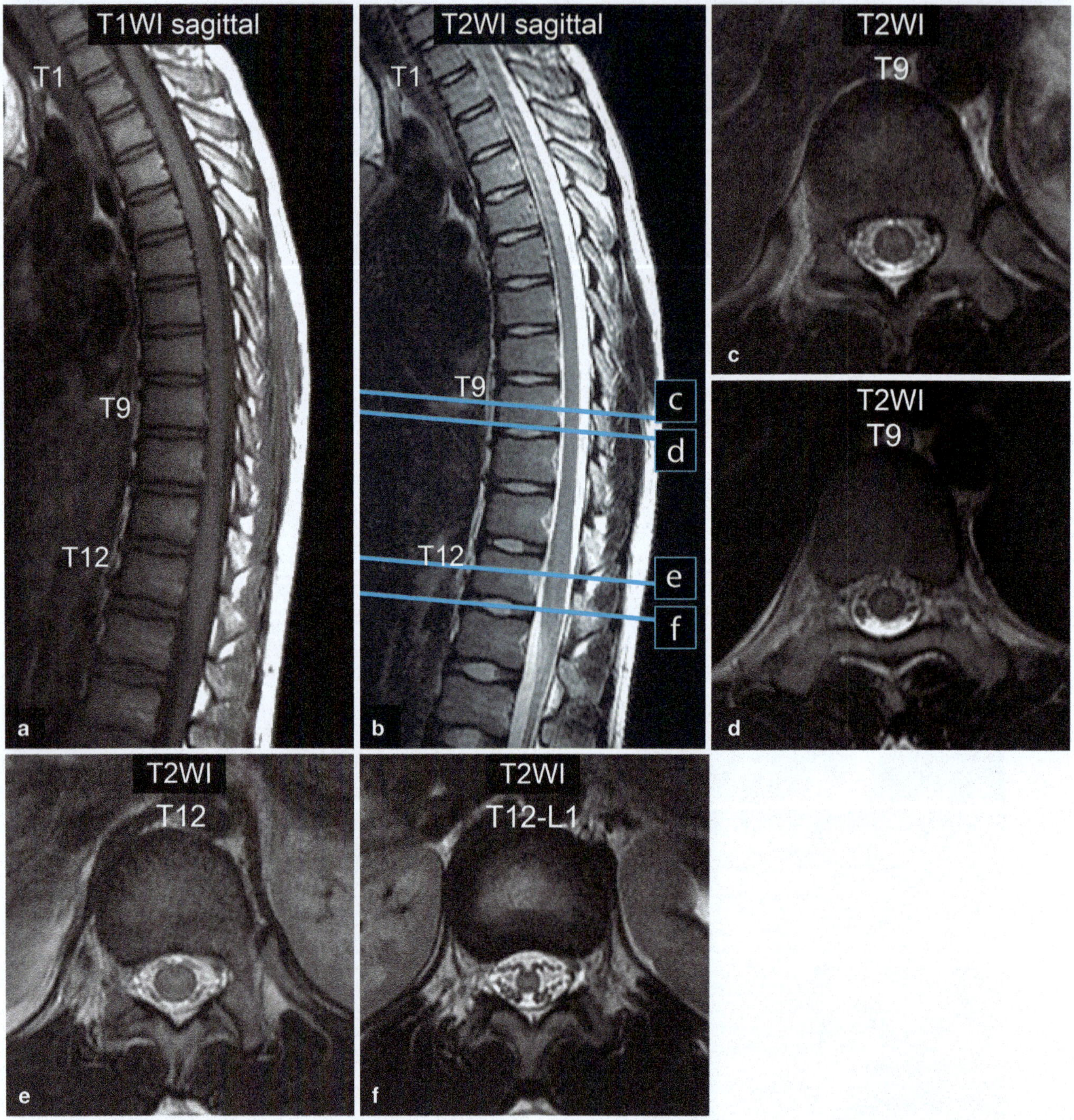

Fig. 8.5 MRI of the normal thoracic spine. (**a**, **b**) T1WI, T2WI, sagittal: the intervertebral discs show hyperintensity on T2WI, the spinal cord is well demonstrated. (**c**, **d**) T2WI, axial: the spinal cord is round on the axial section from T1 to T11 levels, the gray matter in the spinal cord is well demonstrated. (**e**) T2WI: T11 to the T12 level, the spinal cord is called the "conus medullaris," which is slightly enlarged and appears similar to a crab. (**f**) To the L1 level, the spinal cord shrinks and forms filum terminale, and appears similar to a spider

8.2 Spinal Degeneration

Degenerative change of the spine is called degenerative spondylosis, which causes changes in the shape of the vertebral bodies, intervertebral discs, facet joints, and ligaments. The spinal degenerative spondylosis may compress the nerve roots or spinal cord, cause radiculopathy and myelopathy, or cause back pain, soreness, numbness. Many people develop spinal degeneration with age, and in severe cases, surgical correction is required [1–5].

Degenerative spondylosis is not really a disease because people often have degenerative spinal change when they become older. Some people have severe spondylosis, but they do not exhibit symptoms. In contrast, some people experience severe neck pain or lower back pain, but their medical images either do not show spinal degeneration or only mild spinal degeneration that fail to match clinical symptoms.

The following are the anatomical structural changes associated with degenerative spondylosis (Fig. 8.6):

8.2.1 Degenerative Change of Intervertebral Discs

Most cases of degenerative spondylosis are initially caused by a degenerative change in the intervertebral discs, specifically the nucleus pulposus [1].

Normal nucleus pulposus is a gelatinous structure that comprises proteoglycan and 80% water and exhibits high signal intensity in MRI T2WI (Figs. 8.3, 8.4, and 8.5). Each disc in the human spine carries the weight of the body. Due to complex factors such as aging, trauma, or metabolic problems, the nucleus and the annulus fibrosus of disc degenerate over time.

1. **The initial phase of disc degeneration**

   The early disc degeneration can be indicated by MRI only. In a T2WI, the high signal intensity of the nucleus pulposus gradually decreases signal intensity as the nucleus pulposus loses its water content. For this initial phase, a horizontal dark line might appear in the middle of the nucleus pulposus (Figs. 8.7 and 8.15), and a fissure in the annulus. At this stage, the signal changes of the intervertebral discs are observable only on MR images and not X-rays or CT scans.
2. **Disc degeneration:**
   - **Disc bulging out:** Bulging of the intervertebral disc is commonly seen in the lumbar, cervical, and thoracic spines (Figs. 8.7, 8.8, 8.9, 8.10, 8.11, and 8.12). Bulging disc includes diffuse bulging, symmetrical bulging, and asymmetrical bulging. Discs can bulge backward, forward, or laterally. Bulging disc is commonly seen in MRI. In particular, a bulging disc in the sagittal section is extremely similar to the herniation of intervertebral disc (HIVD) and can be distinguished by viewing the intervertebral discs in the axial sections.
   - **Disc height loss:** Disc height decrease occurs as the disc degenerates (Figs. 8.8, 8.10, 8.11, and 8.12). In severe cases of disc degeneration, the disc space narrows severely and even disappear, leading to a condition called block vertebra.
   - **Disc lost water content (dehydration, desiccation, or vacuum phenomenon):** The vacuum in disc means the air in the disc, which is caused by the accumulation of nitrogen gas. The presence of air in a disc is more easily observed in CT than in MR images (Figs. 8.11 and 8.12) and is sometimes observable on X-ray films (Fig. 8.11).
3. **Focal herniation of intervertebral disc (HIVD):**

   HIVD can be diagnosed by using CT (Figs. 8.12 and 8.13) but not X-ray, although CT images are not as clear as MR images (Figs. 8.9, 8.12, 8.14, 8.15, 8.16, 8.17, 8.18, 8.19, and 8.20). Axial sections of CT and MRI must be taken to determine the direction of HIVD. HIVD occurs mostly in the posterior region of the disc and can be divided as the central (Figs. 8.9 and 8.13), paracentral (Figs. 8.12, 8.14, 8.15, 8.16, 8.17, 8.18, and 8.19), foraminal, and extraforaminal regions, with paracentral HIVD being the most common. Anterior HIVD is rare and exhibits no symptoms (Figs. 8.9 and 8.20).

   HIVD is also classified [2] into the following:

- **Protrusion**, in which the annulus is still intact (Figs. 8.9, 8.14, and 8.20). The protrusion part is less than 25% of the whole disc.
- **Extrusion** (a true HIVD), in which a tear in the annulus occurs and the nucleus herniates through this defect (Figs. 8.12, 8.15, 8.16, 8.17, 8.18, and 8.19), the herniated nucleus is still connected to the disc.
- **Extrusion with sequestration**, in which the herniated nucleus is separated from the disc, also named as a "ruptured disc." The sequestered nucleus fragment migrates superiorly or inferiorly (Fig. 8.16). Common cases involve subligamentous sequestration, with occasional reports of transligamentous migration.

  The sagittal sections of CT and MRI scans indicate whether the migration of HIVD is superior or inferior.

  The occurrence of HIVD is not necessarily associated with disc degeneration because some young adults might develop HIVD (Fig. 8.13) with no signs of disc degeneration; their condition may be caused by trauma or unknown reason.

8.2.2 Degenerative Change of Vertebral Bodies

1. **Schmorl's node**: This node is also known as intravertebral herniation, which refers to the herniation of the intervertebral disc through the vertebral body. Such herniation causes deformities in the vertebral end plate (Figs. 8.8, 8.11, 8.14, and 8.21). Schmorl's node is considered to be caused by the degeneration of the intervertebral disc. However, many young adults have Schmorl's node, but disc degeneration does not occur (Fig. 8.22). Schmorl's node is always symptom-free.
2. **Osteophyte (bone spur)**: The vertebral body, specifically the end plate, may develop osteophytes anteriorly, posteriorly, or bilaterally. Anterior osteophytes are easy to assess on X-ray, CT, and MR images (Figs. 8.8 and 8.12). Nevertheless, only the posterior and lateral osteophytes

may compress the nerve roots, thus causing symptoms. Osteophyte in the uncinate process of the cervical vertebral body may cause neuroforamen stenosis (Figs. 8.17 and 8.23) and then compress the cervical brachial nerve and cause cervical radiculopathy.

3. **Degenerative marrow changes (Modic change)**: Degeneration due to pressure on the vertebral body results in degenerative changes in the bone marrow around the end plate. This pathological change is termed the Modic change [3]; it occurs primarily in the end plate, where it may subsequently spread to half of the vertebral body.

   Modic changes can be classified into three types, according to MR images [4] (Fig. 8.24).
   - **Modic I**: It refers to the development of edema, inflammation, and hypervascularity in the bone marrow; Modic type I changes are hypointense on T1WI and hyperintense on T2WI and T2 STIR (Figs. 8.10, 8.25, 8.26, and 8.29). MRI diagnoses of Modic I require careful identification of edema and inflammation in the bone marrow of the vertebral body due to infection (Fig. 8.27).
   - **Modic II**: It refers to the change of bone marrow into a yellow marrow. Modic type II changes are hyperintense on T1WI and T2WI, and its hyperintensity on T2 can be suppressed by T2 STIR (Figs. 8.8, 8.12, 8.21, 8.25, and 8.28).
   - **Modic III**: It refers to the development of sclerosis in and loss of the bone marrow. Modic type III changes are hypointense on T1WI and also hypointense on T2WI and T2 STIR (Fig. 8.29).
   - **Eburnation** in X-rays and CT scans: the bone in the end plate of a degenerating vertebral body is ivory-like hyperdense. This condition is termed **eburnation** (Figs. 8.12, 8.28, and 8.29), which is a type of osteosclerosis and a sign of degenerative change in the vertebral body. Eburnation corresponds to the Modic types II (Figs. 8.12 and 8.28) and III (Fig. 8.29) changes visible in MRI.
4. **Spondylolysis**: It refers to a fracture or defect in the pars interarticularis of the vertebral arch (Figs. 8.8 and 8.30). Spondylolysis is present in approximately 5% of the population, particularly among men and athletes. Most spondylolysis displays no symptoms, and 25% are related to lower back pain. Spondylolysis mostly occurs in L5 (Fig. 8.8) and L4 (Fig. 8.30), rarely occurs in the lumbar vertebrae above L3, and possibly but rarely occurs in the cervical vertebrae. Most spondylolysis is bilateral. Spondylolysis is likely to be accompanied by spondylolisthesis (Figs. 8.8 and 8.30).
5. **Spondylolisthesis**: It typically occurs in the lumbar vertebrae, with a few cases in the cervical vertebrae. Spondylolisthesis refers to the slipping of the upper and lower vertebral bodies. Generally, spondylolisthesis is an anterior or forward slip, known as anterolisthesis (Figs. 8.8, 8.11, 8.26, 8.30, and 8.31). Posterior or backward slippage is termed retrolisthesis (Fig. 8.8). Besides, a rare pattern of lateral spondylolisthesis is described in Fig. 8.32.

   Spondylolisthesis can be classified into the following types according to its causes.
   (a) Spondylolytic spondylolisthesis, which is caused by spondylolysis resulting from the occurrence of a fracture or defect in the pars interarticularis (Figs. 8.8 and 8.30).
   (b) Degenerative spondylolisthesis (Figs. 8.11, 8.26, and 8.31), which is typically comorbid with facet joint degeneration or intervertebral disc degeneration.
   (c) Traumatic spondylolisthesis, which is caused by trauma injuries.
   (d) Pathologic spondylolisthesis, which is caused by infection or malignancy in the spine.
   (e) Congenital spondylolisthesis.

   The grade of spondylolisthesis classified by the degree of the slippage:
   - Grade 1: 20–25% slippage.
   - Grade 2: 25–50% slippage.
   - Grade 3: 50–75% slippage.
   - Grade 4: 75–100% slippage.
   - Grade 5: Greater than 100% slippage.

8.2.3 Facet Joint, Ligamentum, and Spinal Canal Degeneration

1. **Facet joint degeneration** (Figs. 8.31, 8.33, and 8.34): Facet joints degeneration leads to hypertrophic facet joint osteoarthritis (OA), which in turn causes stenosis of the lateral recess and central spinal canal, and neuroforamen. In addition to OA change, facet joint degeneration may associate with the combination of a synovial cyst (Fig. 8.34).
2. **Ligamentum degeneration**
   - **Ligamentum flavum hypertrophy:** The ligamentum flavum connects to the lamina of every two vertebrae from C2 to S1. Ligamentum flavum hypertrophy also causes spinal stenosis (Figs. 8.35 and 8.36).
   - **Ossification of posterior longitudinal ligamentum (OPLL):**The degeneration of the posterior longitudinal ligamentum is commonly found in the cervical spine; Asian people are more likely to suffer from such degeneration. In severe cases, ossification of posterior longitudinal ligamentum (OPLL) occurs (Figs. 8.37 and 8.40). OPLL is a chronic disease that, in severe cases, with compression on the spinal cord, slowly leading to chronic myelopathy.

3. **Spinal stenosis**: It is caused by degenerative spondylosis, which presents in the form of a bulging disc, facet joint OA change, ligamentum flavum hypertrophy, and spondylolisthesis, either alone or collectively. Spinal stenosis includes central canal stenosis (Figs. 8.11, 8.28, 8.31, 8.34, 8.35, 8.36, and 8.38), lateral recess stenosis, and foraminal stenosis (Figs. 8.17, 8.23, and 8.33). Symptoms of spinal stenosis are caused by the compression of the nerve roots or spinal cord. The MRI of severe spinal canal stenosis in the lumbar spine may reveal the redundancy of cauda equina nerves (Fig. 8.38).

8.3 Lumbar Herniation of Intervertebral Discs

Lumbar HIVD can occur alone (typically in young patients) or comorbid with degenerative spondylosis (usually in older patients). In lumbar HIVD, the disc slips into the spinal canal, which compresses the dural sac and nerve root, thus causing sciatica and low back pain. Lumbar HIVD mostly occurs in L4–L5 (Figs. 8.12 and 8.13) and L5–S1 (Figs. 8.14, 8.15, 8.16, and 8.22), sometimes in L3–L4. HIVD in L1–L2 and L2–L3 (Fig. 8.20) is rare. Most instances of lumbar HIVD occur in posterolateral (or posterior paracentral) direction, causing unilateral sciatica. Few cases of posterior central herniation, a condition that induces bilateral sciatica (Fig. 8.13). Anterior HIVD can also occur (Fig. 8.20), but it does not compress the nerve roots and thus presents no symptoms. In several cases, HIVD migrates either superiorly or inferiorly.

8.3.1 Imaging Diagnosis

1. **X-ray:** HIVD diagnosis cannot be achieved with an X-ray.
2. **CT:** A convenient and accurate tool for the diagnosis of lumbar diseases; CT provides a direct view of HIVD in the spinal canal (Figs. 8.12 and 8.13).
3. **MRI:** Scans of the sagittal section provide a direct view of the HIVD and possible superior- or inferior migration of the HIVD, MRI can also reveal if the posterior longitudinal ligamentum is broken or being pushed backward. Compared with CT, MRI allows for the more straightforward classification of HIVD, for example, whether the HIVD is of the protrusion (Fig. 8.14) or extrusion (Figs. 8.15 and 8.16) type. MRI is better than CT to determine sequestration and migration of the herniated nucleus pulposus (Fig. 8.16). However, MRI in the transverse plane is still required to determine the direction of the HIVD (left or right) and to ascertain whether the disc is bulging or not herniation (Figs. 8.7 and 8.11).

8.4 Cervical Spondylosis

Cervical degenerative spondylosis has pathologically similar characteristics with lumbar spondylosis; however, the occurrence of cervical OPLL (Figs. 8.37 and 8.40) is common. Degenerative changes in the vertebral bodies, intervertebral discs, facet joints, and ligaments cause spinal stenosis or neuroforamen stenosis which can result in two typical symptoms (Fig. 8.39):

1. Radiculopathy. This refers to the compression of the nerves and is mostly caused by bulging disc (Fig. 8.9), HIVD (Fig. 8.17), facet joint degenerative osteoarthritis (OA)(Fig. 8.33), and a bone spur of the uncinate process (Figs. 8.17 and 8.23).
2. Myelopathy. This refers to the compression of the spinal cord and is typically caused by HIVD (Figs. 8.18 and 8.19) or OPLL (Fig. 8.37). Symptoms of myelopathy include weakness in the lower extremities, abnormal feelings in the lower half of the body, and loss of urinary or bowel control.

8.4.1 Examination Methods for Cervical Spondylosis

1. **X-ray:** X-ray is the first-line examination method that can be used to observe for bone spurs in the vertebral bodies, and whether the spurs extend into the spinal canal and neuroforamen. The X-ray can also be used to observe changes in the height of the intervertebral discs. However, the spinal cord cannot be observed with an X-ray.
2. **CT:** CT provides a clear view of degenerative changes of vertebral bodies, intervertebral discs, facet joints, ligamentum, and stenosis of the spinal canal and neuroforamina. But CT cannot offer a view of the spinal cord and has thus been supplanted by MRI in most cases.
3. **MRI:** Because a direct view of any degenerative changes in the vertebral bodies, discs, facet joints, ligamentum, and the spinal canal stenosis, neuroforamen stenosis, can also see any compression of the cervical nerve roots and spinal cord, MRI has become the essential diagnostic tool post-X-ray examination.

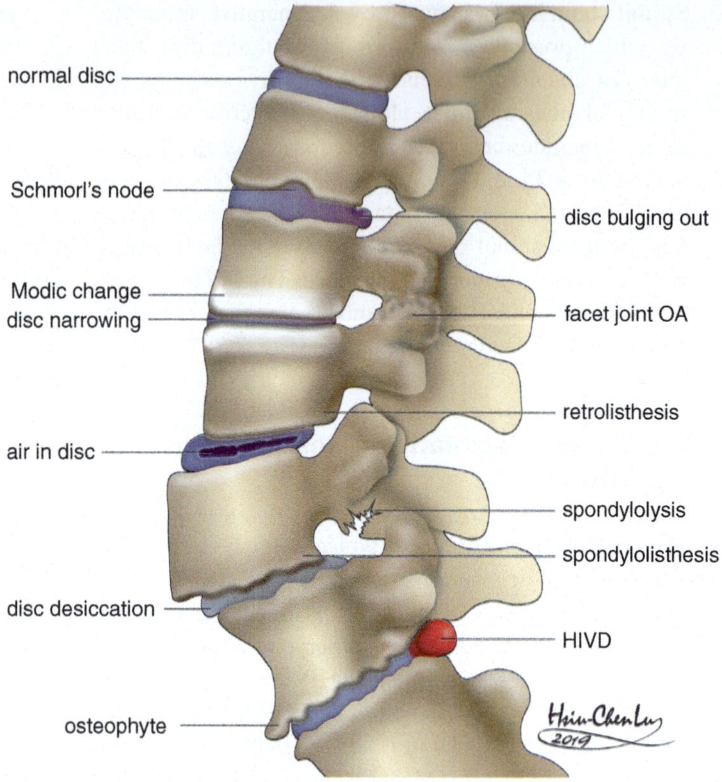

Fig. 8.6 Degenerative spondylosis.
Degenerative spondylosis including:
Intervertebral discs degeneration: reduction of disc height (narrowing of disc space), decreased water-content (disc desiccation), contains air, bulging out, HIVD.
Vertebral bodies degeneration: osteophyte, Modic changes, Schmorl's node.
Facet joint degeneration: osteoarthritis (OA) causes hypertrophy and with osteophytes.
Ligaments degeneration: hypertrophy, calcification, ossification.
Spondylolysis.
Spondylolisthesis, retrolisthesis.
The above degenerative changes cause spinal canal stenosis and neuroforamen stenosis, compress the spinal nerves; in the cervical and thoracic spine may also compress the spinal cord

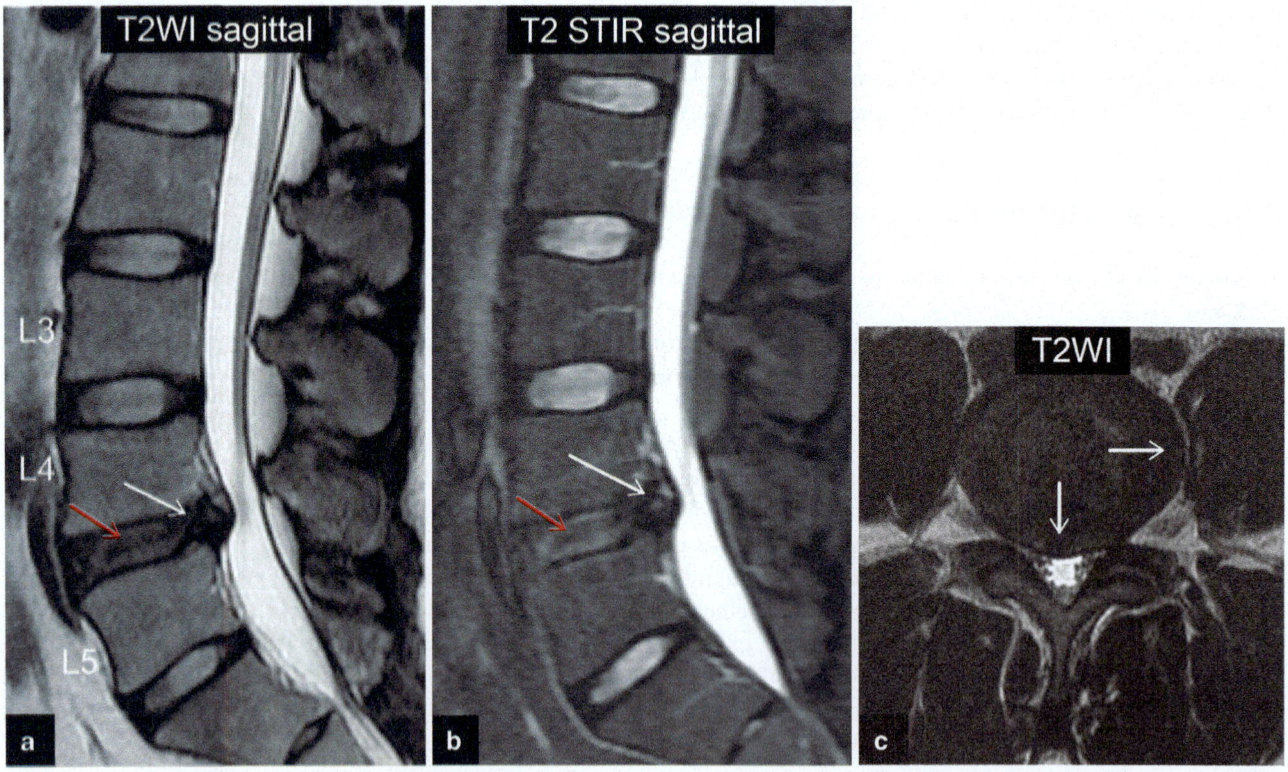

Fig. 8.7 F/31, Intervertebral disc bulging out. (**a**, **b**) MRI, T2WI, T2 STIR: The L4–5 disc shows decreased signal intensity (darker than other discs), indicating the reduction in water content. There is a horizontal dark line (red arrows) in the middle of the nucleus; this is an early sign of disc degeneration. There is also posteriorly bulging out (white arrows), which is a sign of disc degeneration. In the sagittal section, the bulging disc is difficult to distinguish from herniation of intervertebral disc (HIVD); thus, the axial section is needed. (**c**) T2WI, axial section of L4–5: the disc is posteriorly and left laterally bulging out (arrows), indicating that this is not HIVD. The posterior bulging disc compresses the dural sac and bilateral L5 nerve roots, causing lower back pain and numbness

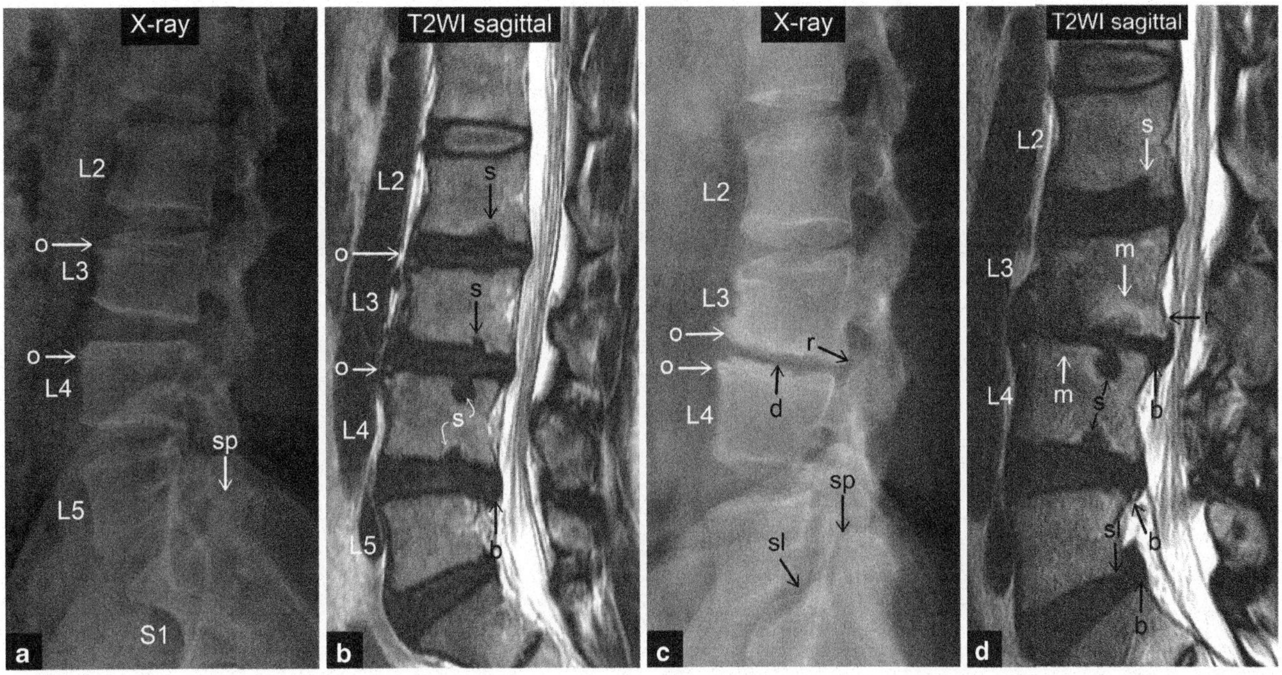

Fig. 8.8 M/53, Degenerative lumbar spondylosis changes in 10 years. Degenerative spondylosis may start young and change slowly. This 53-year-old man has suffered lower back pain for more than 10 years, occasionally sciatica. (**a**) X-ray, when he was 43 years old: small osteophyte (o) on the anterior of L3,4 vertebral bodies, spondylolysis (sp) in L5. (**b**) MRI at the same time, T2WI: In addition to the osteophytes, Schmorl's nodes (s) on the end plates of L2,3,4 vertebral bodies. All the intervertebral discs, except L1–2, show hypointensity, reflecting decreased water content. L4–5 disc bulging out (b). (**c**) X-ray when he was 53 years old: the most significant change is that L3–4 disc space (d) is very narrow, mild retrolisthesis (r) of L3 on L4, spondylolysis (sp) of L5 and mild spondylolisthesis (sl) of L5 on S1. (**d**) MRI at the same time: in addition to the above degenerative changes, observations include Modic II change (m) of L3,4 end plates, severe narrowing and bulging out of L3–4 disc (b), L5-S1 spondylolisthesis (sl), and no change of the Schmorl's nodes (s)

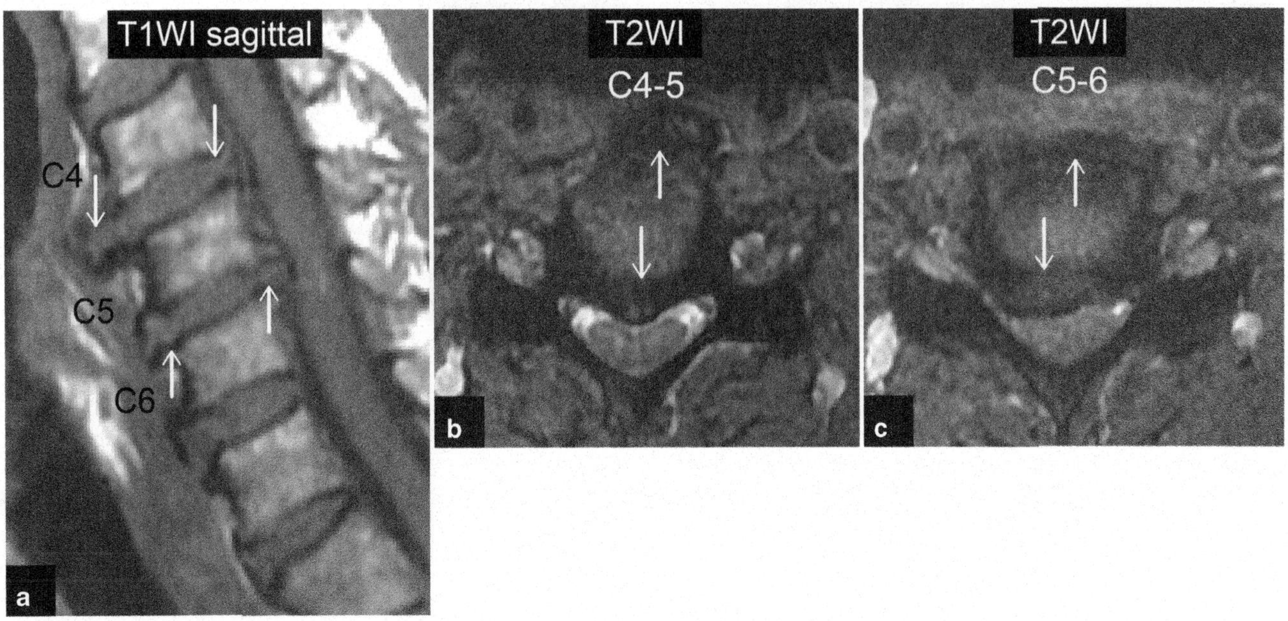

Fig. 8.9 M/56, Cervical spine bulging disc, and anterior herniation of intervertebral disc (HIVD). (**a**) MRI, T1WI, sagittal: The C4–5 intervertebral disc shows severe anterior protrusion (arrow) and posterior protrusion (arrow). Bulging out of the C5–6 intervertebral disc (arrows) is also observed. (**b**) T2WI, axial, C4–5: large anterior HIVD and small posterior HIVD (arrows). (**c**) T2WI, axial, C5–6: anterior and posterior bulging out of disc (arrows), the posterior bulging disc may compress the right C6 nerve root and right-side ventral surface of the spinal cord

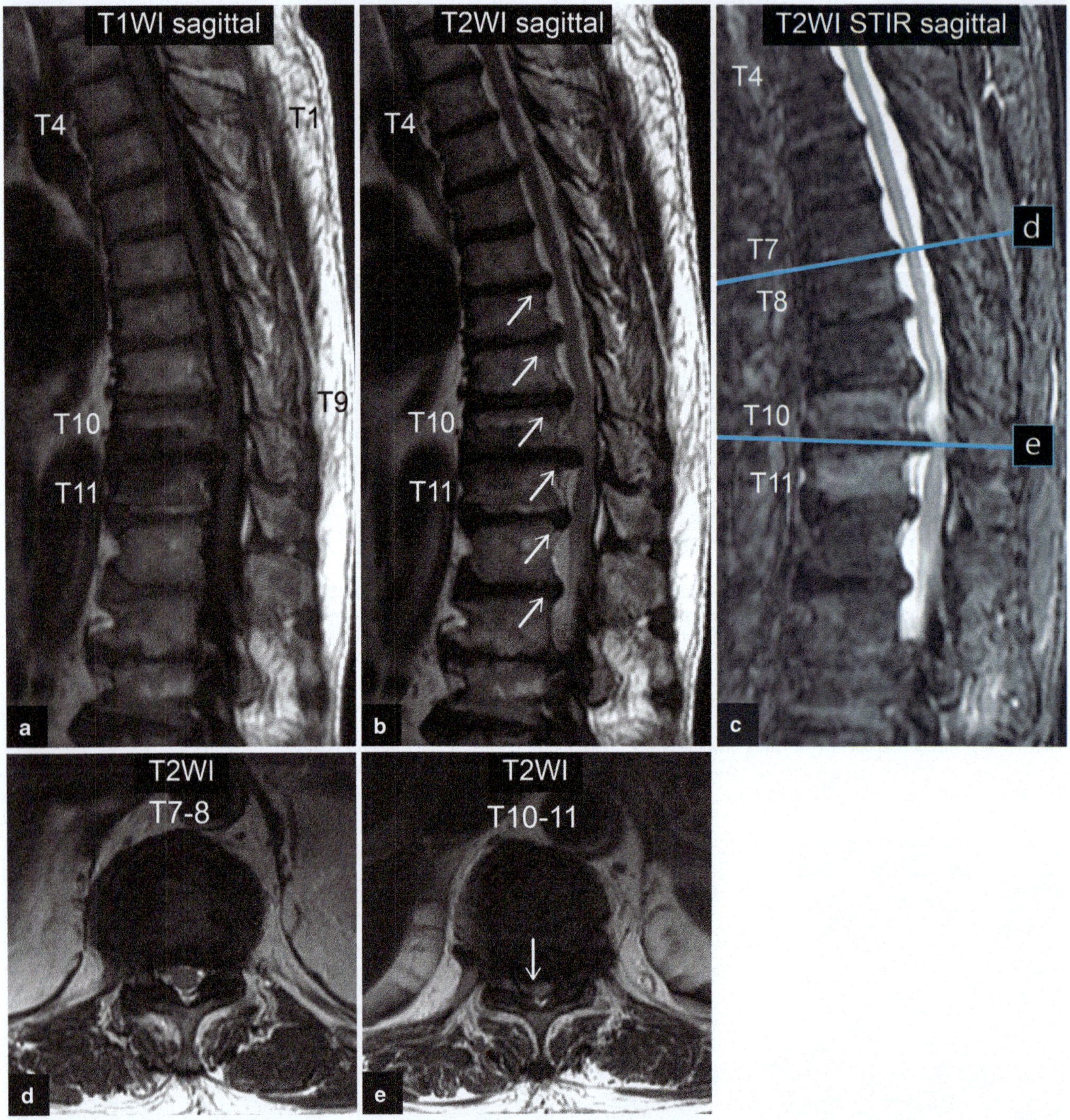

Fig. 8.10 M/59, Severe degenerative spondylosis of the thoracic spine. (**a–c**) MRI, sagittal sections: The T10,11 vertebral bodies show hypointensity on T1WI, hyperintensity on T2 STIR, representing bone marrow edema, this is a Modic I change. Almost every intervertebral disc shows decreased height and bulging out (arrows), reflecting degeneration the discs. (**d**) T2WI, axial section of T7–8: mild bulging out of the disc, the spinal canal is normal, no compression on the spinal cord. (**e**) T2WI, axial section of T10–11: severe bulging out of the disc compresses the spinal cord (arrow)

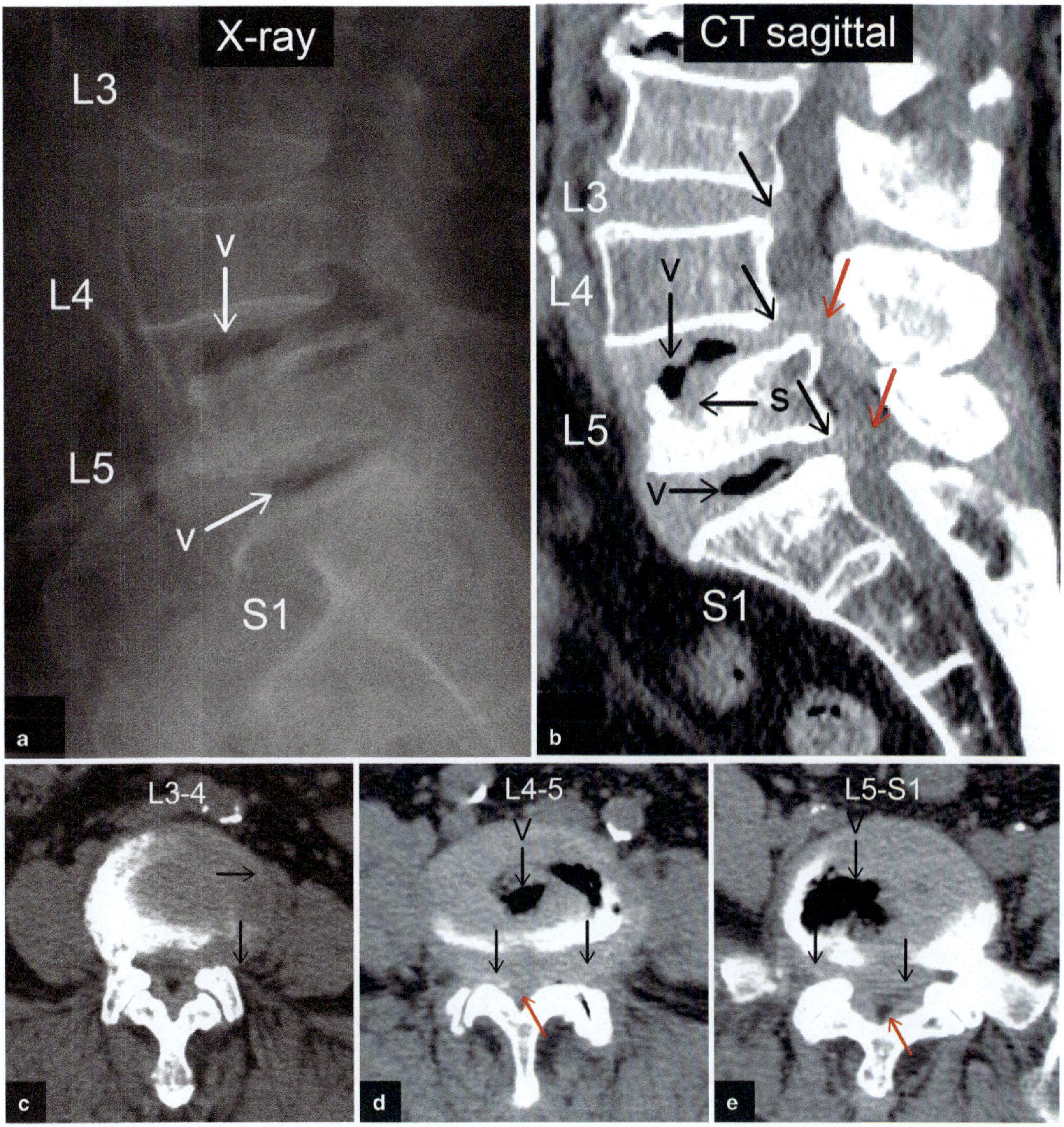

Fig. 8.11 F/74, Disc degeneration, spondylolisthesis, and causes spinal canal stenosis. (**a**) X-ray: Spondylolisthesis of L4 on L5; vacuum (v) is observed in the discs of L4–5 and L5-S1; narrowing of the disc space of L5-S1. (**b–e**) CT: L3–4: disc bulging out (black arrows). L4–5: disc bulging out and with a vacuum (v); spondylolisthesis of L4 on L5, the above causes severe spinal canal stenosis (red arrow). Big bony defect in the superior end plate of L5, the disc herniates into this bony erosion, this is the intravertebral disc herniation, is a big Schmorl's node (s). L5-S1: disc bulging out and with a vacuum (v), the bulging out disc also causes spinal canal stenosis (red arrow). (**f–j**) MRI: the same findings as CT. MRI is better than CT in demonstrating the spinal canal stenosis (red arrows) and Schmorl's node (s), but MRI for vacuum is not as good as CT

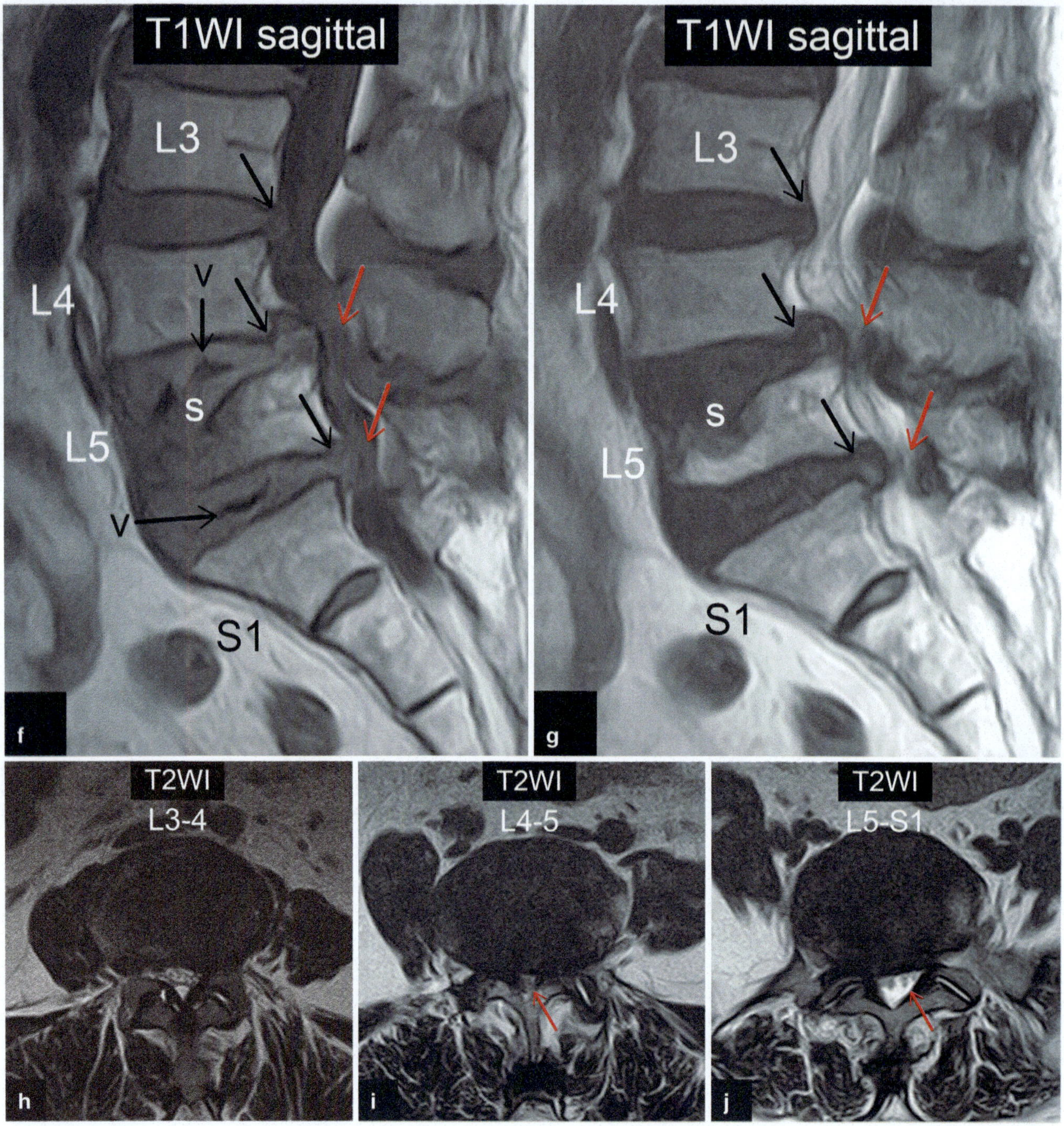

Fig. 8.11 (continued)

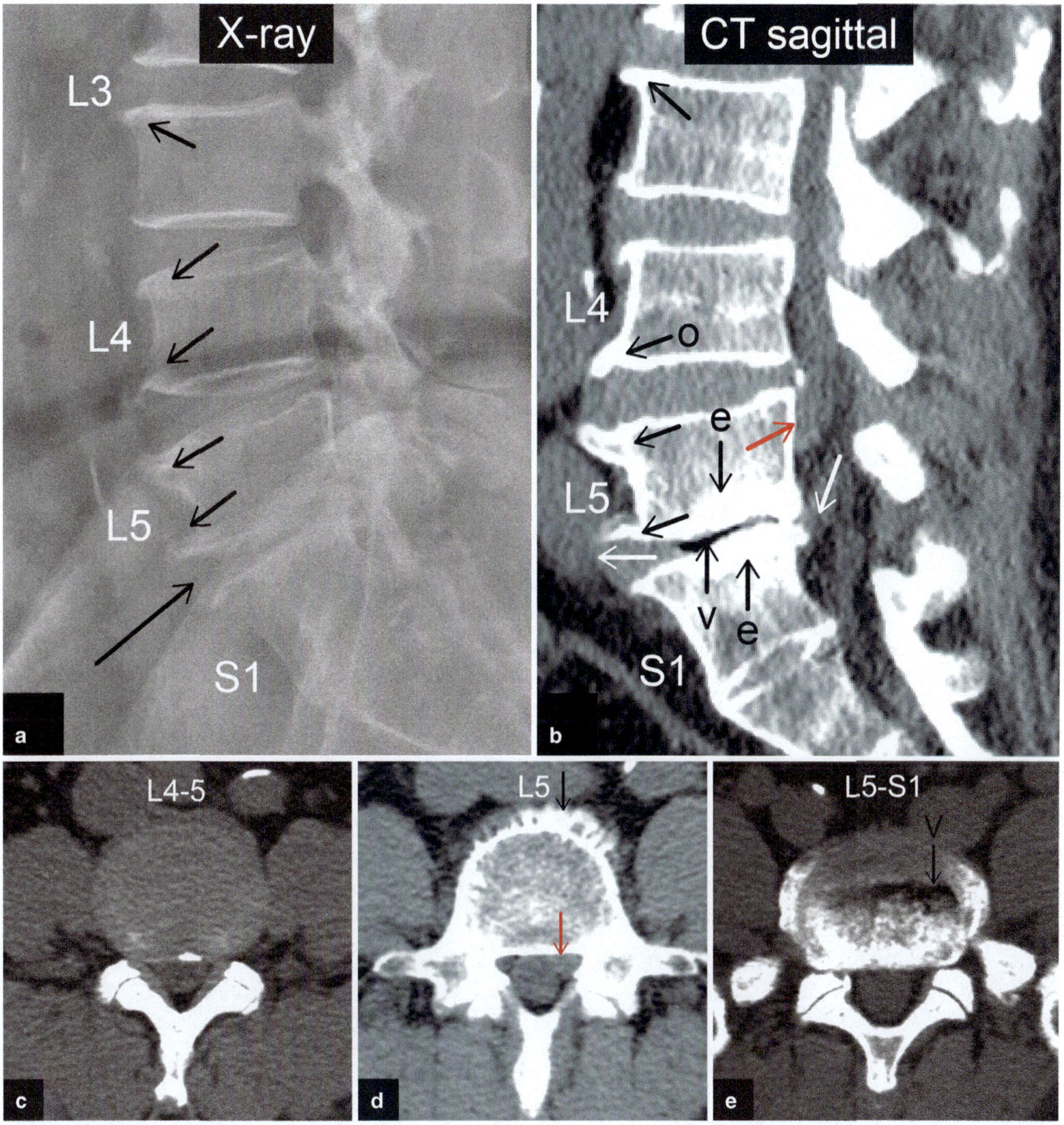

Fig. 8.12 M/68, Degenerative spondylosis of the lumbar spine. This patient suffered left-side sciatica for 1 month. (**a**) X-ray: Only osteophytes (arrows) in every vertebral body are shown. These marginal osteophytes on the end plates of vertebral bodies are caused by disc degeneration. Narrowing of the L5-S1 disc (long arrow), reflecting disc degeneration. (**b–e**) CT: Marginal osteophyte (o) in every vertebral body. L4–5: extrusion (red arrow) in the left-side posterior of L4–5 disc, which is herniation of intervertebral disc (HIVD). It compresses the left L5 nerve root, causing sciatica. L5-S1: severe narrowing, vacuum (v), and bulging out (white arrows) of the L5-S1 disc, reflecting severe degeneration of this disc. Eburnations (e) of the inferior end plate of L5 and superior end plate of S1 are shown. (**f–i**) MRI: L4–5: The same findings as CT. MRI is better than CT in showing the HIVD (red arrow). L5-S1: MRI demonstrates the bulging out of disc (white arrows) but cannot display the vacuum in the disc. Modic type II degeneration (m) of L5, S1 end plates, corresponding to the eburnation shown on CT

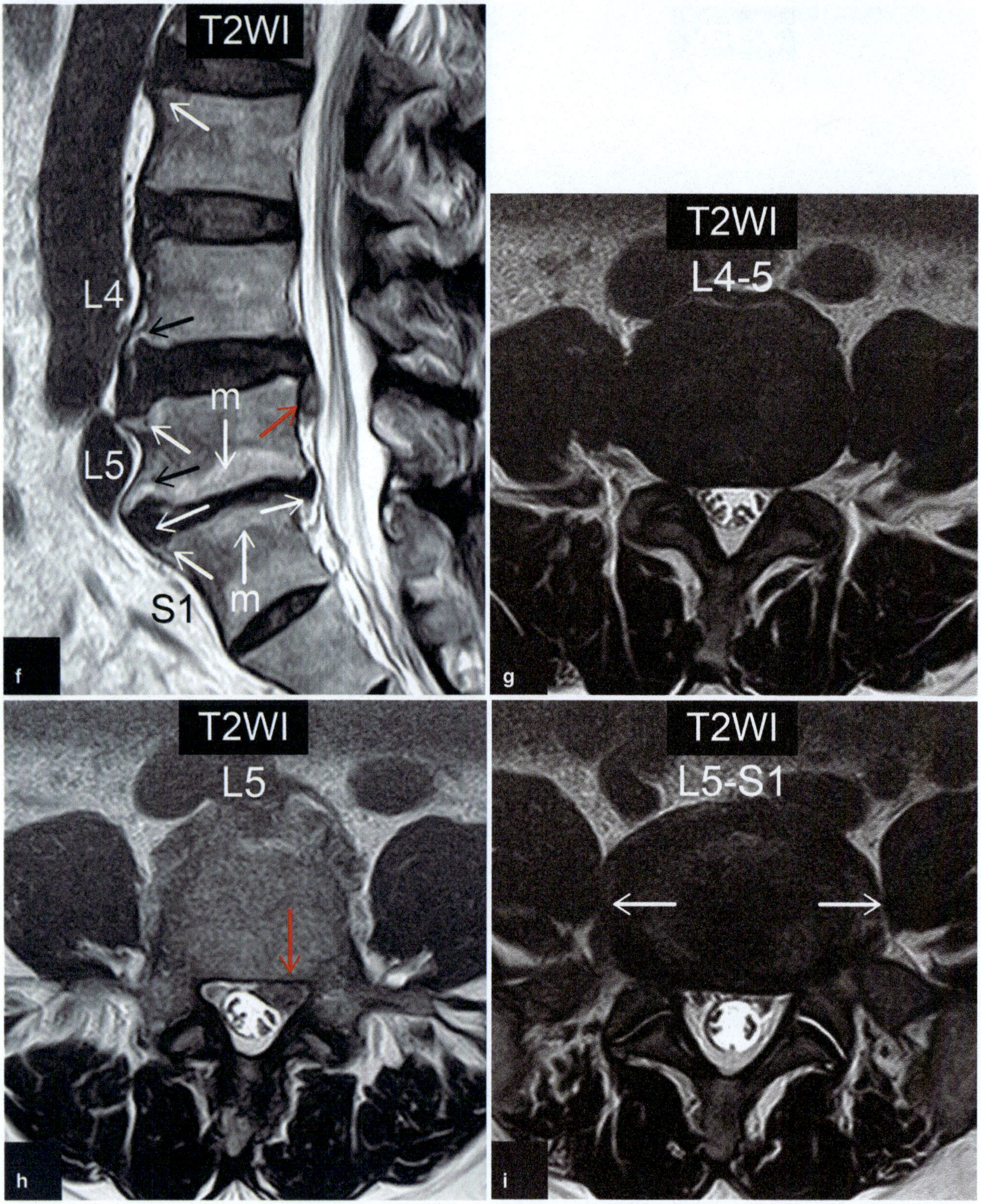

Fig. 8.12 (continued)

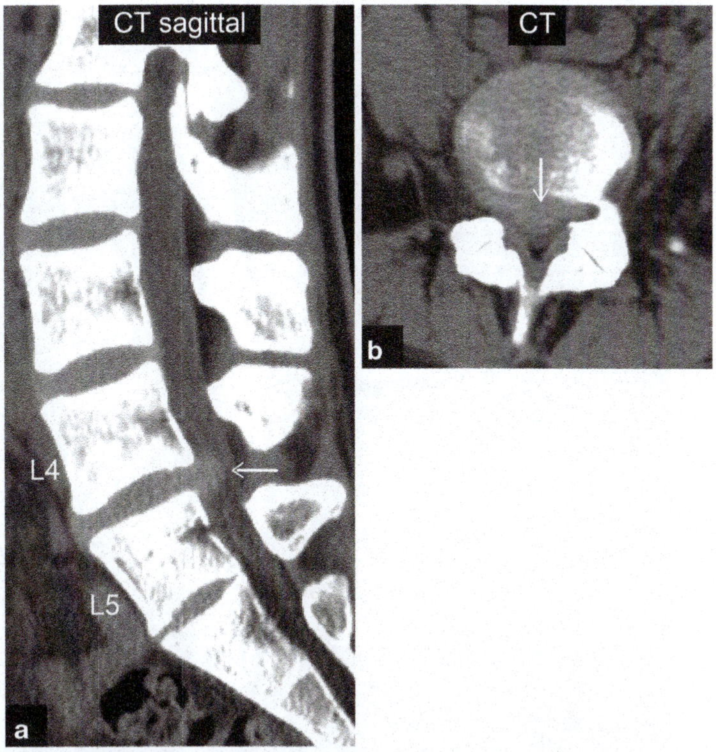

Fig. 8.13 F/20, L4–5 posterior central HIVD. This young lady complained of severe lower back pain and bilateral sciatica for 2 weeks. (**a**) CT, sagittal reconstruction: Posterior protrusion (arrow) of L4–5 intervertebral disc. (**b**) CT, axial section: Posterior central herniation (arrow) of the intervertebral disc (HIVD) compresses the dural sac and bilateral L5 nerve roots

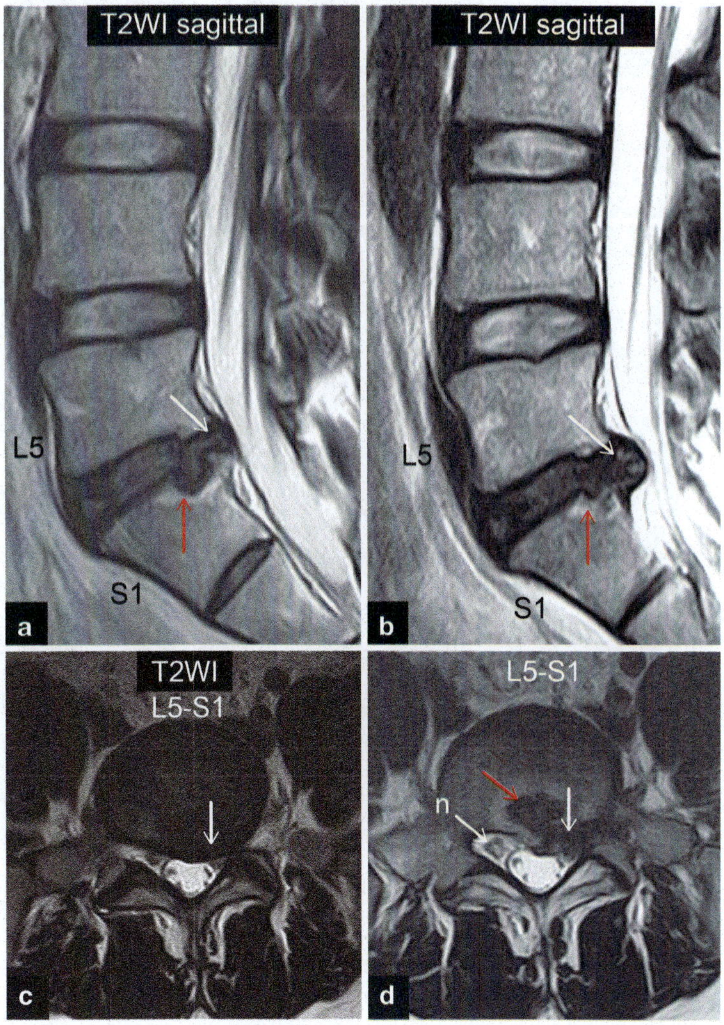

Fig. 8.14 M/37, HIVD, protrusion of disc. This patient suffered lower back pain and left-side sciatica for 3 months. (**a**, **b**) MRI, T2WI, sagittal: The intervertebral discs of L3–4, L4–5 showing hyperintensity and normal height, and L5-S1 disc showing hypointensity (reflecting decreased water content) and posterior protrusion (white arrow), which is a sign of disc degeneration. A defect (red arrow) is observed in the superior end plate of S1; this is intravertebral herniation of disc, and is a Schmorl's node. (**c**, **d**) Axial section: The posterior protrusion of the disc (white arrows) compresses the dural sac and left S1 nerve root. This is HIVD, because the annulus fibrosus is intact; thus, this is a "protrusion" of disc, not "extrusion." The right S1 nerve (n) and epidural fat are apparent, and the left-side S1 nerve and epidural fat are invisible because of obliteration by the HIVD. Schmorl's node in the end plate of S1 (red arrow)

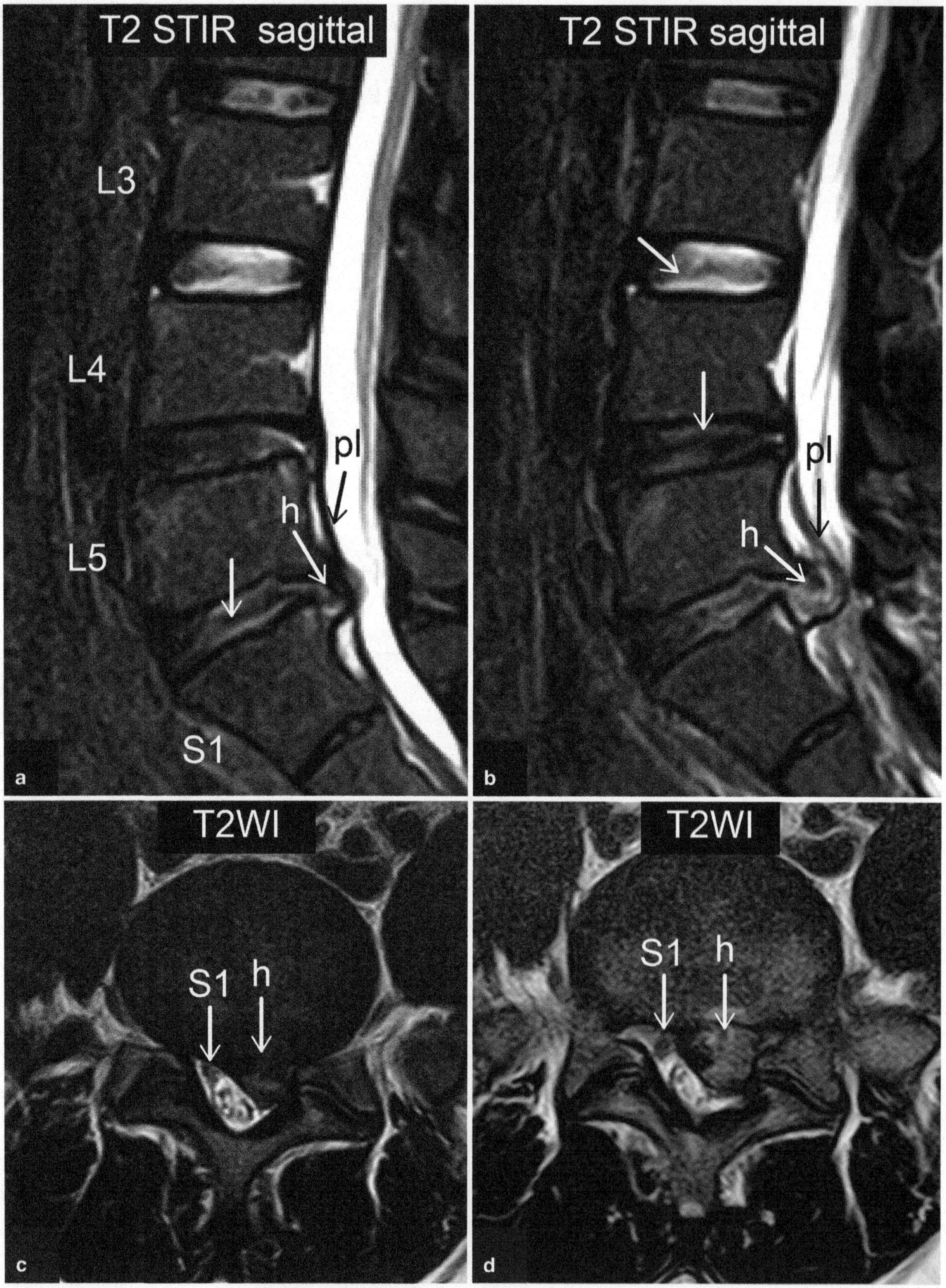

Fig. 8.15 M/41, Disc degeneration, and herniation of intervertebral disc (HIVD). Severe left sciatica after falling 2 months ago. (**a, b**) MRI, T2 STIR, sagittal: Height and signal intensity of L3–4 disc are normal. A linear hypointensity (arrows) in the middle of discs of L3–4, L4–5, and L5-S1 is an early sign of mild degeneration change. The L4–5 disc shows slight bulging out and hypointensity, reflecting decreased water content; these findings reflect the degeneration of this disc. Severe herniation of the L5-S1 disc is shown (h), indicating the tear of the annulus and extrusion of the nucleus pulposus. The posterior longitudinal ligamentum (pl) is compressed and backward displaced. (**c, d**) T2WI, axial sections: Large left posterior paracentral HIVD (h) severely compresses the dural sac and left S1 nerve root. The right S1 nerve root (S1) is normal

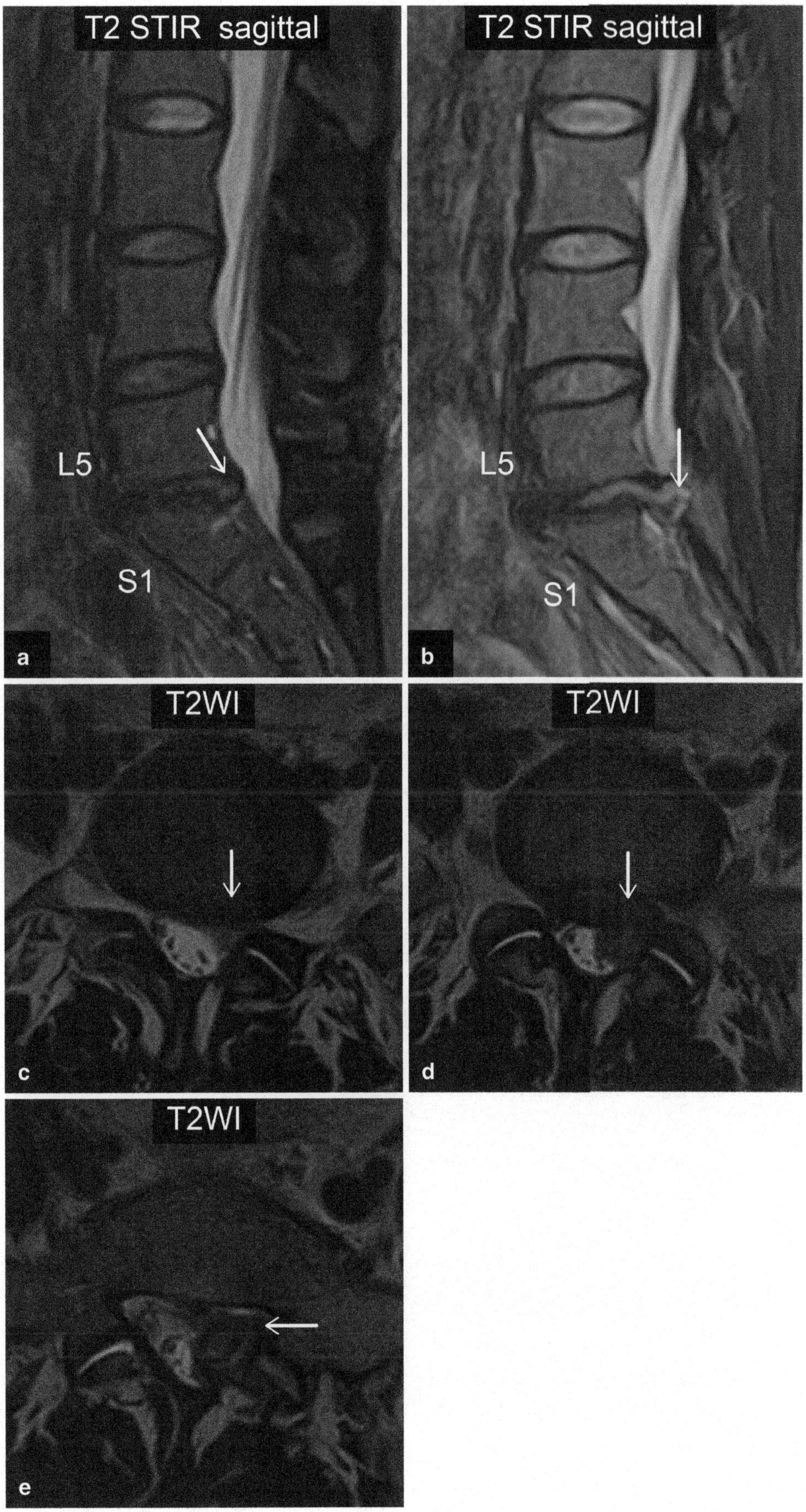

Fig. 8.16 F/45, Herniation of intervertebral disc (HIVD), and ruptured disc. (**a**–**e**) MRI: Decrease height of L5-S1 disc, reflecting disc degeneration. Tear of the annulus; the nucleus pulposus herniates out (arrows) in the left posterior paracentral and shows downward migration. This severe and typical HIVD is disc "extrusion with sequestration," and the herniated nucleus separates from the parent disc

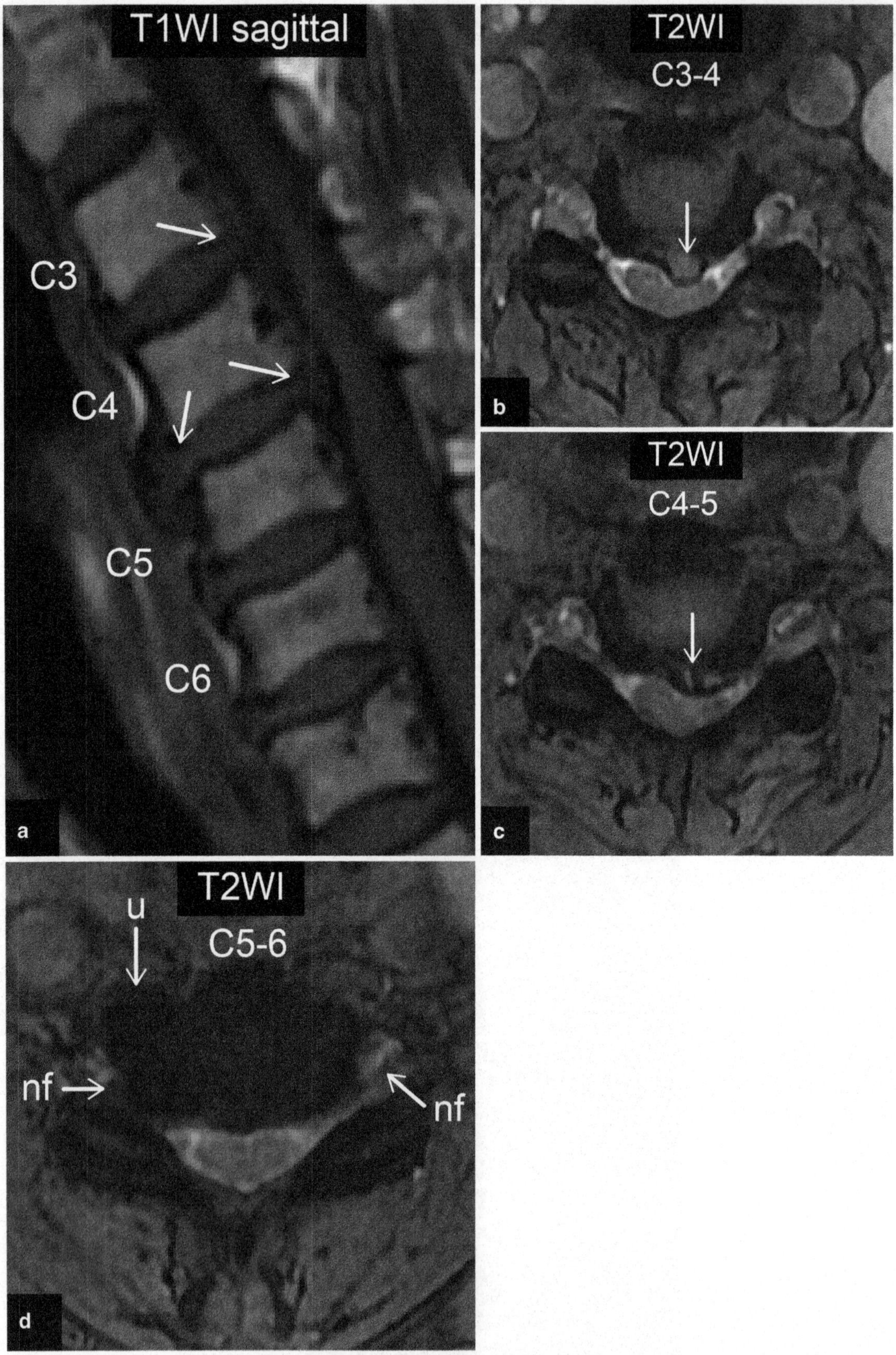

Fig. 8.17 F/71, Cervical herniation of intervertebral disc (HIVD) and neuroforamen stenosis. This patient complained numbness of both arms. (**a**) MRI, T1WI, sagittal: Posterior bulging out of the C3–4 disc (arrow), anterior and posterior bulging out of the C4–5 disc (arrows). (**b, c**) T2WI, axial: Left posterior paracentral HIVDs (arrows) in the C3–4, C4–5 levels compress the left C4, C5 nerve roots and the spinal cord. The HIVD in the C3–4 level is an extrusion of the nucleus pulposus. (**d**) C5–6: Osteophyte of the right uncinate process (u) of C6 causes stenosis of right neuroforamen (nf); the right C5 nerve root may be compressed by the stenosis

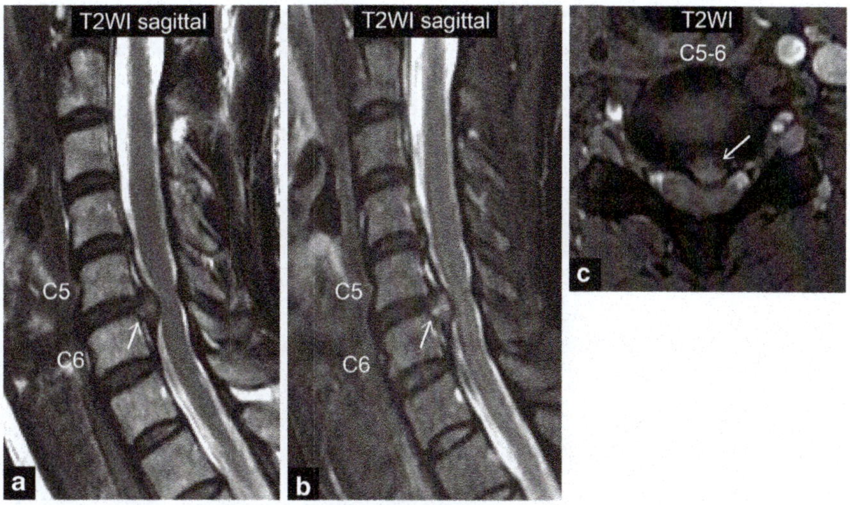

Fig. 8.18 F/46, C5–6 herniation of intervertebral disc (HIVD). This patient complained numbness of the left arm and hand. (**a–c**) MRI: left posterior paracentral HIVD (arrows) in the C5–6 level. The signal intensity of this HIVD is hyperintense; this is an extrusion of the nucleus pulposus. It compresses the left C6 nerve root and left side of the spinal cord

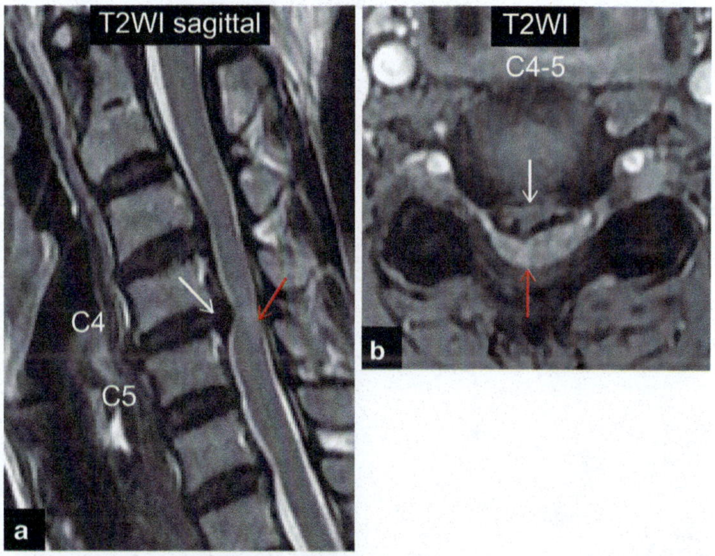

Fig. 8.19 F/44, C4–5 HIVD compresses the spinal cord, causing spinal cord edema. After a cervical spinal injury, this patient suffered numbness of bilateral upper limbs, weakness of lower legs, and urinary incontinence. (**a**) MRI, T2WI, sagittal: Posteriorly bulging out of the C4–5 disc (white arrow), a small area of hyperintensity in the spinal cord (red arrow), which reflects spinal cord edema possibly caused by spinal cord compression by the HIVD. (**b**) T2WI, axial of C4–5: Right-side posterior paracentral extrusion of the disc (white arrow) severely compresses the spinal cord, and a focal hyperintensity (red arrow) in the right side of the spinal cord, indicating focal edema

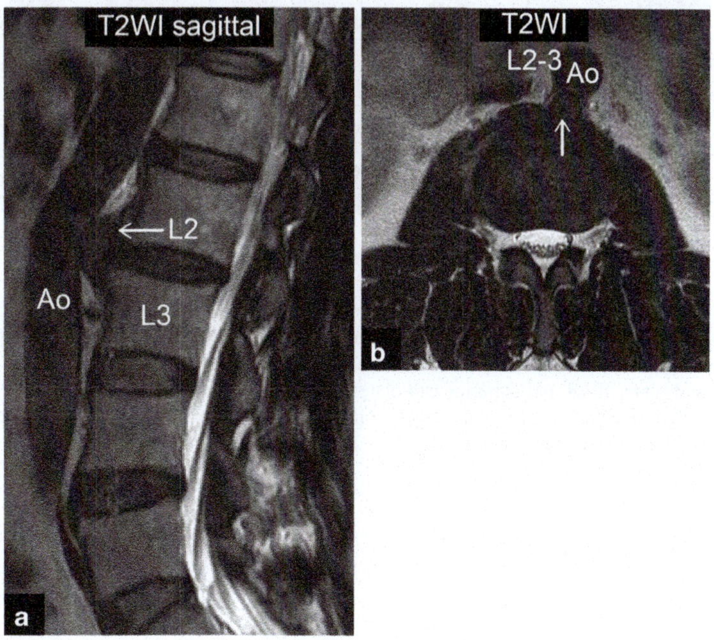

Fig. 8.20 M/45, Lumbar anterior HIVD.. No clinical symptom, MRI of a health check-up. (**a**) T2WI, sagittal: Anterior bulging out (arrow) of the L2–3 intervertebral disc. (**b**) T2WI, axial: anterior protrusion of the disc (arrow), slightly compresses the abdominal aorta (Ao). This is an anterior HIVD. Anterior HIVD is rare and is always asymptomatic

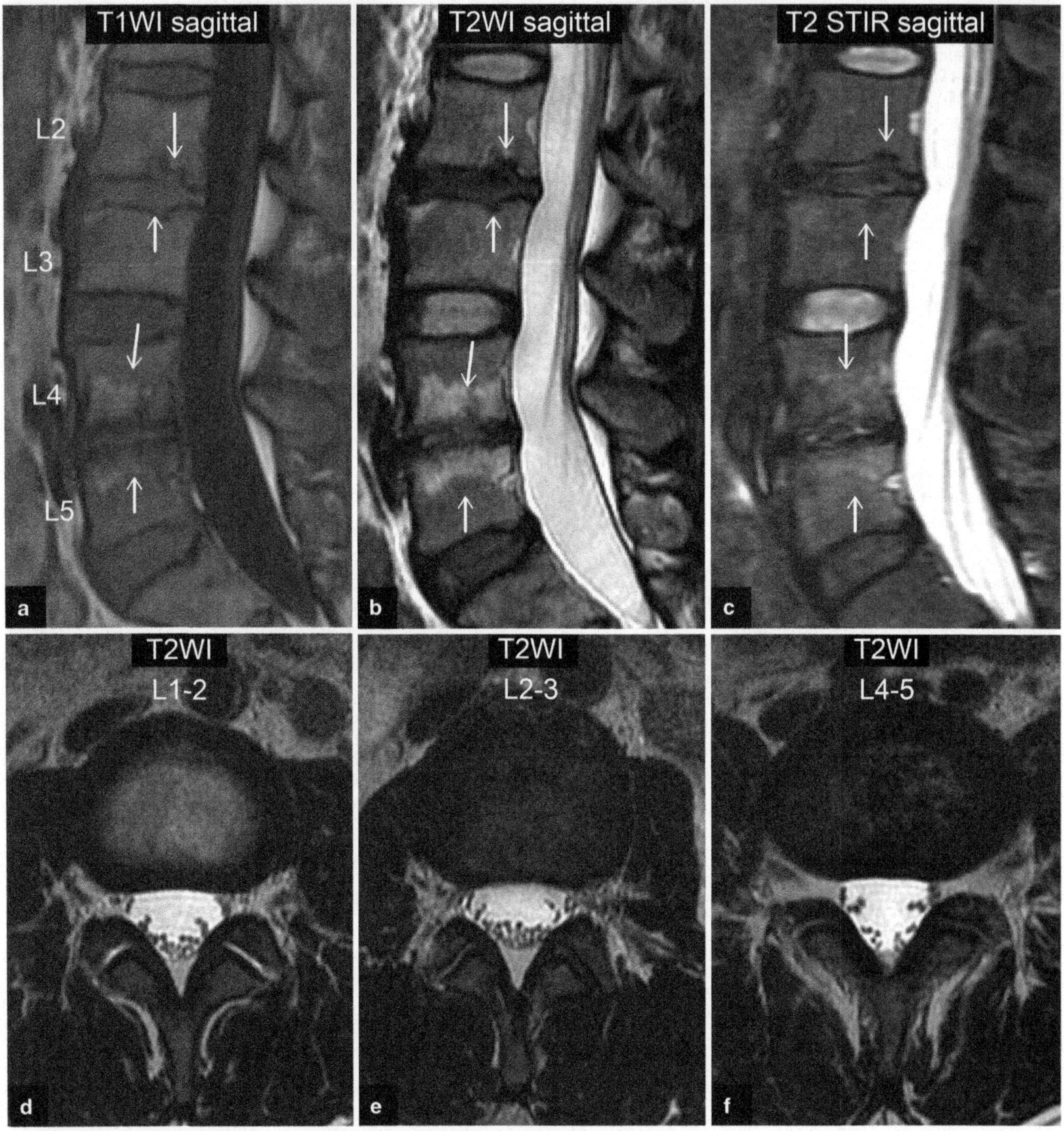

Fig. 8.21 F/36, Lumbar Schmorl's node, and Modic II change. This lady suffered lower back pain for a long time. (**a–c**) MRI, sagittal: Small defects (arrows) in the L2 inferior end plate and L3 superior end plate, and the discs invade the defects, indicating intravertebral herniation of the disc. Thus, these defects are Schmorl's nodes. The inferior end plate of L4 and superior end plate of L5 show hyperintensity on T1WI and T2WI, and suppression on T2 STIR, indicating typical Modic II degenerative change (arrows). Hyperintensity of the L1–2 and L3–4 intervertebral discs on the T2WI and T2 STIR is normal. The L2–3 disc shows hypointensity, reflecting mild degenerative change of the disc; the L4–5 disc shows hypointensity and height reduction, reflecting a severe degenerative change of the disc. (**d–f**) Axial sections: L1–2 disc is hyperintense on T2WI, the L2–3, L4–5 discs are hypointense, but in the axial section, cannot see reduction height of L4–5 disc. No stenosis of the spinal canal

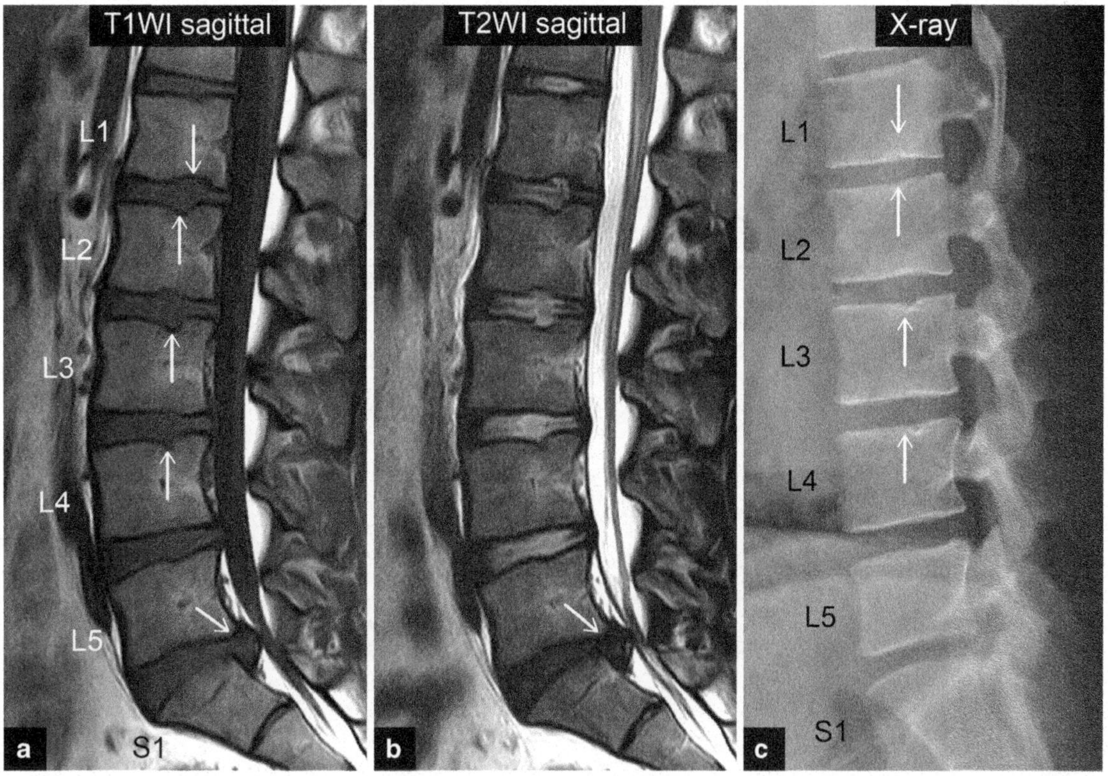

Fig. 8.22 M/21, Lumbar spine Schmorl's node. This patient underwent an MRI examination due to sciatica. (**a, b**) MRI: in addition to a herniation of intervertebral disc (HIVD) (arrow) in L5-S1, defects are incidentally found in the L1–4 end plates, and the discs clearly herniate into these defects. Thus, these are intravertebral herniation of discs, which are typical of Schmorl's nodes. Comment: This patient is young, and the signal intensities of the intervertebral discs from L1 to L4 are normal. Thus, the Schmorl's nodes are unrelated to disc degeneration. (**c**) X-ray: The Schmorl's nodes only show small defects in the L1,2,3,4 end plates (arrows)

Fig. 8.23 F/61, Osteophyte of the uncinate process of the cervical spine. This patient suffered right-hand numbness and pain. (**a**) MRI, T2WI, sagittal: Slight reduction in disc height of C5–6, C6–7. (**b**) MRI, axial section of C4–5: the disc, spinal canal, and bilateral neuroforamina of C4–5 are normal. (**c**) C5–6: Osteophyte formation in the right uncinate process (u) of C6 causes stenosis of right neuroforamen (nf); the stenosis may compress the right C5 nerve root

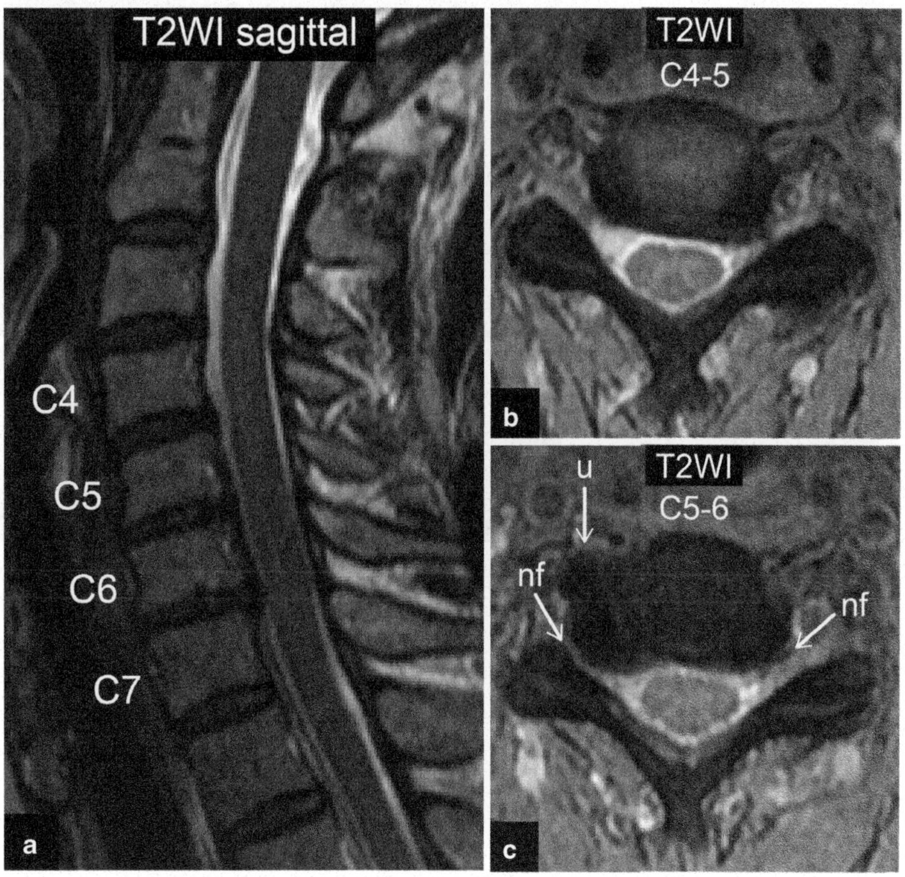

Fig. 8.24 Modic type endplate changes
Modic type I
T1: hypointensity
T2: hyperintensity
T2 STIR: hyperintensity represents bone marrow edema and inflammation
Modic type II
T1: hyperintensity
T2: hyperintensity
T2 STIR: hypointensity represents normal red hematopoietic bone marrow conversion into yellow fatty marrow as a result of marrow ischemia
Modic type III
T1: hypointensity
T2: hypointensity
T2 STIR: hypointensity represents subchondral bone sclerosis

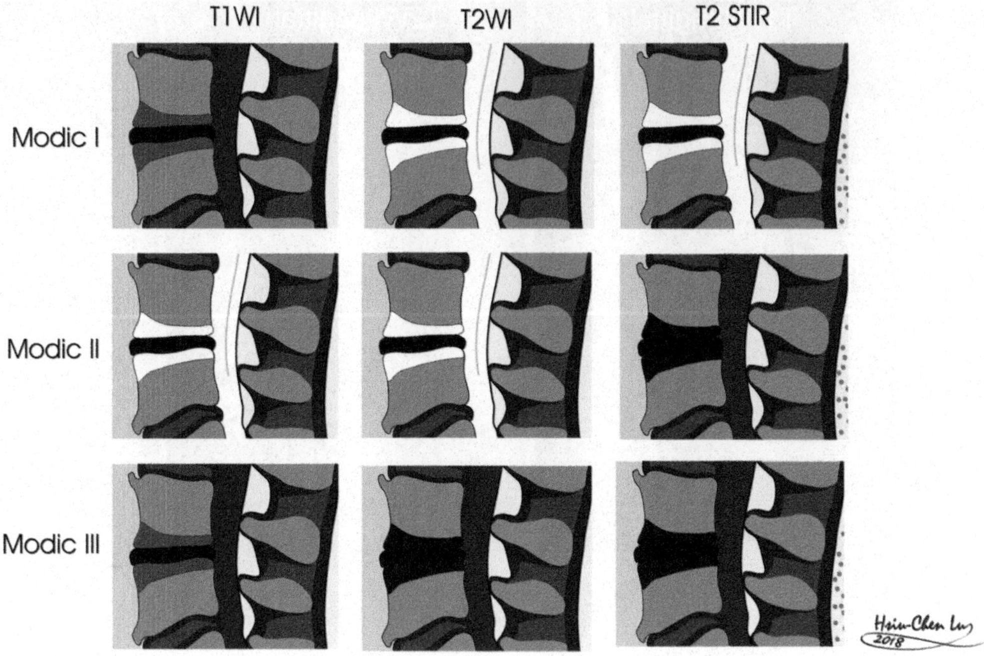

Fig. 8.25 M/60, Modic type I, II degenerations. This patient suffered mild neck pain. (**a**–**c**) MRI: The end plates of C3,4 show mild hypointensity on T1WI, mild hyperintensity on T2WI, hyperintensity on T2 STIR, which is typical Modic type I degeneration, representing bone marrow edema, and inflammation. The signal of the C6,7 end plates shows hyperintensity on T1WI and T2WI, and the signal intensity is suppressed on T2 STIR, which indicates typical Modic type II degeneration, representing red hemopoietic bone marrow conversion into yellow fatty marrow

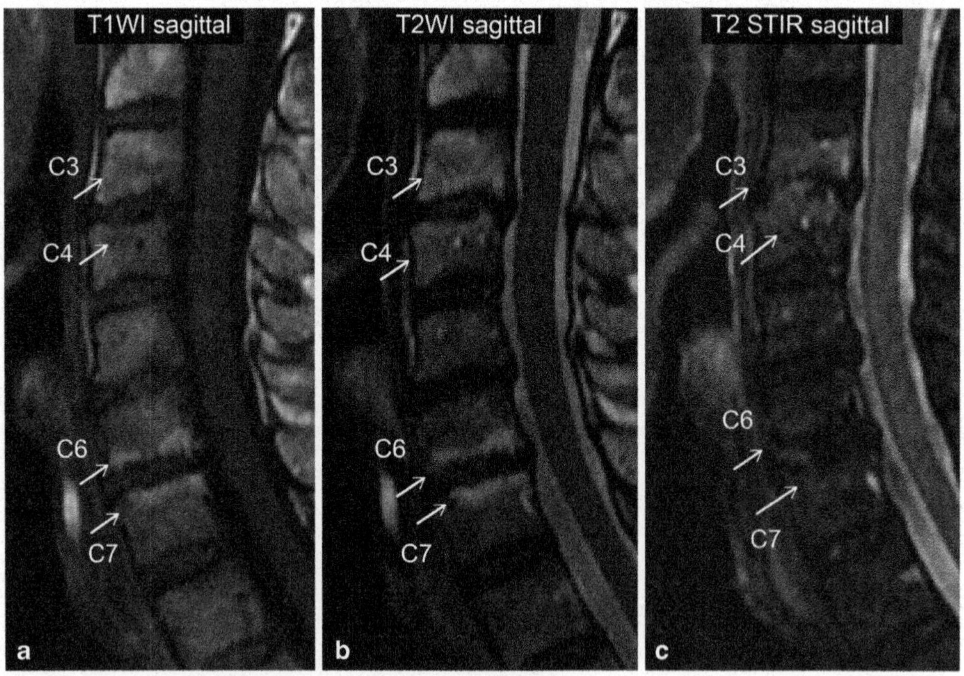

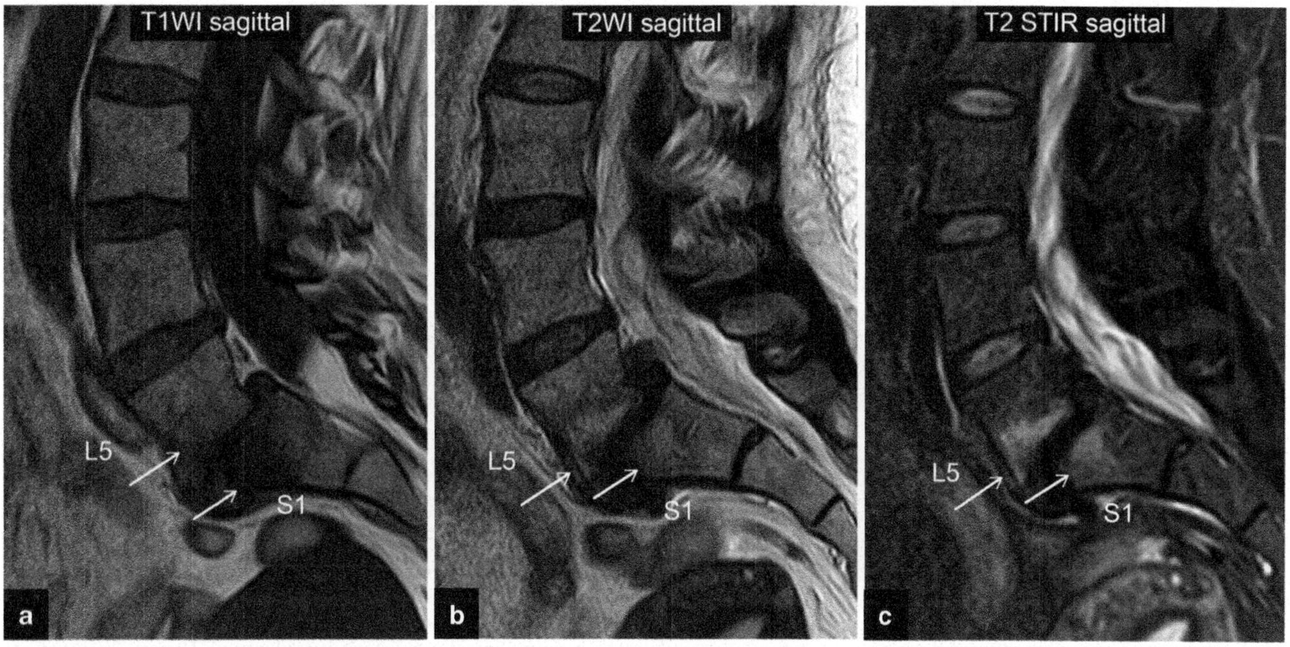

Fig. 8.26 F/40, Spondylolisthesis of L5 on S1 and Modic I degeneration. This patient suffered chronic low back pain and exaggeration in recent months. (**a–c**) MRI: Spondylolisthesis of L5 on S1; the L5-S1 disc is very narrow and desiccation (dehydration), reflecting severe disc degeneration. The inferior end plate of L5 and superior end plate of S1 show hypointensity on T1WI, mild hyperintensity on T2WI, and hyperintensity on T2 STIR, which is a Modic type I degeneration, representing bone marrow edema and inflammation

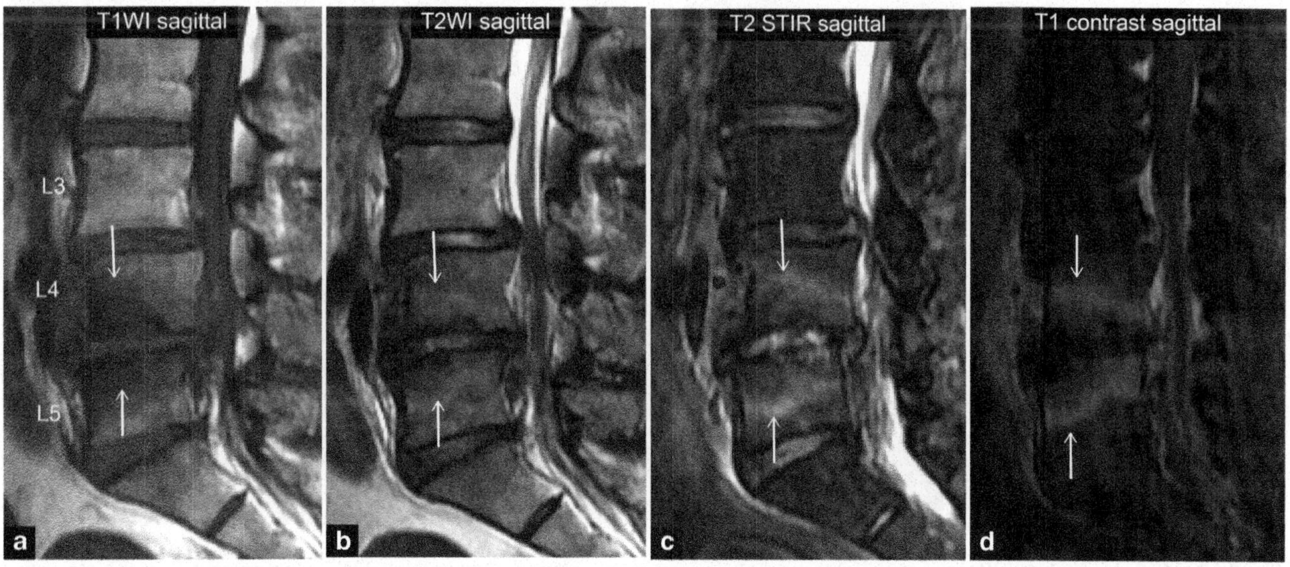

Fig. 8.27 F/51, Lumbar disc bulging, and osteomyelitis. This patient suffered severe lower back pain for 2 weeks. (**a–c**) MRI: Mild spondylolisthesis of L3 on L4; narrowing and bulging out of discs of L3–4, L4–5. The inferior half of L4 and superior half of L5 vertebral bodies show hypointensity on T1WI and hyperintensity on T2WI and T2 STIR. The features are similar to Modic type I degeneration, but the involving areas are larger than the end plates. Thus, a specific cause of bone marrow edema and inflammation was considered, and intravenous contrast medium (Gd-DTPA) was administrated. (**d**) Contrast T1WI: The above areas are enhanced by contrast medium, suggesting inflammation. The patient received L3–4, L4–5 diskectomies, and underwent a biopsy of L4,5 vertebral bodies; pathology proved osteomyelitis

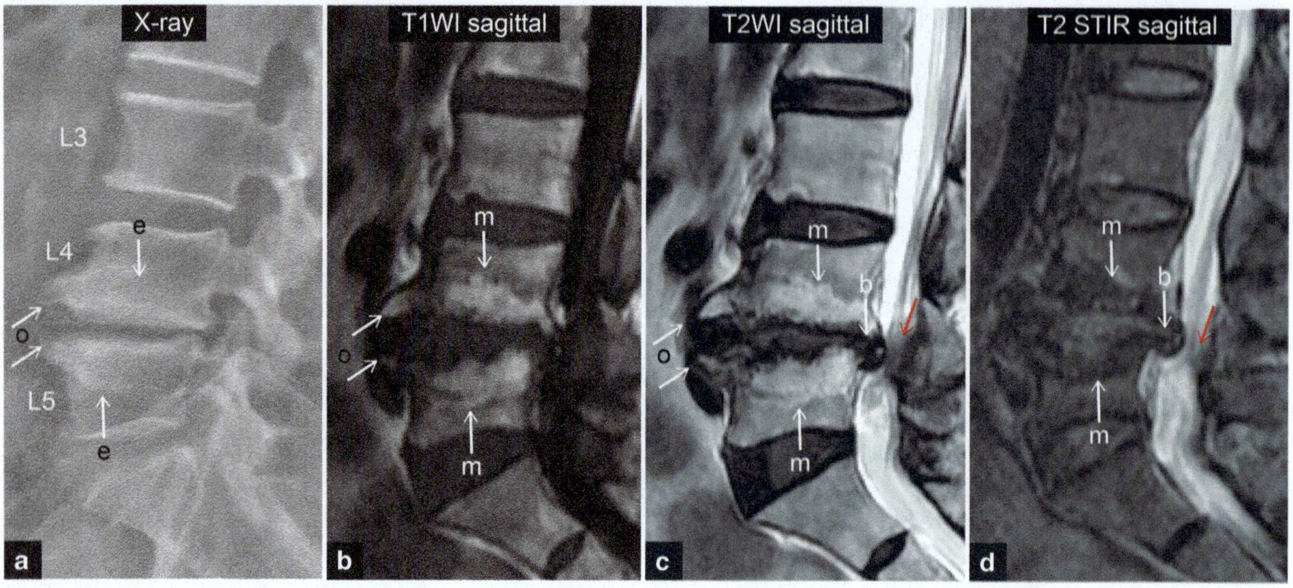

Fig. 8.28 F/74, Lumbar 4,5 degenerative change with osteophytes and Modic II change. This patient suffered chronic low back pain for several years. (**a**) X-ray: Severe degenerative change of L4–5 vertebral bodies, with osteophyte (o), reduction of disc height, eburnation (e) of the end plates. (**b–d**) MRI: L4–5-disc height reduction and bulging out (b), which causes spinal canal stenosis (red arrow). Hyperintensity of end plates of L4,5 on T1WI, T2WI is suppressed to be hypointensity on T2 STIR, which is a typical Modic type II degeneration (m)

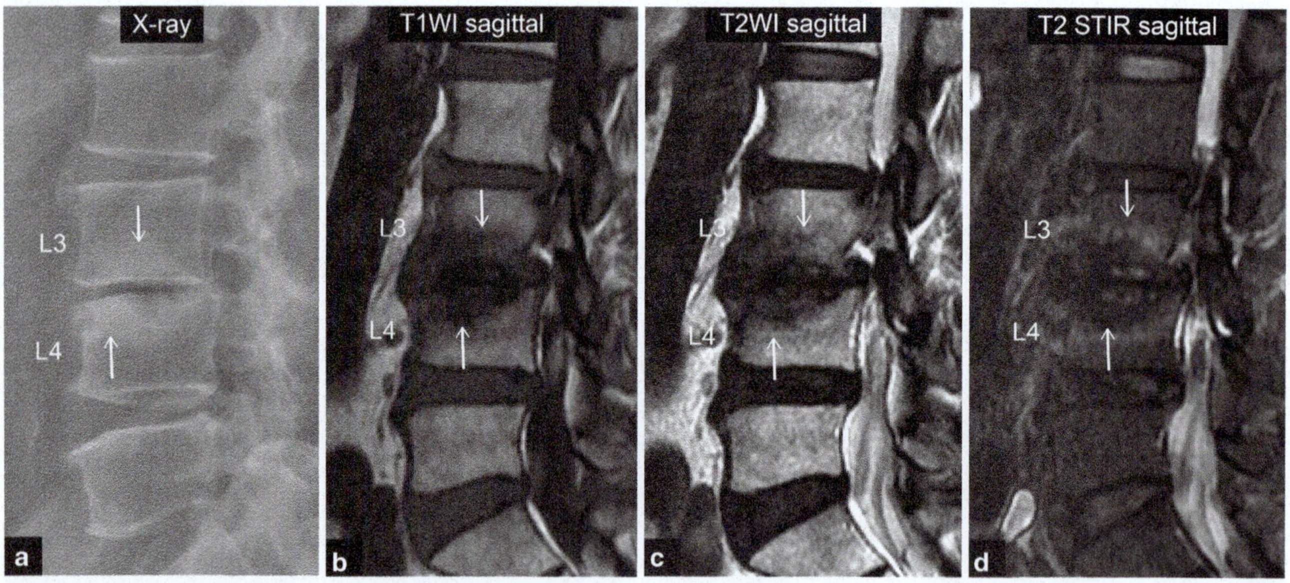

Fig. 8.29 M/63, Modic I and III degenerative changes. This patient suffered low back pain for many years. (**a**) X-ray: Severe degeneration of L3–4 disc with very narrowing of disc space, eburnation (arrows) of the L3, L4 end plates. (**b–d**) MRI: The end plates of L3, L4 show hypointensity (arrows) on T1WI, corresponding to the eburnation shown on X-ray. Most of these areas show hypointensity (arrows) on T2WI and T2 STIR, indicating Modic III change and representing bone marrow sclerosis change. Margins of these areas show hyperintensity on T2WI and T2 STIR, indicating Modic I change

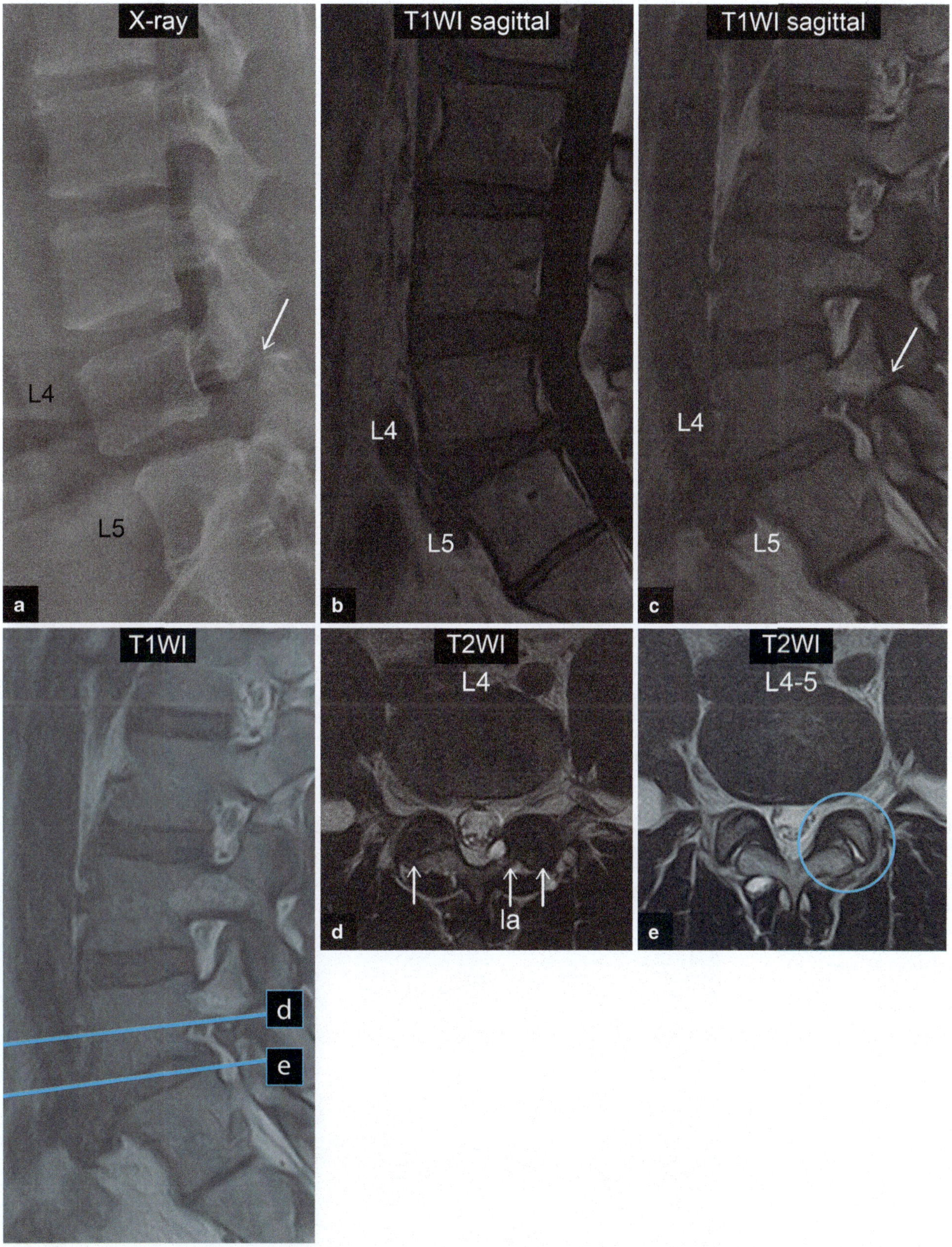

Fig. 8.30 M/30, Spondylolysis, and spondylolisthesis. (**a**) X-ray: An old fracture in the inferior articular process of L4 (arrow); this is spondylolysis. Mild spondylolisthesis of L4 on L5. (**b**, **c**) MRI, T1WI: Same findings as X-ray. MRI displays slight bulging out of the L4–5 disc, no spinal canal stenosis. (**d**, **e**) MRI, T2WI, axial section: Spondylolysis is symmetrical old fractures and hypertrophy of bilateral articular processes (arrows in **d**), easily confusing with the facet joints (blue circles in **e**). The facet joints have joint space with fluid and can be used as a difference. The axial image must be read with a careful comparison with sagittal views. *la* lamina

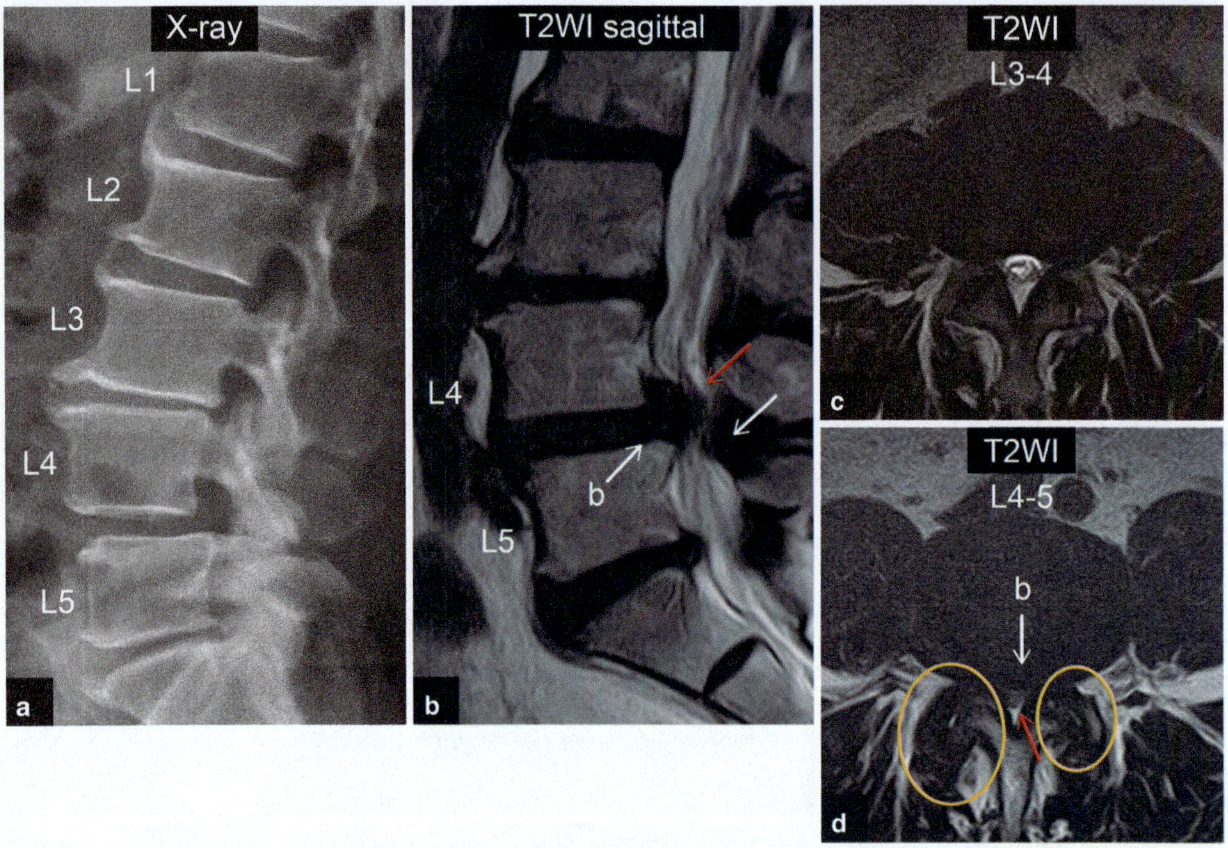

Fig. 8.31 M/63, Spinal canal stenosis. (**a**) X-ray: Degenerative spondylosis of the lumbar spine, with marginal osteophytes in every lumbar vertebral body; narrowing of disc spaces of L3–4, L5-S1; spondylolisthesis of L4 on L5. The X-ray cannot show the condition of the spinal canal. (**b**–**d**) MRI, T2WI: The L4–5 level shows bulging out of the disc (b), degenerative change with hypertrophy of bilateral facet joints (white arrow in **b** and yellow circles in **d**) and spondylolisthesis, the above three factors cause severe spinal canal stenosis (red arrow). The spinal canal in the L3–4 level is normal

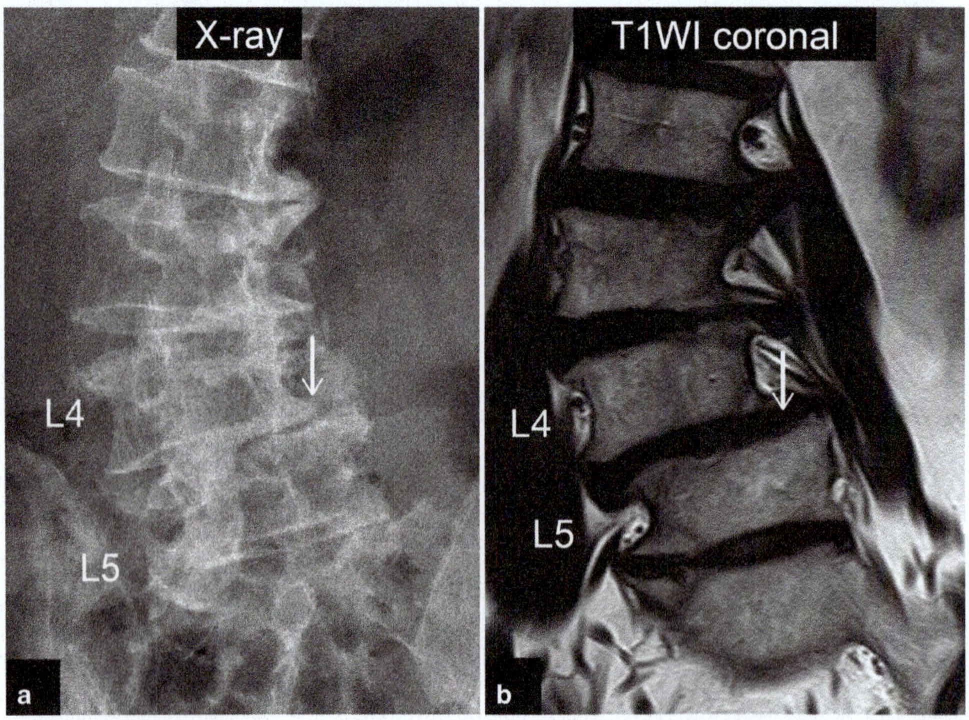

Fig. 8.32 M/82, Lateral spondylolisthesis. (**a**) X-ray. (**b**) MRI: Severe degenerative spondylosis of lumbar spine, osteophytes in every lumbar vertebral body, narrowing of every intervertebral disc, scoliosis of the lumbar spine. There is right-side lateral spondylolisthesis of L4 on L5 (arrow)

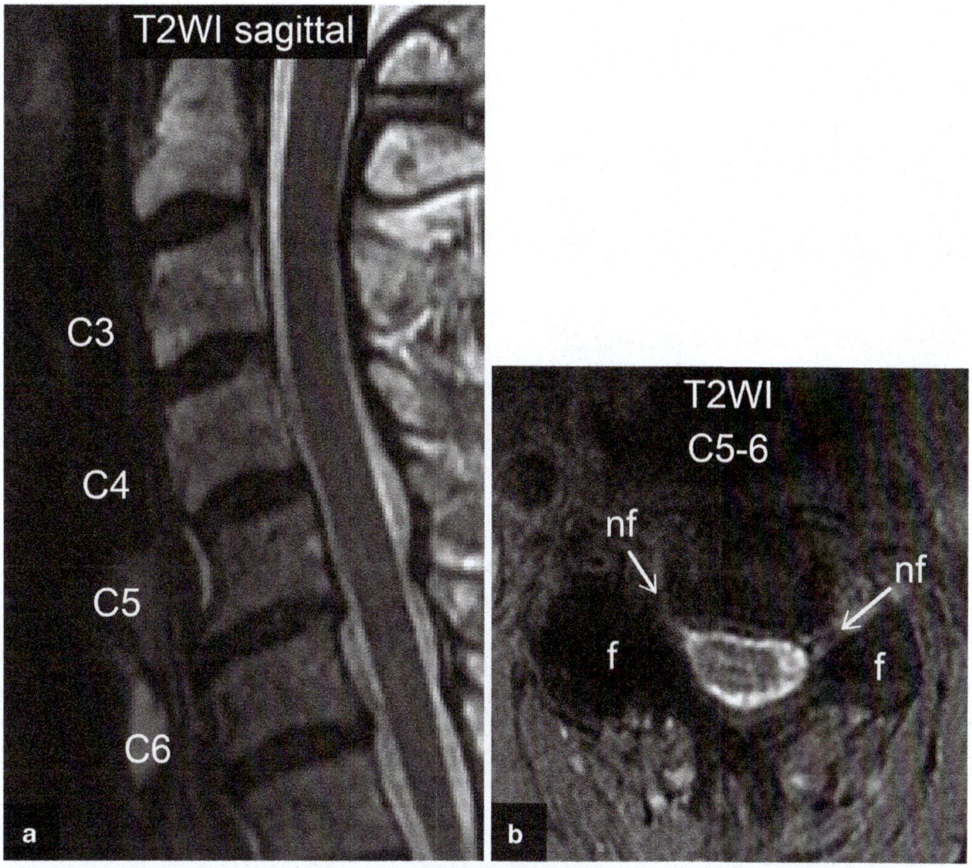

Fig. 8.33 F/50, Degenerative OA change of facet joint. The patient suffered right-hand numbness for several months. (**a**) MRI, T2WI sagittal: Only shows reduction in disc height of C5–6 disc. (**b**) C5–6, axial: The right facet joint (f) showing very hypertrophy and with osteophytes, this is degenerative osteoarthritis (OA) and causes stenosis of right neuroforamen (nf). The right C5 nerve root in the neuroforamen may be compressed and cause right cervical radiculopathy

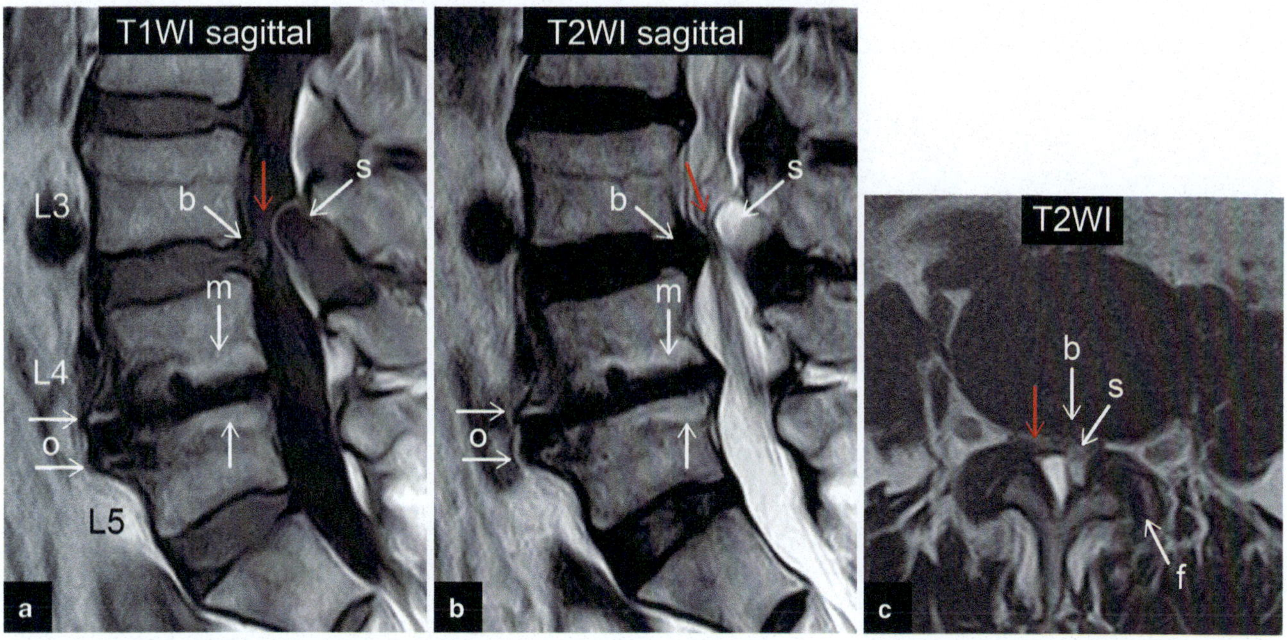

Fig. 8.34 F/66, Facet joint OA change and associated with a synovial cyst. This patient suffered long-term low back pain. (**a**, **b**) MRI, T1WI, T2WI, sagittal sections: Posterior bulging out of the L3–4 disc (b) and synovial cyst (s) arising from the left facet joint. These two factors cause spinal canal stenosis (red arrow). The L4,5 vertebral bodies show marginal osteophytes (o) and Modic type II change (m), reduction height, and desiccation of the L4–5 intervertebral disc, but no stenosis of the spinal canal in the L4–5 level. (**c**) Axial section of L3–4: OA change of the left facet joint (f), associated with a synovial cyst (s), and bulging disc (b), the above three factors cause spinal canal stenosis (red arrow)

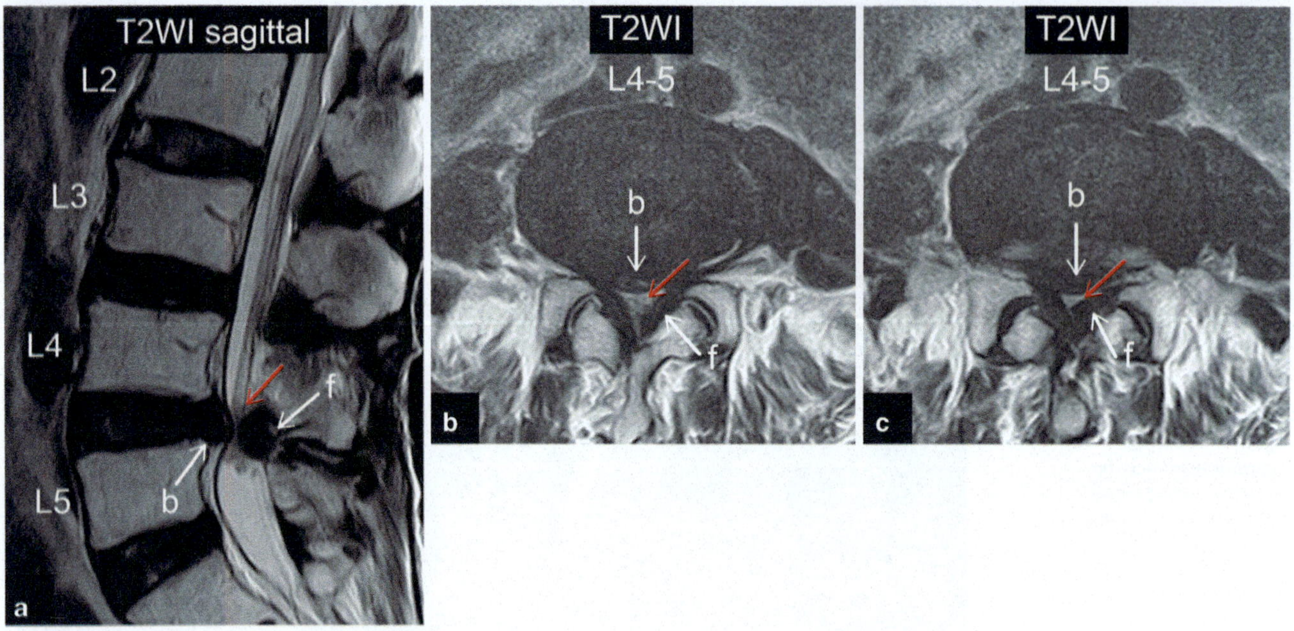

Fig. 8.35 M/82, Severe spinal canal stenosis. This patient suffered low back pain and intermittent claudication, clinically suspected he has spinal canal stenosis. (**a**) MRI, T2WI, sagittal: Bulging out of the L4–5 disc (b), hypertrophy of ligamentum flavum (f), the two factors cause severe spinal canal stenosis (red arrow). (**b**, **c**) Axial sections: Demonstrate severe spinal canal stenosis (red arrow) of L4–5 level, caused by disc bulging (b) and hypertrophy of ligamentum flava (f)

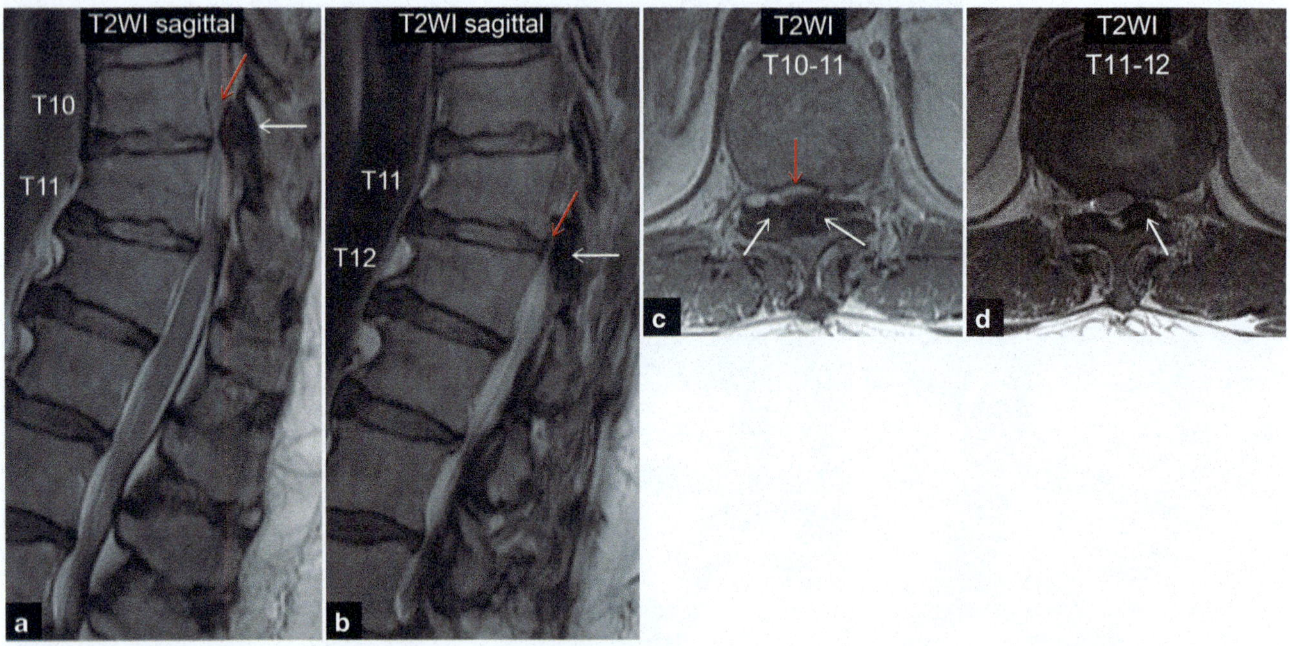

Fig. 8.36 M/48, Hypertrophy of ligamentum flava, compress the spinal cord. This patient suffered both lower legs weakness and numbness below the umbilicus after a spinal injury. (**a**, **b**) MRI, T2WI, sagittal: Hypointense lesions (white arrows) in the posterior of the spinal canal of the T10–11 and T11–12 levels cause severe stenosis of the spinal canal (red arrows). (**c**) Axial section of the T10–11 level: Hypertrophy of the bilateral ligamentum flava (arrows) causes spinal canal stenosis (red arrow), severely compressing the spinal cord. (**d**) T11–12 level: Hypertrophy of the left ligamentum flavum (arrow) slightly compresses the spinal cord

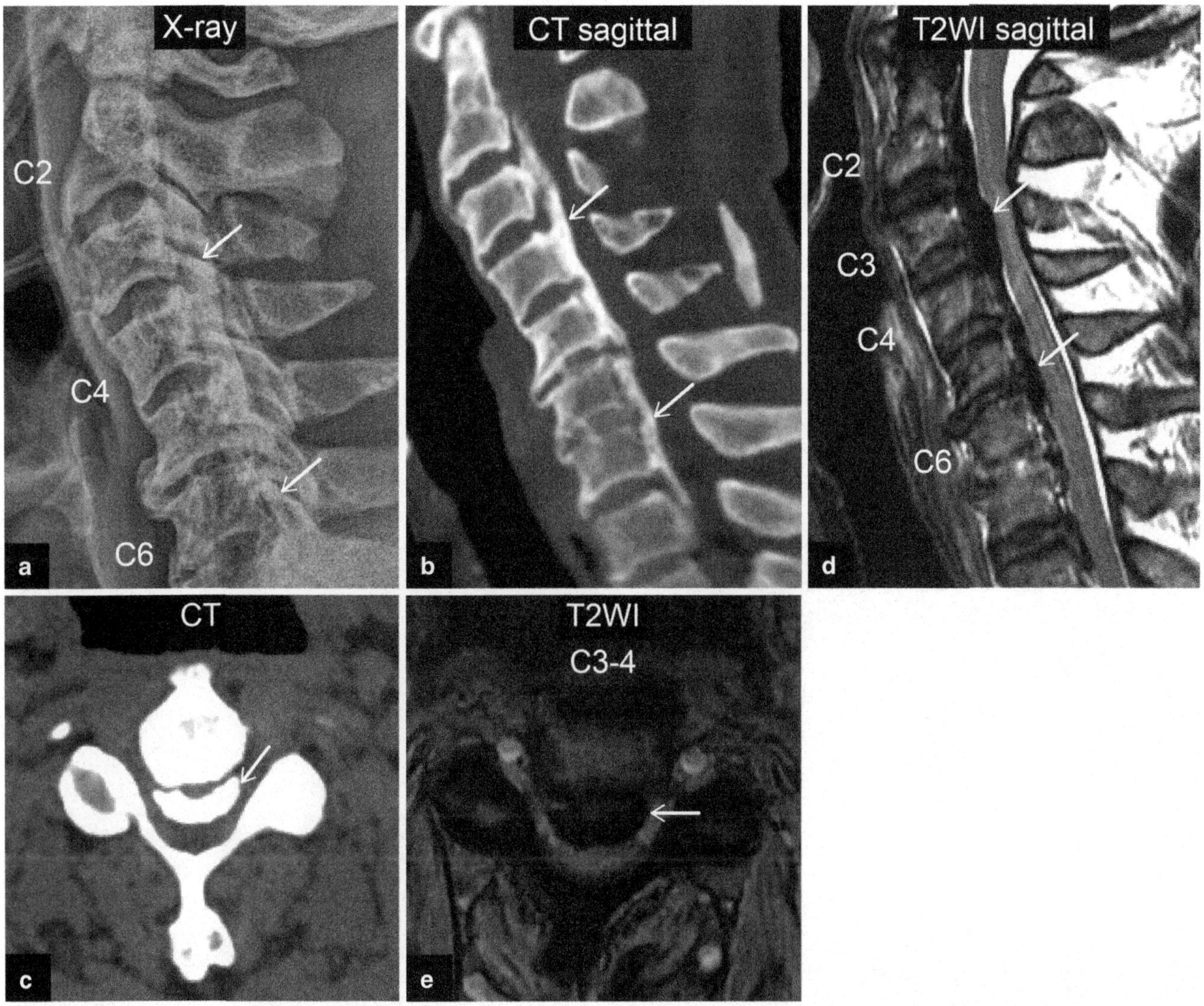

Fig. 8.37 M/75, OPLL. This patient suffered long-term spastic weakness of both lower legs. (**a**) X-ray: Degenerative spondylosis of the cervical spine with osteophytes in every vertebral body, and ossification of the posterior longitudinal ligamentum (OPLL) (arrows). (**b**) CT, sagittal reconstruction: Clearly demonstrates the OPLL (arrows) from the C2 to the T1 level. (**c**) CT, axial section: The OPLL (arrow) occupies half of the spinal canal; thus, the spinal cord is compressed and causes myelopathy symptoms. (**d**) MRI, T2WI, sagittal: The OPLL (arrows) is hypointense on T2WI, and it compresses the spinal cord in the C3–4 level. (**e**) MRI, axial, C3–4: The OPLL (arrow) occupies half part of the spinal canal, and it compresses the spinal cord

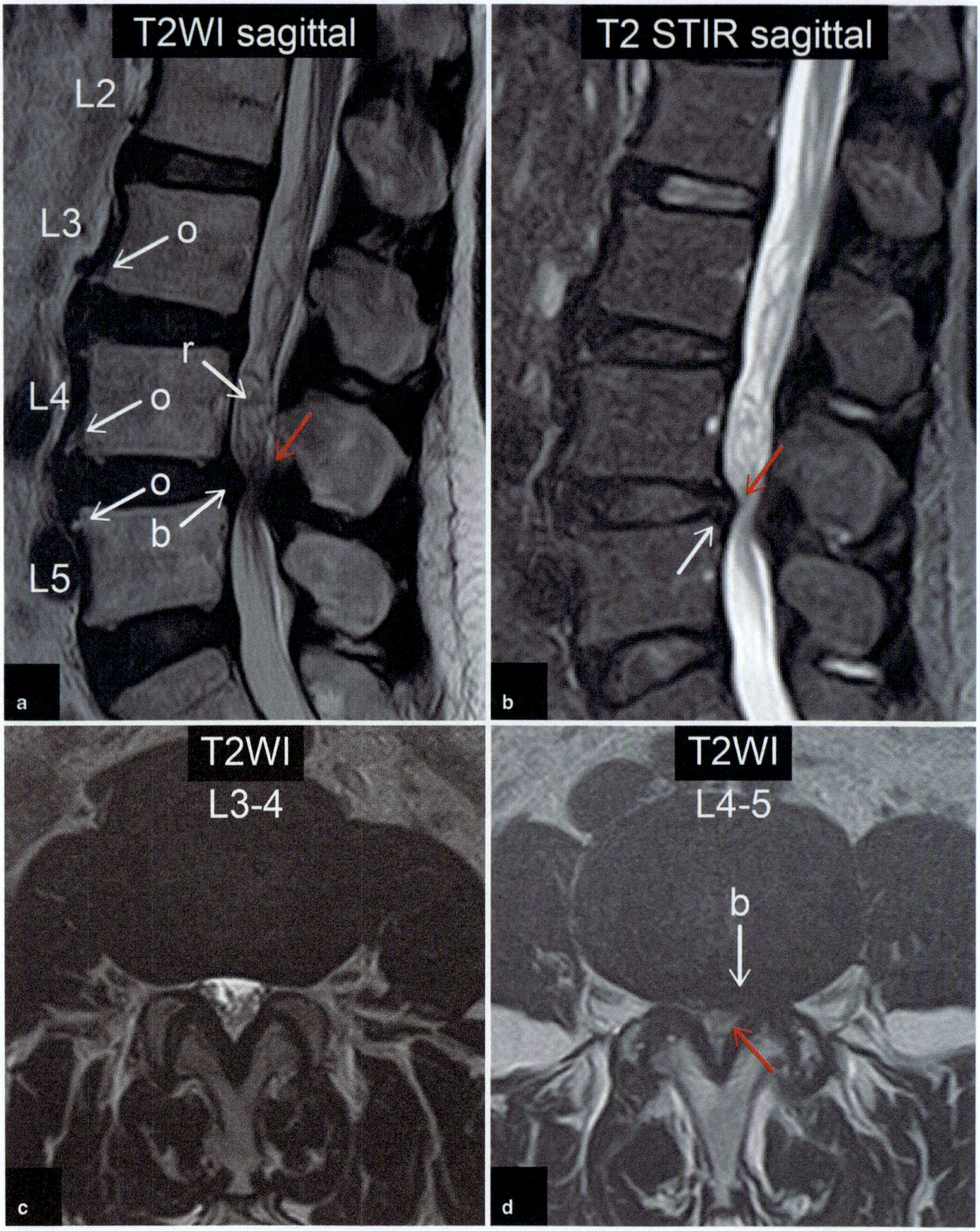

Fig. 8.38 F/63, Spinal canal stenosis causes redundancy of cauda equina nerves. This patient suffered long-term low back pain, numbness of both legs, a sign of claudication. (**a**, **b**) MRI, sagittal sections: Degenerative change in the L3,4,5 vertebral bodies with osteophytes (o). Bulging out of the L4–5 disc (b) causes spinal canal stenosis (red arrow). Redundancy of the caudal equina nerves (r) occurs above the L4–5 level because of spinal canal stenosis. (**c**, **d**) Axial sections: The spinal canal in the L3–4 level is normal; the cauda equina nerves are visible in the dural sac. Spinal canal stenosis (red arrow) occurs in the L4–5 level due to bulging disc (b); the cauda equina nerves are invisible

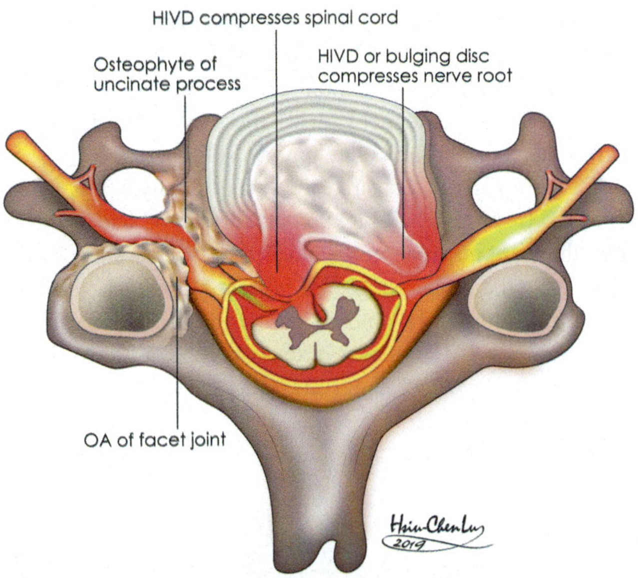

Fig. 8.39 Cervical radiculopathy and myelopathy. The following etiologies may cause cervical nerve and spinal cord compression and produce cervical radiculopathy and myelopathy symptoms. (**a**) Disc: HIVD or bulging disc, directly compresses the nerve root or spinal cord, causes radiculopathy or myelopathy. (**b**) Facet joint: DJD (degenerative joint disease) or named OA (osteoarthritis), causes joint hypertrophy because of osteophyte formation. (**c**) Uncinate process: osteophyte formation. (**b** and **c**) cause stenosis of neuroforamen, compressing the nerve root, and cause radiculopathy

8.5 Diffuse Idiopathic Skeletal Hyperostosis (DISH)

Diffuse idiopathic skeletal hyperostosis (DISH) or Forestier disease (Fig. 8.40) occurs mostly in older men. Ranked in order of commonality, the thoracic, cervical, and lumbar spines are where ossification of the anterior longitudinal ligamentum typically occurs. The X-ray can indicate the continual ossification of at least four vertebrae, and that the intervertebral discs are generally normal. DISH is likely to be accompanied by OPLL.

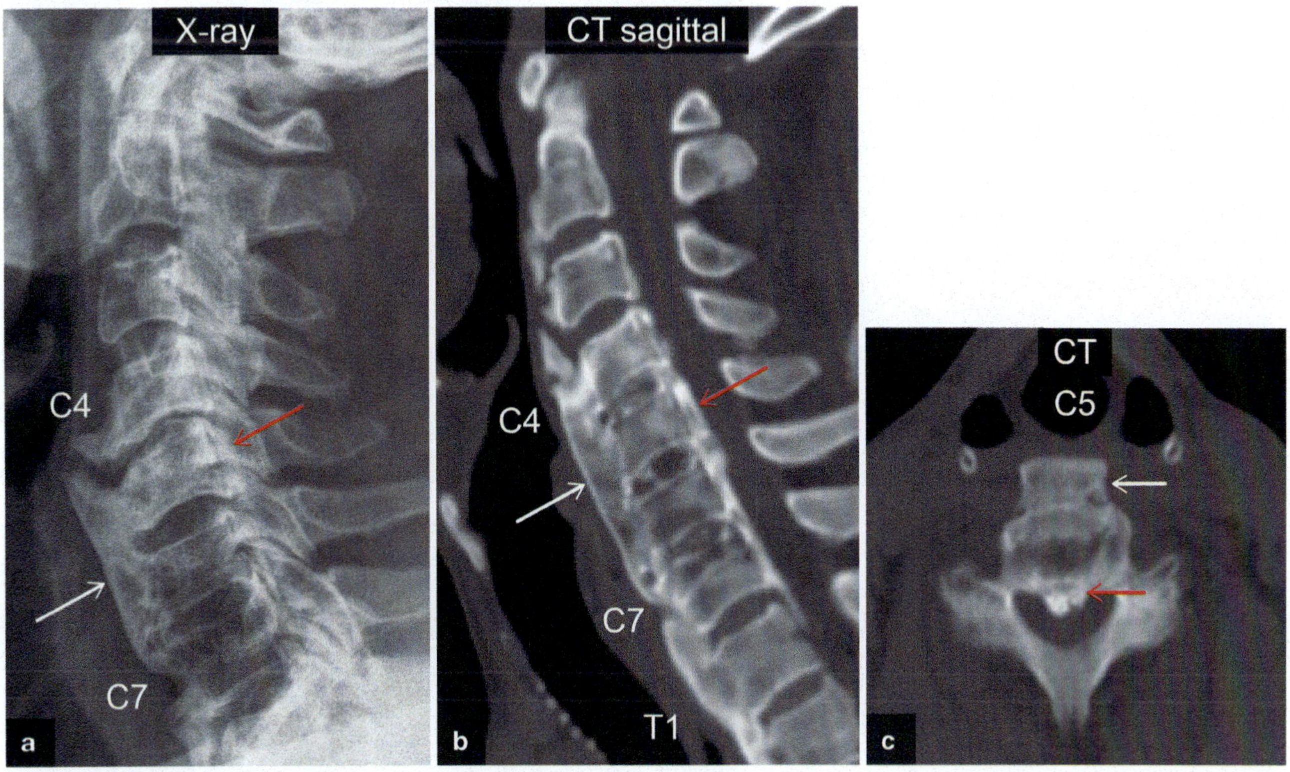

Fig. 8.40 M/76, DISH, and OPLL. (**a**) X-ray: Abnormal plate-like bone structures (white arrow) are found in front of the C4 to C7 vertebral bodies; these structures are ossifications of the anterior longitudinal ligamentum, indicating typical diffuse idiopathic skeletal hyperostosis (DISH). Suspicious OPLL (red arrow) is observed in the spinal canal. (**b**) CT, sagittal reconstruction: DISH (white arrow) extends from C4 to T2 and OPLL (red arrow) in the spinal canal. (**c**) CT, axial, C5 level: DISH (white arrow) in front of the C5 vertebral body and the OPLL (red arrow) in the spinal canal

8.6 Ankylosing Spondylitis

Ankylosing spondylitis (AS) is the most common form of spondyloarthritis, which also includes psoriatic arthritis and Reiter syndrome.

AS mainly involves the sacroiliac (SI) joints and the whole spine.

Discussions on imaging of AS typically focus on "bamboo spine," which is a typical AS-induced change that is identified using X-ray (Fig. 8.41). Bamboo spine results from syndesmophytes-induced vertebral body fusion, which causes the spine to lose its flexibility and to exhibit a squarish shape; these, in turn, result in ankylosis of the vertebral column.

The AP view of the lumbar on X-rays (Fig. 8.41) can indicate the disappearance of the bilateral SI joints and a thick white line in the center of the spine, which is termed the "dagger sign." The dagger sign is caused by syndesmophytes of the supraspinous and interspinous ligaments.

CT can clearly demonstrate the syndesmophyte (Fig. 8.42), followed by X-rays and MR images (Figs. 8.42 and 8.43). In fact, the bamboo spine in AS develops at a later stage of the disease. In the earlier stage, AS presents Romanus lesion or anterior discitis in the anterior corner of the vertebral body. Both X-ray and MRI images of the condition feature a shiny-corner sign (Figs. 8.42 and 8.43) [6].

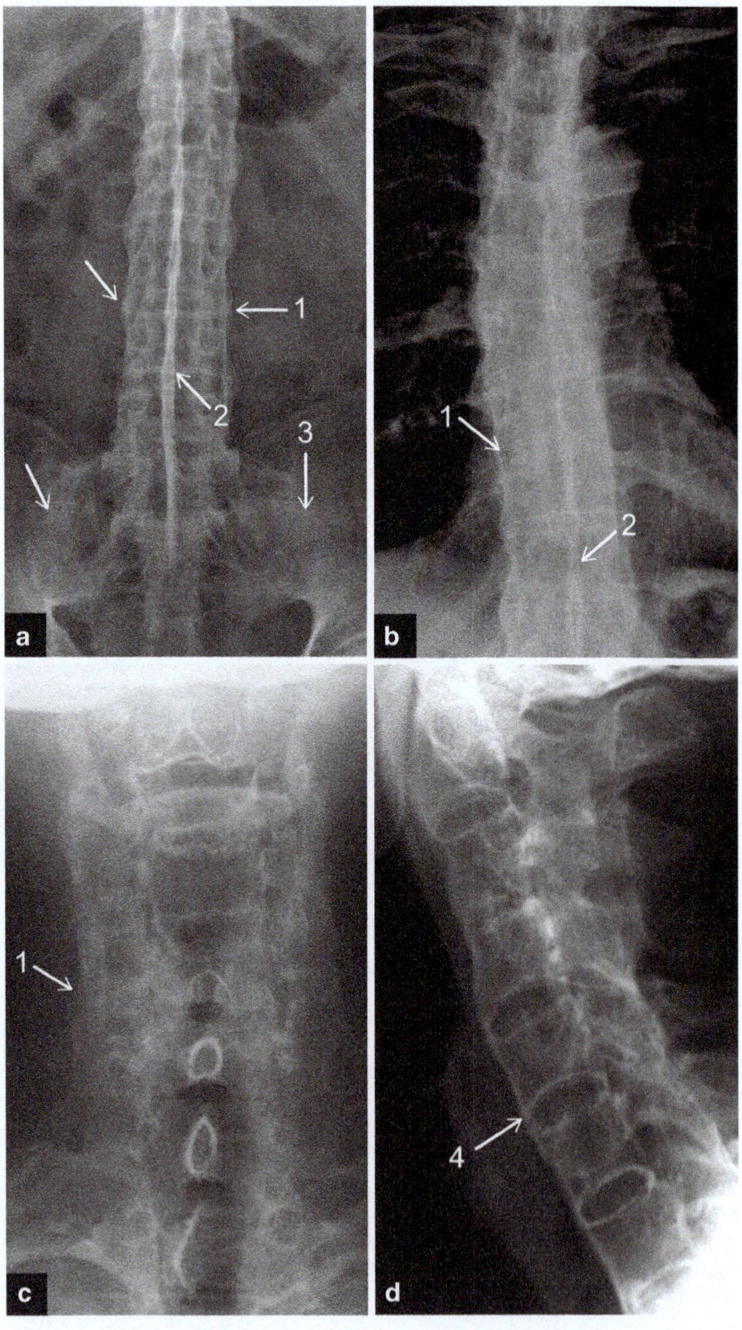

Fig. 8.41 M/60, Ankylosing spondylitis (AS). (**a**) X-ray of L-spine: There is bilateral marginal syndesmophyte (1), making the spine like a bamboo spine. There is a dagger sign (2) in the middle of the spine, which is caused by the ossification of the ligaments of the spinous process. The bilateral SI joints also lose joint spaces and fuse together (3). (**b**) X-ray of T-spine: The bilateral marginal syndesmophyte (1) and dagger sign (2) are noted. (**c, d**) X-ray of C-spine: The bilateral marginal syndesmophytes (1) are seen, but no dagger sign. On the lateral view, the anterior syndesmophyte (4) is visible

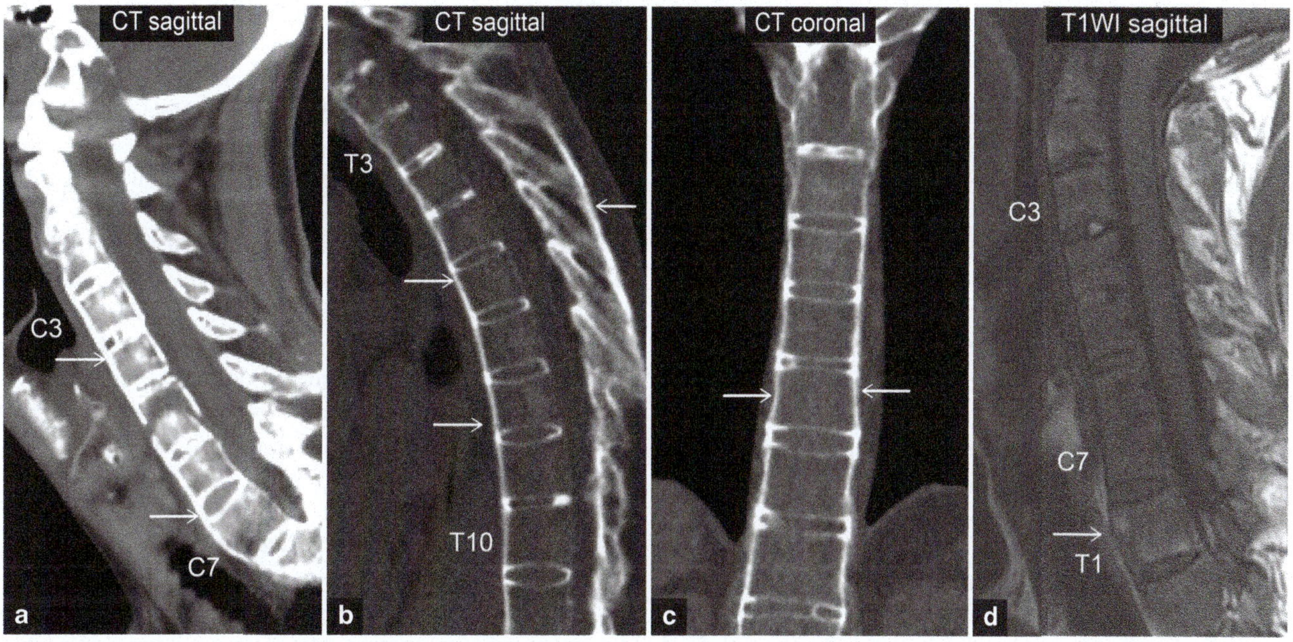

Fig. 8.42 M/75, Ankylosing spondylitis (AS). (**a–c**) CT: The anterior and bilateral marginal syndesmophytes of the cervical and thoracic spines are connected in straight lines (arrow), making the spine appear similar to a bamboo spine. (**d**) MRI, T1WI sagittal: Anterior syndesmophytes show only a small line, which is not clearly demonstrated as in CT. A small hyperintensity in the anterior corner of the T1 vertebral body is a shiny-corner sign (arrow), indicating focal spondylitis

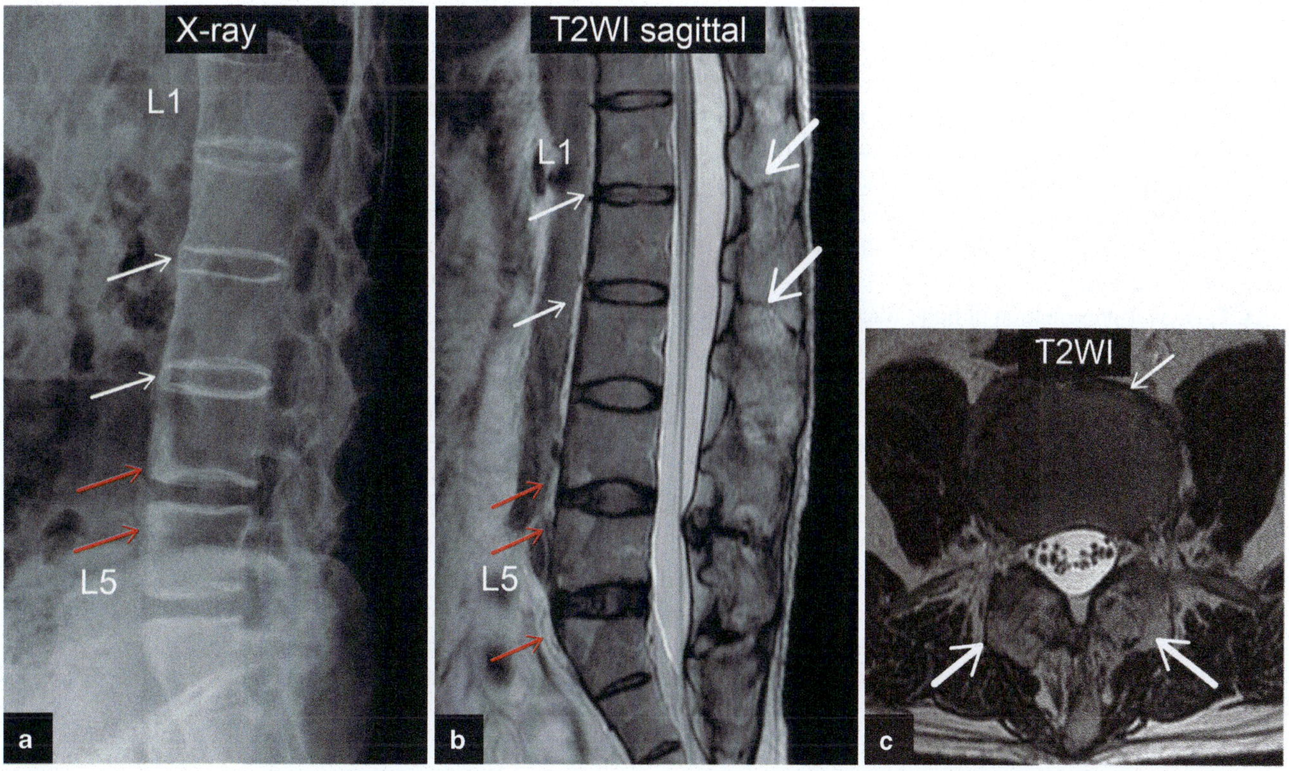

Fig. 8.43 M/46, Ankylosing spondylitis (AS). (**a**) X-ray: Anterior syndesmophytes connect in a straight line (white arrows). Increased density of the anterior corners of L4,5 vertebral bodies; they are the shiny-corner sign (red arrows) due to focal spondylitis. (**b**) MRI, T2WI: The small line indicates anterior syndesmophytes (white arrows), which is not as apparent as X-ray. Shiny-corner sign (red arrows) is observed in the anterior of the L4,5, S1 vertebral bodies. Syndesmophytes (thick arrows) in the interspinous ligaments of every spinous process. (**c**) T2WI, axial: The anterior syndesmophyte (arrow) is visible but hard to be recognized. Hypertrophic change of the bilateral facet joints and lost joint spaces (thick arrows)

8.7 Spinal Injury

8.7.1 Spinal Fractures

For cases of spinal fracture, examining the shape changes caused by the fracture of the vertebral body is crucial. The spinal fracture can be classified into the following types according to the mechanism of fracture [7, 8].

1. Flexion compression fracture causes wedge compression fracture (Figs. 8.44 and 8.48).
2. Axial compression fracture causes burst fracture (Fig. 8.45).
3. Flexion-distraction fracture causes displacement of fracture fragments (Figs. 8.46 and 8.47).

In addition to the fractures of the vertebral bodies, attention must be paid to the fractures of the posterior elements, such as the facet joints, spinous process, and lamina. We must observe the presence or absence of epidural or subdural hematoma in the spinal canal and the compression, edema, and hemorrhage of the spinal cord.

8.7.2 Imaging Diagnostic Methods

X-ray: As the first-line examination tool for spinal injuries, X-rays can indicate the presence or absence of fracture and dislocation in the spine, as well as injuries in other parts of the body. However, X-ray is difficult to differentiate new from old vertebral fractures (Figs. 8.44 and 8.48). X-ray cannot make a diagnosis of occult fracture that does not significantly change the shape of the vertebral body (Figs. 8.44 and 8.47).

CT: A clear presentation of bone fractures is afforded by CT. Multislice CT can quickly reconstruct the sagittal and coronal planes, even 3D images. The reconstructions of these images are conducive to the assessment of bone fractures and separation (Figs. 8.45, 8.46, and 8.47). However, CT cannot reveal edema or hemorrhage in the spinal cord.

MRI: MRI is crucial for the diagnosis of spinal fracture; MRI is especially sensitive to implicit occult fractures that do not significantly deform the vertebral bodies (Figs. 8.44 and 8.47). MRI is the only method that can provide an assessment of the spinal cord (Figs. 8.46 and 8.47). MRI is also most sensitive to traumatic edema in the peripheral soft tissues of the spine.

Because acute fracture is accompanied by bone marrow edema, T1WI signals in MRI are hypointense. Thus, the observation of T1WI images is crucial (Figs. 8.44, 8.45, 8.46, 8.47, and 8.48). T2WI signals are hyperintense but insufficiently sensitive, whereas T2 STIR images are more explicit than T2WI images regarding the signal change due to bone marrow edema.

After the acute period, vertebral bodies continue to collapse and deform, but the signal gradually returns to normal, i.e., T1WI signals are hyperintense, and T2WI and T2 STIR signals are hypointense. Because old vertebral body fractures are height-decreased and deformed, unlike MRI, X-ray and CT differentiate new from old fractures in the vertebral bodies with difficulty (Figs. 8.44 and 8.48).

8.7.3 Osteoporotic Vertebral Fracture

Osteoporosis is a common geriatric problem, particularly among menopausal women. Minor trauma injuries in people with osteoporosis can cause a bone fracture, mostly in the vertebral body (Figs. 8.44 and 8.48), proximal femur, distal radius, and proximal humerus, of which vertebral fractures are often overlooked [9].

The osteoporosis-induced spinal fracture generally occurs in the vertebral body; these fractures can be distinguished into wedge, biconcave, and crush fractures. Attention must be paid to shape changes, and particularly to the changes in MRI signals. Hypointense T1WI signals are the most sensitive, and its combination with hyperintense T2STIR signals allows for a definitive diagnosis of acute compression fracture. Although an occult fracture exhibits no deformity in the vertebral body, a diagnosis of compression fracture can be achieved if changes in MRI signals occur (Fig. 8.44).

Currently, compression fractures are treated with vertebroplasty. Older adults often develop fractures over time. For these adults, a comparison between current and previous X-rays and CT scans allows clinicians to distinguish between new and old fractures. However, in the absence of previous X-ray and CT results, MRI must be used to distinguish between old and new vertebral fractures (Figs. 8.44 and 8.48).

In the case of an osteoporotic compression fracture, attention must be paid to pathological fracture, which is a type of compression fracture that is caused by malignancy in the vertebral body. (see the following Sect. 8.8).

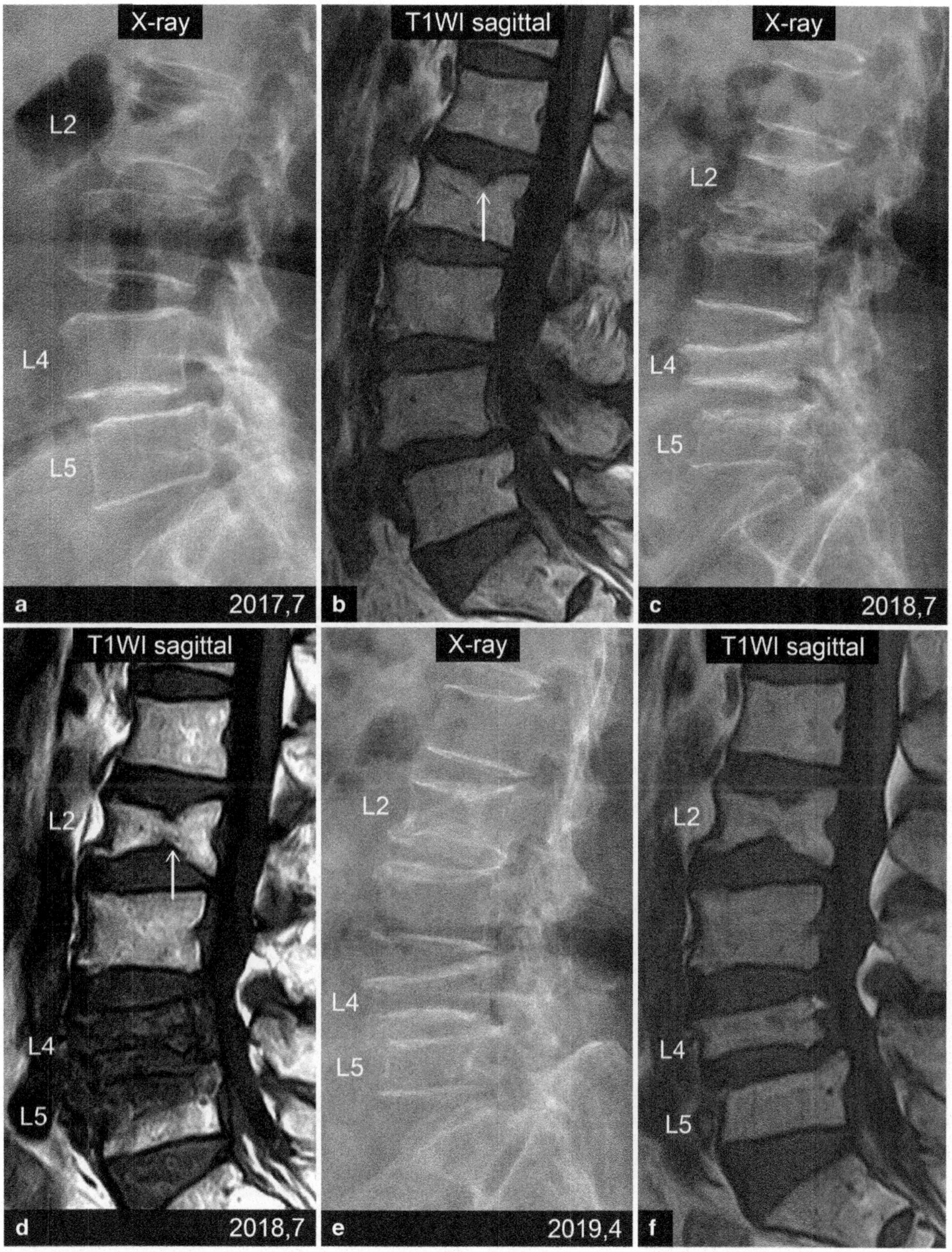

Fig. 8.44 F/64, Compression fractures, acute, and old. This woman has osteoporosis and suffered severe low back pain after a fall. (**a, b**) X-ray and MRI: Mild spondylolisthesis of L4 on L5, a small Schmorl's node (arrow) in the superior end plate of L2 vertebral body, no fracture is noted. 1 year later, more severe low back pain after another fall. (**c**) X-ray: Significantly decreased the body height of the L4 vertebral body, indicating wedge compression fracture. The L2, L5 vertebral bodies also show slightly reduced body height. (**d**) MRI, T1WI: Decreased body height and hypointense L4 vertebral body represent acute compression fracture. Hypointensity is observed in the superior half of the L5 vertebral body, indicating compression fracture. Surface depressions appear in the inferior (arrow) and superior end plates of L2 vertebral body and the discs herniate into them, creating defects known as Schmorl's nodes. The body height of the L2 vertebral body is reduced, but the signal intensity is not changed, indicating the absence of acute compression fracture. This patient received conservative treatment, and symptoms subsided. Follow-up X-ray and MRI were performed 9 months later. (**e, f**) X-ray and MRI: In X-ray, the shape of the L2,4 vertebral bodies (**e**) is the same as 9 months ago (**c**), but in the present MRI (**f**), the signal intensity of L4,5 vertebral bodies restore to be normal because they changed to be old fractures, which is different from the MRI 9 months ago (**d**). Comment: Acute and chronic compression fractures cannot be easily distinguished in X-ray images, but the signal change on T1WI in MRI shows that the lost signal intensity (change to be hypointense due to bone marrow edema) is an acute fracture, whereas the signal intensity restores to hyperintensity is a chronic fracture

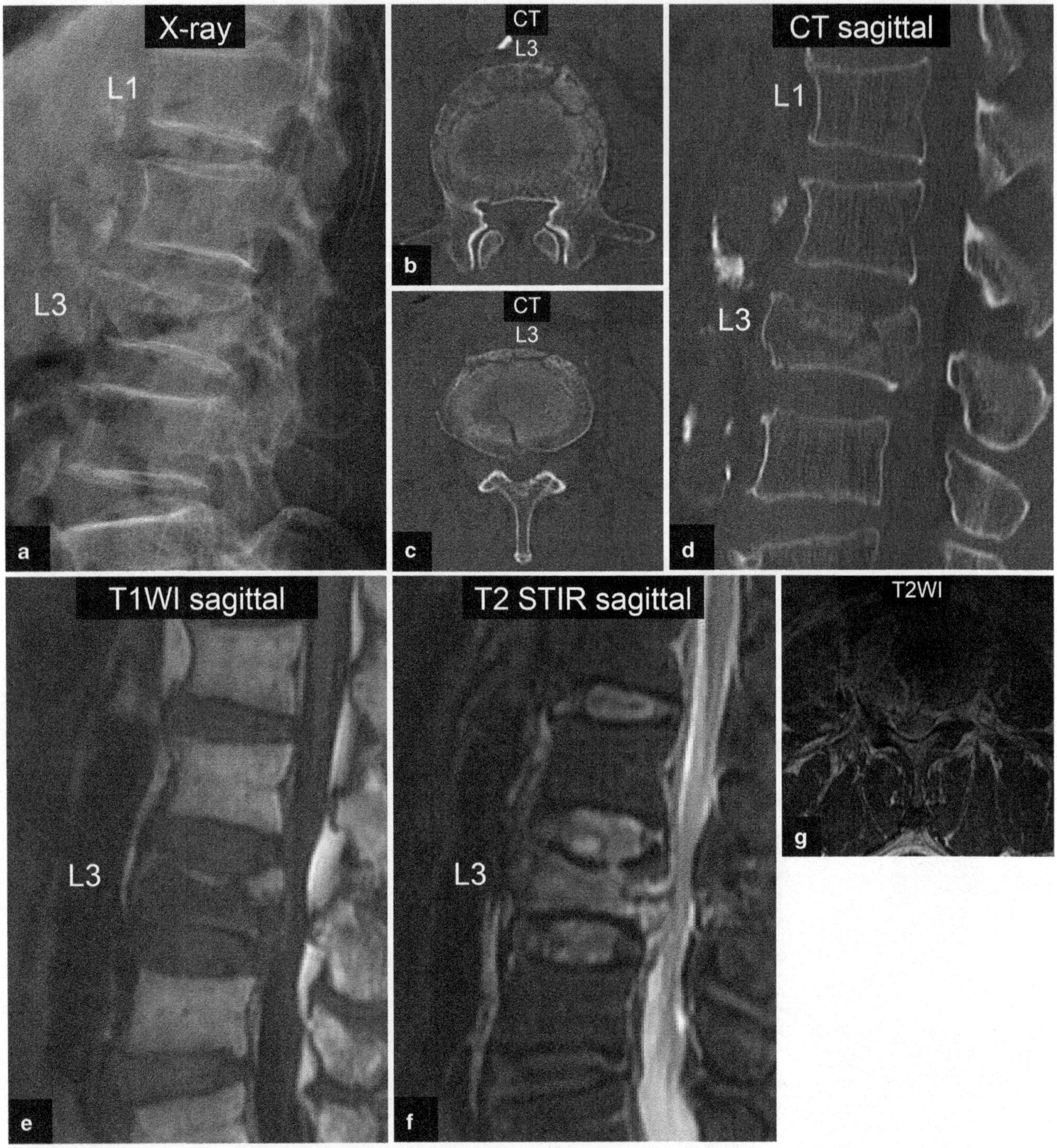

Fig. 8.45 M/70, L3 burst fracture. This patient suffered severe low back pain after a traffic accident. (**a**) X-ray: Reduction of the height of the L3 vertebral body and a concave in the middle, which is a significant compression fracture. (**b, c**) CT, axial sections: Several vertical and transverse fracture lines, reflecting that this is a burst fracture. (**d**) CT sagittal reconstruction: Clearly shows the fractures than X-ray and the vertebral body backward displacement into the spinal canal. (**e, f**) MRI: The L3 vertebral body shows hypointensity on T1WI and hyperintensity on T2 STIR, representing acute compression fracture with bone marrow edema. (**g**) MRI, the axial section does not clearly show the fractures as the axial section of the CT scan

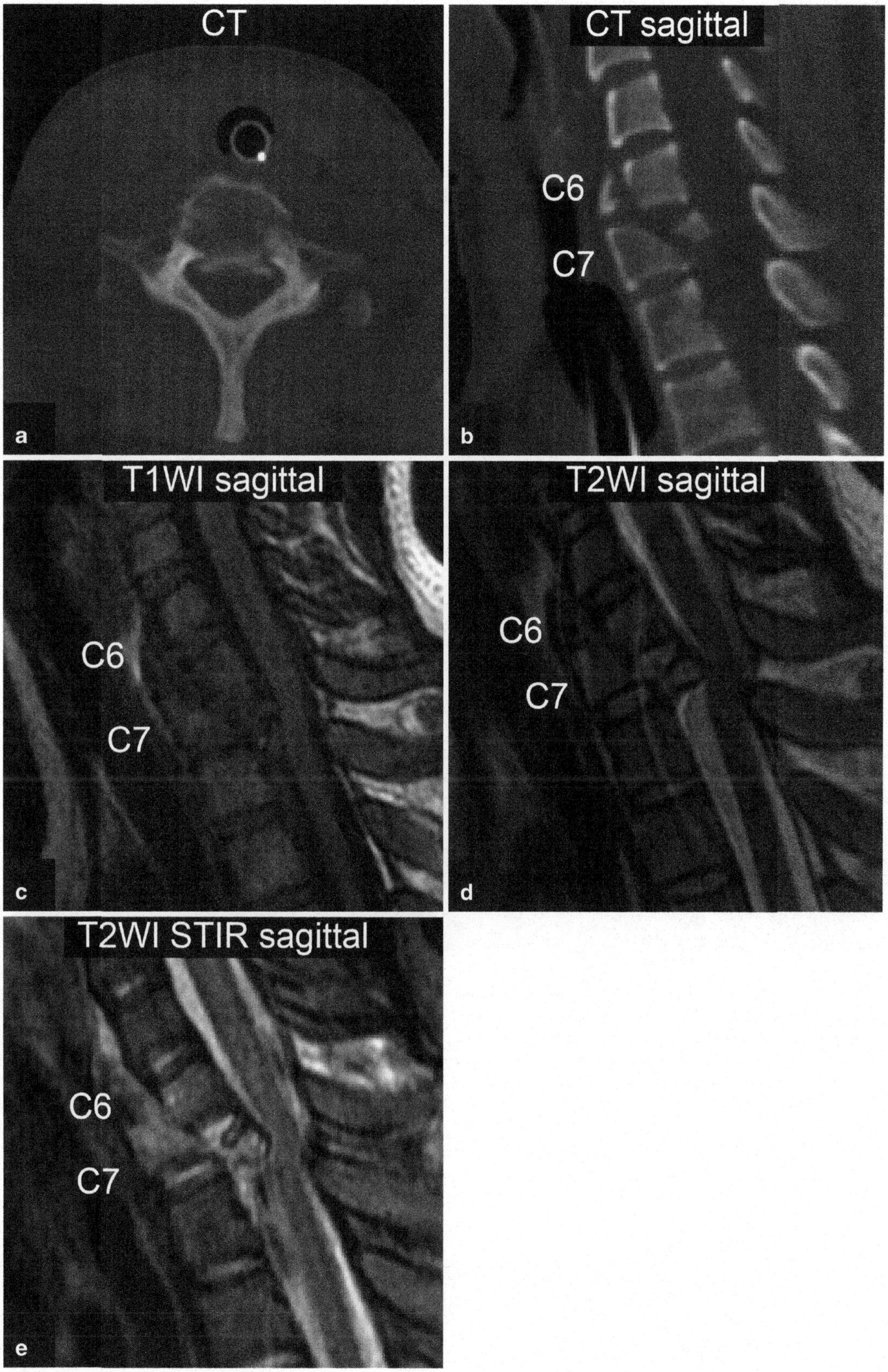

Fig. 8.46 F/21, Flexion-distraction fracture. This patient suffered quadriplegia after a traffic accident with a cervical spine injury. (**a**, **b**) CT, axial, and sagittal reconstruction: Fractures and displacement of the anterior portion of C6 and posterior portion of C7 vertebral bodies occur. The fracture fragment of C7 posteriorly moves into the spinal canal. CT cannot show the spinal cord. (**c**–**e**) MRI: Fractures are not necessarily more precise than CT, but MRI shows that the C7 fracture fragment backward shifts in the spinal canal and slightly compresses the spinal cord, the no signal change of the spinal cord indicates no edema or hemorrhage

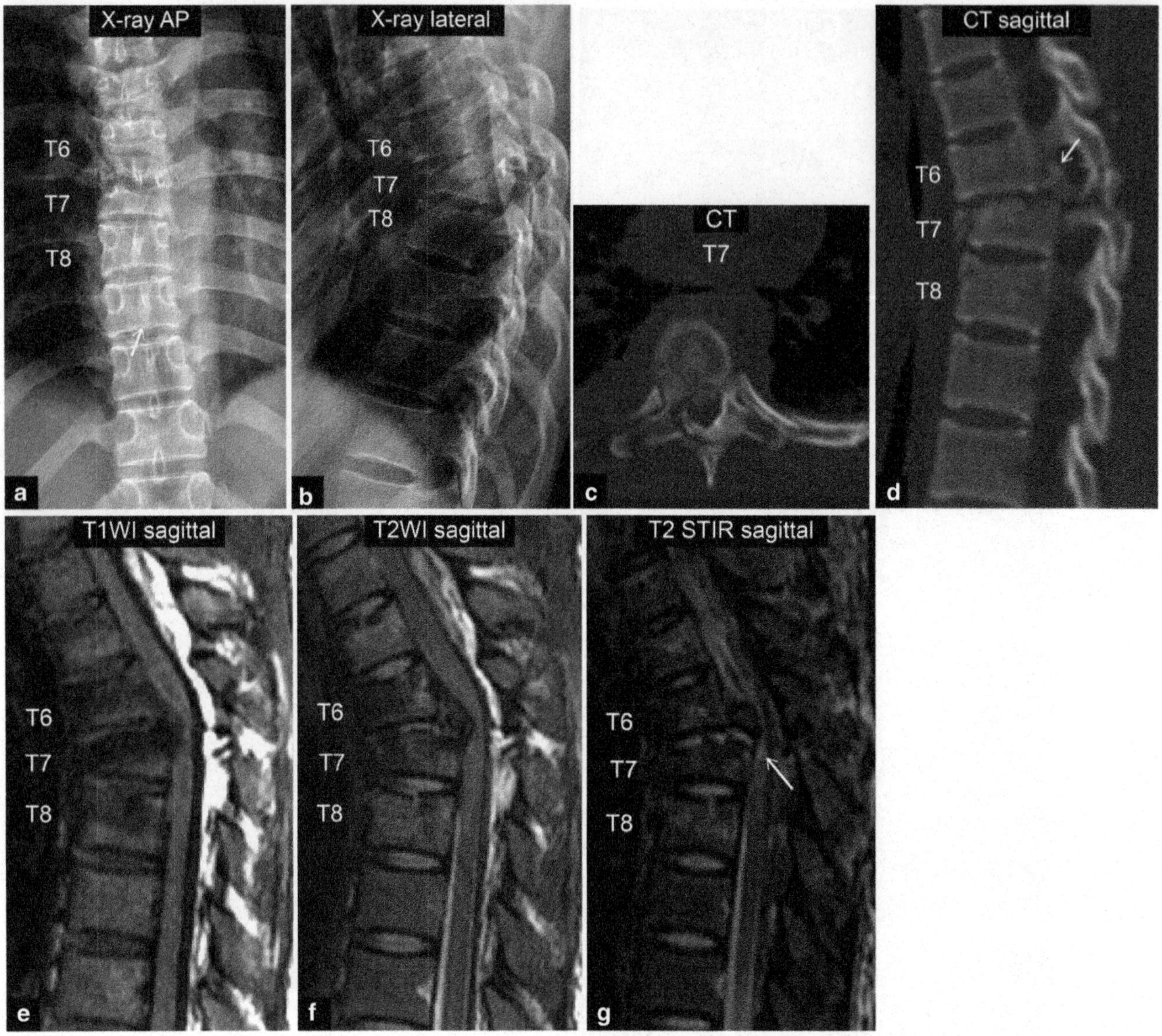

Fig. 8.47 M/27, Flexion-distraction fracture.. This patient suffered paraplegia after a traffic accident. (**a**, **b**) X-ray: In the AP view, the T6,7 intervertebral disc space is not clear. In the lateral view, the T7 vertebral body shows a wedge shape, reflecting acute compression fracture. (**c**) CT: Several fractures occur in the posterior column of the T7 vertebral body, including fractures in the lamina, transverse process, and spinous process, and distraction of the vertebral body. (**d**) CT, sagittal reconstruction: Bony fractures occur in the anterior of T7,8 vertebral bodies, a posterior fracture fragment of T7 embeds in the spinal canal (arrow), and other fractures of the posterior column of T7, spondylolisthesis of T6 on T7. CT can precisely demonstrate the condition of fractures but cannot evaluate the situation of the spinal cord. (**e**–**g**) MRI: There is a reduction in body height and signal change of the T7 vertebral body, reflecting acute compression fracture. No significant decrease in body height but with the signal change of T6,8, so also have fractures. The fracture fragment backward embeds into the spinal canal and severely compresses the spinal cord, which shows focal hyperintensity on T2 STIR and reflects spinal cord edema (arrow)

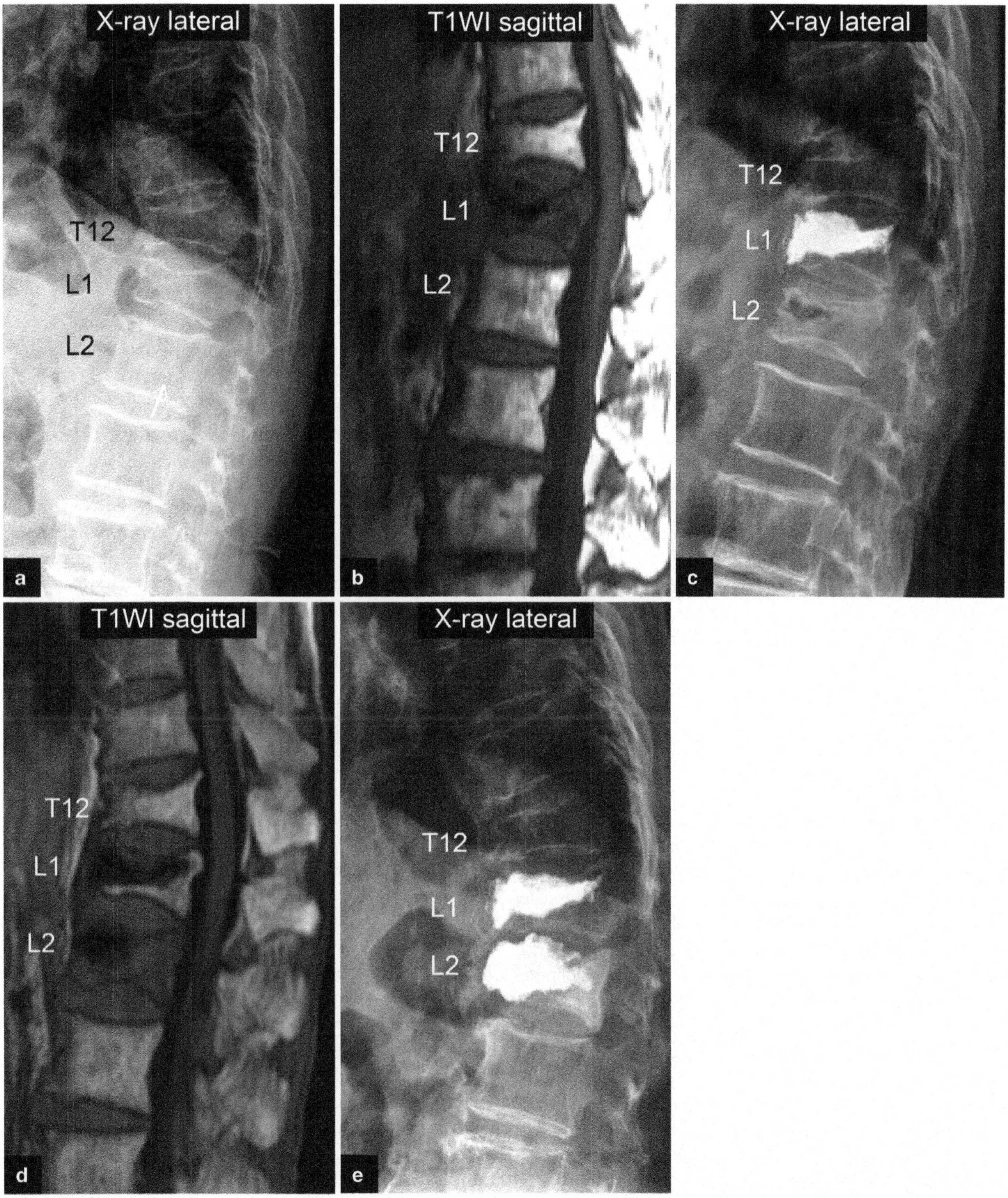

Fig. 8.48 F/87, Osteoporosis, and repeat compression fractures. This patient has osteoporosis and has fallen many times. This time, the patient suffered severe low back pain after a fall. (**a**) X-ray: Wedge shape and reduction in body height of T12, L1 vertebral bodies, represent compression fractures, but X-ray cannot distinguish new or old fractures. (**b**) MRI, T1WI: The L1 vertebral body shows hypointensity, representing bone marrow edema due to acute fracture. No change in the signal intensity of the T12 vertebral body, indicating old compression fracture. The patient received vertebroplasty of L1. 3 years later, another fall caused severe low back pain again. (**c**) X-ray: Still old fracture of T12, cement retention in L1 vertebral body due to vertebroplasty, reduction in L2 vertebral body, indicating a new compression fracture. (**d**) MRI, T1WI: The lost signal intensity of the L2 vertebral body, MRI confirms this is acute compression fracture with bone marrow edema. The L1 also shows hypointensity because of cement retention in the vertebral body. (**e**) X-ray after vertebroplasty: Cement retention in the L1, L2 vertebral bodies

8.8 Spinal Tumors

Spinal tumors can be classified into three types according to the anatomical location of the tumor [10]:

1. **Intramedullary tumors**
   - The most common intramedullary tumors are ependymoma (Fig. 8.49) and astrocytoma (Fig. 8.50), and a few cases are hemangioblastoma. Ependymoma is common in adults, and astrocytoma occurs mostly in children and young adults [11].
   - The intramedullary tumor is accompanied by syringomyelia (Fig. 8.50), and the spinal cord above and below the tumor may have a cyst (Fig. 8.49).
   - In young adults, ependymoma may develop in the filum terminale at the end of the spinal cord in the lumbar spine (Fig. 8.51).
   - Filum terminale also develops into rare tumors, such as paraganglioma and primitive neuroectodermal tumor (PNET). Because the lumbar spine does not have spinal cord, tumors of the filum terminale are also a type of intradural tumor.
2. **Intradural extramedullary tumors** and **intradural tumors**
   - The most common intradural extramedullary tumors are meningioma growing from the spinal dura (Figs. 8.52, 8.53, and 8.54) and schwannoma growing from the nerve root (Figs. 8.55, 8.56, and 8.57) [12]. Meningioma is typically situated in the thoracic spine and mostly occurs in middle-aged women; it may contain calcifications (Fig. 8.54).
   - Spinal schwannomas mainly grow in the cervical and lumbar spine. Specifically, intradural extramedullary schwannoma grows in the cervical region, and intradural schwannoma grows in the lumbar region because the lumbar spine does not have a spinal cord. Schwannoma can easily penetrate the spinal dura and grow along with the nerve roots toward the neuroforamen and along the paravertebral direction, forming a dumbbell shape (Figs. 8.55 and 8.56). Schwannoma can also be completely extradural, and even paravertebral (Fig. 8.58). Because schwannoma is a slow-growing tumor, it easily erodes the adjacent bones (Fig. 8.56). Schwannoma is mostly solid and tends to exhibit cystic change (Fig. 8.57).
   - Some kind of intracranial tumors may spread to the spinal canal by CSF seeding; this is another kind of intradural tumor (Fig. 8.59).
3. **Extradural tumors**

   Extradural tumors can develop in the following locations.

   (a) The spinal canal, including arachnoid cyst (Fig. 8.60), lymphoma, and hemangioma (Fig. 8.61). The perineural cyst is also commonly found in the sacrum (Fig. 8.62) and lumbar spine.

   (b) The vertebral body, where cancer metastasis is the most common and most important (Figs. 8.63, 8.64, 8.65, 8.66, and 8.67). Primary tumors include a few malignant tumors (e.g., hemangiopericytoma) and benign tumors (e.g., hemangioma). Primary tumors in the sacrum are typically chordoma (Fig. 8.68).

   Malignant tumors in the vertebral body may cause compression fracture, which is a pathological fracture (Figs. 8.66 and 8.67) [13] that may compress the spinal cord, causing paralysis.

Spinal tumors are not associated with any specific symptoms. Clinical signs include back pain, numbness, weakness in the arms and legs, and other symptoms of radiculopathy or myelopathy, which are similar to the symptoms of degenerative spondylosis. Therefore, spinal tumors are often clinically considered as degenerative spondylosis (Figs. 8.52, 8.53, and 8.58) or spinal trauma injuries (Fig. 8.65) and do medical imaging, then the spinal tumors are identified. Spinal tumors are suspected only when a patient presents clear signs of myelopathy. Hence, medical imaging is imperative for the diagnosis of spinal tumors. In imaging, MRIs are the most crucial; however, X-rays are generally the first-line diagnostic tool although CTs are occasionally performed.

X-ray: Intramedullary and intradural tumors are undetectable with X-rays. In cases of vertebral body tumors, X-rays can indicate osteolytic (Figs. 8.63 and 8.66) or osteoblastic changes. In cases of osteolysis, attention must be paid to the presence or absence of pedicles (Fig. 8.63) on X-ray AP views. Attention should be paid to whether the compression fracture is a pathological fracture (Fig. 8.66).

CT: A clear view of osteolytic (Figs. 8.63 and 8.64) and osteoblastic changes (Fig. 8.64) is afforded by CT. However, for soft tissue mass, the clarity of CT is inferior to that of MRI. In contrast to MRI, CT cannot provide clear images of intramedullary tumors of the spinal cord and other tumors compressing the spinal cord. In some cases, tumor calcification can be observed with CT but not with MRI (Fig. 8.54).

MRI: As the most crucial tool for the examination of spinal tumors, particularly intramedullary tumors, MRI indicates spinal cord swelling (Figs. 8.49 and 8.50) and signal changes. When the gadolinium contrast agent is injected, the tumor is enhanced and necrosis is visible. MRI can indicate edema and syringomyelia which may be associated with spinal cord tumors (Fig. 8.50).

In cases of an intradural extramedullary tumor, according to the widening of the CSF space above and below the tumor (CSF space-widening sign), it indicates the spinal cord is compressed by the tumor (Figs. 8.52, 8.53, and 8.54).

MRI provides a clear view of the extradural tumor located inside and outside of the spinal canal (Figs. 8.55 and 8.56) as well as the extent to which the tumor has invaded the bone of the vertebral body (Figs. 8.56, 8.63, 8.64, 8.65, 8.66, and 8.67).

In cases of a compression fracture, attention must be paid to the presence or absence of paravertebral soft tissue mass and epidural mass in the spinal canal. The compression fracture associated with paravertebral or epidural mass is often caused by malignancy (Figs. 8.66 and 8.67). When necessary, a contrast agent can be used to prevent a misdiagnosis of osteoporotic fracture.

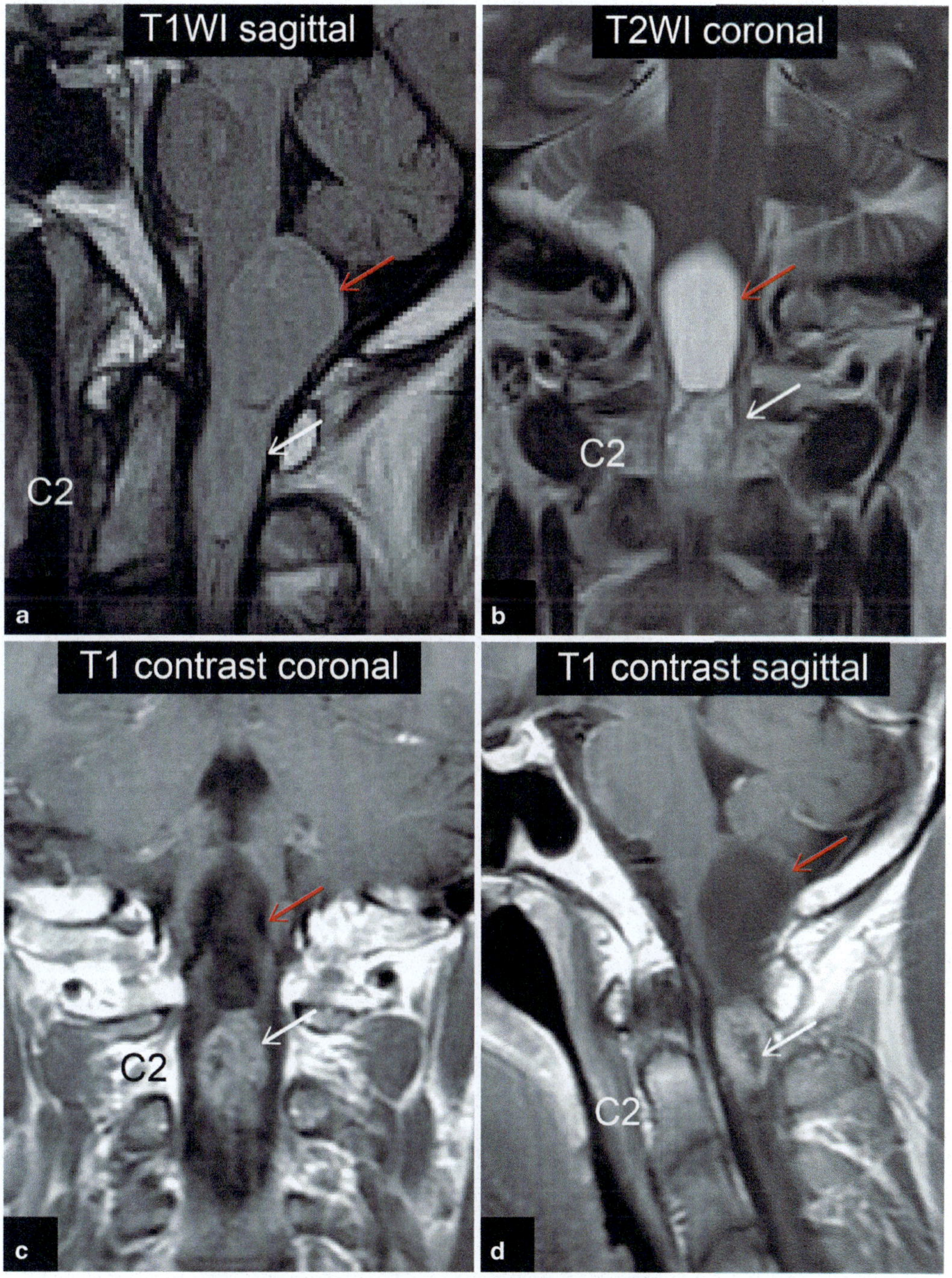

Fig. 8.49 M/30, Spinal cord ependymoma. This patient complained of dizziness and left-hand numbness, weakness. (**a**) MRI, T1WI, sagittal: A tumor mass (white arrow) in the spinal cord, C1–2 level, and extending upward to the medulla oblongata (red arrow). (**b**) MRI, T2WI, coronal: The superior part shows homogeneous hyperintensity, is cystic content (red arrow). The inferior part is soft tissue mass (white arrow). (**c**, **d**) Contrast T1WI: The inferior part (white arrows) has well-enhancement and with some central necrosis. No contrast enhancement of the superior cystic part (red arrow). For such type of intramedullary tumor, ependymoma should be the first consideration followed by astrocytoma because this patient is an adult. Surgical removal of this tumor, pathology proved to be ependymoma, WHO Gr-II

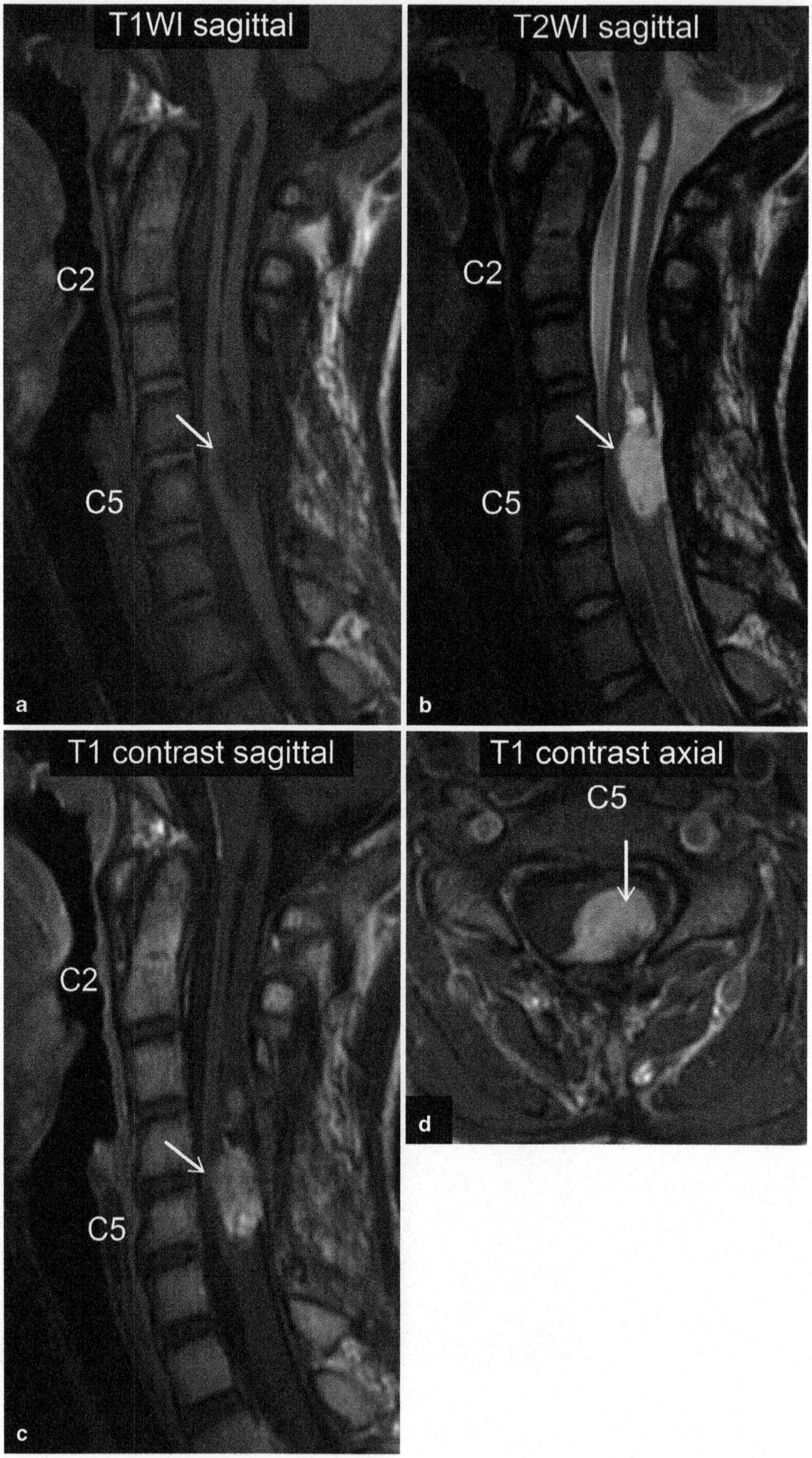

Fig. 8.50 M/13, Spinal cord astrocytoma. This boy complained of four limb weakness and numbness for several months. (**a**, **b**) MRI: The spinal cord shows swelling in the C4–5 level and contains a tumor (arrow), which shows hypointensity on T1WI and hyperintensity on T2WI. Syringomyelia is observed in the spinal cord from C1 to C4 and upward to the medulla oblongata. (**c**, **d**) Contrast T1WI: Homogeneous enhancement of the tumor occurs in the C4–5 level and combines with syringomyelia above it. For this intramedullary tumor, the first consideration should be astrocytoma, followed by ependymoma because this patient is a child. After surgical removal of this tumor, pathology proved to be low-grade fibrillary diffuse astrocytoma (WHO grade II)

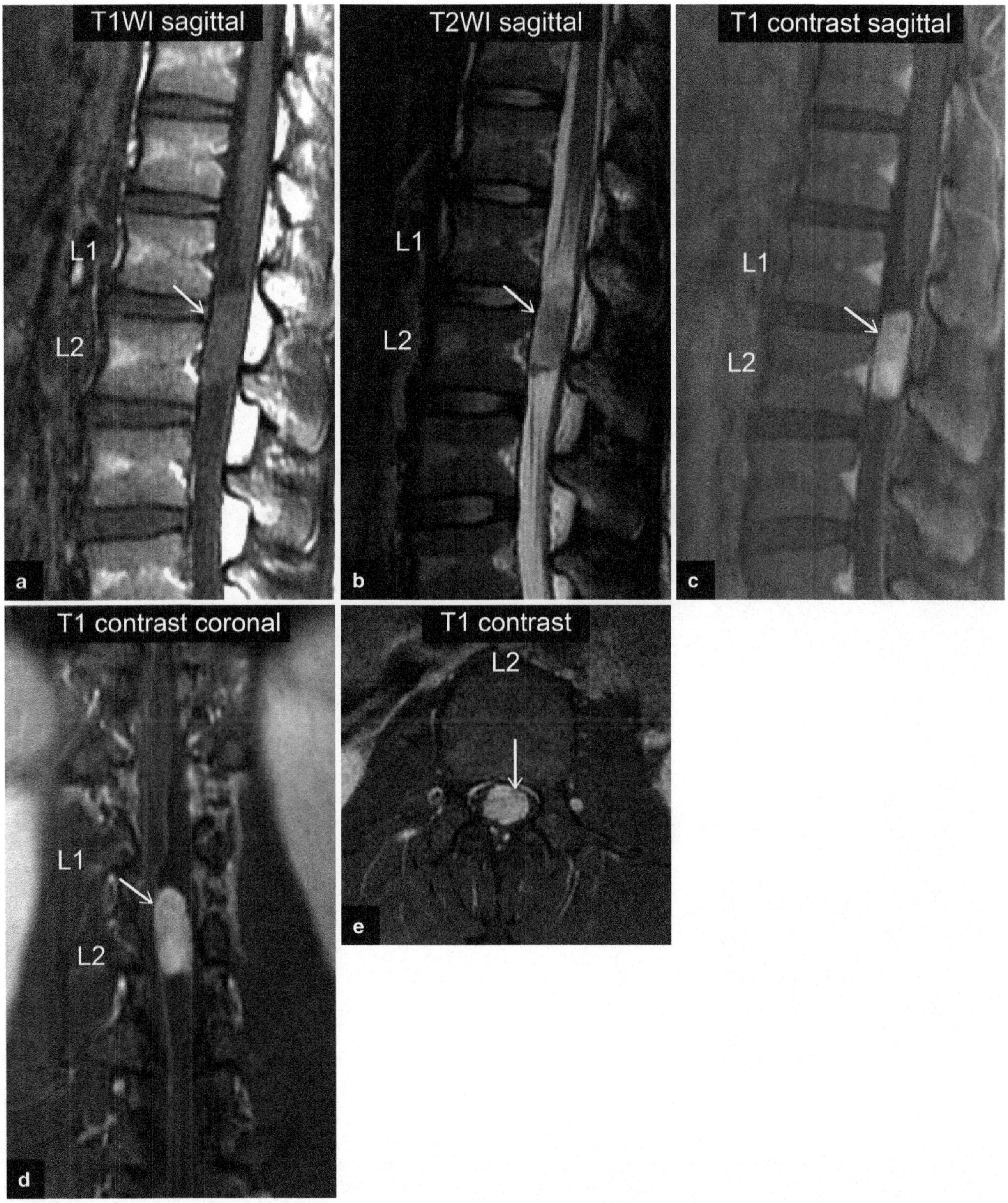

Fig. 8.51 M/17, Filum terminale ependymoma. This patient complained of weakness of both legs and lower back pain for 2 months. (**a–e**) MRI: Soft tissue tumor mass (arrows) in the L1–2 level, indicating an intradural tumor. Contrast T1WI shows good and homogeneous enhancement. Young people have a tumor in this location, an ependymoma arising from the filum terminale should be considered. Surgical removal of this tumor and pathology proved to be filum terminale ependymoma, Gr-II

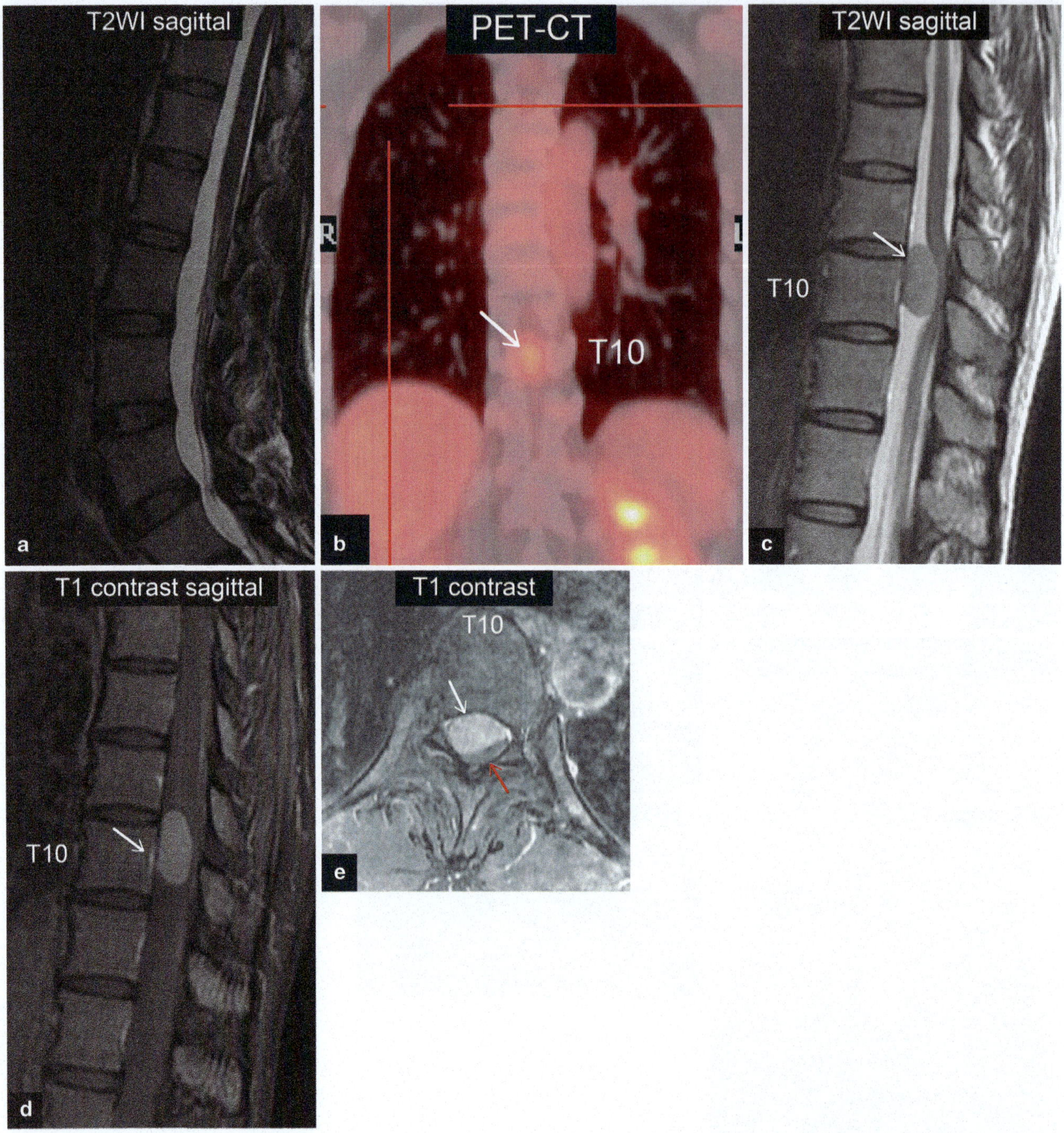

Fig. 8.52 F/44, T-spine meningioma. This patient suffered severe low back pain for several months. (**a**) MRI of the lumbar spine: The clinician considered she had degenerative spondylosis of the lumbar spine and thus arranged an MRI examination. However, results showed no significant abnormality. (**b**) PET-CT was performed a month later: A high-signal lesion in the T10 level (arrow). PET is sensitive for detecting an intense hypermetabolism tumor but is unsuitable for the outline of a tumor and peripheral anatomies. Thus, another MRI of the thoracic spine was performed. (**c**–**e**) MRI: a tumor (white arrow) in the T10 level, there is a widening of CSF space above and below this tumor (CSF space-widening sign), reflecting this is an intradural extramedullary tumor. It shows homogeneous contrast enhancement, and the spinal cord is severely compressed and backward displaced (red arrow). For a middle-aged woman, an intradural extramedullary tumor in the thoracic spine is first considered to be a meningioma. Surgical removal of this tumor and pathology proved to be a meningioma

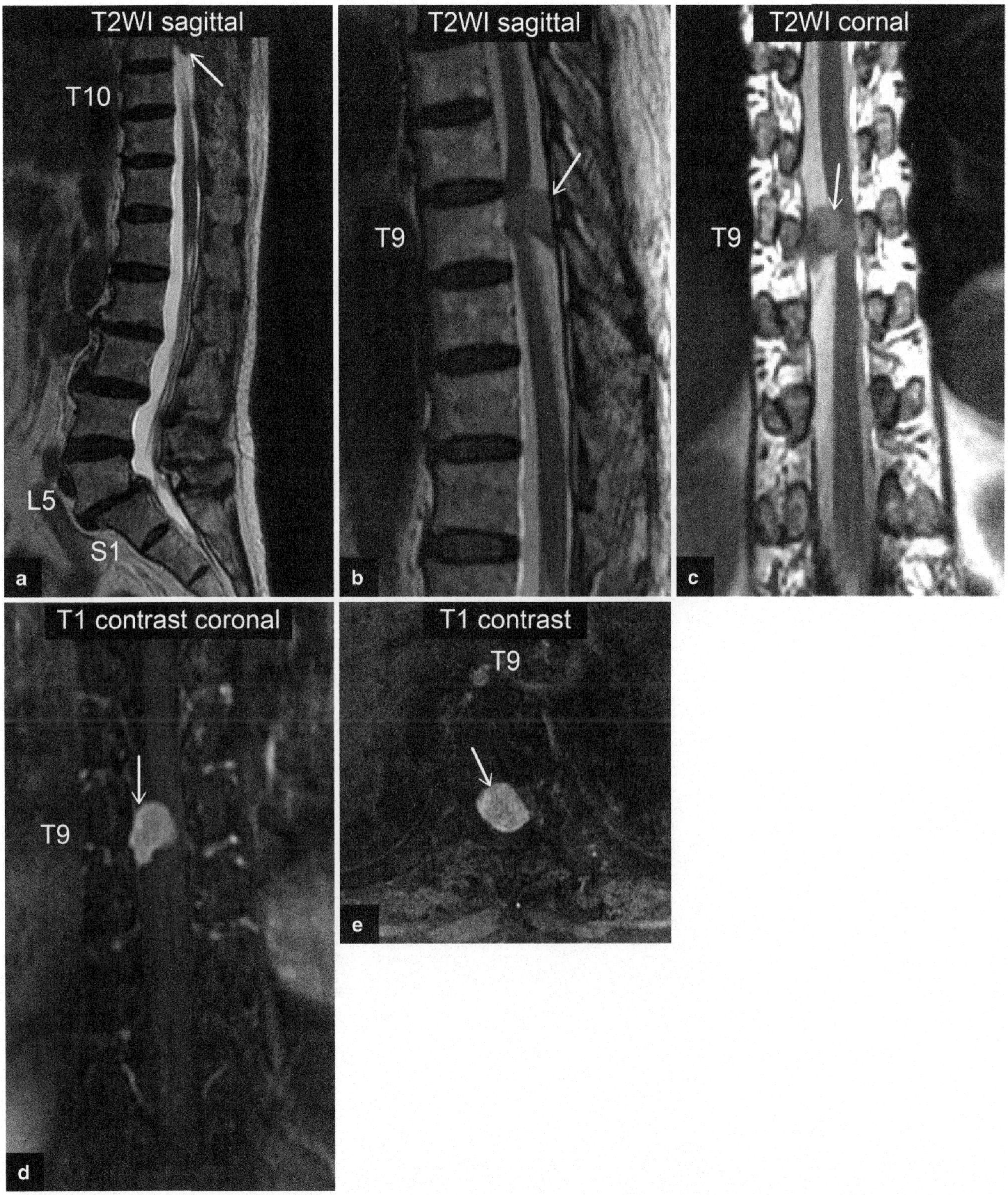

Fig. 8.53 F/73 T-spine meningioma. This patient suffered severe low back pain for several months. The clinician considered she had degenerative spondylosis of the lumbar spine and thus arranged an MRI examination. (**a**) MRI: Spondylolisthesis of L5 on S1 is found. However, the radiologist found a suspicious mass lesion at the T9 level (arrow). Thus, a repeat MRI for the thoracic spine was performed. (**b**–**e**) MRI: There is a typical intradural extramedullary tumor (arrows) in the T9 level, with excellent contrast enhancement, which compresses the spinal cord, the spinal cord is anteriorly and left side laterally displaced. An adult woman has a thoracic intradural extramedullary tumor; meningioma is first considered. Surgical removal of this tumor and pathology proved to be a meningioma

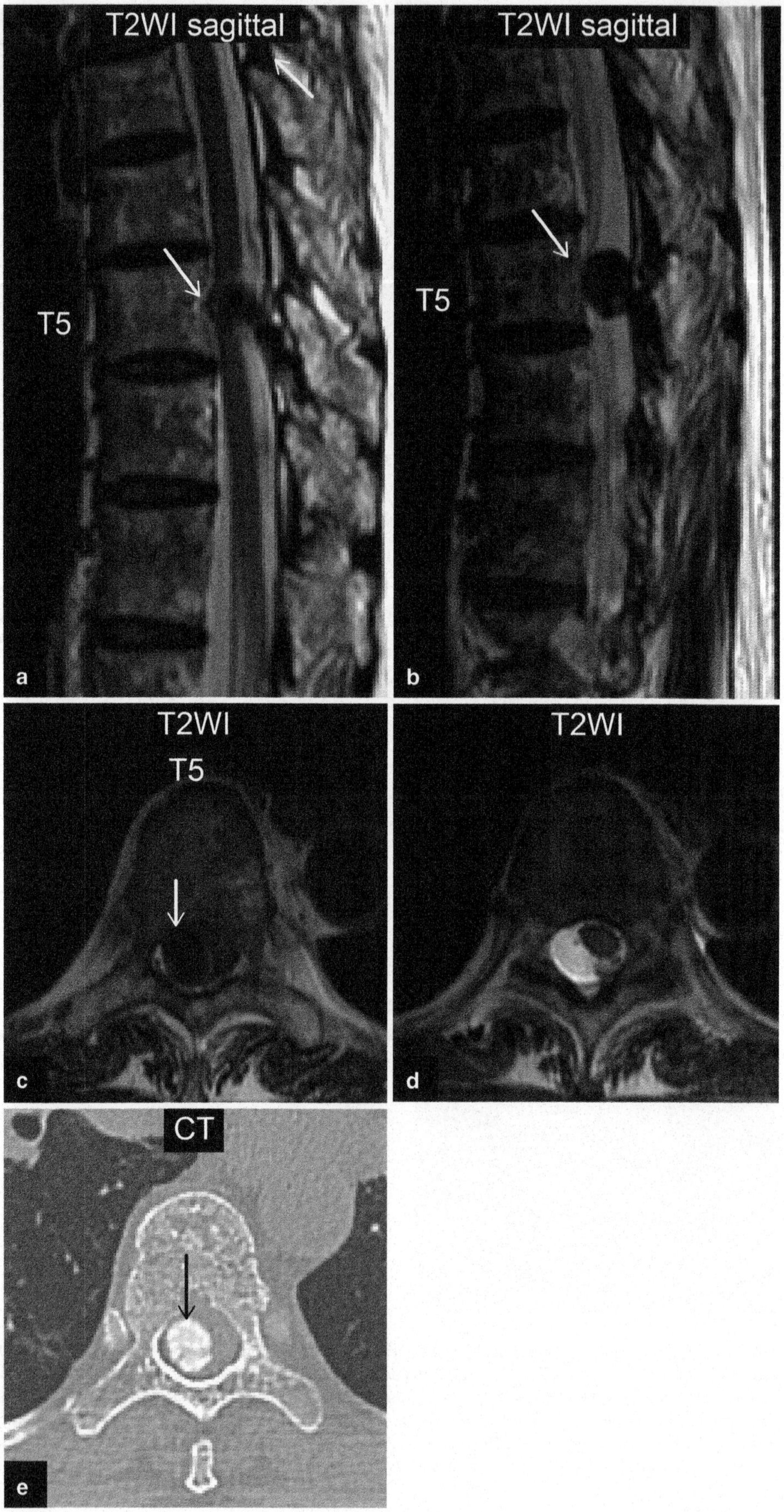

Fig. 8.54 F/64, Calcified meningioma. This patient complained about upper back pain and numbness of lower limbs for several months. (**a–d**) MRI: A hypointense mass (arrows) is found in the T5 level, which compresses the spinal cord. A "CSF space-widening sign" appears above and below this tumor, indicating an intradural extramedullary tumor. The signal intensity of this tumor is very low (dark) and hence should be considered a calcified meningioma. (**e**) CT (this patient received a CT of the lung 2 months ago): Total calcification of this tumor mass is noted. Surgical removal of this tumor and pathology proved to be a meningioma containing abundant psammoma bodies

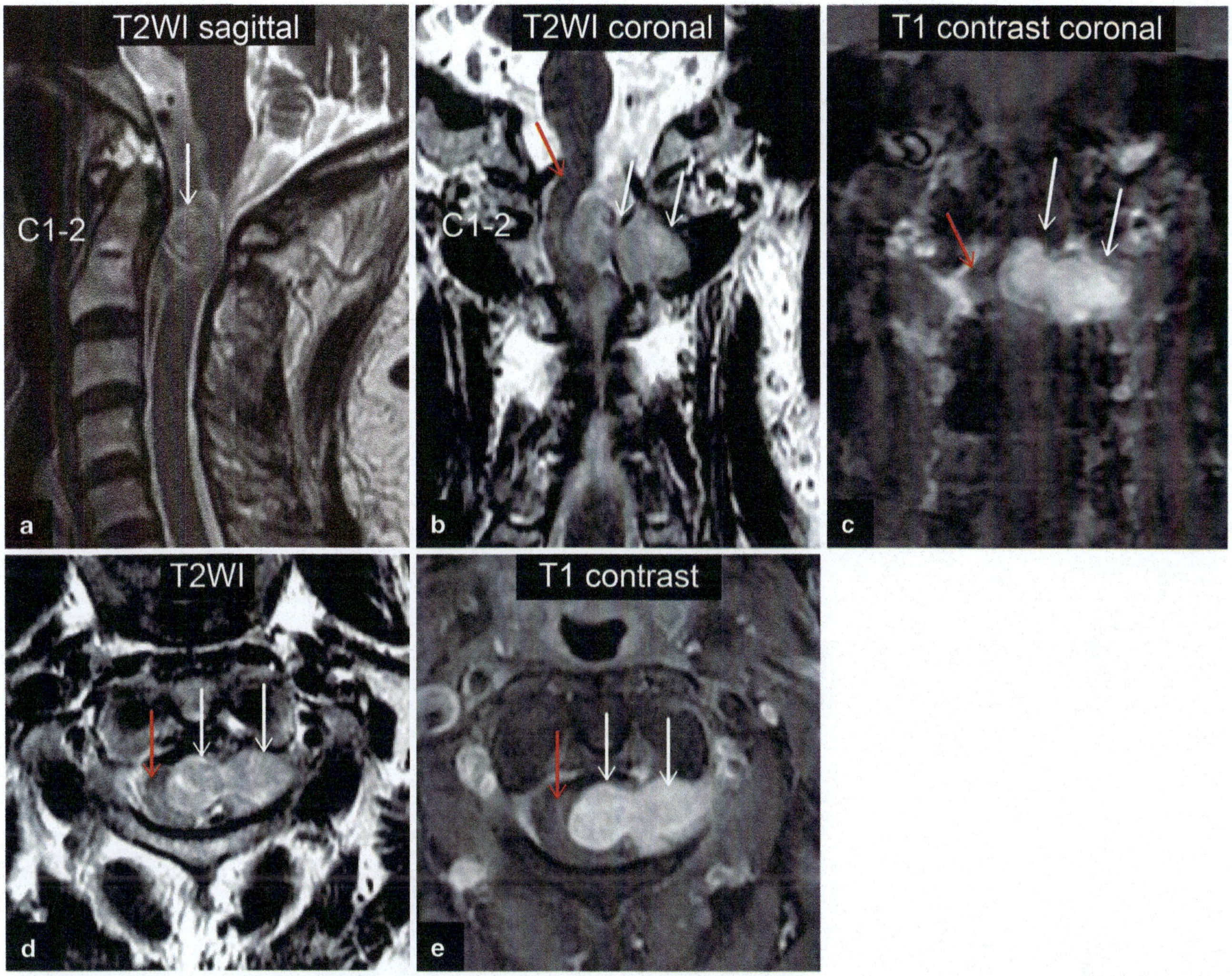

Fig. 8.55 F/73, Cervical spine schwannoma. This patient suffered neck pain and gradual weakness of both lower legs. (**a–e**) MRI: A tumor mass (white arrows) is found in the spinal canal, C1–2 level, and compresses the spinal cord (red arrow). Half of this tumor is in the spinal canal, and another half extends out via the neuroforamen, forms as a dumbbell shape, showing a typical schwannoma. Surgical removal of this tumor and pathology proved to be a schwannoma

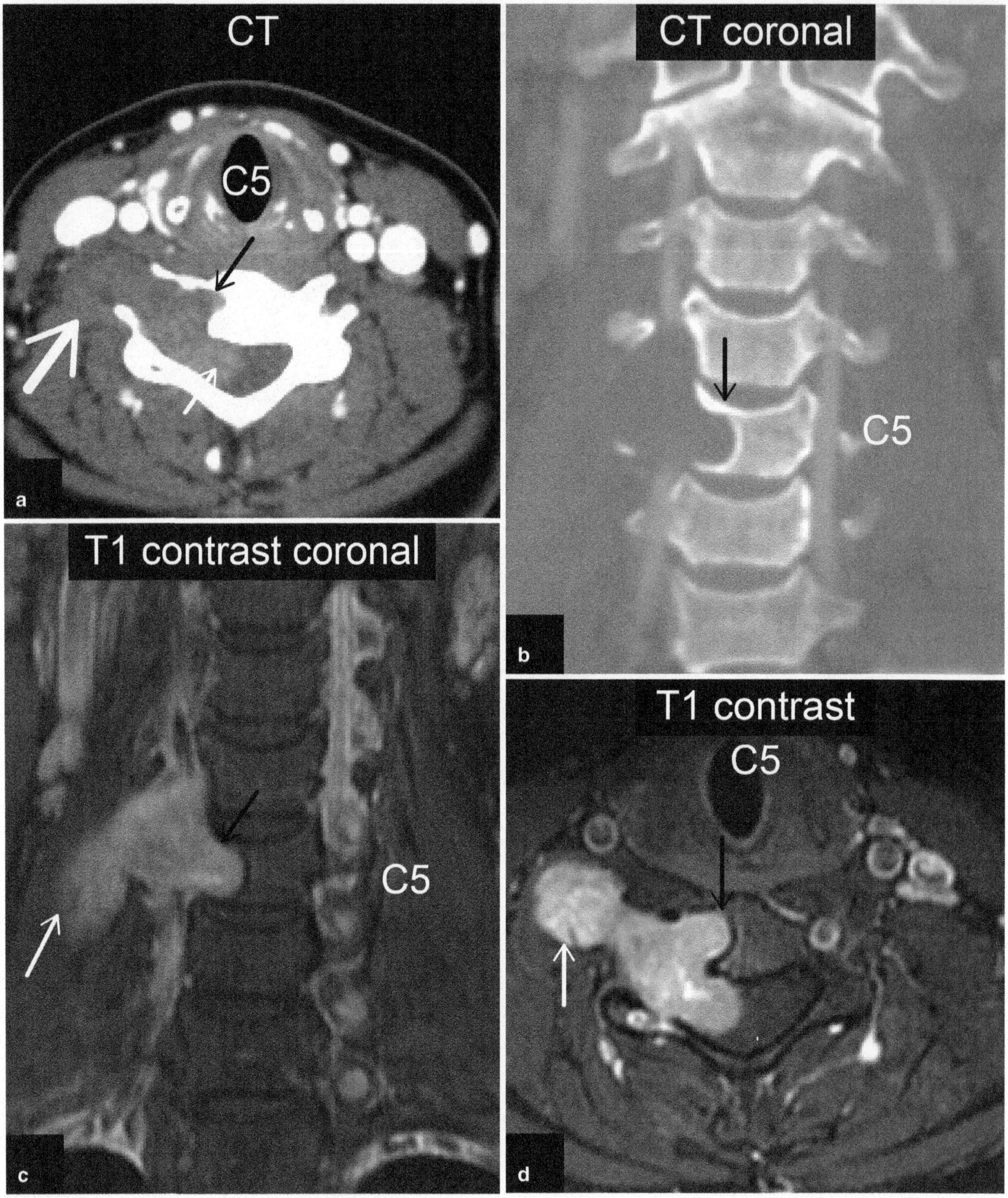

Fig. 8.56 F/28, Cervical schwannoma. The patient touched a lump in her right neck. She went to see an otolaryngologist and did this CT examination. (**a**) Contrast CT, C5 level: A soft tissue mass (thick arrow) is observed in the right-side neck, with mild contrast enhancement. Widening of the right neuroforamen and peripheral bony erosion (black arrow) is observed. A tumor in the spinal canal (thin white arrow) appears similar to a spinal canal tumor and extends to the paravertebral space via the neuroforamen. (**b**) CT, coronal reconstruction, bone window: The margin of the erosion (arrow) on the C5 vertebral body is smooth; this finding hints that it is a slow-growing tumor mass with gradual bony erosion. (**c**, **d**) MRI, contrast T1WI: Well-enhanced tumor mass, intradural, and with extradural extension via the neuroforamen, as dumbbell shape (arrows), indicating a typical schwannoma of the cervical nerve. Surgical removal of this tumor and pathology proved to be a schwannoma

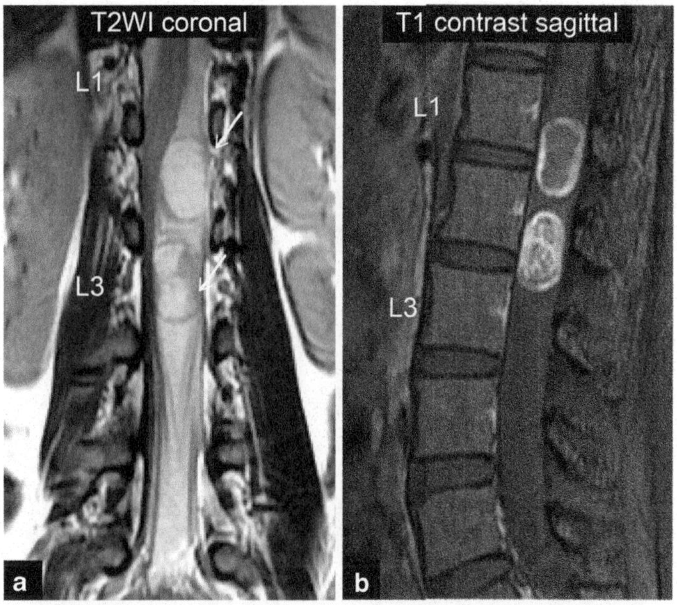

Fig. 8.57 F/37, Lumbar schwannoma. This patient complained of low back pain and numbness for several months. (**a**) MRI, T2WI: Two tumor masses (arrows) in the spinal canal, L1–3 level. (**b**) Contrast T1WI: The upper tumor mass shows rim enhancement, reflecting the complete central cystic change. The inferior tumor mass has some irregular cystic change. The outer margins of these tumors are smooth. For intradural tumors with a cystic change in the lumbar spine, the first consideration is schwannoma. Surgical removal of these tumors and pathology proved to be schwannomas

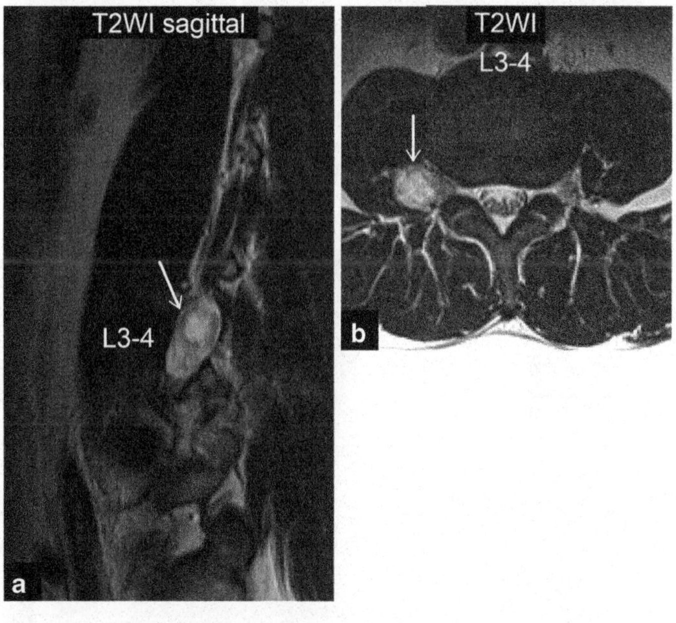

Fig. 8.58 M/48, Paravertebral schwannoma. This patient complained of lower back pain with radiation to the right lower leg; the symptom is like sciatica; thus, HIVD was suspected. (**a**, **b**) MRI: A tumor mass is found outside the right neuroforamen of L3–4. A tumor in this location should consider an extradural schwannoma. Surgical removal of this tumor and pathology proved to be schwannoma

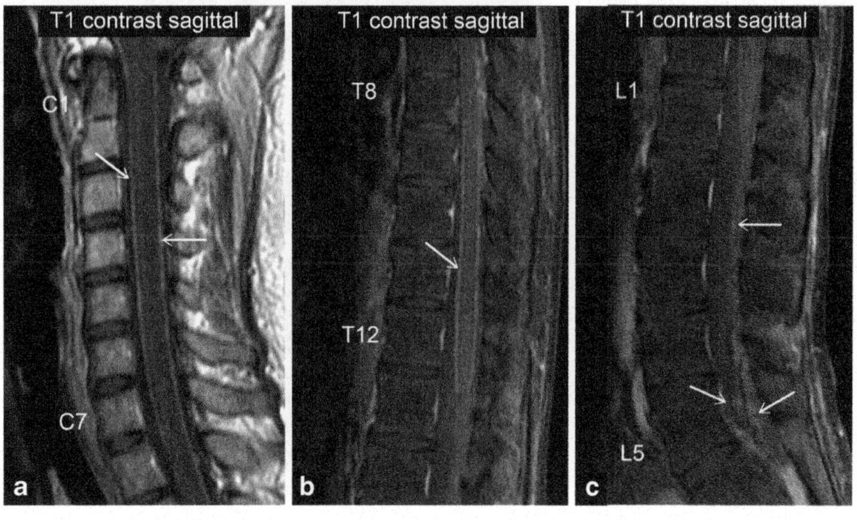

Fig. 8.59 F/26, Spinal seeding by intracranial malignancy. The patient had an intracranial malignant tumor. (**a**, **b**) Contrast T1WI, cervical and thoracic spine: Linear enhancement (arrows) is found on the surface of the cervical and thoracic spinal cord, representing infiltration with malignant tumor cells. (**c**) Contrast T1WI, lumbar spine: Nodular enhancement is observed on the cauda equina nerves (arrows), representing tumor cell infiltration on the nerves

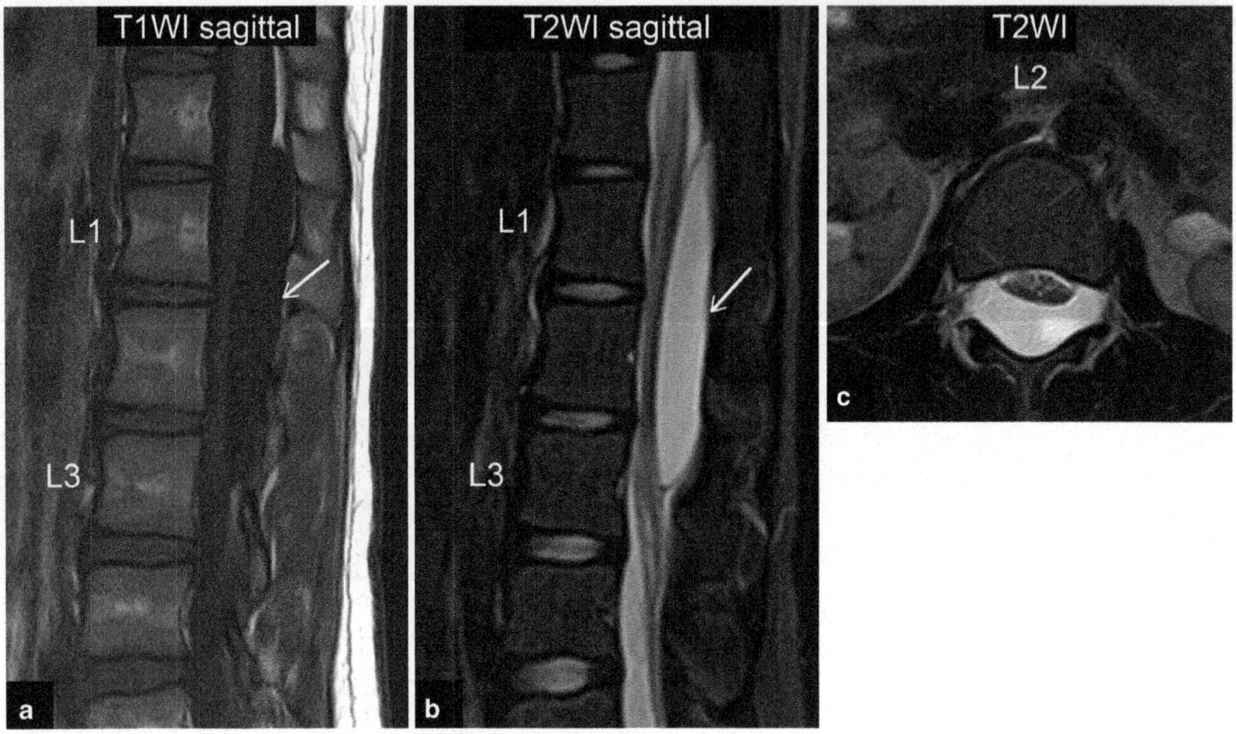

Fig. 8.60 F/16, Arachnoid cyst. This girl suffered low back pain for several months. (**a**–**c**) MRI: A long-shape cystic mass in the posterior of the spinal canal, L1–L3 levels, compressing the dural sac, which is anteriorly displaced. This is an epidural cyst. Surgical removal of this mass and pathology proved to be an arachnoid cyst

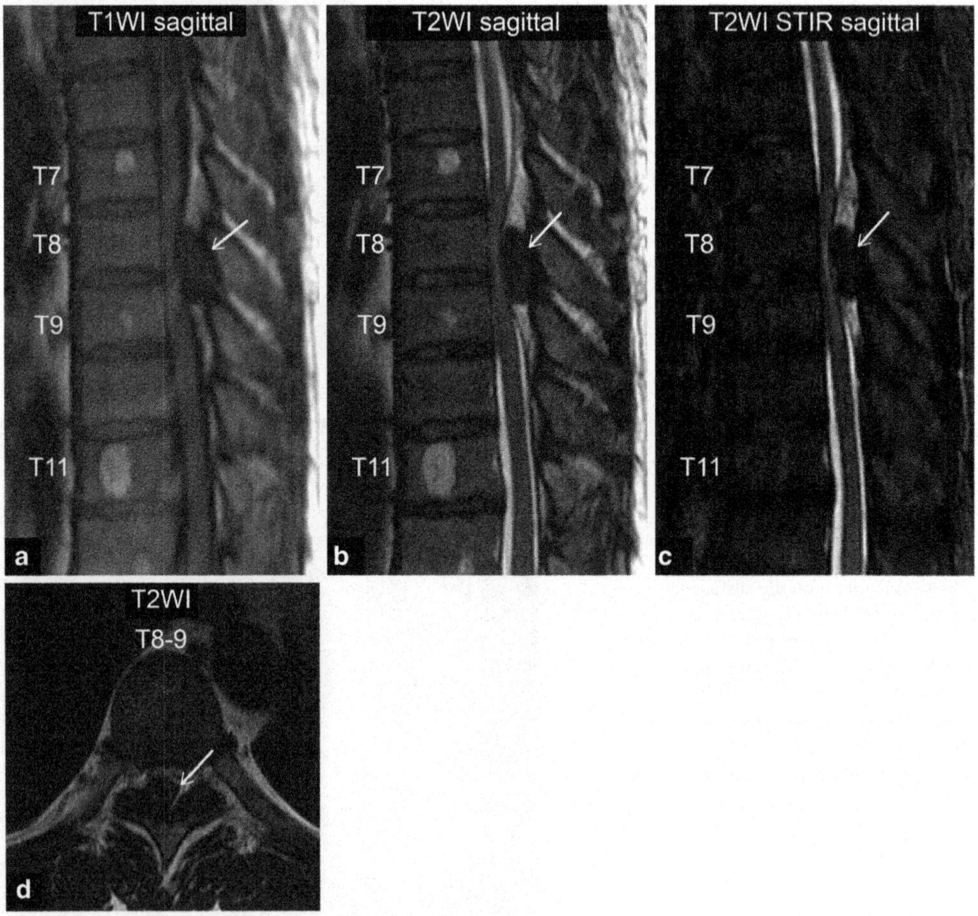

Fig. 8.61 M/45, Cavernous hemangioma. This patient suffered back pain for a long time. (**a**–**d**) MRI: A tumor mass (arrows) in the posterior epidural space of the spinal canal in the T8–9 level. It shows hypointensity on T1WI and T2WI; the outer margin is smooth. It compresses the spinal cord. Hyperintense lesions appear in the T7 and T11 vertebral bodies, and the signal intensity can be suppressed on T2 STIR, indicating bone marrow fatty change and is asymptomatic. Surgical removal of the epidural tumor and pathology proved to be a cavernous hemangioma

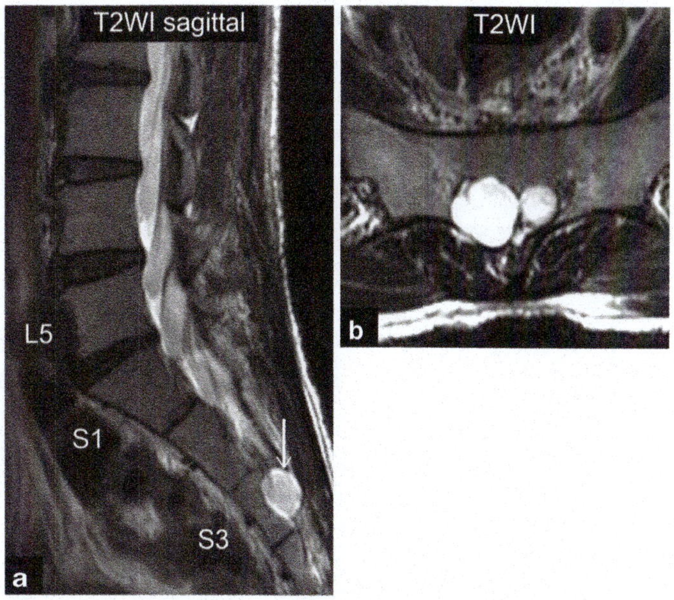

Fig. 8.62 M/47, Perineural cyst (Tarlov cyst). MRI: Two cysts in the spinal canal of the S3 level. The right cyst causes bony erosion of peripheral bones. These are a typical perineural cyst, also named Tarlov cyst, and are usually asymptomatic

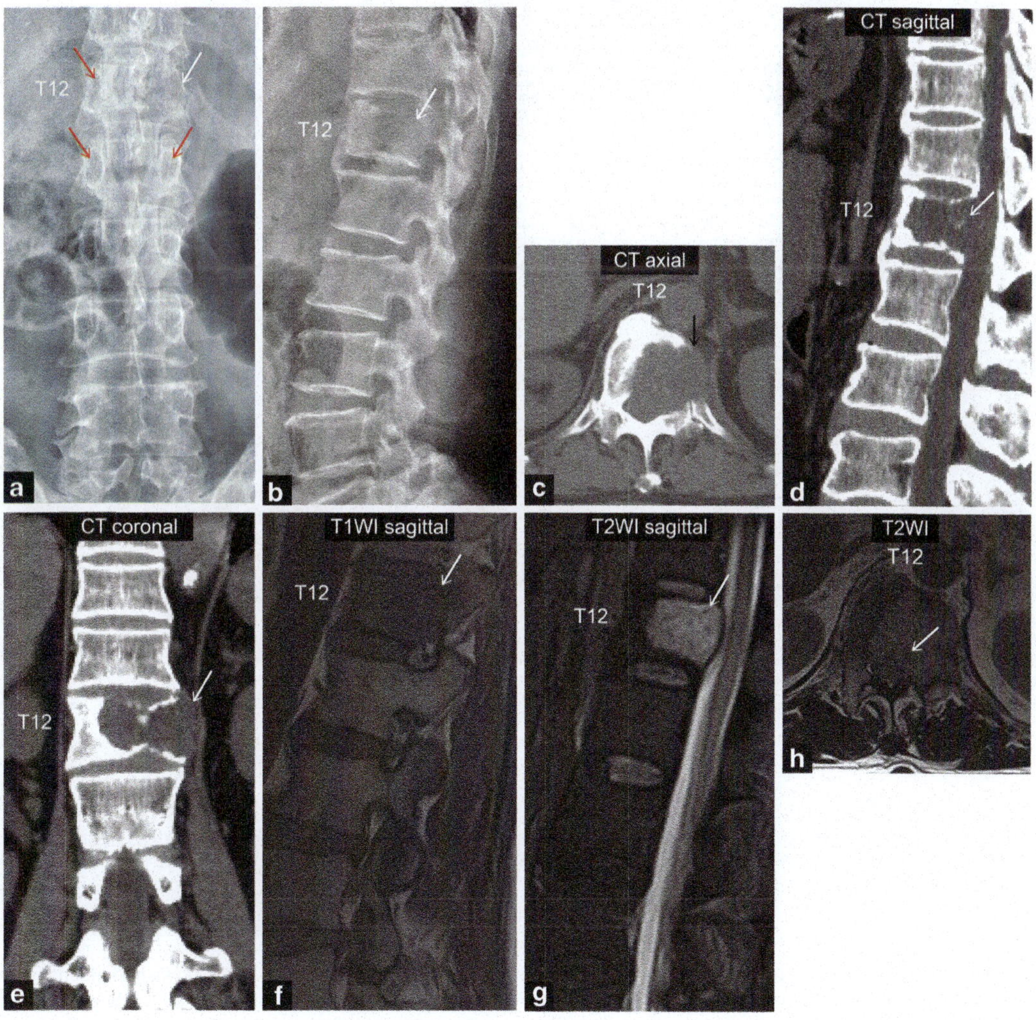

Fig. 8.63 M/67, Hepatoma with spinal metastasis. A hepatoma patient suffered severe back pain for a week. (**a**, **b**) X-ray: Red arrows in (**a**) indicate the pedicles of the vertebral body. The left pedicle of T12 is invisible (white arrow), which is the "lost pedicle sign", and radiolucent density in the left half of T12 vertebral body, for a cancer patient, the findings are highly suspected bony metastasis. (**c**–**e**) CT: About two-thirds of the T12 vertebral body shows osteolysis, and with soft tissue mass replacement (arrow), so this is osteolytic metastasis. (**f**, **g**) MRI: Most of the T12 vertebral body shows hypointensity on T1WI, hyperintensity on T2WI, represents osteolysis, and replaced by soft tissue mass (arrows). (**h**) MRI, axial section: Can see the soft tissue mass invades into the spinal canal (arrow)

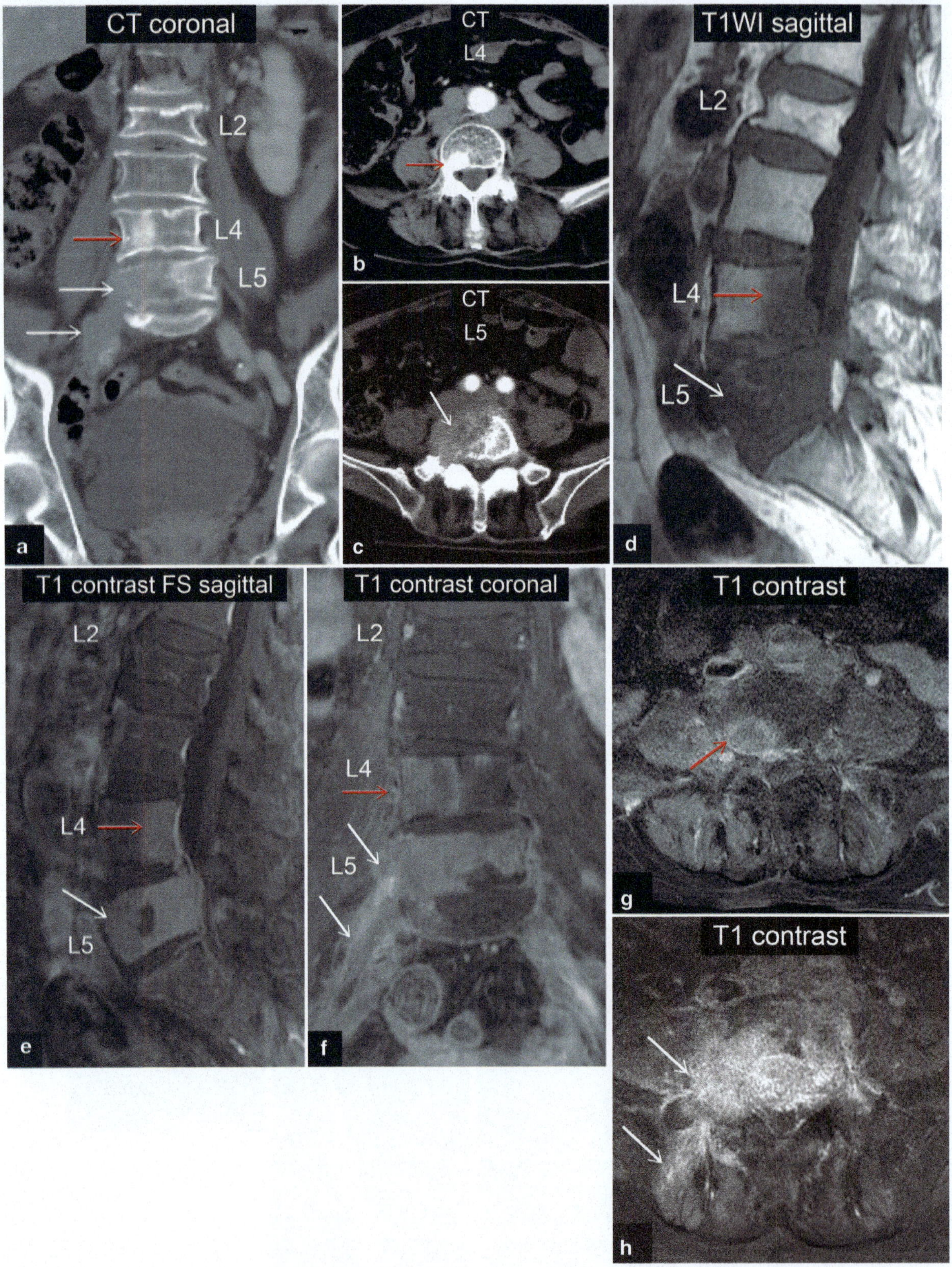

Fig. 8.64 F/86, Osteoblastic, and osteolytic metastases. This patient has ureteral carcinoma and suffered severe low back pain and right sciatica. (**a–c**) CT: L2 compression fracture; hyperdensity in the right side of the L4 vertebral body; suspect osteoblastic metastasis (red arrow). Osteolysis and soft tissue mass replacement in the right side of the L5 vertebral body; the soft tissue mass downward extends (white arrow); this is osteolytic metastasis. (**d–h**) MRI: Normal signal intensity of the L2 vertebral body, indicating old compression fracture. The right side of L4 and the L5 vertebral body shows hypointensity on T1WI, which are enhanced by contrast medium; all are bony metastases; thus, MRI cannot distinguish osteoblastic (red arrows) and osteolytic (white arrows) metastases. Note: (**e**, **f**) T1WI with fat suppression (FS) after contrast medium, normal bone marrow is suppressed and appears hypointensity, the hyperintensities in L4,5 vertebral bodies are metastases. All the osteoblastic, osteolytic metastases and soft tissue mass are enhanced to be hyperintense

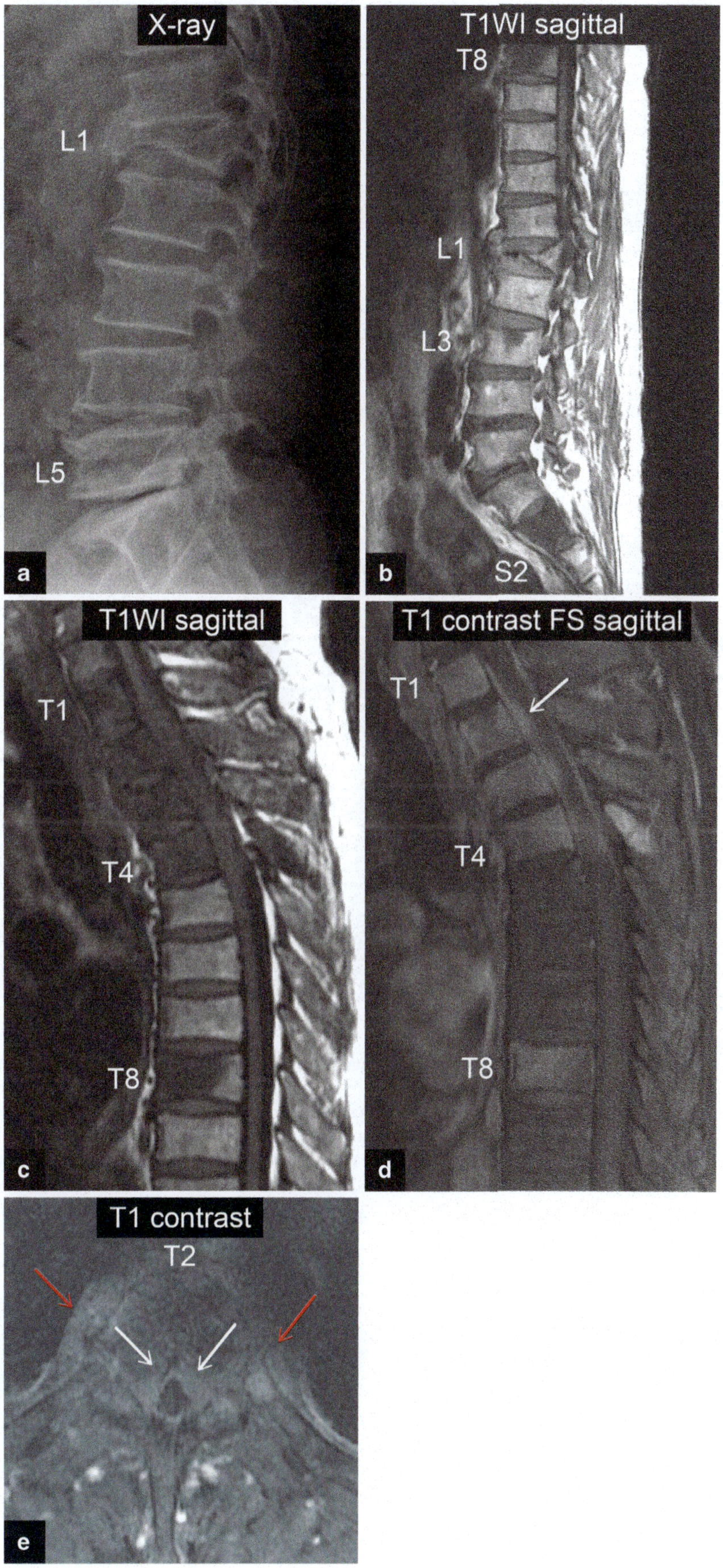

Fig. 8.65 M/71, Multiple spinal metastases. This patient suffered weakness of both legs and felt down, followed by paraplegia. (**a**) X-ray: Severe compression fracture of the L1 vertebral body and degenerative spondylosis with osteophytes in every lumbar vertebral body. However, the above are chronic diseases and cannot explain the clinical symptom of paraplegia after a fall. (**b**) MRI, T-L spine, T1WI: No signal change in L1 vertebral body, indicating old compression fracture. Hypointensities of S2, L3, and T8 vertebral bodies indicate possible osteolyses. (**c**) MRI, T-spine, T1WI: The T8 and T1–4 vertebral bodies losing normal signal intensity show hypointensity on T1WI. These are osteolyses, for so many levels of osteolyses of vertebral bodies, we should consider spinal metastases. (**d**) Contrast T1WI with fat suppression: The signal intensity of healthy vertebral bodies bone marrow is suppressed, and the T8 and T1–4 vertebral bodies show enhancement, representing osteolyses, and some soft tissue mass (arrow) invades into the spinal canal, compresses the spinal cord. (**e**) Contrast T1W, axial section: An epidural mass (white arrows) compresses the spinal cord, the clinical symptom of paraplegia is a type of myelopathy caused by this spinal cord compression. Paravertebral masses (red arrows) are also observed. Surgical decompression was performed, and biopsy proved to be poorly differentiated carcinoma, metastatic with an unknown origin

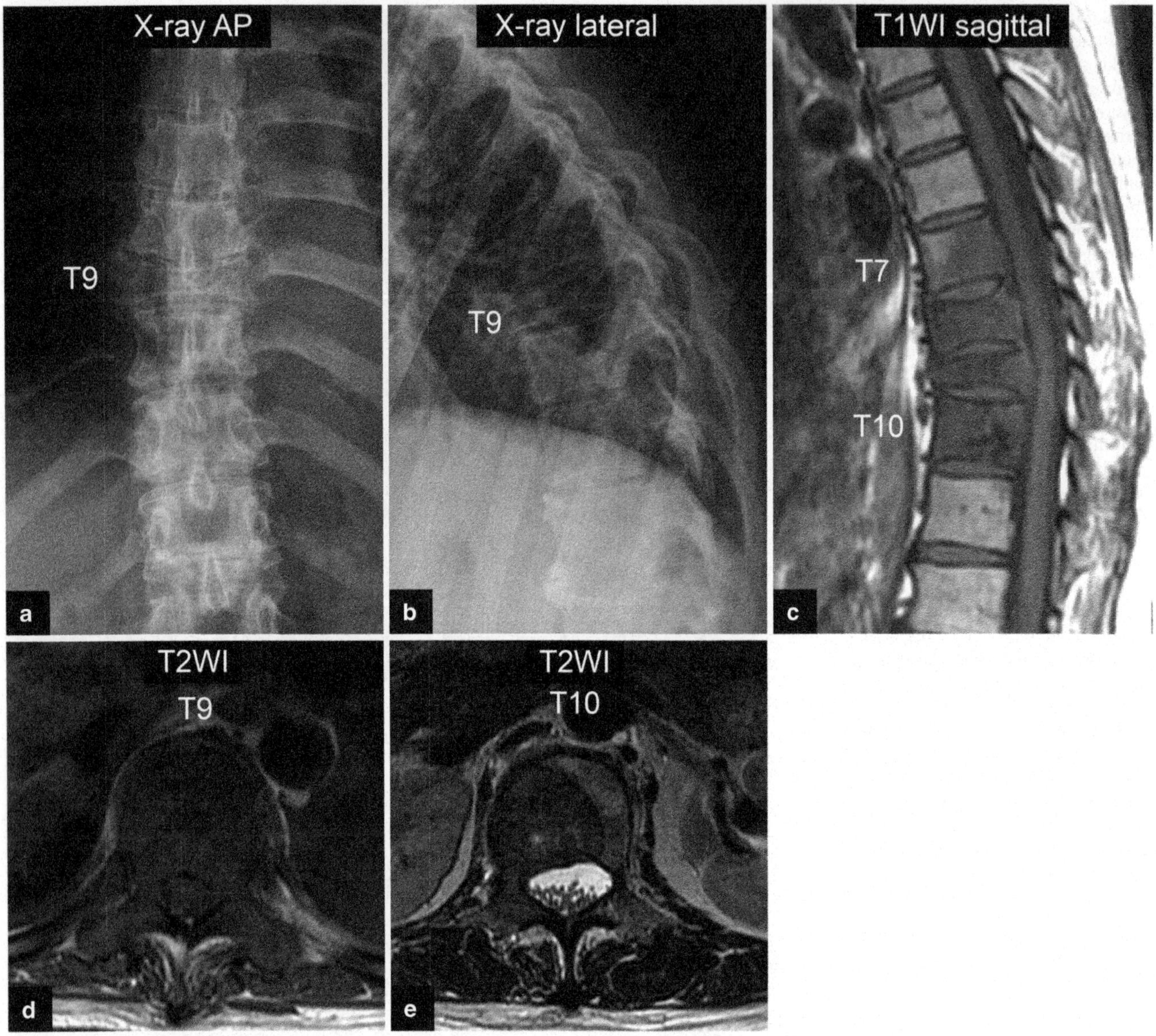

Fig. 8.66 F/41, Lung cancer with spinal metastases. This lung cancer patient suffered severe back pain. (**a**, **b**) X-ray: Compression fracture of the T9 vertebral body and lost bilateral pedicles suspected due to metastasis. (**c**) MRI, T1WI: Reduction in the height and shows hypointensity of T9 vertebral body, and slightly compresses the spinal cord, this is a pathological fracture due to osteolytic metastasis. The T7,8,10 vertebral bodies show hypointensity, indicating osteolytic metastases. A mild pathological fracture of T8 also occurs. Every intervertebral disc is normal. (**d**, **e**) T2WI, axial: No significant soft tissue mass in the above osteolytic areas. The pathology of the biopsy revealed lung cancer with spinal metastases

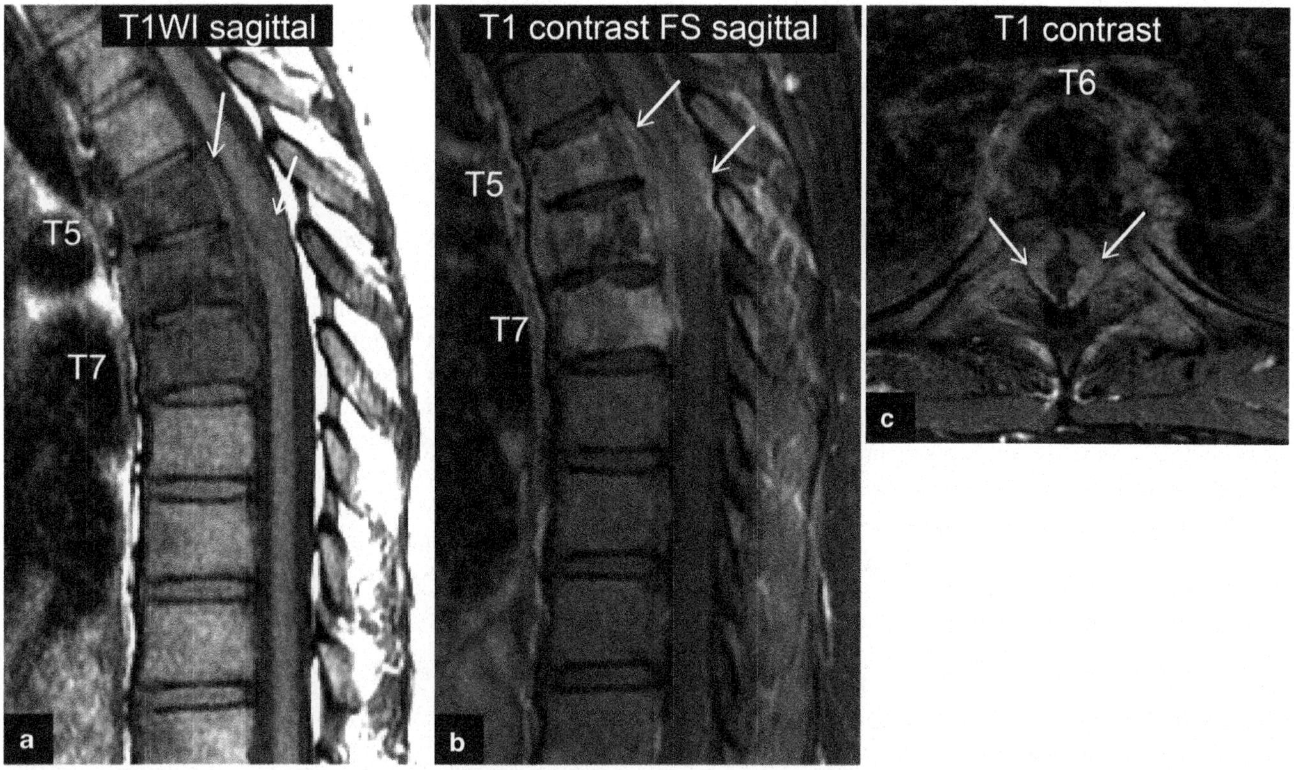

Fig. 8.67 F/39, Breast cancer with thoracic spinal metastases. This breast cancer woman suffered back pain and weakness of both legs. (**a**) MRI, T1WI: Hypointensity of the T5,6,7 vertebral bodies and with some soft tissue mass in the spinal canal (arrows). Slight reduction in body height of T5 vertebra indicates a mild pathological fracture. (**b**) Contrast T1WI: Enhancement of the T5–7 vertebral bodies by contrast medium, and some soft tissue masses (arrows) in the spinal canal are enhanced; the soft tissue masses compress the spinal cord. (**c**) Contrast T1, axial section: The epidural soft tissue masses (arrows) compress the spinal cord, explaining the weakness of both legs

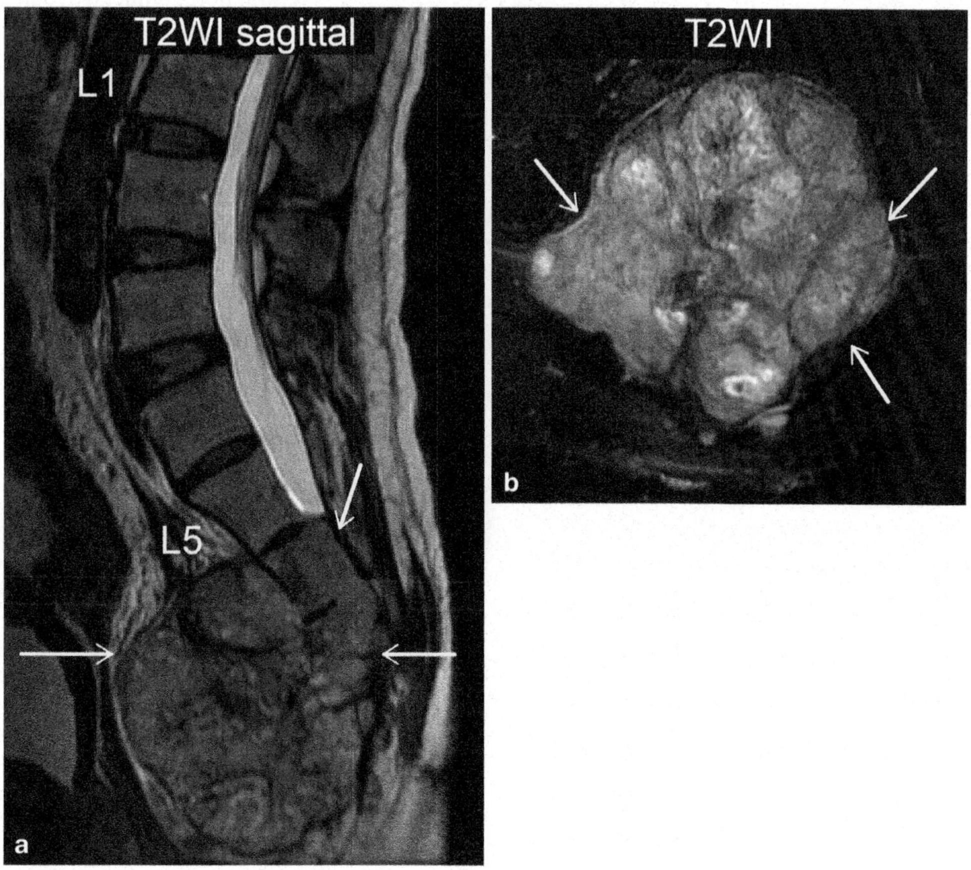

Fig. 8.68 M/50, Sacrum chordoma. This patient suffered long-term buttock pain. (**a**, **b**) MRI, T2WI: A big soft tissue mass (arrows) invades the sacrum, this is a typical chordoma. Surgical removal of this tumor, and pathology proved to be chordoma

8.9 Inflammatory Diseases of the Spine

8.9.1 Vertebral Osteomyelitis and Discitis

Spinal infections include infection of the vertebral body (osteomyelitis) and intervertebral disk (discitis or diskitis) caused by bacteria (including mycobacteria). Spondylodiscitis (or spondylodiskitis) is when two adjacent vertebral bodies and an intervertebral disc are infected (Figs. 8.69 and 8.70). In some cases, the spondylodiscitis is associated with paravertebral soft tissue and muscle infection (Fig. 8.69), and even paravertebral abscess formation (Fig. 8.71), and may also cause epidural empyema in the spinal canal (Fig. 8.70). This epidural empyema and paravertebral soft tissue infections can spread upward and downward to other vertebrae. A few cases involve an initial infection of paravertebral soft tissue, and sometimes muscle infections, followed by an inflammation of the adjacent vertebral body (Fig. 8.71).

Spondylodiscitis must be diagnosed according to clinical symptoms (e.g., fever and leukocytosis). X-rays are inaccurate because of only minor changes. MRI is the optimum method for diagnosis. If MRI cannot be performed, CT can also provide accurate diagnosis [14].

The diagnosis of spondylodiscitis must be distinguished from the vertebral body's malignant tumor, particularly spinal metastasis. In both conditions, the involved vertebral bodies show hypointensity on T1WI, hyperintensity on T2WI, and be enhanced by contrast media; both may associate with paravertebral soft tissue masses and may have a pathological fracture. The main distinctions between spondylodiskitis and spinal metastasis are as follows: (1) ***Metastasis may spread to different vertebral bodies, even skip for several levels*** (Fig. 8.65)***; (2) If metastasis is in continuous vertebral bodies, the intervertebral disc is not affected*** (Figs. 8.65, 8.66, and 8.67)***; (3) For osteolytic metastasis, the bone structure may be replaced by soft tissue mass*** (Figs. 8.63 and 8.64)***. While, spondylodiscitis may be in continuous vertebral bodies and often associate with discitis of their intervertebral disc*** (Figs. 8.69 and 8.70)***, no soft tissue mass to replace the infected area of the vertebral body.***

8.9.2 Spinal Cord Inflammation (Myelitis)

Myelitis refers to spinal cord inflammation. The causes of spinal cord inflammation are mostly unknown. The most common transverse myelitis is possibly related to autoimmune disorders or viral infection (Figs. 8.72 and 8.73).

MRI is the only diagnostic tool available for diagnosing myelitis. A T2WI image indicates the presence of long high-signal lesions across many vertebral levels (Fig. 8.72) and an occasional presence of a localized high signal (Fig. 8.73). Multiple sclerosis (MS) is occasionally misdiagnosed as myelitis; the imaging distinction is that MS lesions are present at more than one vertebral level and at different time points (Fig. 8.74).

8.9.3 Viral Myelitis

The most common viral myelitis is enteroviral myelitis, which is caused by enterovirus 71. Enteroviral myelitis commonly involves the bilateral ventral horns of the spinal cord. The transverse section of a T2WI image indicates symmetrical high-signal lesions (Figs. 8.75 and 8.76). Clinically, enteroviral myelitis causes diplegia [15]. A few cases of enteroviral myelitis exhibit only unilateral invasion of the ventral horn, clinically causing monoplegia [16].

Poliomyelitis is extinct in developed countries and Taiwan. Some people aged more than 50-year-old might have poliomyelitis during childhood. When MRI is performed on polio patients with permanent unilateral limb disabilities for the diagnosis of some other condition, residual lesions in the spinal cord are often found, typically in the unilateral ventral horn (Fig. 8.77).

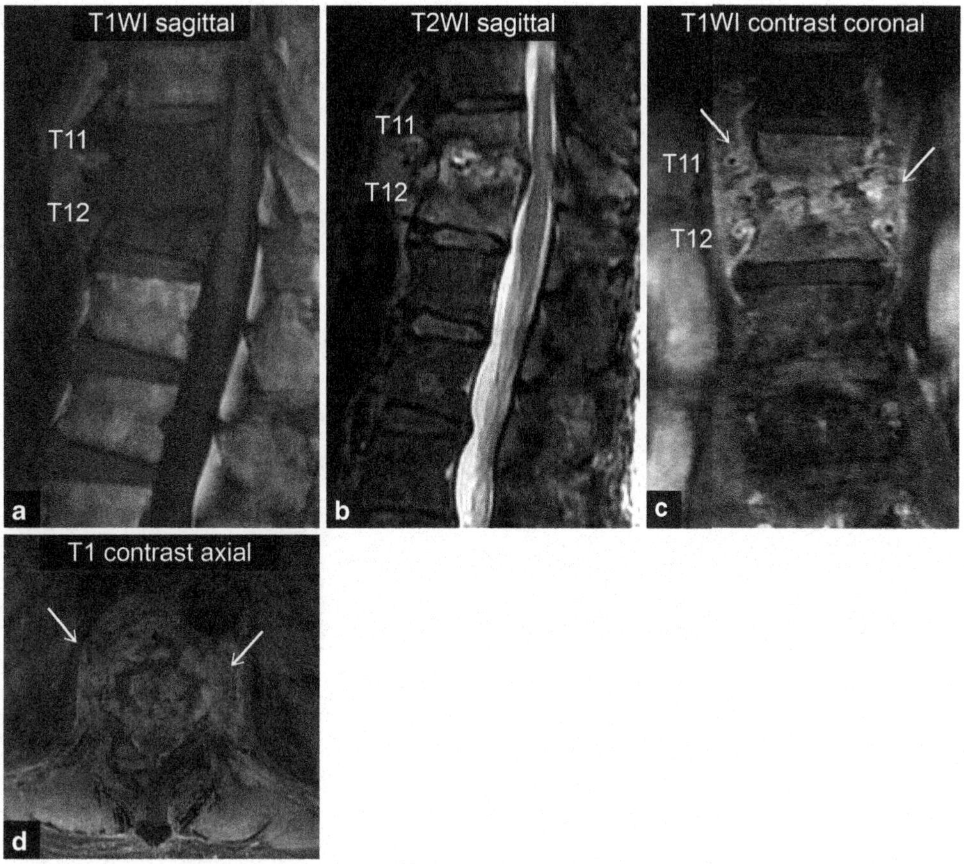

Fig. 8.69 M/75, Osteomyelitis, and discitis (spondylodiscitis). This patient suffered severe back pain and fever. (**a**, **b**) MRI: The T11,12 vertebral bodies show hypointensity on T1WI and hyperintensity on T2WI, whereas the intervertebral disc shows bright (strong hyperintense) on T2WI. (**c**, **d**) Contrast T1WI: the T11,12 vertebral bodies, and their intervertebral disc are enhanced by contrast medium; some paravertebral inflammatory soft tissue (arrows) is also shown, indicating osteomyelitis associated with discitis (spondylodiscitis). Because the disc is also involved, so ruling out spinal metastasis

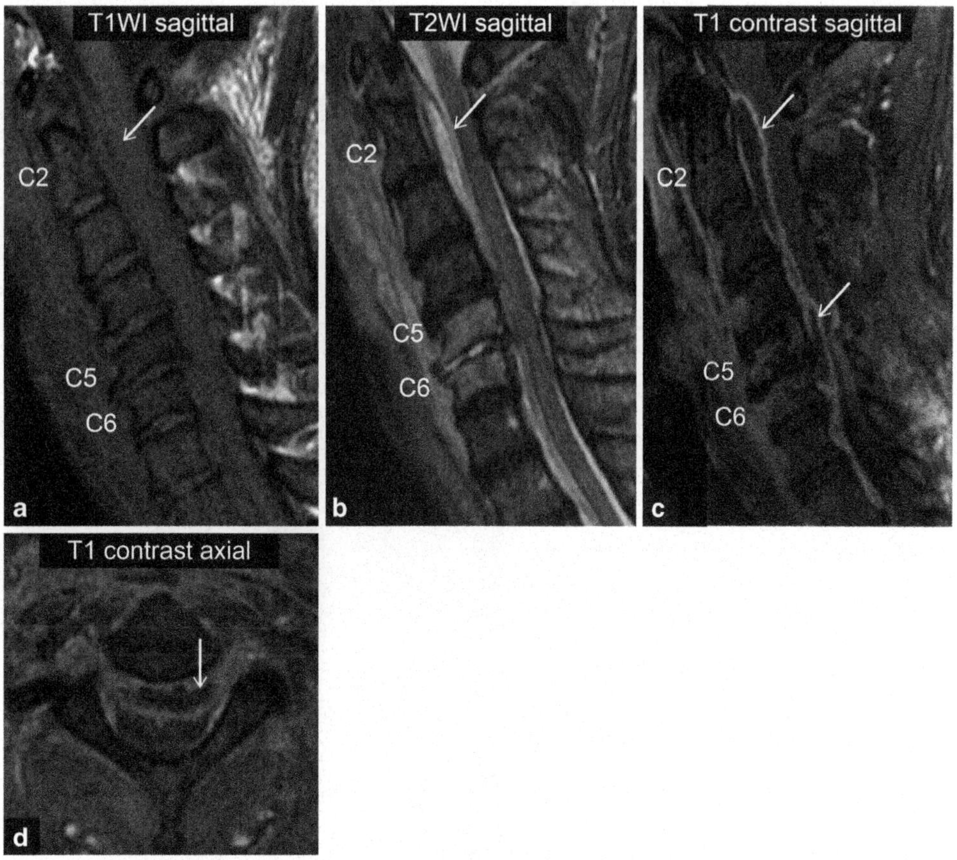

Fig. 8.70 M/49, Osteomyelitis associated with epidural empyema. This patient suffered neck pain, four limb weakness, and fever. (**a**, **b**) MRI: The C5,6 vertebral bodies show hypointensity on T1WI, hyperintensity on T2WI, their intervertebral disc is also hyperintense. The findings are reflecting spondylodiscitis. Epidural effusion (arrow) also occurs behind the C2–3 level. (**c**, **d**) Contrast T1WI: The C5,6 vertebral bodies are enhanced, and epidural effusion from C1 to C6 is also enhanced, indicating epidural empyema (arrows)

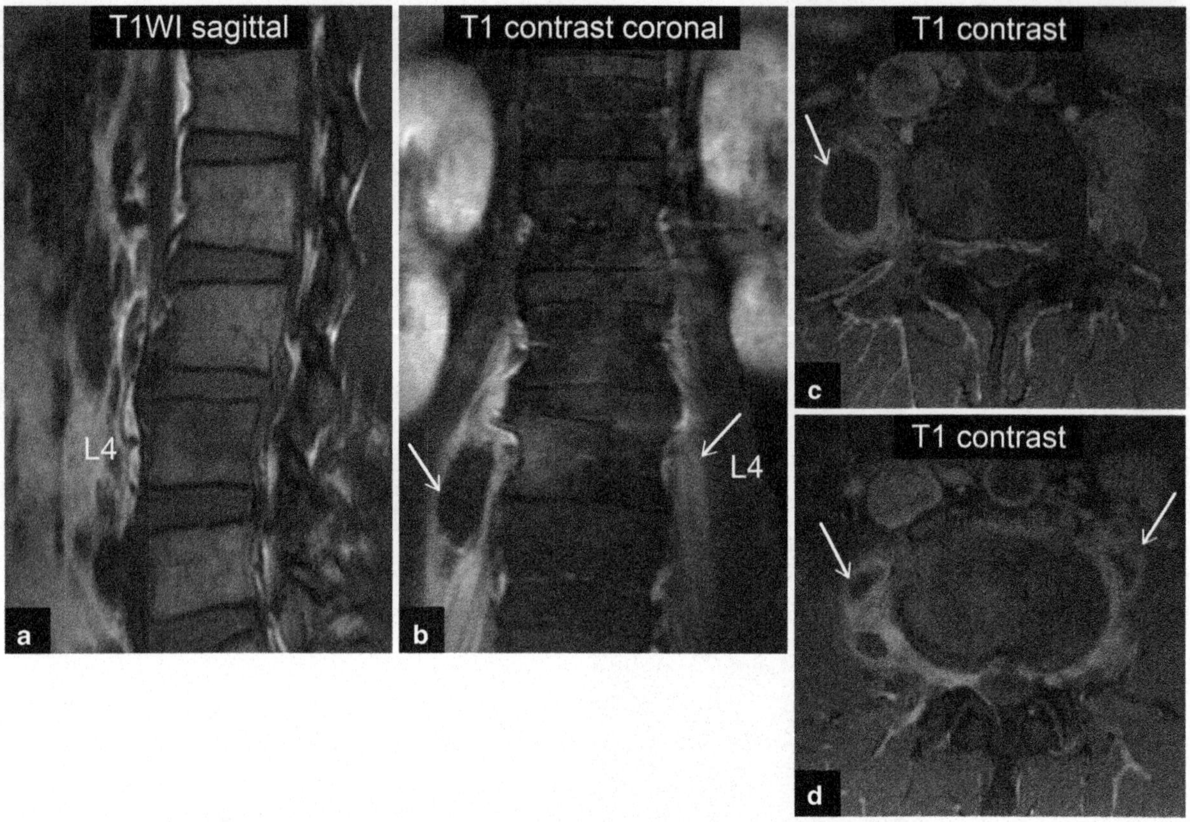

Fig. 8.71 M/34, Psoas muscle abscess. This patient suffered severe low back pain and fever. (**a**) MRI, T1WI: Hypointensity of the L4 vertebral body. (**b**) Contrast T1WI, coronal: Enhancement is observed on the right side of the L4 vertebral body and the bilateral psoas muscles (arrows) and an abscess in the right. (**c**, **d**) Contrast T1WI, axial sections: Abscesses (arrows) are observed in the bilateral psoas muscles. This case is a severe infection of bilateral psoas muscles and caused osteomyelitis of the L4 vertebral body

Fig. 8.72 F/27, Transverse myelitis. This SLE patient suffered a sudden onset of paraplegia. (**a**) MRI, T2WI sagittal: Long-shape hyperintensity (arrow) in the spinal cord. (**b**) T2W, axial: Hyperintensity in the middle of the spinal cord involving the gray matter, indicating acute myelitis. For an SLE patient, this condition is a type of transverse myelitis

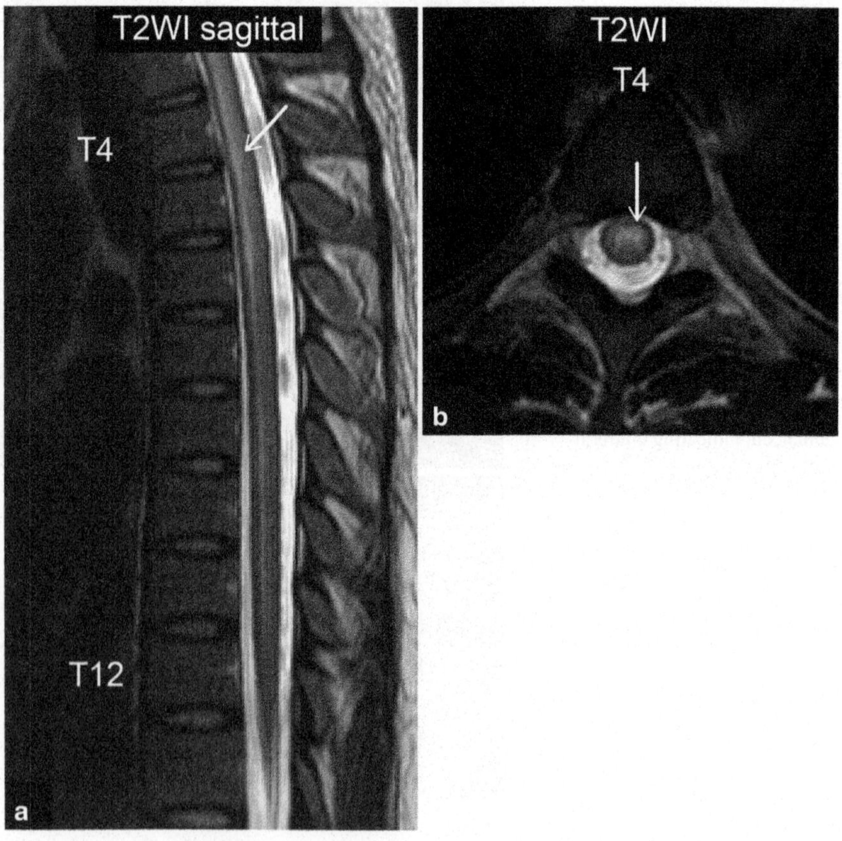

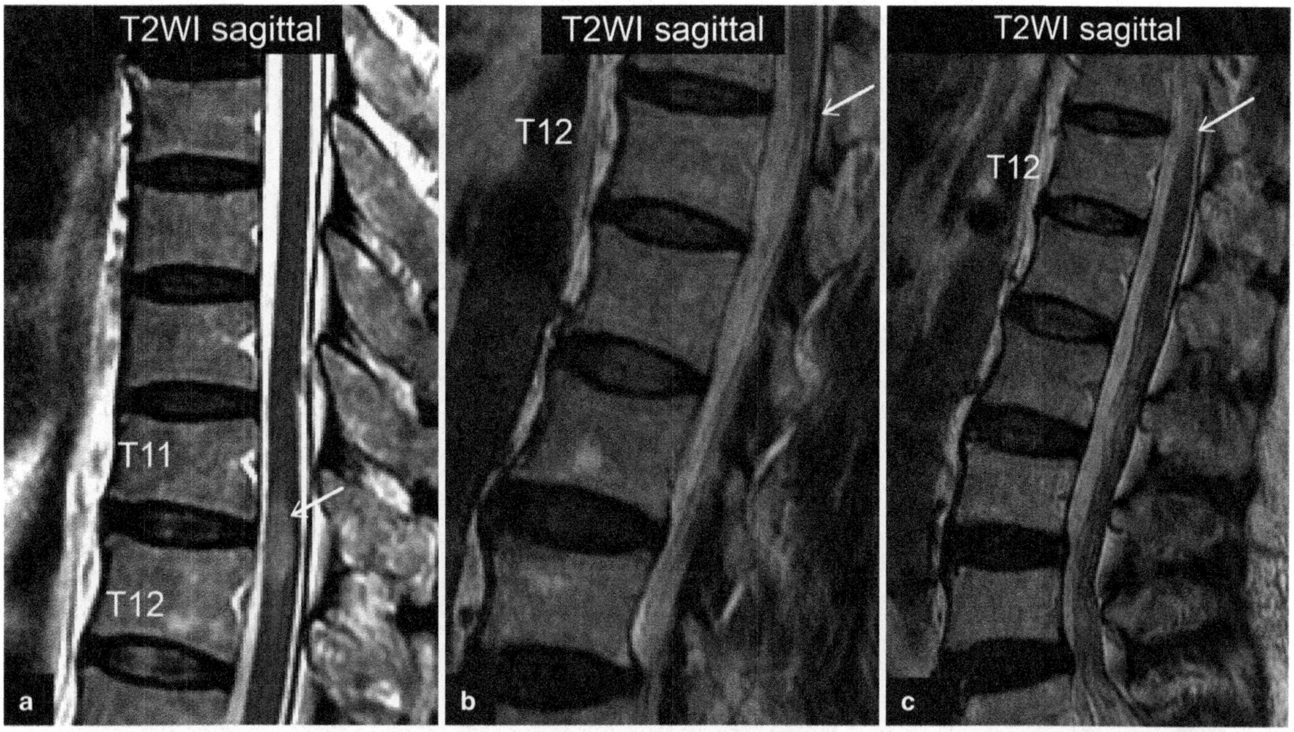

Fig. 8.73 M/64, Acute myelitis. This patient suffered a sudden onset of paraplegia, urine, and stool incontinence. (**a**) MRI, T2WI: A focal hyperintense lesion (arrow) in the spinal cord of the T11–12 level cannot distinguish if it is myelitis or an intramedullary tumor. The clinical symptoms persisted; follow-up with an MRI was performed half a year later. (**b**, **c**) MRI, T2WI: Focal atrophy (arrow) of the spinal cord in the T11–12 level; thus, this is myelitis, not a tumor

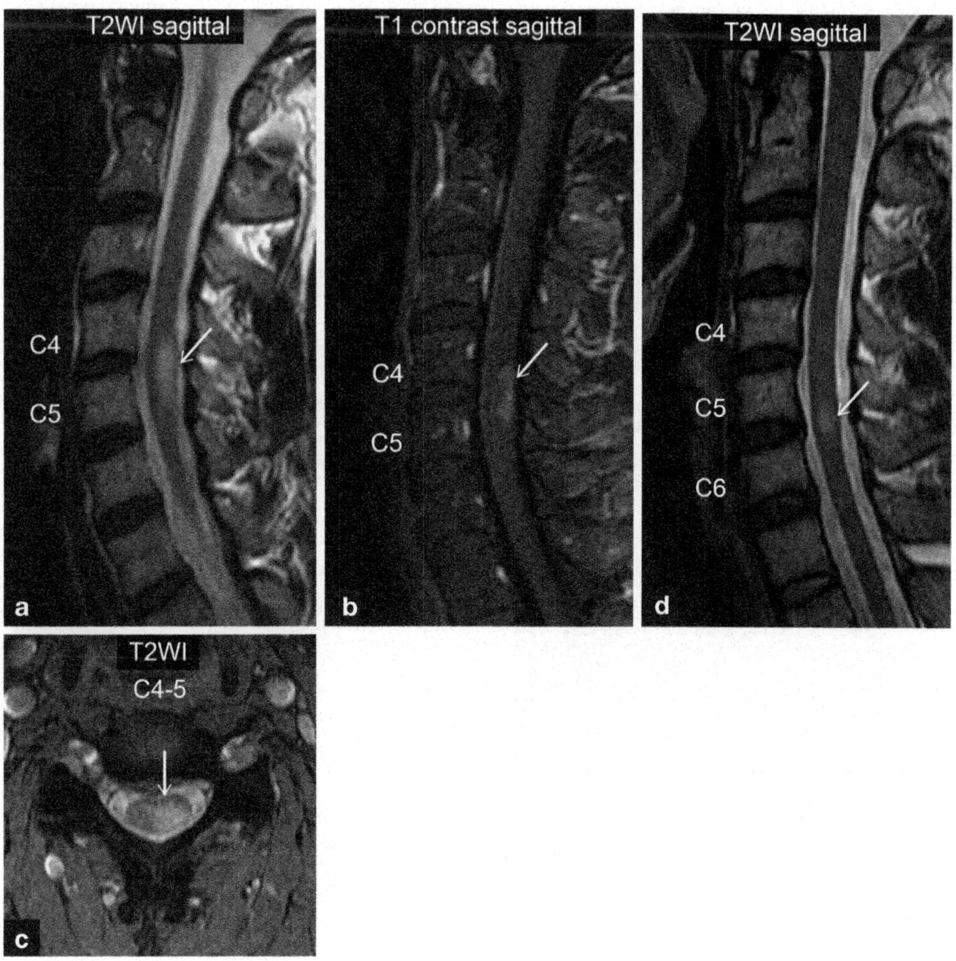

Fig. 8.74 M/38, Multiple sclerosis (MS). This patient suffered weakness of both lower legs and numbness of both arms. (**a**–**c**) MRI: T2WI shows a hyperintense lesion (arrows) that appeared on the left side of the spinal cord, C4–5 level. Some enhancement (arrow in **b**) by contrast medium is observed. (**d**) Follow-up MRI, T2WI: Disappearance of the lesion in the C4–5 level and a new hyperintense lesion (arrow) in the C5–6 level. It repeatedly produces lesions at different locations in the spinal cord, which is characteristic of MS

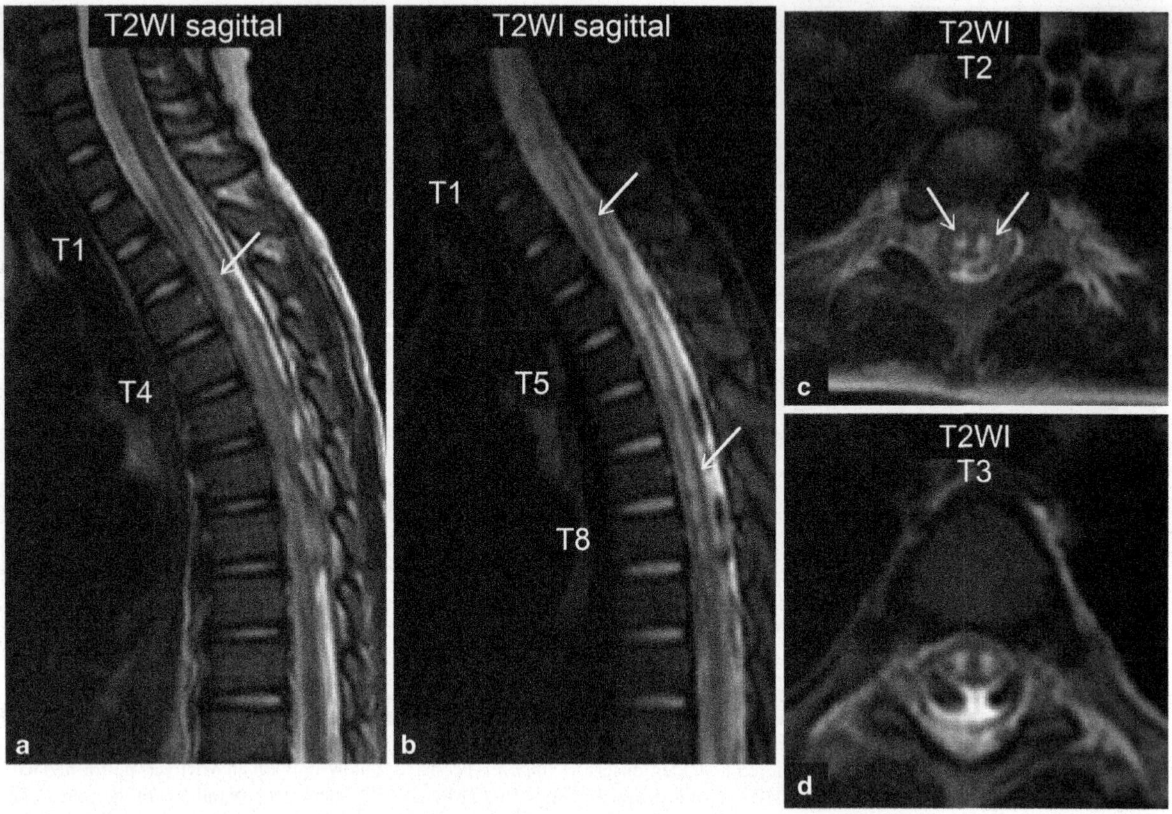

Fig. 8.75 F/4, Enteroviral myelitis. This girl had a hand–foot–mouth disease, with fever, and sudden onset of paraplegia. (**a**, **b**) MRI, T2WI: long hyperintense lesion (arrows) in the spinal cord at the T1–8 level, indicating myelitis. (**c**, **d**) T2WI, axial sections: Symmetrical hyperintense lesions (arrows) appear on both sides of the ventral horn, indicating typical enteroviral myelitis caused by enterovirus 71

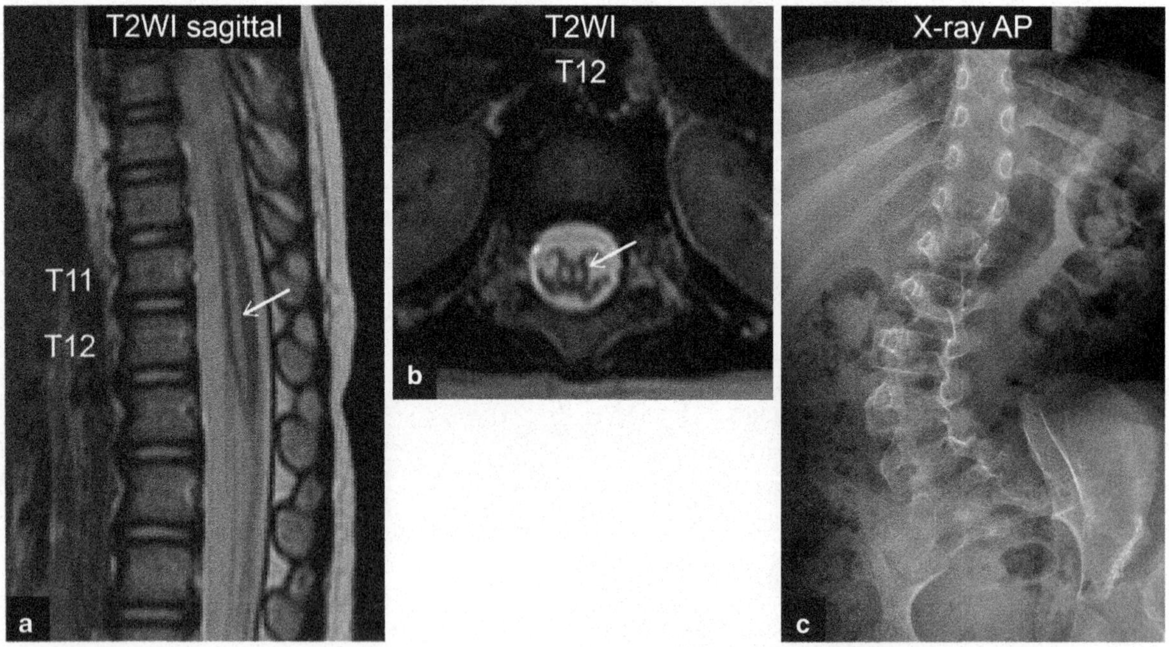

Fig. 8.76 F/9m, Enteroviral myelitis. This girl suffered fever, herpangina, and sudden onset of paraplegia. (**a**) MRI, T2WI: A linear hyperintense lesion (arrow) appeared in the conus medullaris, indicating myelitis. (**b**) T2WI, axial section: Symmetrical hyperintense lesions (arrow) on both sides of the ventral horn. This is a typical enteroviral myelitis caused by enterovirus 71. This patient suffered long-term paraparesis since this acute episode of myelitis. (**c**) KUB took at 9-year-old: KUB shows severe scoliosis of the T-L spine, which is a sequela of myelitis

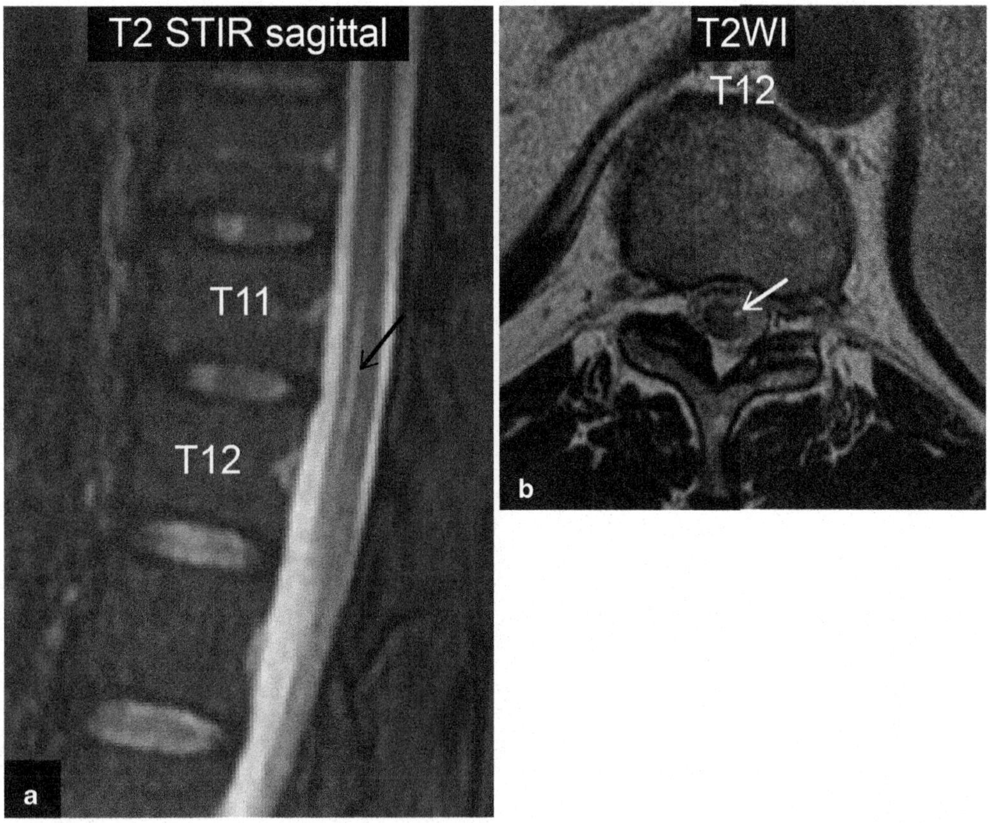

Fig. 8.77 M/62, Sequela lesion of poliomyelitis. The patient was infected with polio at childhood age, and then the left lower extremity was weakened and became atrophic. An MRI on 62 years old for healthy examination. (**a**) MRI, T2WI, sagittal section: A small linear hyperintense lesion is found in the spinal cord at the T11–12 level. (**b**) MRI, T2WI, axial section: A small hyperintense lesion is found on the left-side ventral horn of the spinal cord

References

1. Kushchayev SV, et al. ABCs of the degenerative spine. Insights into Imaging. 2018;9:253–74.
2. Fardon DF, et al. Lumbar disc nomenclature: version 2.0: recommendations of the combined task forces of the North American Spine Society, the American Society of Spine Radiology and the American Society of Neuroradiology. Spine J. 2014;14:2525–45.
3. Modic MT, et al. Degenerative disk disease: assessment of changes in vertebral body marrow with MR imaging. Radiology. 1988;166:193–9.
4. Zhang YH, et al. Modic changes: a systematic review of the literature. Eur Spine J. 2008;17:1289–99.
5. Nouri A, et al. Magnetic resonance imaging assessment of degenerative cervical myelopathy: a review of structural changes and measurement techniques. Neurosurg Focus. 2016;40(6):E5.
6. Hermann KGA, et al. Spinal changes in patients with spondyloarthritis: comparison of MR imaging and radiographic appearance. Radiographics. 2005;25:559–69.
7. Parizel PM, et al. Trauma of the spine and spinal cord: imaging strategies. Eur Spine J. 2010;19:S8–17.
8. Khurana B, et al. Traumatic thoracolumbar spine injuries: what the spine surgeon wants to know. Radiographics. 2013;33:2031–46.
9. Lenchik L, et al. Diagnosis of osteoporotic vertebral fractures: importance of recognition and description by radiologists. AJR. 2004;183:949–58.
10. Gebauer GP, et al. Magnetic resonance imaging of spine tumors: classification, differential diagnosis, and spectrum of disease. J Bone Joint Surg Am. 2008;90:146–62.
11. Koeller KK, Shih R. Neoplasms of the spinal cord and filum terminale: radiologic-pathologic correlation. Radiographics. 2000;20:1721–49.
12. Koeller KK, Shih R. Intradural extramedullary spinal neoplasms: radiologic-pathologic correlation. Radiographics. 2019;39:468–90.
13. Jung HS, et al. Discrimination of metastatic from acute osteoporotic compression spinal fractures with MR imaging. Radiographics. 2003;23:179–87.
14. Modic MT, et al. Vertebral osteomyelitis: assessment using MR. Radiology. 1985;157:157–66.
15. Shen WC, et al. MR imaging findings of enteroviral encephalomyelitis: an outbreak in Taiwan. AJNR Am J Neuroradiol. 1999;20:1889–95.
16. Shen WC, et al. MRI of enterovirus 71 myelitis with monoplegia. Neuroradiology. 2000;42:124–7.

Index

W.-C. Shen, *Diagnostic Neuroradiology*, https://doi.org/10.1007/978-981-15-4051-6

The manufacturer's authorised representative in the EU is Springer Nature Customer Service Centre GmbH, Europaplatz 3, 69115 Heidelberg, Germany. If you have any concerns regarding our products, please contact ProductSafety@springernature.com

Printed and bound by CPI Group (UK) Ltd, Croydon, CR0 4YY
30/09/2026
02225268-0003